MEDICAL RADIOLOGY

Diagnostic Imaging and Radiation Oncology

Springer
Berlin
Heidelberg
New York
Barcelona
Hong Kong
London
Milan
Paris
Singapore
Tokyo

J. N. Bruneton (Ed.)
in collaboration with B. Padovani and M.-Y. Mourou

Radiological Imaging of Endocrine Diseases

With Contributions by

S. Agostini · M. André · E. Baechler Sadoul · J.-M. Bartoli · M. Belaidi · B. Benoit
O. Bernard · A. Bleuse · L. Boyer · P. Bret · J. M. Bruel · J. N. Bruneton · P. Brunner
F. Bussière · J. N. Buy · F. Calabro · C. Calvet · S. Chanalet · P. Chevallier · J. M. Cucchi
I. Damarey · A. Daneman · J. Darcourt · T. de Baere · J. Drouillard · F. Durand · O. Durieux
A. Gangi · V. Gense · A. Geoffray · M. Ghossain · M. Gray · A. Grimaud · D. Jeanbourquin
V. Juhan · R. Lecesne · T. Livraghi · O. Louis · C. Maestro · A. Maubon · P. Y. Marcy
J.-F. Merrer · G. Michelozzi · M.-Y. Mourou · M. Osteaux · B. Padovani · J. Pradel · C. Raffaelli
A. Ravel · Y. Robert · A. Roche · N. Rocourt · J. P. Rouanet · C. Roy · J. L. Sadoul · D. Samama
S. Schiavoni · J. Tramalloni · F. Tranquart · D. Vadrot · J.F. Viallet

Translated by N. Reed-Rameau

Series Editor's Foreword by

A.L. Baert

Preface by

B. Cavinet

With 253 Figures in 432 Separate Illustrations, 46 in Color

Springer

J.N. BRUNETON, MD
Professor, Centre Régional de Lutte contre le Cancer
Centre Antoine-Lacassagne
33, Avenue de Valombrose
F-06189 Nice Cedex 2
France

MEDICAL RADIOLOGY · Diagnostic Imaging and Radiation Oncology

Continuation of
Handbuch der medizinischen Radiologie
Encyclopedia of Medical Radiology

ISBN-13: 978-3-642-64200-5
e-ISBN-13: 978-3-642-59965-1
DOI: 10.1007/978-3-642-59965-1

Library of Congress Cataloging-in-Publication Data. Radiological imaging of endocrine diseases/ J.N. Bruneton (ed.) in collaboration with B. Padovani and M.-Y. Mourou; with contributions by S. Agostini... [et al.] ; foreword by B. Cavinet p. cm. -- (Medical radiology) Includes bibliographical references and index. ISBN 3-540-64843-7 (alk. paper) 1. Endocrine glands--Diseases--Imaging. I. Bruneton, J.N. II. Padovani, B. (Bernard) III. Series. [DNLM: 1. Endocrine Diseases--radiography. 2. Endocrine Diseases--diagnosis. 3. Diagnostic Imaging. 4. Diagnostic Techniques, Endocrine--instrumentation. WK 140 R129 1999] RC649.R29 1999 616.4'0754--dc21 DNLM/DLC for Library of Congress 98-44275 CIP

Typesetting: Best-set Typesetter Ltd., Hong Kong

SPIN: 106 607 89 21/3135 - 5 4 3 2 1 0 - Printed on acid-free paper

Foreword

Radiological imaging of endocrine diseases has not, in the past, always received all the attention it deserves in the literature, as evident from the limited number of comprehensive modern textbooks currently available. Endocrinological diseases typically involves several different organ systems and anatomical areas of the human body, and the knowledge on these diseases is frequently spread over numerous different journals and textbooks.

Moreover, as in many other areas of medicine and surgery, great progress has been achieved during recent years in the field of endocrinology due to the development of new and more sophisticated methods for bio-assay of hormones and related substances. Parallel to that biochemical development, the new cross-sectional radiological imaging methods have provided us with totally new possibilities for morphological and functional visualization of the causes and effects of endocrinological disorders as well as for the clinical evaluation of the results of medical therapy.

For all these reasons we believed that the time had come to prepare a comprehensive book covering all important radiological aspects of endocrine diseases and providing an update on the latest insights in this field. As series editor I am very grateful that Pofessor J. N. Bruneton accepted the challenge of preparing and editing such a volume.

Professor Bruneton, an outstanding radiologist with a wide range of interests, is a well-known international expert on various problems related to endocrinological imaging. He is the author of French and English textbooks on this topic as well as on other aspects of radiology and a very much appreciated lecturer and teacher at national and international meetings.

Professor Bruneton was able to engage an outstanding group of widely known experts, mainly from France but also from other countries. Their excellent contributions cover the various aspects and problems related to endocrine disorders very appropriately.

Radiologists involved in the different subspecialties, but also general radiologists, will find this volume of great value for their daily work. The book is also aimed at clinical endocrinologists, internists and others involved in the treatmend of endocrine disorders. It will provide them with an excellent update on the radiological aspects of the disease they are dealing with in their clinical practice.

The attractive technical presentation and the high quality of printing and reproduction of photographic material contribute, together with the outstanding level of the scientific content, to the excellence of this book.

As editor of the series Medical Radiology I hope that this volume will – like earlier volumes – be well received by my colleagues in many fields of medicine. I would welcome any constructive criticism.

Leuven — Albert L. Baert

Preface

Endocrinology was long considered solely the domain of anatomy and physiology, restricted to study of the structure and internal secretions of the endocrine glands.

In the 1960s, this concept was revolutionized by advances in biochemistry. Radioimmunology and associated techniques allowed identification of hormones, their origins (no longer limited to the endocrine glands), and their targets. Biological diagnosis of endocrine disorders had a profound effect on medical management: treatment planning and surgical indications could be based on biochemical data that proved pertinent at a stage where today's so-called conventional imaging procedures were generally noncontributory.

The past two decades have been marked by progress in medical imaging and image processing. The benefits provided by computed tomography, ultrasound, magnetic resonance imaging, and scintigraphic techniques in endocrinology are all the more impressive as these methods were previously of limited utility in this area. Imaging and biochemical techniques have gradually been combined in procedures for localization of even minute lesions (e.g. imaging-guided hormone assays). These developments have obviously influenced treatment planning in endocrinology. The endocrine surgeon now works not only with a positive diagnosis, but also with knowledge of the exact location of the abnormal gland or intraglandular abnormality. Medical endocrinology has had to adapt to the new information obtained with modern imaging modalities, one example being the need for specific approaches to fortuitously discovered abnormalities in endocrine glands ("incidentalomas").

Interventional radiology has played a pioneering role in endocrinology, in particular thanks to radionuclide treatment of thyroid disease. Although not yet as spectacular in endocrinology as in other fields such as cardiovascular disease, such therapies have become routine practice since the 1960s.

Increased awareness of the systemic manifestations of endocrine disorders has necessitated modifications in medical management. For example, treatment of mild yet authentic primary hyperparathyroidism in elderly patients, a much more frequent pathology than previously thought even only two or three decades ago, is now based on the extent of lesions demonstrated by imaging, and in particular bone involvement.

Written by specialists in the field, the 18 chapters of this book cover the numerous applications of modern medical imaging to endocrinology. The impact of imaging data on treatment planning and follow-up of endocrine diseases is discussed along with potential complications of therapy. This book will be highly appreciated by specialists in both medical imaging and medical and surgical endocrinology. It should also prove valuable to those working in fields such as gynecology, urology, rheumatology, neurology, cardiology, and internal medicine, who deal directly with the consequences of endocrine disorders. Owing to continuing developments in imaging and their impact on the practice of endocrinology, updates of this book will no doubt be welcomed just as enthusiastically as this first edition.

Nice

BERTRAND CANIVET

Contents

1 Pituitary Gland

F. Calabro, S. Chanalet, P. Chevallier, G. Michelozzi, M.-Y. Mourou, B. Padovani,
C. Raffaelli, and S. Schiavoni

CONTENTS

F. Calabro, G. Michelozzi, S. Schiavoni, Ospedale S. Corona, Pietra Ligure (S.V.), Italy
S. Chanalet, B. Padovani, C. Raffaelli, Service de Radiodiagnostic, Hôpital Pasteur, 30 avenue de la Voie Romaine, BP 69, 06002 Nice, France
P. Chevallier, Service de Radiologie, Hôpital de l'Archet, Route de St. Antoine de Ginestière, 06012 Nice, France
M.-Y. Mourou, Service de Radiologie, Centre Hospitalier Princess Grace, Avenue Pasteur, 98000 Monaco

1.1 Imaging Techniques

S. Chanalet and B. Padovani

1.1.1 Introduction

Magnetic resonance imaging (MRI) has become the neuroradiological modality of choice for initial evaluation of the sellar region. Computed tomography (CT), carotid angiography, venous sampling for hormone assays, scintigraphy, and intraoperative ultrasound (US) are still used or have been developed as second-line procedures to refine tissue characterization of sellar masses.

1.1.2 Magnetic Resonance Imaging

MRI is the first-line technique for assessment of pituitary adenomas and other pathologies of the sellar region, in particular tumors. It has numerous advantages: absence of ionizing radiation, direct multiplanar imaging capabilities without patient mobilization, markedly better contrast resolution than CT, and much better tissue characterization. The sensitivity of MRI is over 90% for the detection of microadenomas (Davis et al. 1987a; Elster 1993a). MRI also permits optimal assessment of the sellar region, in particular the optic tracts, the chiasmatic cistern, and the floor of the third ventricle. The cavernous sinuses are also well visualized, although MRI cannot always affirm tumor involvement, especially in the case of pituitary adenomas.

Apart from absolute contraindications such as pacemakers, ferromagnetic vascular clips, and intraocular metallic foreign bodies, the major limitation of MRI is its poor evaluation (compared to CT) of minimal bone erosion of the sellar cavity and small calcifications.

Standard MR protocols for the sellar region include T_1-weighted sequences before and after gadolinium injection and T_2-weighted sequences. Gradient-echo sequences (GRE) are made less accurate by the bony septa and air in the sphenoidal sinuses, which cause artifacts. Spin-echo (SE) sequences are thus preferred. Most machines now operate with fast SE sequences.

Technical parameters typically include a section thickness of 3mm, a field of view of 20 cm, and a matrix of 512 or 256 × 256. Imaging is usually performed in the sagittal and coronal planes (Fig. 1.1). Axial views are sometimes helpful for large lesions.

Dynamic sequences have been used by a number of investigators to assess microadenomas (Davis et al. 1994; Kucharczyk et al. 1994a; Bartynski and Lin 1997). Bartynski and Lin (1997) reported an 11%–14% increase in the detection of microadenomas with dynamic sequences and a normal dose of gadolinium. In their study, contrast was administered 30s before the start of scanning and was continued for 90s during a conventional SE sequence (total duration, 120–190s.). Pre- and post-contrast T_1-weighted volumetric sequences (three-dimensional Fourier transformation, 3D FT) with slices 1mm thick improve the detection of very small lesions (Girard et al. 1994; Stadnick et al. 1994a). Fat-suppression techniques are occasionally useful to refine tissue characterization.

The role of the various MRI techniques is discussed as a function of specific pathologies in the following sections.

1.1.3 Computed Tomography

The introduction of CT considerably improved exploration of the sellar region thanks to the dynamic assessment of pituitary vascularity it allowed. CT was rapidly superceded by MRI, however. The sensitivity of both techniques increases with the size of the adenoma. CT is 1.5 to two times less sensitive than MRI for adenomas smaller than 5mm (Buchfelder et al. 1993), but it remains useful for pathologies of the bony walls of the sella turcica, for patients in whom MRI is contraindicated, and for refinement of tissue characterization by localization of small intratumoral calcifications in sellar masses.

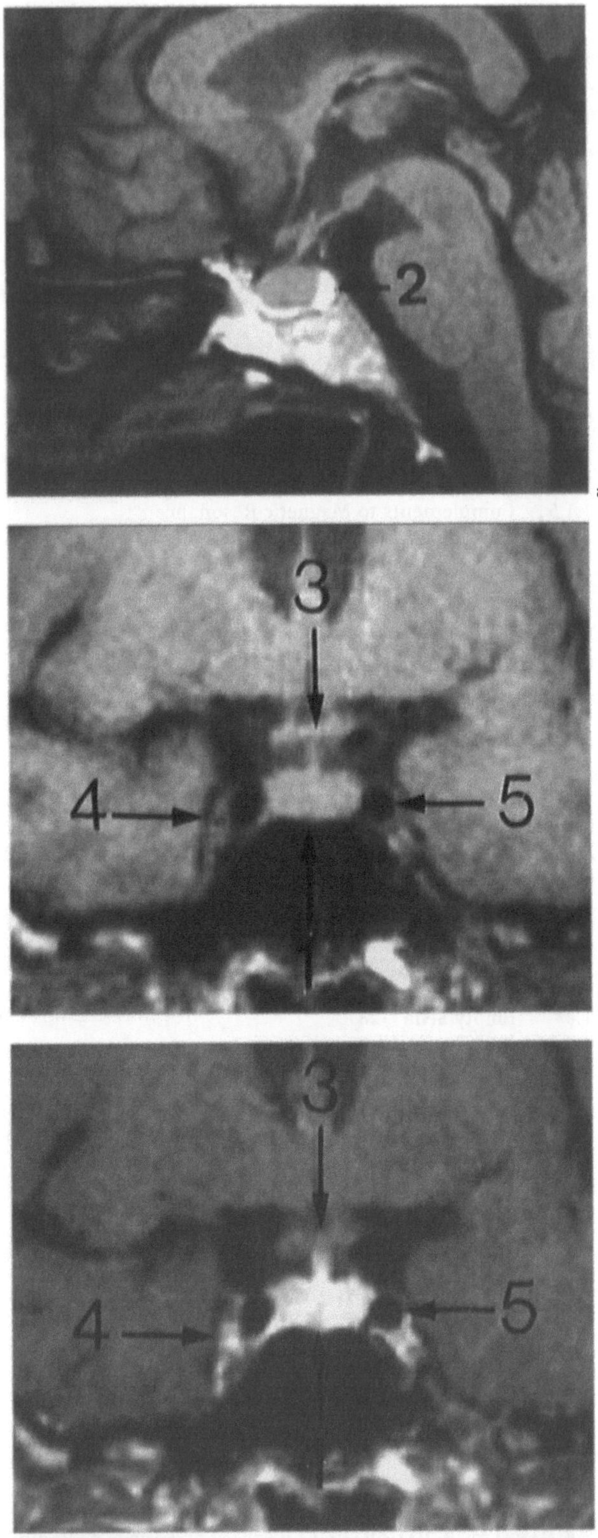

a b c

Fig. 1.1a–c. MRI of a normal sella turcica. **a** Sagittal T_1-weighted scan. **b** Unenhanced coronal T_1-weighted scan. **c** Enhanced coronal T_1-weighted scan. *1*, anterior pituitary; *2*, posterior pituitary; *3*, optic chiasma; *4*, cavernous sinus; *5*, intracavernous internal carotid artery

1.1.4 Bilateral Carotid Angiography

Angiographic differentiation between intrasellar meningiomas and pituitary adenomas has proven impossible because their vascular flow patterns are often identical. Bilateral carotid angiography was formerly performed preoperatively to search for intrasellar aneurysms and arteriovenous malformations. Today, these differential diagnoses can usually be ruled out by MRI.

1.1.5 Complements to Magnetic Resonance Imaging

Depending on the type of lesion and the series, MRI has a false-negative rate of up to 40%. The false-positive rate for pituitary adenomas is as high as 10%. A number of specialized techniques have been developed to compensate for the insufficiences of MRI.

1.1.5.1 Petrosal Venous Sampling

This technique is used essentially for workup of Cushing's syndrome. Imaging studies demonstrate an adenoma in less than 60% of all patients with pituitary Cushing's disease (Mampalam et al. 1988; Kaye and Crapo 1990; Buchfelder et al. 1993). Furthermore, half of all patients with Cushing's syndrome due to ectopic adrenocorticotropic hormone (ACTH) secretion have clinical manifestations suggesting a pituitary origin (Findling and Tyrell 1986; Howlet et al. 1986; Kaye and Crapo 1990). The endocrinologic tests used to distinguish Cushing's syndrome of pituitary origin from ectopic Cushing's syndrome are often nondiscriminatory (Findling and Tyrell 1986; Tabarin et al. 1991). Finally, "incidentalomas" responsible for false-positive imaging errors are extremely common (Parent et al. 1981; Mampalam et al. 1988).

Rationale. The venous drainage of the anterior pituitary lobe is to the cavernous sinuses, which are interconnected by three venous sinuses that pass through the sella turcica: the anterior, posterior, and inferior intercavernous sinuses. The surface of the pituitary gland is covered by two venous plexuses that drain laterally into one of the intercavernous sinuses or directly into the cavernous sinuses. These plexiform networks receive small pituitary veins that emerge directly from the anterior lobe. Each half of the pituitary gland thus drains towards the homolateral cavernous sinus under normal physiologic conditions, i.e., in the absence of stasis or flow reversal that can be provoked by a Valsalva maneuver, for example (Doppman et al. 1984). The cavernous sinuses drain primarily into the inferior petrosal sinuses.

Technique and Indications. Bilateral puncture of the common femoral vein allows selective catheterization of the two inferior petrosal sinuses (Fig. 1.2). Timed samples are taken before and after injection of corticotrophin releasing factor (CRF) through a peripheral venous catheter. The indications for petrosal venous sampling include the following:

- Cushing's syndrome with a discordance between imaging findings and endocrinologic tests (Doppman et al. 1984; Snow et al. 1988; Oldfield et al. 1991).
- For certain authors, pituitary Cushing's syndrome, with or without a demonstrable adenoma. When an adenoma is visualized, venous sampling permits differentiation from an incidentaloma. If no adenoma is demonstrated, petrosal venous sampling helps to guides hemihypophysectomy (Doppman et al. 1984; Landolt et al. 1986).

Results. Petrosal venous sampling is considered positive when the central/peripheral gradient is over

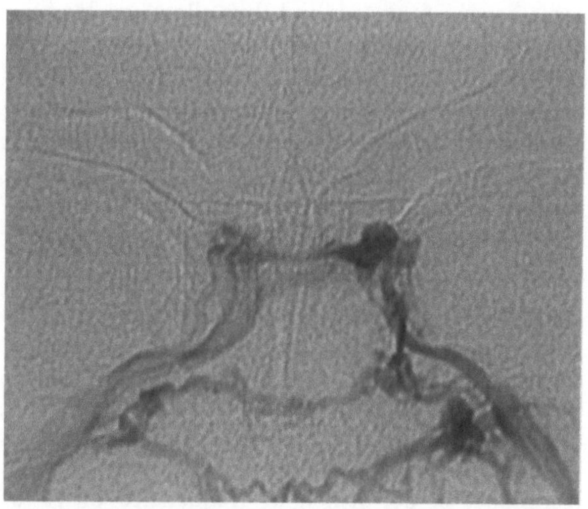

Fig. 1.2. Phlebographic verification of catheter positioning for petrosal venous sampling

2 at baseline and/or after stimulation (OLDFIELD et al. 1991). The test is considered positive for lesion lateralization when the ratio of the right side to the left side is 1.4 (OLDFIELD et al. 1991; BESSAC et al. 1992).

Using these criteria, and provided catheterization is of good quality and the protocol is followed carefully, petrosal venous sampling is universally considered to have excellent specificity for differentiation of ectopic and pituitary secretion (DOPPMAN et al. 1984; LANDHOLT et al. 1986; OLDFIELD et al. 1991; TABARIN et al. 1991; BESSAC et al. 1992). In contrast, this method is often considered unreliable for lateralization of adenomas (TABARIN et al. 1991; BESSAC et al. 1992). OLDFIELD et al. (1991), for example, reported a specificity of only 70%.

Petrosal venous sampling has also been used for assessment of acromegaly (DOPPMAN et al. 1990). However, as acromegaly is usually not diagnosed until an advanced stage, microadenomas are infrequent in this pathology (only 13% of patients). Mixed growth hormone (GH)/prolactin (PRL)-secreting adenomas are much more common (26% of patients) (DOPPMAN et al. 1990). Catheterization of the petrous sinuses allows early diagnosis of acromegaly. When feasible, surgery is more effective than medical therapy.

1.1.5.2 Scintigraphy

Scintigraphy using an ^{123}I-labeled somatostatin analogue as a tracer has also been used for investigation of acromegaly. ^{123}I-labeled Tyr3-octreotide binds to somatostatin receptors and thus allows exploration of numerous endocrine neoplasia expressing this receptor. This technique has been proposed for detection and functional characterization of GH-secreting pituitary adenomas. In their study of 15 patients with acromegaly, Ur et al. (1992) found a close correlation between pituitary uptake and the reduction in the concentration of GH, reflecting the therapeutic response to somatostatin therapy.

1.1.5.3 Intraoperative Ultrasound

Intraoperative ultrasound, an as yet experimental technique, is performed at frequencies of 10 or 15 MHz with a mechanical transducer 11mm in diameter attached to a 15-cm probe. The probe is inserted following transsphenoidal resection of the anterior wall of the sella turcica. Adenomas smaller than 5mm in diameter appear hypoechoic, whereas those over 5mm tend to be hyperechoic. Accurate localization of the adenoma is possible in over 60% of cases. Although intraoperative ultrasound may demonstrate the cavernous sinuses and the intracavernous carotid arteries, it cannot depict minimal invasion of the internal wall of the cavernous sinuses. The major drawback of the technique is its high false-negative rate: in one series of 14 patients, only seven adenomas were correctly visualized (Doppman et al. 1994).

1.1.5.4 Conclusion

The superiority of MRI over CT is today widely acknowledged for detection of pituitary adenomas and for staging of macroadenomas. Complementary techniques such as petrosal venous sampling often provide useful data. Promising results have also been obtained using novel markers (labeled CRF) for scintiscanning. Development of small electronic probes for intraoperative ultrasound should improve image quality and permit color Doppler analysis.

1.2 Pituitary Adenomas

G. MICHELOZZI, F. CALABRO, and S. SCHIAVONI

1.2.1 Introduction

Pituitary adenomas are the most common tumors of the sellar region and represent 10%–15% of all intracranial neoplasms (ELSTER 1993b; KOVACS et al. 1995). Practically all pituitary tumors arise in the anterior lobe. Prolactinomas predominate, accounting for approximately 50%–60% of all pituitary adenomas. Peak incidence is between the ages of 30 and 50years; there is no sex predilection (MIYANOHARA et al. 1993; HALL et al. 1994).

These benign tumors are generally slow growing; malignant degeneration is rare. They may be asymptomatic or cause syndromes of hormone excess, sometimes with clinical signs and symptoms related to mass effect on adjacent structures (particularly the optic tracts), with or without secondary hypopituitarism.

Diagnosis of pituitary adenomas is made primarily by sophisticated imaging techniques such as MRI and CT. MRI is the procedure of choice for identification of pituitary tumors, whereas CT is currently a complementary modality.

Neuroradiologically, pituitary adenomas are classified by size. Lesions smaller than 10mm are termed microadenomas, while those with a diameter over 10mm are referred to as macroadenomas.

1.2.2 Pathologic Anatomy

Pituitary adenomas are generally solid, well-defined lesions that are usually separated from the normal pituitary gland by a capsule or pseudocapsule. Dimensions vary. These lesions may be firm and homogeneous or characterized by cystic degeneration and/or hemorrhage (OSTROV et al. 1989; LAZARO et al. 1994). Ischemia and hemorrhage may occur spontaneously or may be secondary to medical therapy (YUSEM et al. 1989). Bleeding, in particular, is more frequent with PRL-secreting adenomas, nonfunctioning adenomas, and after bromocriptine therapy. Three hypotheses have been proposed to explain bleeding inside pituitary tumors: (1) outgrowing of blood supply by the expanding tumor, (2) presence of the foramen diaphragmatis sellae that impairs the blood supply, and (3) an increase in intracapsular pressure (LAZARO et al. 1994).

Although pituitary adenomas are almost always histologically benign, they may be locally invasive and characterized by a rapid cellular growth rate, cellular pleomorphism, and invasion of adjacent structures (especially the cavernous sinus). Aggressive tumors have a less favorable prognosis, probably because complete resection is difficult. Malignant degeneration is extremely rare, however, and is associated with distant metastases (SCHEITHAUER et al. 1986b; MARIUZZI et al. 1987).

Functioning pituitary adenomas are generally diagnosed when they are still small and have a well-defined capsule. Large lesions are encountered, however, especially in the elderly. The mass effect exerted by these space-occupying lesions compresses the surrounding structures, particularly the optic chiasm, the pituitary gland, the hypothalamus, the third ventricle, and the cavernous sinuses. Erosion of the sellar floor and the skull base may also occur.

Traditionally, pituitary adenomas have been classified on the basis of staining features into acidophilic (30%), basophilic (5%), and chromophobic adenomas. This classification does not reflect their functional or nonfunctional nature, however. A new and more sophisticated classification based on electron microscopy and immunohistochemical staining distinguishes hormonally active adenomas (75%) from clinically nonfunctional adenomas. Functioning adenomas are further differentiated by the hormone they produce. PRL-secreting adenomas (50%–60%) and GH- and ACTH-secreting tumors (THORNER et al. 1992; TAMAKI and YONEZAWA 1993; KOVACS et al. 1995) predominate. Adenomas producing thyroid-stimulating hormone (TSH), follicle-stimulating hormone (FSH), and luteinizing hormone (LH) are much less common (MARIUZZI et al. 1987). The higher incidence of hyperprolactinemia is not due exclusively to PRL-producing adenomas. Elevated PRL levels may also result from a loss of hypothalamic inhibitory signals due to interference by the tumor mass or another pathology ("stalk section effect"; SMITH and LAWS 1994). Around 10%–15% of all pituitary adenomas secrete multiple hormones (SCHEITHAUER et al. 1986a; KOVACS et al. 1995). These plurihormonal lesions may be composed of a single cell type secreting two or more different hormones simultaneously or two or more cell types each secreting a single hormone. Acidophilic, basophilic, and chromophobic adenomas may be functionally inactive (nonfunctional): the tumor cells may not produce any hormone, they may secrete minimal amounts of hormone insufficient to cause clinical signs, or they may produce a biologically inactive hormone subunit that is unable to interact with the specific receptors (KOVACS et al. 1995). A nonfunctioning adenoma may also represent the terminal stage of a previously secretory adenoma.

As mentioned previously, pituitary adenomas are classified at neuroradiological examination as micro- or macroadenomas (LUNDIN and BERGSTROM 1992). There are currently no imaging features allowing differentiation of the various types of adenomas (GUY et al. 1991; KOBAYASHI et al. 1994; WU and THOUMAS 1995).

1.2.3 Clinical Presentation

The clinical manifestations of pituitary adenomas depend on the hormone or hormones produced, the extent of impairment of normal pituitary gland function, tumor size, and any extrasellar extension. Microadenomas are often asymptomatic. They may be fortuitous discoveries at autopsy (14%–27%) or incidental findings (10%–20%) in patients without clinically significant pituitary disorders who undergo neuroradiological examination (especially MRI) for other purposes (Parent et al. 1981; Chacko and Chandy 1992; Elster 1994b; Hall et al. 1994; Teramoto et al. 1994). Functioning adenomas may cause symptoms due to hormone excess or mass effect correlated with tumor size. The signs and symptoms of hormone overproduction depend on the hormone or hormones secreted. Prolactinomas cause galactorrhea and hypogonadism (amenorrhea in females; impotence, decreased libido, gynecomastia, and testicular atrophy in males; Lundin et al. 1992b). GH-secreting adenomas cause acromegaly or gigantism, while ACTH-secreting adenomas cause Cushing's disease or Nelson's syndrome. Extremely rare TSH- and gonadotropin-secreting tumors cause hyperthyroidism and hypogonadism, respectively. However, hyperplasia of TSH- and ACTH-secreting cells is more often due to hypofunction of the target gland (hypothyroidism and hypoadrenocorticism) (Wolansky et al. 1996).

Nearly 10%–15% of all pituitary tumors are mixed adenomas that secrete multiple hormones. GH–PRL is the most common combination, but GH–TSH, ACTH–PRL, and GH–PRL–TSH tumors are also frequent.

In contrast to microadenomas, macroadenomas usually exert mass effect. Extrasellar tumor growth compresses and displaces the adjacent structures, especially the optic chiasm (Arita et al. 1993), the anterior portion of the third ventricle, and/or the cavernous sinus (Ahmadi et al. 1985; Scotti et al. 1988). Compression of the normal pituitary gland may cause hypopituitarism (Mariuzzi et al. 1987). Functioning adenomas, especially those secreting PRL in young adults and females and ACTH-producing tumors in both sexes, are usually detected when still small because they cause typical endocrine manifestations. Other pituitary adenomas, such as those secreting PRL in adult males and nonfunctioning tumors, are not discovered until they become large and alter function of the juxtasellar structures (especially the optic chiasm) or the pituitary gland due to compression (Chacko and Chandy 1992). Nonfunctioning adenomas do not produce quantitatively or qualitatively active hormones. Prolactinomas may be asymptomatic or cause nonspecific symptoms such as loss of libido, impotence, or testicular atrophy; these complications are sometimes underestimated because they are also age related.

Although infrequent, pituitary apoplexy is a serious complication of acute hemorrhage or, less often, infarction of the adenoma (Rolih and Ober 1993; Lazaro et al. 1994). The clinical picture may be silent or mild or may be sudden in onset and fulminant. The severity of manifestations varies. Symptoms include severe headache (often frontal and bitemporal), diplopia, depression of consciousness, hypo- or panhypopituitarism, meningeal irritation due to subarachnoid hemorrhage, and exacerbation of preexistent symptoms (Rossitch et al. 1992; Anderson and Afshar 1993). Fortunately, intratumoral hemorrhage often occurs without such a dramatic syndrome and is discovered incidentally (Ostrov et al. 1989) or is suggested by the presence of hemosiderin deposits (Lazaro et al. 1994). Pituitary apoplexy must be distinguished from a leaking aneurysm and acute meningitis (Ostrov et al. 1989).

1.2.4 Neuroradiological Features

The neuroradiological approach to the pituitary gland has changed remarkably during the past decade. Today, MRI is the imaging modality of choice for the diagnosis of pituitary disease (Davis et al. 1987b; Baleriaux et al. 1990; Johnson et al. 1992; Webb et al. 1992: Elster et al. 1993a; Brechtelsbauer et al. 1996). Despite its lower cost, CT currently plays only a complementary role; its sensitivity is not as good as MRI, and considerable radiation exposure may occur if follow-up studies are required. Conventional radiography of the pituitary sella is used solely for intraoperative verifications. Tomography of the pituitary sella is no longer performed. Once the mainstay for preoperative evaluation of the circle of Willis, cerebral arteriography has seen its indications decline because noninvasive techniques such as MR angiography and CT angiography can adequately assess the gross vascular anatomy of the sellar and parasellar regions (Barrou et al. 1997). Petrosal venous sampling is not yet routine practice; the technique is currently limited to patients with false-negative MRI examinations despite high serum hormone levels. Petrosal venous sampling may assist diagnosis of occult microadenomas, especially those secreting ACTH. It can also predict the location of an adenoma within the pituitary gland because venous drainage of each half of the gland occurs preferentially to the ipsilateral cavernous sinus (ELSTER 1993a; DE HERDER et al. 1994).

Literature data vary concerning the sensitivity and specificity of MRI for the detection of pituitary microadenomas (POJUNAS et al. 1986; KULKARNI et al. 1988; NEWTON et al. 1989; LUNDIN et al. 1991; BUCHFELDER et al. 1993; STADNIK et al. 1994).

The development of new pulse sequences (pre- and postcontrast T_1-weighted SE, T_2-weighted turbo spin-echo (TSE), GRE, dynamic and volumetric T_1-weighted sequences) has improved MR depiction of very small lesions. Today, precontrast MRI is considered just as sensitive as contrast-enhanced CT (STADNIK et al. 1994a). The diagnostic accuracy of MRI is further increased (to over 90%) by intravenous gadolinium administration (DAVIS et al. 1987b; STEINER et al. 1989; ELSTER 1993b; WU and THOUMAS 1995).

Compared to CT, MRI is radiation free and allows multiplanar analysis without requiring modification of patient positioning. The higher sensitivity of MRI is achieved by optimal spatial resolution that provides exquisite anatomic delineation of the pituitary region and can demonstrate an adenoma's relations to the anterior and posterior pituitary and the pituitary stalk (MARK et al. 1991; SUMIDA et al. 1994b). MRI can also accurately demonstrate the relations of the tumor to the optic chiasm, the cavernous sinus, the third ventricle, and the vessels of the circle of Willis (MARK et al. 1984; HIROHATA et al. 1992; ARITA et al. 1993; ELSTER et al. 1993b). Focal areas of necrosis, cystic degeneration, and hemorrhage within pituitary adenomas are also readily depicted. Intratumoral bleeding is particularly well demonstrated, even when minimal and/or subacute or chronic. In comparison, CT cannot distinguish necrosis and cystic degeneration from chronic hematoma.

MRI does, however, have limitations for assessment of focal erosion of the sellar floor, especially if minimal, and for detection of intratumoral calcifications. Although infrequent, calcifications are useful for differentiation of pituitary adenomas from other pituitary pathologies (especially craniopharyngioma). MRI is not sensitive enough to depict acute bleeding within the tumor and/or into the subarachnoid spaces.

MRI of the sellar region generally relies on coronal and sagittal T_1-weighted SE sequences before and after gadolinium administration. Thin slices are used (2–3 and 3–5 mm for micro- and macroadenomas, respectively), generally with a small field of view (20 cm) and high resolution (256+512). Axial scans are indicated only for macroadenomas. Although some authors consider postcontrast T_1-weighted SE sequences superfluous if the pituitary adenoma has already been demonstrated on unenhanced scans, gadolinium is useful for both micro- and macroadenomas (STADNIK et al. 1992; ELSTER 1994). Microadenomas within the pituitary gland, for example, are usually more conspicuous (HAMON-KERAUTRET et al. 1994). For macroadenomas, gadolinium improves delineation of the normal pituitary that can be spared during surgery (STEINER et al. 1994).

Standard T_1-weighted SE sequences can be completed by other pulse sequences. Coronal dynamic MRI during contrast injection is particularly helpful for evaluation of microadenomas (DAVIS et al. 1994). Coronal T_2-weighted TSE sequences are performed increasingly frequently, despite their relatively low sensitivity. The actual value of such sequences remains controversial; despite excellent anatomic resolution and only moderate flow-dependent artifacts, these sequences depict only 30%–50% of all microadenomas due to their high intensity signal. In contrast, T_2-weighted GRE imaging can demonstrate posthemorrhagic hemosiderin deposits as focal areas of low signal intensity.

Additional data may be obtained with volumetric postcontrast T_1-weighted images, fat-suppression techniques, three-dimensional turbo FLASH, and angiographic sequences (FINELLI and KAUFMAN 1993; DAVIS et al. 1994; GIRARD et al. 1994; KUCHARCZYK et al. 1994a; STADNIK et al. 1994a).

1.2.5 Microadenomas

Microadenomas are pituitary tumors with a diameter of less than 10mm. Along with direct demonstration of a focal area of signal alteration within the pituitary gland, MRI may reveal indirect signs: convexity of the superior aspect of the pituitary gland, erosion of the pituitary floor, asymmetry of the cavernous sinuses, and deviation of the pituitary stalk.

1.2.5.1 Direct Signs

Focal Area of Signal Alteration. A total of 80%–95% of all microadenomas are accurately detected and localized by MRI (Figs.1.3, 1.4). On T_1-weighted sequences, the majority image as a focus of low signal intensity relative to the surrounding pituitary gland (POJUNAS et al. 1986; ELSTER et al. 1993a). The more extensive any degenerative changes, the lower the signal intensity. However, a hypointense focus in the pituitary gland does not necessarily correspond to a microadenoma. Similar hypointense foci are also seen in healthy individuals. CHONG et al. (1994) observed such hypointense foci on T_1-weighted images in approximately 40% of healthy subjects, although they were generally smaller and less hypointense than microadenomas. Focal hypointensity on T_1-weighted images may also correspond to another pituitary pathology, especially cystic lesions (ELSTER 1993a).

Pituitary microadenomas are usually best depicted on enhanced MR images; they stand out as relatively unenhanced, well-defined focal areas on scans obtained immediately after intravenous gadolinium injection. The normal pituitary tissue enhances more rapidly than the adenoma. This particular enhancement behavior is even more conspicuous on dynamic sequences (DAVIS et al. 1987a; NEWTON et al. 1989; MIKI et al. 1990), which improve diagnostic accuracy (COLOMBO et al. 1994). Pituitary microadenomas usually enhance more slowly than the normal pituitary tissue; when tumor enhancement peaks, enhancement of the normal gland has usually already faded. A microadenoma may thus be visible as a hyperintense focus on delayed scans (about 30–60min after contrast injection) (NEWTON et al. 1989; STADNIK et al. 1992; SUMIDA et al. 1994; YUH et al. 1994).

Nearly 10% of all microadenomas are difficult to detect on pre- or postcontrast scans because they enhance just as rapidly as the normal parenchyma.

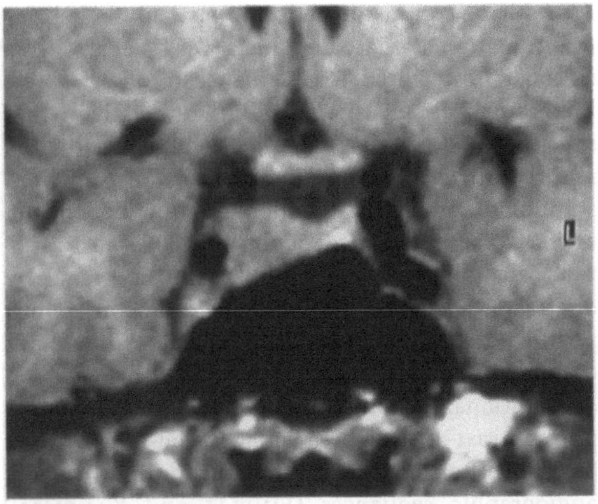

a

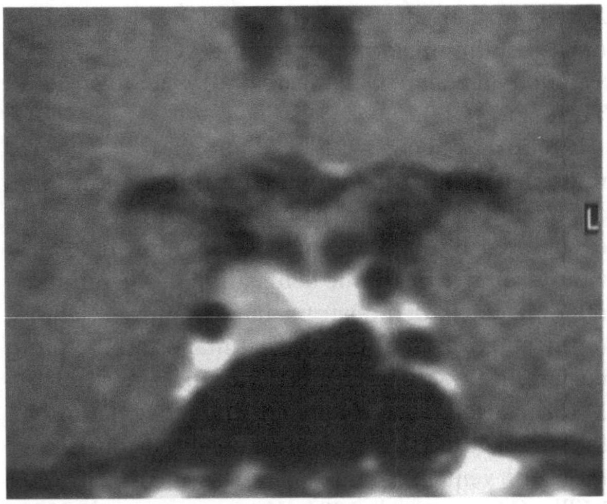

c

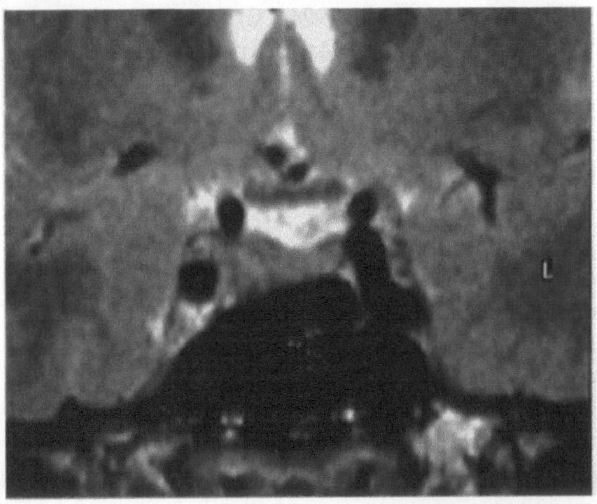

b

Fig. 1.3a–c. Prolactin (PRL)-secreting pituitary microadenoma. **a** Unenhanced coronal T_1-weighted SE sequence. **b** Coronal T_2-weighted turbo spin-echo (TSE) sequence. **c** Dynamic sequence during gadolinium injection. On the T_1-weighted sequence (**a**) and the first unenhanced dynamic image (**c**), the microadenoma lateralized on the right is directly visible as a zone of relatively low signal intensity compared to the pituitary tissue; the low signal intensity is more conspicuous during and after gadolinum injection (**c**). On the T_2-weighted TSE images (**b**), the microadenoma has a relatively inhomogeneous high signal intensity. Indirect signs of this microadenoma include the convexity of the superior aspect of the pituitary gland, collapse of the sellar floor, and minimal deviation of the neural stalk. Note the early invasion of the right cavernous sinus

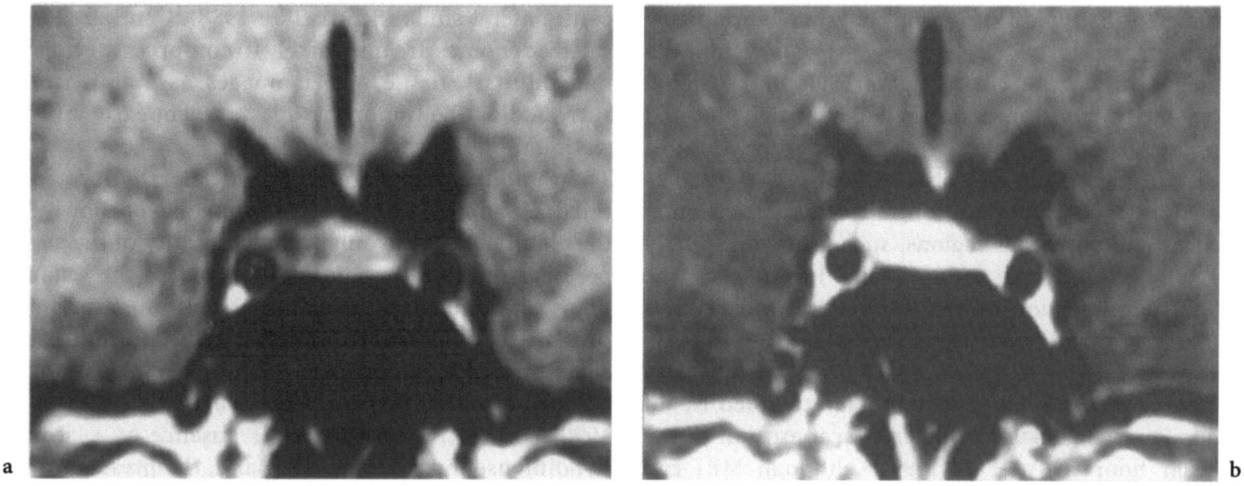

Fig. 1.4a,b. Prolactin (PRL)-secreting pituitary microadenoma. a Unenhanced coronal T_1-weighted SE sequence. b Contrast-enhanced coronal T_1-weighted SE image. This hypointense microadenoma lateralized on the right on the unenhanced T_1-weighted image appeared inhomogeneously hyperintense after gadolinium injection. No signs of sellar floor collapse. Minimal blistering is apparent on the superior aspect of the pituitary gland

Several means have been proposed to reduce the frequency of false-negative studies, including dynamic sequences (Scheithauer et al. 1986; Miki et al. 1990; Finelli and Kaufman 1993; Davis et al. 1994; Kucharczyk et al. 1994b) and injection of only half the usual dose of contrast agent (Davis et al. 1991). Despite their low diagnostic accuracy, T_2-weighted TSE images may allow detection of microadenomas as focal areas of high signal intensity (Elster 1993a,b; Jack et al. 1994; Mukherji et al. 1994).

Cystic-necrotic degeneration and chronic hematoma are usually depicted as a hyperintense focus within a tumor on T_2-weighted TSE images. The microadenoma has usually already been identified as a focus of hypointensity (cystic degeneration) or hyperintensity (necrosis) on T_1-weighted images. Subacute and chronic intratumoral bleeding images as a spontaneous bright signal on both T_1-weighted SE and T_2-weighted TSE sequences. After contrast administration, the intensity fades following enhancement of the normal pituitary tissue (Hamon-Kerautret et al. 1994).
On rare occasions, multiple hypointense foci have been detected in the pituitary gland. Autopsy in such cases revealed the presence of multiple microadenomas.

Location of the Signal Alteration. The various cell types in the anterior pituitary are distributed in a well-defined manner. Lactotrophs and somatotrophs occur predominantly in the lateral wings. Corticotrophs, thyrotrophs, and gonadotrophs tend to be centrally located. The characteristic locations of the different cell types are well correlated with the location of certain pituitary microadenomas. PRL- and GH-secreting adenomas, for example, are generally found in the lateral part of the pituitary gland (Buchfelder et al. 1993; Elster 1993a).

1.2.5.2 Indirect Signs

The predominantly lateral location of certain microadenomas explains the frequency of ancillary findings despite their small dimensions. These indirect signs include focal convexity of the superior aspect of the pituitary, erosion of the sellar floor, tilting of the pituitary stalk, and occasionally asymmetry of the cavernous sinus (Figs.1.3, 1.4) (Ahmadi et al. 1990; Wu and Thoumas 1995).

Convexity of the Superior Surface of the Pituitary Gland. In the normal adult, the pituitary gland is spherical or flat. The height varies but is always less than 8 mm. The average width is 10–12 mm, and the anteroposterior diameter is usually about 8 mm. The upper aspect of the gland is usually flat or minimally concave downward, but is always symmetrical (Wiener et al. 1985). The presence of a microadenoma may cause a slight focal elevation of the superior aspect of the pituitary gland on the same side as the tumor (Fig. 1.3; Davis et al. 1987b). In contrast, global convexity of the superior aspect of the gland is typical of normal physiologic pituitary hyperplasia during adolescence, pregnancy, and the postpartum period (Elster et al. 1990, 1991). Global convexity may also correspond to a medially located microadenoma. Convexity of the superior aspect of the pituitary gland may also be due to the particular anatomic configuration of the otherwise normal sellar and parasellar regions, such as a congenitally small sella turcica or a medial location of the cavernous portion of the internal carotid arteries ("kissing carotids") (Elster 1993a).

Sloping of the Sellar Floor. Pressure exerted by an adenoma may cause ipsilateral focal erosion of the sellar floor (Guy et al. 1991). Although MRI can detect changes in the sellar floor, minimal erosion is best defined by CT. Moreover, the presence of a well-aerated sphenoidal sinus makes MR detection of bony erosion even more difficult. A nonpathologic slope of the sellar floor may be congenital or related to a sphenoid sinus septum (Wu and Thoumas 1995).

Tilt of the Pituitary Stalk. A pituitary adenoma may displace the pituitary stalk from its normal midline position. Deviation generally occurs to the side opposite the adenoma. Displacement of the pituitary stalk may also be due to a congenitally eccentric location of the pituitary gland or to eccentric insertion of the infundibulum on the gland. On rare occasions, a paradoxical and ipsilateral tilt of the pituitary stalk is observed secondary to sloping of the sellar floor and/or tumor shrinkage in response to medical treatment (Ahmadi et al. 1990; Wu and Thoumas 1995). Overall, however, tilting of the stalk is of little value for detection and localization of pituitary adenomas.

Asymmetry of the Parasellar Regions. The lateral location of numerous pituitary tumors, especially PRL- and GH-secreting adenomas, may cause unilateral contour deformities such as an eccentric bulge toward the ipsilateral cavernous sinus. Depiction of lateral bulging is generally improved by contrast administration. True invasion of the ipsilateral cavernous sinus is also possible (Peck et al. 1988; Hirohata et al. 1992; Barrou et al. 1997). MRI prediction of cavernous sinus invasion is often difficult because the dural membrane separating the pituitary cavity from the cavernous sinus is not always easy to visualize. The only features suggestive of early invasion of the cavernous sinus are asymmetry in size and signal intensity relative to the contralateral sinus (Scotti et al. 1988). Centrally located adenomas are more likely to compress the normal pituitary tissue, which images as a thin rim surrounding the tumor that may prevent early infiltration of the cavernous sinuses.

These indirect signs are typical of laterally located microadenomas. Tumors in the medial portion of the gland may cause only slight convexity of the superior aspect and/or minimal erosion of the sellar floor; tilt of the pituitary stalk is usually absent. The presence of two or more of these nonspecific indirect signs strongly suggests the diagnosis, especially if serum hormone levels are elevated (Ahmadi et al. 1990; Hall et al. 1994). In the absence of a clear hypointense focus within the gland, the presence of only one sign is not diagnostic for pituitary microadenoma (Yusem et al. 1989).

At CT, microadenomas may image as a low-density focus; they are often visible only on postcontrast scans. Dynamic CT improves diagnostic accuracy and may demonstrate the pituitary tuft (Bonneville et al. 1993). Indirect signs are sometimes present, but are always less conspicuous than with MRI, except for erosion of the sellar floor.

1.2.6 Macroadenomas

MRI is the imaging modality of choice for these pituitary tumors measuring 10mm or more. Its high spatial resolution and multiplanar imaging capabilities allow precise anatomic and topographic delineation of the entire region. Tumor size, shape, location, extension, and relations to the juxtasellar structures are all well depicted, as are modifications in internal architecture (Lundin et al. 1991; Elster 1993a). CT can also demonstrate macroadenomas, but lacks resolution for definition of tumor relations with adjacent structures (especially the optic tracts). In addition, CT cannot characterize the internal structure of the tumor itself. In contrast, CT is more sensitive than MRI for demonstration of bone changes and intratumoral calcification (Lundin et al. 1991).

1.2.6.1 Signal Features

On T_1-weighted SE sequences, solid macroadenomas are usually isointense to the brain parenchyma and relatively hypointense to the anterior pituitary, if still visible. On T_2-weighted TSE images, they appear isointense or slightly hyperintense (Kobayashi et al. 1994). Controversy exists as to whether the homogeneous signal pattern of macroadenomas on T_1- and especially T_2-weighted images is actually correlated with their solid consistency (Weissbuch 1986; Snow et al. 1990). After contrast administration, tumor enhancement is generally homogeneous, although not as intense as that of the normal pituitary gland (Sumida et al. 1994).

Changes in intratumoral signal intensity are due essentially to necrosis, cystic degeneration, hemorrhage, posthemorrhage hemosiderin deposits, and calcifications. Except for calcifications, MRI is usually superior to CT for detection of intratumoral architectural alterations.

Necrosis and cystic degeneration (see Fig .1.7) are visible as one or more focal areas of different size, with a low T_1 signal and a high T_2 signal. The signal intensity on T_2-weighted sequences depends essentially on the protein concentration and the fluid content (free water) in these areas. Use of paramagnetic contrast agents accentuates the hyposignal: the solid components of the tumor enhance, whereas degenerative areas do not (Nakamura et al. 1988).

The signal intensity of an intratumoral hematoma depends on its age and the strength of the magnetic field (Barkovich and Atlas 1988; Lazaro et al. 1994). In the acute stage, bleeding is usually not visible on MRI; occasionally, it is depicted as a hypointense focus on T_2-weighted images. In contrast, acute bleeding is usually well demonstrated by CT as an area of focal hyperdensity. Subacute and chronic intratumoral hemorrhage are always spontaneously hyperintense on both T_1- and T_2-weighted images. CT cannot distinguish subacute and chronic hemorrhage from necrosis or cystic degeneration. On postcontrast T_1-weighted SE images, the spontaneously hyperintense signal corresponding to hemorrhage fades, as previously described for microadenomas. Both cystic and hemorrhagic masses may contain fluid levels (see Fig. 1.8). Intratumoral calcifications are rare and are seen predominantly with PRL- and GH-secreting tumors (Webster et al. 1994).

Posthemorrhagic hemosiderin deposits appear as hypointense foci and are most conspicuous on T_2-weighted sequences.

As mentioned previously, MRI has limited value for detection of calcifications, especially microcalcifications. Larger calcifications may be identified as a hyposignal on T_1-weighted sequences. Intrasellar aneurysms have a similar low-intensity signal because of the signal void created by flowing blood. Differential diagnosis may be improved by T_2-weighted GRE imaging and MR angiography (Holland et al. 1985; Davis et al. 1987b).

1.2.6.2 Size and Extension

Pituitary macroadenomas vary in size from 10mm to several centimeters (Scheithauer et al. 1986; Lundin and Pedersen 1992). Small macroadenomas (10–12 mm) may remain confined within the pituitary sella, even after enlargement of the pituitary cavity itself. These intrasellar macroadenomas have MRI features similar to those of microadenomas, except for their size and indirect signs, which are accentuated (Fig. 1.5). Once the lesion diameter exceeds 13–15 mm, contiguous spread occurs outside of the sellar cavity to adjacent structures, in particular to the suprasellar cisterns, the sphenoidal sinus, and the cavernous sinus. Anterosellar and retrosellar spread are less common (Fig. 1.6–1.8).

Best recognized on postcontrast scans because it enhances more than the macroadenoma, the anterior pituitary is compressed and deformed. When still visible, it tends to be sickle or club shaped and is displaced to the periphery of the adenoma, especially laterally or superiorly (Steiner et al. 1994; Sumida et al. 1994a). Extremely large macroadenomas over 20mm may prevent clear demonstration of the anterior pituitary, the posterior pituitary, and the pituitary stalk (Lundin and Bergstrom 1992; Steiner et al. 1994). In particular, the bright signal on precontrast T_1-weighted images corresponding to the posterior pituitary may be displaced, even outside of the sellar cavity (Colombo et al. 1987; Brooks et al. 1989).

Juxtasellar Extension. This kind of extension depends on the anatomic and topographic features of the sellar and parasellar regions and the intrinsic characteristics of the tumor itself (growth rate, infiltrative behavior).

Slowly growing adenomas are generally round or bilobar, while rapidly growing adenomas tend to be asymmetrical and/or multilobar. Although histologically benign, some pituitary adenomas have invasive and infiltrative features (Scotti et al. 1988) and may spread in all directions.

Suprasellar Extension. Contiguous spread toward the suprasellar cisterns is initially prevented by the

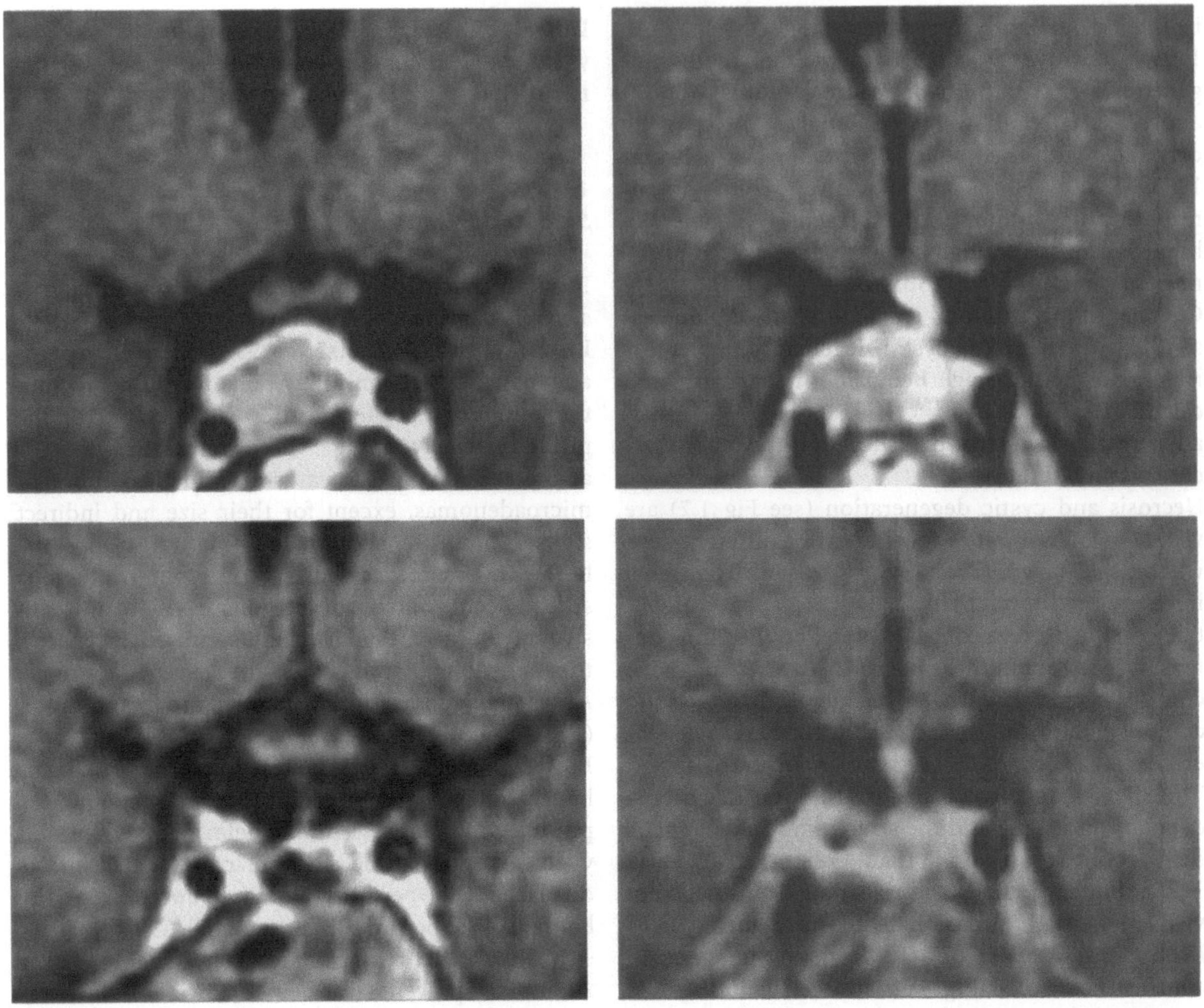

Fig. 1.5a–d. Growth hormone (GH)-secreting pituitary macroadenoma. **a,b** Contrast-enhanced coronal T_1-weighted SE sequence. Postoperative recurrence: expanding lesion occupying the right lateral and median portion of the sellar cavity with early suprasellar extension. The adenoma appears hypointense relative to the pituitary parenchyma. Note the convexity of the superior aspect of the pituitary gland, contralateral deviation of the neural stalk and the residual pituitary tissue, and minimal compression on the right parasellar sinus. The suprasellar optic tracts are not compressed. **c,d** Contrast-enhanced coronal T_1-weighted SE sequence. Postoperative control after 3months: complete ablation of the pituitary adenoma with postsurgical median and paramedian intrasellar hypointensity. The signs of mass effect on the residual pituitary gland and the neural stalk are no longer visible. Postsurgical inflammatory changes are visible in the sphenoid sinus

fibrous diaphragm of sella turcica. As it enlarges, the adenoma progressively causes slight upward convexity of the diaphragm of sella turcica before ultimately entering the suprasellar region through the widened foramen diaphragmatis sellae. The Bonneville classification (Bonneville et al. 1986), which distinguished three grades of suprasellar extension, has been supplanted by the SIPAP (suprasellar, infrasellar, parasellar, anterior, posterior) system (Edal et al. 1997), which differentiates five grades of cranial growth. Grade 0 is characterized by the absence of extrasellar tumor extension. Grades 1 and 2 correspond to bulging of the tumor within the suprasellar cisterns, without (grade 1) or with (grade 2) extension to the inferior aspect of the optic chiasm. Grade 3 corresponds to cranial dislocation of the optic chiasm with initial deformation of the third ventricle. Grade 4 is characterized by the obstruction of one or both interventricular foramina, resulting in hydrocephalus. Spread toward the suprasellar cisterns may be accompanied by anterior, posterior, or lateral extension. In contrast to CT, MRI accurately defines tumor relations with the adjacent structures, which may be displaced (especially the optic tracts, the third ventricle, and the vessels of the circle of Willis).

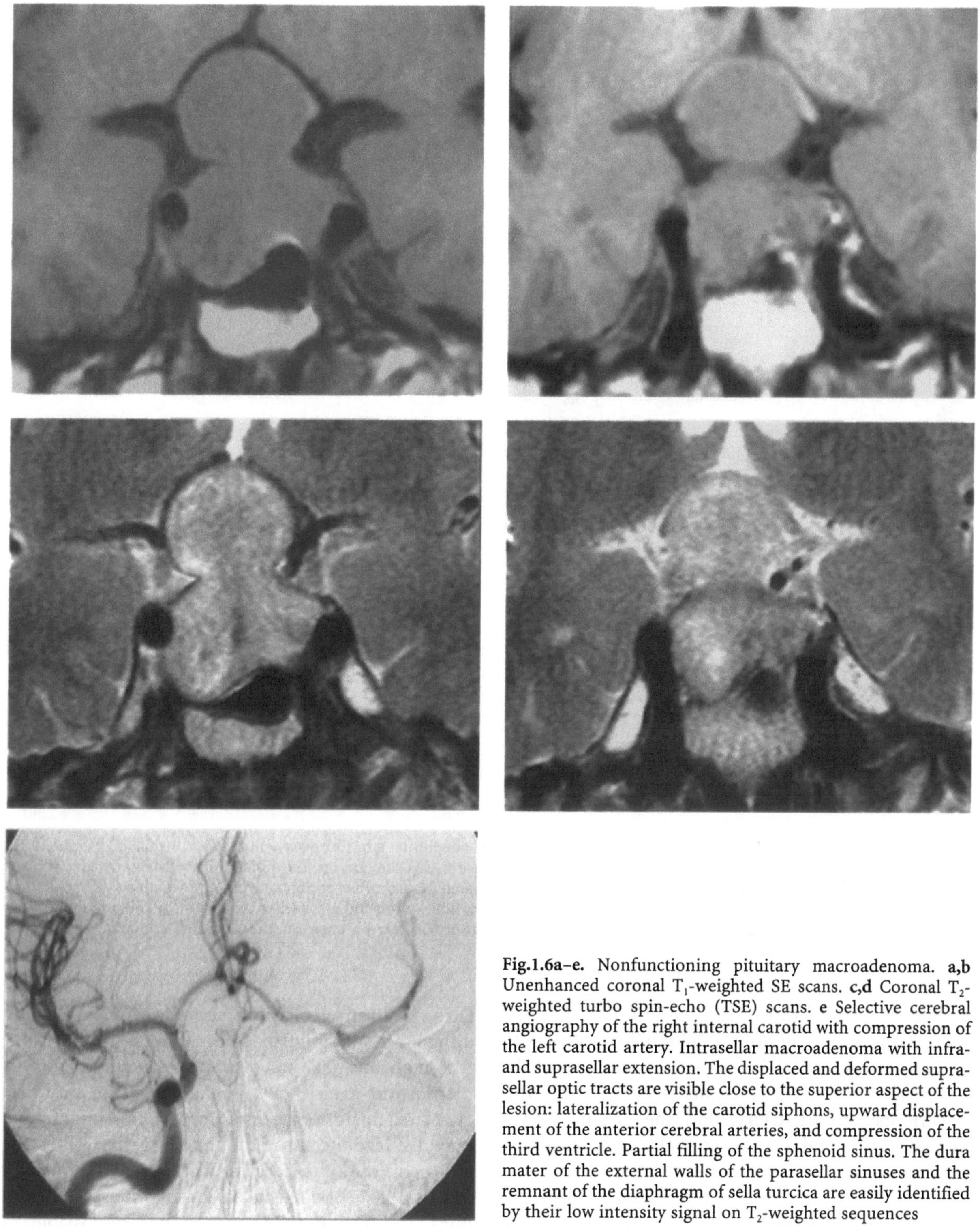

a b c d e

Fig. 1.6a–e. Nonfunctioning pituitary macroadenoma. **a,b** Unenhanced coronal T_1-weighted SE scans. **c,d** Coronal T_2-weighted turbo spin-echo (TSE) scans. **e** Selective cerebral angiography of the right internal carotid with compression of the left carotid artery. Intrasellar macroadenoma with infra- and suprasellar extension. The displaced and deformed suprasellar optic tracts are visible close to the superior aspect of the lesion: lateralization of the carotid siphons, upward displacement of the anterior cerebral arteries, and compression of the third ventricle. Partial filling of the sphenoid sinus. The dura mater of the external walls of the parasellar sinuses and the remnant of the diaphragm of sella turcica are easily identified by their low intensity signal on T_2-weighted sequences

Parasellar Extension. Parasellar extension involving the cavernous sinus is frequent. It may be unilateral or bilateral and may correspond to compression or various degrees of invasion of the cavernous sinus. Parasellar extension is classified in five grades based on relations with the medial or lateral tangent to the carotid siphon (grade 0 and 2, respectively) or to the carotid line (grade 1). Extension beyond the lateral tangent and encasement of the intracavernous carotid artery correspond to grades 3 and 4, re-

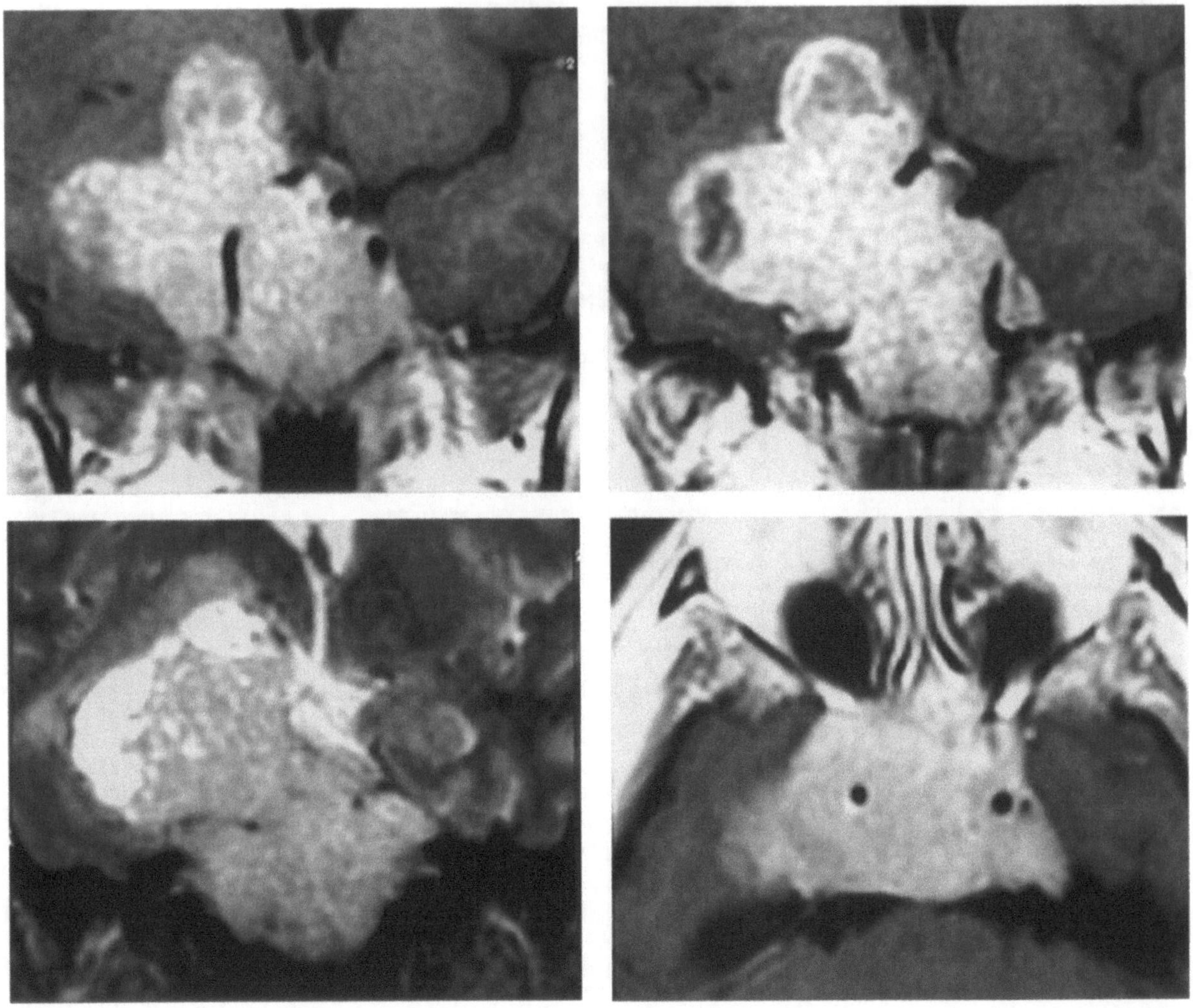

a b

c d

Fig. 1.7a–d. Invasive prolactin (PRL)-secreting pituitary macroadenoma. **a,b** Contrast-enhanced coronal T_1-weighted SE sequences. **a,b** This macroadenoma with polycyclic contours had invaded the body of the sphenoid and the parasellar sinuses bilaterally. **c** Coronal T_2-weighted turbo spin-echo (TSE) sequence. **d** Contrast-enhanced axial T_1-weighted SE sequence. Encasement of the carotid siphons is visible as a reduction in caliber. Note the retrosellar extension of the adenoma. This essentially solid tumor containing peripheral cystic-necrotic zones is hypointense on the T_1-weighted images (**a,b**) and hyperintense on the T_2-weighted sequences (**c**)

spectively (Edal et al. 1997). Optimum imaging of the parasellar regions is obtained with GRE sequences, which reliably depict the anatomy of the cavernous sinus. The venous spaces, the intracavernous carotid artery, and the cranial nerves (especially III and V) are especially well delineated (Daniel et al. 1985,1988).

The lateral dural membrane of the caverous sinus is usually clearly identified on pre- and especially on postcontrast T_1- and T_2-weighted SE sequences. The medial dural membrane separating the cavernous sinus from the pituitary gland is rarely well delineated. Recognition of initial infiltration of the parasellar region is thus usually difficult (Scotti et al. 1988; Daita et al. 1995).

Early infiltration of the cavernous sinus is usually difficult to distinguish from simple compression. Although the position of the cavernous portion of the carotid artery varies relative to the pituitary gland, extrinsic compression on the cavernous sinus may displace the carotid siphon laterally, with widening of the intercarotid distance (Hirsch and Frank 1988; Scotti et al. 1988). In other cases, early dural infiltration is difficult if not impossible to detect. Although rarely present, the rim sign (presence of normal pituitary tissue around the periphery of the tumor) may help rule out infiltration. In contrast, extensive tumor invasion of the cavernous sinus results in encasement of the carotid siphon, although generally without causing

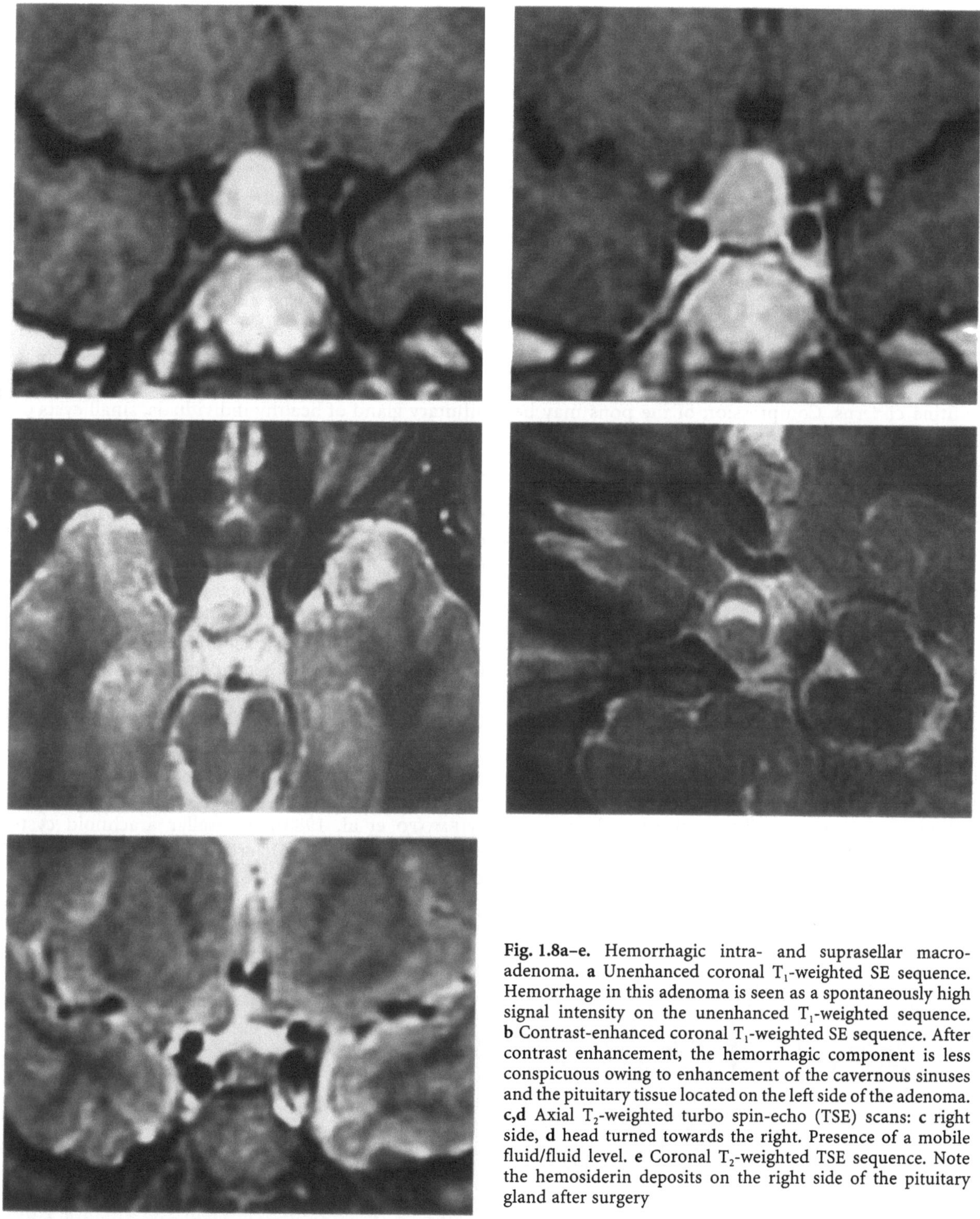

Fig. 1.8a–e. Hemorrhagic intra- and suprasellar macroadenoma. **a** Unenhanced coronal T_1-weighted SE sequence. Hemorrhage in this adenoma is seen as a spontaneously high signal intensity on the unenhanced T_1-weighted sequence. **b** Contrast-enhanced coronal T_1-weighted SE sequence. After contrast enhancement, the hemorrhagic component is less conspicuous owing to enhancement of the cavernous sinuses and the pituitary tissue located on the left side of the adenoma. **c,d** Axial T_2-weighted turbo spin-echo (TSE) scans: **c** right side, **d** head turned towards the right. Presence of a mobile fluid/fluid level. **e** Coronal T_2-weighted TSE sequence. Note the hemosiderin deposits on the right side of the pituitary gland after surgery

occlusion, unlike parasellar meningiomas. Owing to their location in the lateral compartment of the cavernous sinus, cranial nerves III–VI are less affected by pituitary adenomas than by other parasellar pathologies.

Infrasellar, Posterior, and Anterior Extension. Infrasellar spread towards the sphenoidal sinus is always secondary to erosion of the sellar floor. Grade 0 corresponds to the absence of erosion or minimal erosion of the sellar floor. Grades 1 and 2 correspond to initial bulging and extensive penetration of the sphenoidal sinus, respectively. Further extension in anteroinferior or posterocaudal directions may involve the rhinopharynx, the ethmoidal cells, the nasal cavities, and the clivus (LUNDIN et al. 1991; EDAL et al. 1997). Anterior spread towards the anterior cranial fossa may occur if the tumor extends beyond the tuberculum sellae.

Retrosellar Extension. This kind of extension (Fig. 1.9) generally occurs after initial cranial growth of the tumor that spreads secondarily beyond the dorsum sellae. Less often, erosion of the dorsum sellae results in posterior development of the macroadenoma toward the interpeduncular and prepontine cisterns. Compression of the pons may be accompanied by compression, displacement, and encasement of the basilar artery (EDAL et al. 1997). Posterior and anterior extension of macroadenomas are usually both classified in two grades (0 and 1).

1.2.6.3 Sellar Cavity

Pituitary macroadenomas always alter the size and shape of the sellar region: modifications include enlargement of the pituitary cavity (or complete destruction in extreme cases) and erosion or lysis of the dorsum sellae, the posterior and anterior clinoid processes, and/or the tuberculum sellae. Bone changes are usually readily visualized both on standard radiographs and on CT scans. On MRI, these architectural alterations are demonstrated by disappearance of the hypointense signal of the cortical bone and the hyperintense signal of the bone marrow. Tumor infiltration of the bone tissue also results in enhancement on postcontrast sequences (Edal et al. 1997). In advanced disease with complete destruction of the pituitary cavity, a phantom cavity may be seen.

1.2.7 Differential Diagnosis

The main differential diagnoses for microadenomas include hypointense foci detected incidentally in the pituitary gland of healthy individuals, small cysts of the pars intermedia, and tumors of the posterior pituitary. Microscopic abscesses and micrometastases are exceptional (BERGER et al. 1986; ELSTER 1993b; REUL et al. 1995). Macroadenomas must be differentiated from a wide variety of pathologies, including all of the space-occupying lesions of the sellar and parasellar regions (SENER and JINKINS 1991; SAUTNER et al. 1993; YU et al. 1995). Expanding lesions may be of primary intrasellar origin with secondary extrasellar extension or of primary extrasellar origin with secondary invasion of the sellar cavity (SUMIDA et al. 1994b). The most frequent nonadenomatous sellar lesions are meningioma of the diaphragm of sella turcica and the tuberculum sellae, Rathke cleft cyst (NEMOTO et al. 1988), intrasellar arachnoid cysts (NOMURA et al. 1996), craniopharyngioma, chordoma, metastasis, lymphocytic hypophysitis

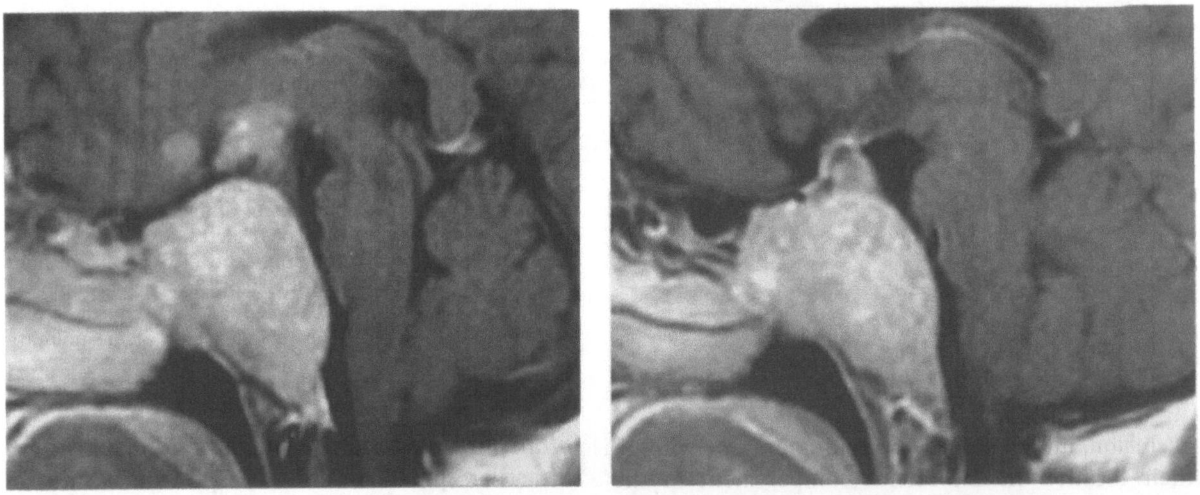

a b

Fig. 1.9a,b. Compact invasive macroadenoma. Contrast-enhanced sagittal T_1-weighted SE sequences. This invasive adenoma has spread anteroinferiorly toward the rhinopharynx, the ethmoid, and the nasal cavities. Disappearance of the sellar cavity (phantom sella)

(Baskin et al. 1982; Ahmadi et al. 1995), plasmacytoma of the clivus, and sphenoidal sinus mucocele and pyocele with sellar extension (Clarke et al. 1992). Careful evaluation of the signal intensity of a space-occupying lesion usually permits differential diagnosis by MRI. However, supplemental CT scans may be required to demonstrate calcifications and/or focal erosion (Holland et al. 1985; Lundin et al. 1991).

Vascular disease of the sellar and parasellar regions is usually readily demonstrated by MRI. Intrasellar aneurysm, intrasellar trigeminal artery, and carotid–cavernous fistulae usually display typical MRI features, and the diagnosis can usually be confirmed by carotid angiography (Kayath et al. 1991; Elster 1993a).

1.2.8 Therapy and Follow-Up

Three treatment options are available for pituitary adenomas: medical therapy, surgery, and radiation therapy.

1.2.8.1 Medical Therapy

Drug therapy is the standard first-line treatment for pituitary microadenomas, preoperative macroadenomas, and nonsurgical macroadenomas. It is administered postoperatively to patients who have had subtotal tumor resection and patients with persistently high serum hormone levels (especially PRL or GH) (Lundin et al. 1992a; Plockinger et al. 1994). Prolactinomas are treated with non-ergot dopamine receptor agonists such as bromocriptine and cabergoline. Somatostatin and somatostatin analogues such as octreotide are used for GH- and TSH-secreting adenomas and nonfunctioning adenomas (Bevan et al. 1992; Sy et al. 1992; Chanson et al. 1993; Delgrange et al. 1996). The response of pituitary adenomas to medical treatment depends on the presence of specific cell receptors such as dopamine D_2 receptors and sex steroid receptors (SSR) in the tumor. The presence of SSR can be confirmed by 111-indium octreotide scintigraphy (De Bruin et al. 1992; Van Royen et al. 1996). Somatostatin analogues have also been used to treat ACTH- and FSH/LH-producing adenomas, although results have been less satisfactory (Warnet 1992). Combination regimens including bromocriptine and somatostatin analogues are generally used for plurihormonal adenomas, in particular GH–PRL and TSH–PRL tumors (Cremonini et al. 1992; Sadoul et al. 1992; Verhoeff et al. 1993).

Medical therapy lowers serum hormone levels and shrinks the tumor mass (Sy et al. 1992; Gancel et al. 1994). The two effects are usually not correlated, however; the reduction in serum levels is usually more rapid and of greater amplitude. Complete disappearance of a pituitary adenoma followed by reexpansion of the pituitary gland has been described (Fassbender et al. 1992). The literature also contains several reports of resistance or intolerance to bromocriptine (Schwarzstein et al. 1993).

The spectrum of intratumoral changes varies considerably, depending on the type of medical treatment. Bromocriptine and its analogues induce conspicuous ischemic and hemorrhagic degenerative phenomena associated with perivascular and interstitial fibrosis, whereas somatostatin analogues do not (Ezzat et al. 1994; Kreft et al. 1996).

Medical therapy is effective in producing symptomatic improvement, whether due to excess hormone secretion or mass effect (including hypopituitarism) (Van't Verlaat et al. 1990; Elster et al. 1993a; Paoletti et al. 1994).

Few complications are encountered with medical therapy. Cerebrospinal fluid (CSF) rhinorrhea may occur after drug-induced shrinkage of an invasive adenoma that has eroded the sellar floor, resulting in creation of an empty sella (Pascal-Vigneron et al. 1994). These CSF fistulae require surgical closure. A transient collection of intrasellar air is an infrequent complication: shrinkage of the macroadenoma in response to medical therapy allows air to penetrate the sellar cavity through the eroded sellar floor. Surgery is usually not required because these fistulae close spontaneously and the air is resorbed (Fagel et al. 1986). Other adverse effects are usually transient, with the exception of an increased frequency of asymptomatic cholelithiasis (Sadoul et al. 1992; Chanson et al. 1993).

1.2.8.2 Surgery

Surgery is currently the treatment of choice for adenomas refractory to medical therapy, GH- and ACTH-secreting microadenomas, plurihormonal adenomas, and lesions responsible for rapidly progressive neurological symptoms (especially visual disorders). The surgical approach (transsphenoidal or frontal) depends on the size, anatomic relations, and invasiveness of the tumor and the anatomy of the sellar and parasellar regions (DINA et al. 1993). These regions are best assessed by MRI. Complementary CT provides important anatomic details concerning pneumatization of the sphenoidal sinus, the presence and location of the thin sphenoidal septa, and the condition of the sellar floor (thinning or complete erosion) (SNOW et al. 1990).

1.2.8.3
Radiation Therapy

Radiation therapy is today reserved as second-line treatment after medical therapy. Indications include inoperable adenomas, invasive and only partially resected tumors, and persistence of high hormone levels after surgery (MOBERG et al. 1991; FISHER et al. 1994; TSANG et al. 1994).

1.2.8.4
Follow-Up

MRI is helpful to assess response to medical and radiation therapy and for postoperative follow-up. The efficacy of medical therapy, for example, is apparent as a reduction in tumor size and intratumoral modifications (WEISSBUCH 1986; YUSEM et al. 1989; LUNDIN et al. 1992a; BENESCH et al. 1995). Thanks to the absence of ionizing radiation, follow-up by MRI is also possible during pregnancy (after the third

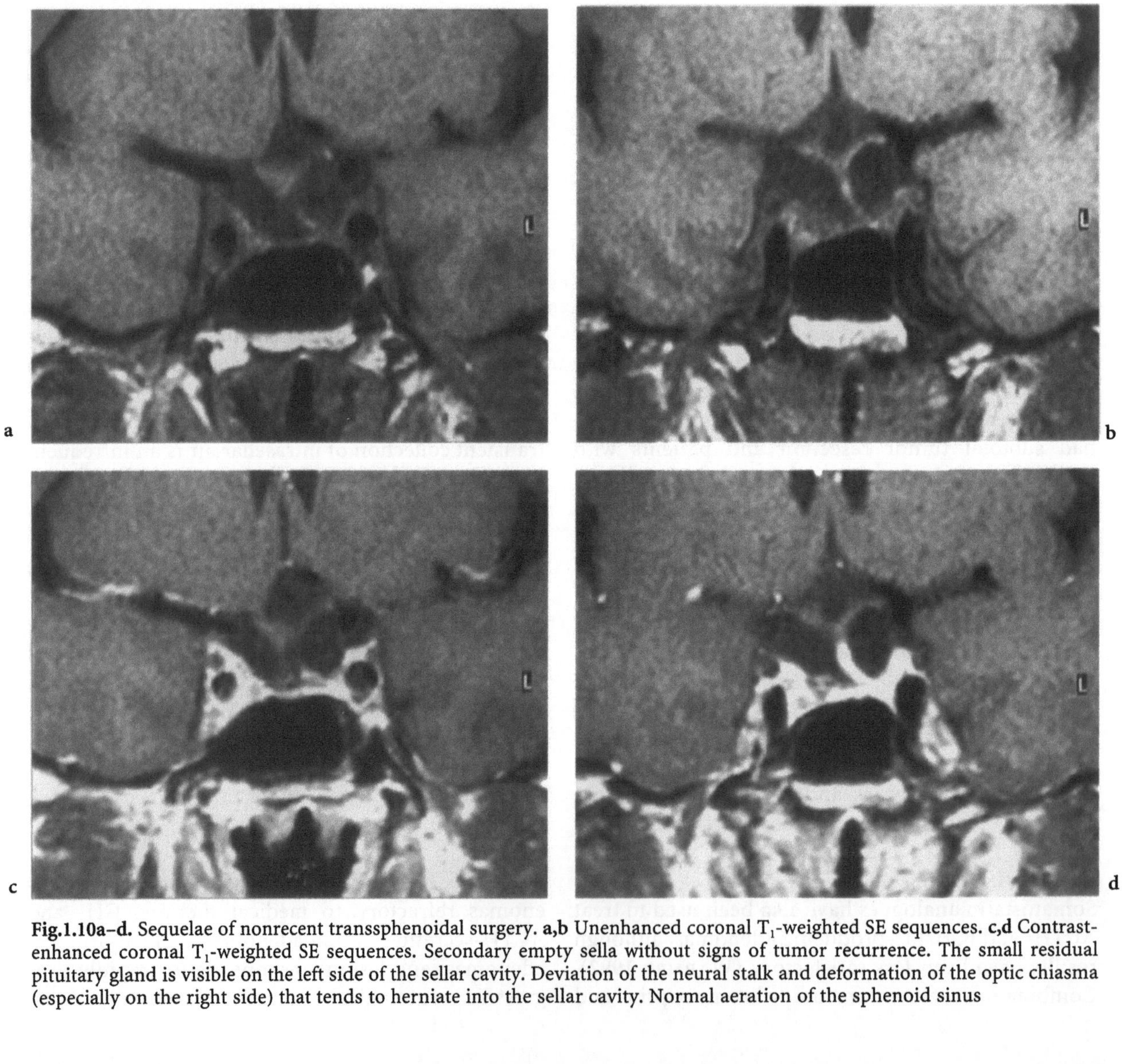

Fig.1.10a–d. Sequelae of nonrecent transsphenoidal surgery. **a,b** Unenhanced coronal T_1-weighted SE sequences. **c,d** Contrast-enhanced coronal T_1-weighted SE sequences. Secondary empty sella without signs of tumor recurrence. The small residual pituitary gland is visible on the left side of the sellar cavity. Deviation of the neural stalk and deformation of the optic chiasma (especially on the right side) that tends to herniate into the sellar cavity. Normal aeration of the sphenoid sinus

month and without contrast administration) and the postpartum period.

The MRI appearance of the postoperative sella depends on the surgical approach, the presence of residual tumor, the extent of lesions caused by the macroadenoma, and the type and amount of graft material (STEINER et al. 1992; KREMER et al. 1996). MRI also provides additional information on the pituitary gland, its reexpansion, and its location. Complete reexpansion of the pituitary gland is seldom seen (Fig. 1.10), whereas the frequently deformed optic chiasm slowly returns to its former position (HALD et al. 1992; STEINER et al. 1994). Herniation of the optic chiasm into a secondary empty sella may occur postoperatively or as a complication of medical treatment (KAUFMAN et al. 1989; DINA et al. 1993).

Following transsphenoidal surgery, the sphenoidal sinus and the sellar cavity are partially or completely filled with various types and amounts of graft materials (gelatin foam, muscle, fat; Spongostan, Ferrosan, Copenhagen) in order to prevent bleeding and CSF rhinorrhea.

During the immediate postoperative period, MRI cannot distinguish graft materials from residual tumor or normal pituitary tissue as they have similar signal intensities. Furthermore, graft materials (especially Spongostan) often showing inflammatory changes may also mimic recurrent tumor (STEINER et al. 1992). After a variable interval (about 3months), graft materials are partially resorbed and replaced by scar tissue. Residual tumor (Fig. 1.11) or recurrence is then more easily depicted by MRI. Because of postoperative reorganization, only

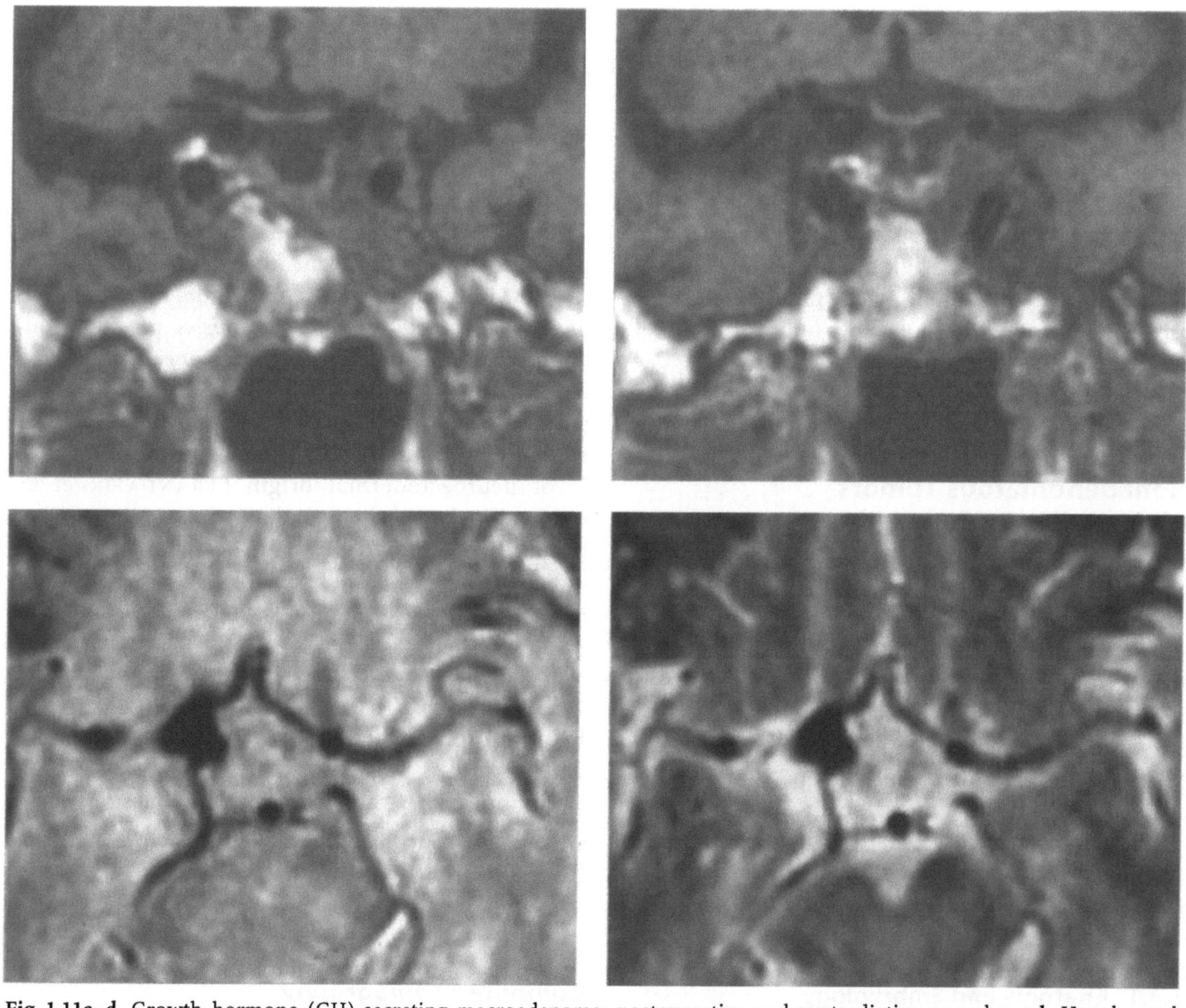

a b c d

Fig. 1.11a–d. Growth hormone (GH)-secreting macroadenoma: postoperative and postradiation sequelae. **a,b** Unenhanced coronal T_1-weighted SE sequences. Tumor infiltration of the left parasellar sinus. **c,d** Axial T_2-weighted SE density proton (DP) sequences. Partially empty sella. Diffuse thickening of the cranial vault due to acromegaly. Presence of an aneurysm of the right carotid siphon intrasellar relapse can be seen, possibly associated with cranial, posterior, or parasellar extension. Infrasellar and anterior spread are rarely visible.

The reduction in the cellular growth rate and intratumoral modifications produced by radiation therapy result in progressive shrinkage. However, irradiation has similar effects on adjacent structures: potential iatrogenic lesions include radionecrosis of the optic chiasm and secondary hypopituitarism (Van Effenterre and Boch 1993; Zaugg et al. 1995). Other long-term complications are cerebral ischemia (Fisher et al. 1993), aneurysm (Mortiyama et al. 1992), and various neoplasms (e.g., meningiomas, gliomas) (Tamura et al. 1992).

1.2.9 Conclusion

Thanks to the absence of ionizing radiation, its high spatial resolution, and multiplanar imaging capabilities without patient mobilization, MRI is the imaging modality of choice for the pituitary gland. MRI is superior to CT for both detection and follow-up (during and/or after treatment) of microadenomas and macroadenomas. CT essentially plays a complementary role by providing information on bone changes and calcification. Arteriography and petrosal venous sampling are now only occasionally employed.

1.3 Nonadenomatous Tumors of the Sellar Region

S. Chanalet, C. Raffaelli, and P. Chevallier

Pituitary adenomas account for the great majority of tumors of the sellar region (approximately 15% of all intracranial tumors). However, due to embryologic and anatomical particularities, tumors of numerous other origins also affect this region. Some of these sellar lesions are diagnosed solely on the surgical specimen. In other cases, their features on preoperative imaging studies suggest the diagnosis and may even modify the therapeutic approach.

1.3.1 Anatomy and Embryology

The sella turcica is a deep transverse depression in the basisphenoid that contains the pituitary gland (hypophysis) and the lower portion of the neural stalk (infundibulum). Posteriorly, it is bounded by the posterior clinoid processes and the quadrilateral plate of the clivus. Anteriorly, it is bounded by the anterior clinoid processes and the jugum sphenoidale. The posterior and anterior walls and floor of the sella turcica are made up of cortical bone whose thickness varies with the degree of pneumatization of the sphenoidal sinus. The roof of the sella turcica is formed by a small ring-shaped fold of dura mater, the diaphragm of sella turcica, which presents an opening for passage of the neural stalk. Upon the roof rests the chiasmatic cistern, which contains the optic chiasm and the initial portion of the neural stalk. Immediately above lie the hypothalamus and the recess of infundibulum of the third ventricle. The lateral walls of the sella turcica are formed by the cavernous sinuses, which are covered by folds of dura mater and contain the carotid siphon and venous plexuses. The oculomotor nerves (cranial nerves III, IV, and VI) and the first two branches of the trigeminal nerve (V1 and V2) are lodged in the external wall. The trigeminal ganglion, lying within Meckel's cavity (trigeminal cavity), is situated in the posteroexternal part of the cavernous sinuses.

The bony structures of the base of the skull, and in particular the clivus, result from endochondral ossification. The superior extremity of the notochord lies at the level of the clivus. The anterior pituitary (adenohypophysis) is classically considered to develop from a diverticulum of the stomodeum, Rathke's pouch, whose distal portion disappears. Recently, however, it has been suggested that Rathke's pouch is of neuroectodermal origin (Trandafir et al. 1990). The posterior pituitary lobe (neurohypophysis) is formed by an extension of the hypothalamus derived from the diencephalic neuroectoderm.

1.3.2 Examination Techniques

Techniques for the investigation of nonadenomatous sellar tumors differ slightly from standard procedures for pituitary adenomas.

1.3.2.1 Computed Tomography

CT remains of considerable interest for investigation of nonadenomatous tumors of the sellar region. Pre-

and postcontrast scans are obtained in both the coronal and axial planes. Bone window studies are indispensable for analysis of the sellar walls. CT is particularly useful for demonstration of small calcifications that are invisible on MRI.

1.3.2.2
Magnetic Resonance Imaging

Standard sagittal and coronal views are often completed by axial scans with T_2- or T_1-weighted sequences with and without contrast enhancement.

1.3.2.3
Bilateral Carotid Angiography

Bilateral carotid angiography is an invasive technique that is sometimes useful for the neurosurgeon for mapping purposes. It also allows assessment of potential tumoral hypervascularity.

1.3.3
Results

The nonadenomatous tumors encountered in the sellar region are the result of the anatomical and embryologic particularities described above.

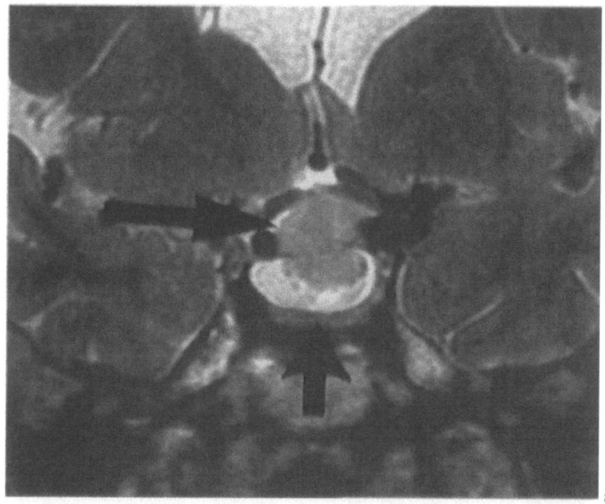

a

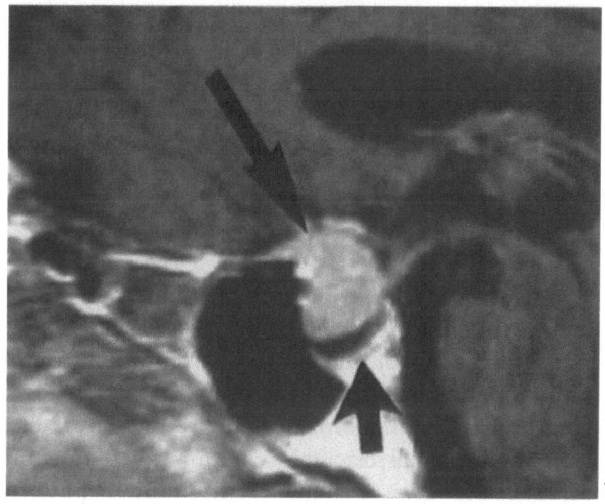

b

Fig. 1.12a,b. Meningioma of the diaphragma sellae (*large arrows*). The pituitary gland (*small arrows*) is compressed against the bottom of the sella turcica by the entrapped cerebrospinal fluid (CSF). **a** Coronal T_2-weighted sequence. **b** Contrast-enhanced sagittal T_1-weighted sequence

1.3.3.1
Meningiomas

Meningiomas of the sellar region are benign tumors occurring in middle-aged adults and account for one third of all intracranial meningiomas. Two thirds of all cases occur in women. These lesions can be divided into:

- Presellar meningiomas, which can develop at the level of the olfactory sulci, the jugum, the optic sulcus, the anterior clinoid process, or the meningeal sheaths of the optic nerves
- Meningiomas of the diaphragm of sella turcica (Fig.1.12)
- Retrosellar meningiomas of the dorsum sellae
- Laterosellar meningiomas involving the cavernous sinuses, the trigeminal cavity, or the internal portion of the sphenoid crest

All of these meningiomas may present an intrasellar extension.

Pure intrasellar meningiomas are rare (Michael and Paige 1988). On CT, these usually isodense or discretely hyperdense masses often contain calcifications of variable size. After contrast injection, these lesions enhance intensely. On MRI, the tumor signal varies, but is usually homogeneous; it is generally isointense on both T_1-weighted and T_2-weighted sequences and enhances intensely after contrast injection. Enhanced CT and MR both have a sensitivity close to 100% (Dietemann et al. 1992).

Care must be taken to detect anomalies of bone insertion. Hyperostosis is best visualized by CT, while blistering of the roof of the sphenoidal sinus

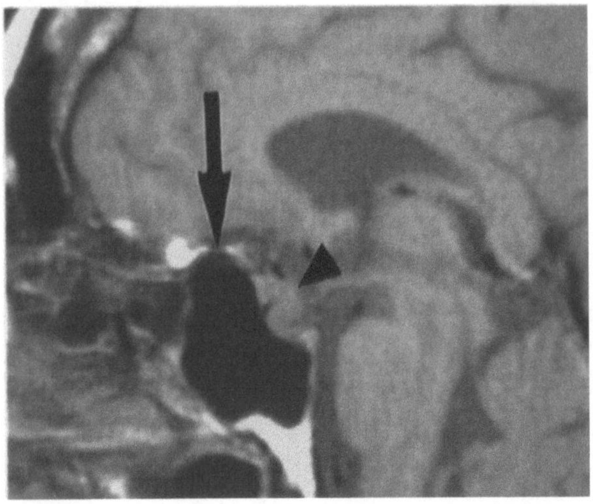

Fig. 1.13. Blistering of the jugum sphenoidale. Sagittal T_1-weighted scan: extensive elevation of the roof of the sphenoidal sinus (*arrow*) associated with an intrasellar meningioma of the optic sulcus (*arrowhead*)

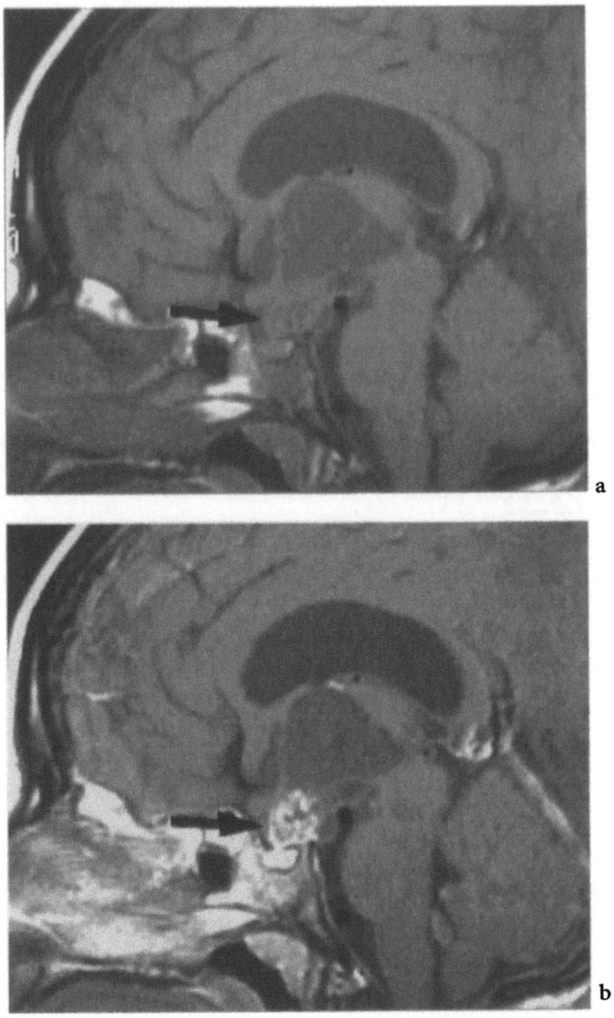

Fig. 1.14 a,b. Craniopharyngioma: sagittal T_1-weighted sequences. **a** Unenhanced. **b** Contrast-enhanced. Large suprasellar tumor invading the third ventricle: the cystic components are slightly more intense than the cerebrospinal fluid (CSF); the tissue component (*arrows*) enhanced after injection to reveal low-density areas consistent with calcification

(Fig. 1.13) is visible in 70% of meningiomas of the jugum sphenoidale (Dietemann et al. 1992). These signs are diagnostic and allow differentiation from a pituitary adenoma in cases of intrasellar extension. Laterosellar meningiomas often present an extension to the small circumference of the tentorium cerebelli that gives a characteristic "fantail" pattern on axial scans. Large meningiomas of the diaphragm of sella turcica may be confused with a pituitary adenoma when the normal pituitary gland is displaced to the bottom of the sella turcica and cannot be distinguished from the tumor, even on T_2-weighted sequences.

1.3.3.2 Neurilemmomas

Neurilemmomas (neurinomas) of the sellar region usually involve the trigeminal nerve, in particular the trigeminal ganglion and its branches (Yuh et al. 1988). These tumors are generally encountered in neurofibromatosis (NF)-2. Neurilemmomas along the intracavernous portion of the oculomotor nerves are rare. On CT, these tumors are usually isodense and enhance homogeneously after contrast injection. The tumor signal on MR is usually homogeneous and isointense on T_1-weighted sequences, hyperintense on T_2-weighted sequences, and enhances intensely after contrast injection. These lesions have a tendency to extend along the course of the nerves through the foramina of the skull base, which they enlarge; such enlargement is highly suggestive of the diagnosis.

1.3.3.3 Craniopharyngiomas

Craniopharyngiomas (Rathke's pouch tumors) are benign congenital tumors that account for 3% of all cerebral tumors and 17% of all supratentorial tumors in children. These supra- and/or intrasellar tumors arise from remnants of Rathke's pouch. The location of these tumors has been explained by embryonal rotation of the anterior pituitary that places the cell in a posterosuperior position.

Craniopharyngiomas consist of three components in varying proportions: a vascular solid component that enhances after contrast injection, a cystic component, and a calcified component (Fig. 1.14). Calcification is best demonstrated by CT; it may not be visible on MRI (DIETEMANN et al. 1992). The solid component enhances on both CT and MR. The signal intensity of the cysts depends on their protein, cholesterol crystal, or methemoglobin content (DIETEMANN et al. 1992). On T_1-weighted sequences, the signal can range from a low-intensity signal that is generally higher than that of CSF to a signal of very high intensity (Fig. 1.15). On T_2-weighted sequences, the signal intensity is usually higher than that of CSF (Amadi et al. 1992). Enhancement of the cyst wall after injection of contrast material facilitates diagnosis of isodense or isointense cysts.

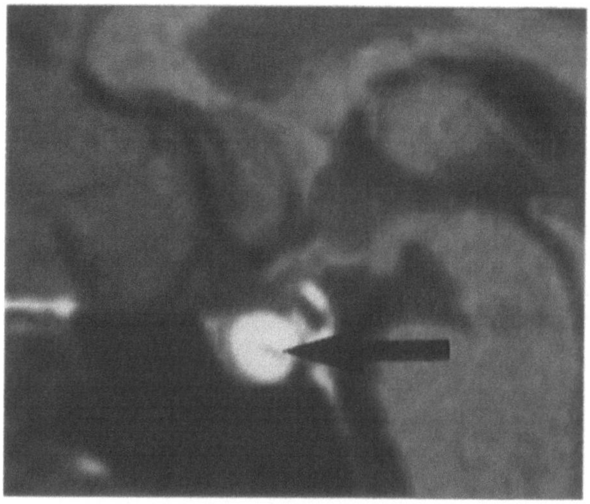

Fig. 1.15. Intrasellar craniopharyngioma: sagittal T_1-weighted sequence. The cystic components were spontaneously hyperintense. Note the small tissue component (*arrow*)

1.3.3.4 Rathke's Cleft Cysts

Presumably derived from persistence of the intrasellar extremity of Rathke's pouch, Rathke's cleft cysts are intrasellar cysts that may show suprasellar extension. Their appearance on imaging studies depends on their contents. They are often spontaneously hyperintense on T_1-weighted sequences or isointense (Fig. 1.16). They usually do not enhance after injection of contrast material or exhibit only thin peripheral enhancement (ELSTER 1993a). These imaging features are similar to those of pituitary colloid cysts and cysts of the pars intermedia, which are more frequent.

1.3.3.5 Gliomas

Gliomas can occur in the chiasma and the optic tract, the infundibulum, or the hypothalamus and are associated with NF-1 in 20%–50% of cases (LOES et al. 1991). Pilocytic astrocytomas predominate (grade I). These tumors can produce changes in skull markings on plain skull X-rays (erosion of the optic sulcus, enlargement of the optic foramina) (DIETEMANN et al. 1992). Gliomas appear iso- or hypodense on CT and enhance in 60% of cases. These tumors often contain cysts. MRI is the imaging modality of choice for these lesions because it can demonstrate tumor spread to the optic tract (optic nerve and optic tract roots).

1.3.3.6 Epithelial Cysts

Epidermoid and dermoid cysts are formed by the inclusion of ectodermal elements at the time of neural tube closure.

Epidermoid cysts, also referred to as cholesteatomas, predominate in the parasellar regions. Their internal wall is lined by a keratinizing stratified pavementing epithelium containing layers of keratin. These cysts have irregular linings and tend to spread into the subarachnoid spaces. On imaging studies, epidermoid cysts can be difficult to distinguish from arachnoid cysts because their CT density and MR signal are very similar to those of CSF (DIETEMANN et al. 1992).

Dermoid cysts are well-demarcated, lobulated, extracerebral masses located near the midline. They contain lipids and may present extensions and calcifications. Dermoid cysts are most frequent in the sellar region and can extend into the subarachnoid spaces. Their lipid content facilitates diagnosis

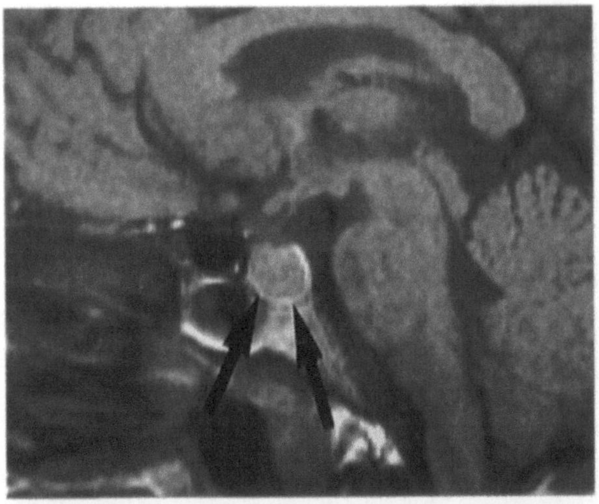
a

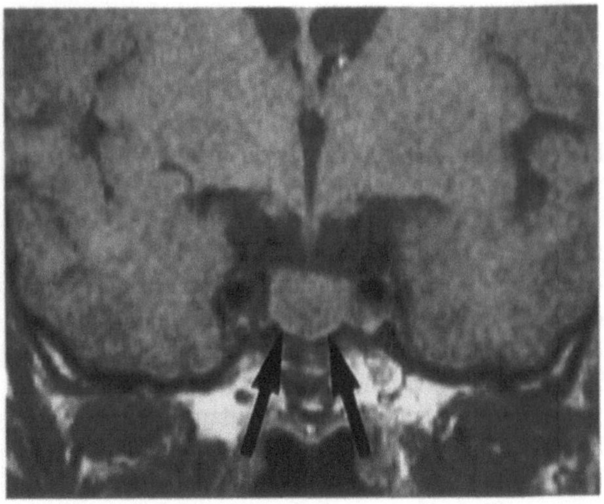
b

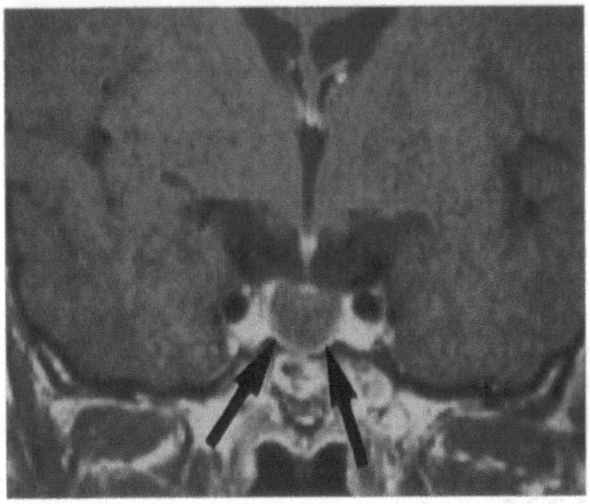
c

Fig. 1.16a–c. Rathke's pouch cyst. **a** Sagittal T_1-weighted scan. **b** Coronal T_1-weighted sequence. **c** Contrast-enhanced coronal T_1-weighted sequence. Round, nonenhancing isointense intrapituitary mass. The enhanced normal pituitary tissue is visible at the periphery of the cyst (*arrows*)

(negative density on CT, high-intensity signal on T_1-weighted MR sequences; Fig. 1.17).

1.3.3.7 Lipomas

Lipomas are congenital fatty lesions that are located on the midline, on the floor of the third ventricle. They have a negative density on CT and appear hyperintense on T_1-weighted MR sequences. Their MR signal is annuled on fat-saturation sequences (Fig. 1.18).

1.3.3.8 Arachnoid Cysts

Arachnoid (leptomeningeal) cysts are frequent in the parasellar regions. These well-circumscribed lesions with smooth and sometimes even rectilinear contours displace the cerebral parenchyma. Their density and signal are homogeneous and identical to those of CSF (Dietemann et al. 1992).

1.3.3.9 Hypothalamic Hamartomas

These occasionally large, benign tumors consist of a collection of more or less organized nerve tissue in an ectopic site. Situated on the floor of the third

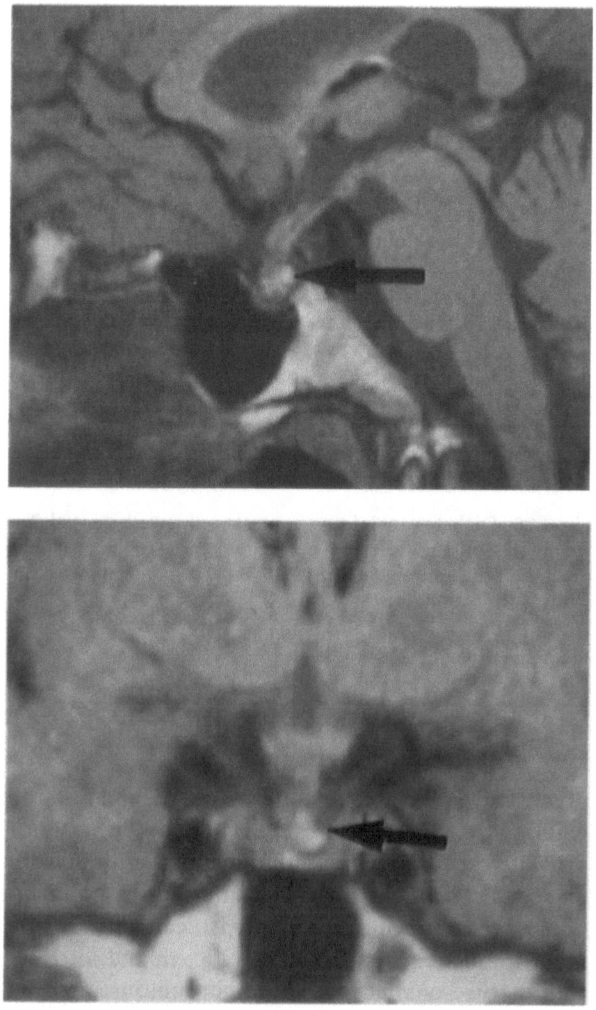

a

b

Fig.1.17a,b. Intrasellar dermoid cyst. **a** Sagittal T_1-weighted sequence. **b** Coronal T_1-weighted sequence. Heterogeneous spontaneously hyperintense lobular mass (*arrows*) located above the anterior pituitary

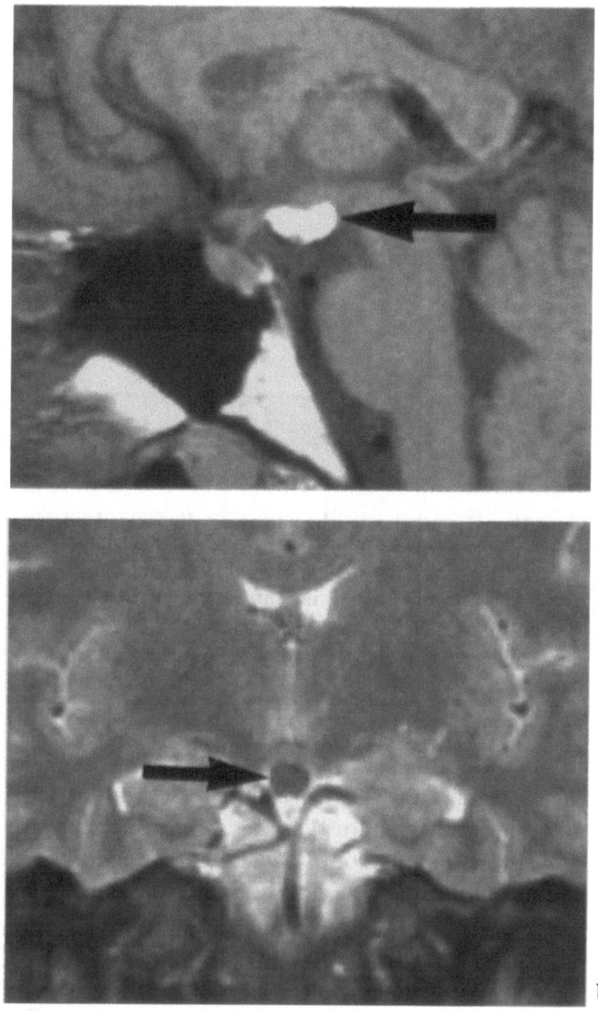

a

b

Fig.1.18a,b. Lipoma of the floor of the third ventricle. **a** Sagittal T_1-weighted sequence. **b** Coronal T_2-weighted sequence with fat saturation. This homogeneous mass was hyperintense on T_1-weighted images and extremely hypointense on the fat saturation sequence (*arrows*)

ventricle, between the neural stalk and the mamillary bodies (Boyko et al. 1991), these sessile or pedunculated lesions manifest clinically by isosexual precocious puberty. On imaging studies, hypothalamic hamartomas have regular contours; they are homogeneous and have a signal identical to that of the gray matter on T_1-weighted sequences. They are often hyperintense on T_2-weighted sequences (Fig. 1.19). Hypothalamic hamartomas usually do not enhance after injection of contrast material.

1.3.3.10
Rare Tumors

Choristomas (granular cell tumor, primary tumor of the neurohypophysis) are intrasellar tumors that can spread along the neural stalk. They are usually isointense on T_1-weighted sequences and hyperintense on T_2-weighted sequences. Intense, inhomogeneous enhancement is the rule after contrast injection.

Germinomas or germ cell tumors (intracranial seminomas) are midline tumors. The hypothalamo-pituitary region is the second most frequent site of these tumors after the pineal body. They often

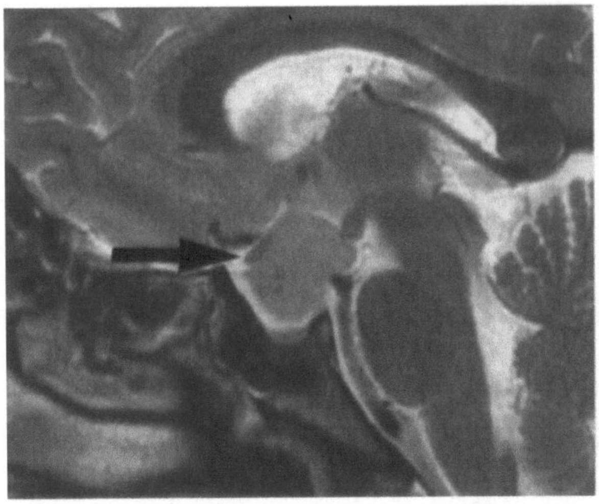

Fig. 1.19. Hypothalamic hamartoma discovered during workup for precocious puberty. Sagittal T_2-weighted sequence. This well-delimited, discretely hyperintense homogeneous mass on the floor of the third ventricle displaced the optic chiasma anteriorly (*arrow*)

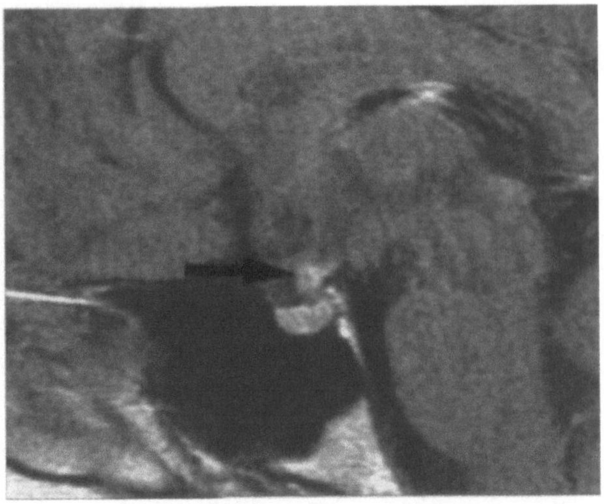

Fig. 1.20. Diabetes insipidus: contrast-enhanced sagittal T_1-weighted sequence. Heterogeneous thickening of the proximal portion of the neural stalk (*arrow*) that was hyperintense after contrast injection. Histiocytosis X

metastasize to the CSF, spreading into the ventricles and the subarachnoid spaces. Germinomas are typically isointense on T_1-weighted sequences and slightly hyperintense on T_2-weighted images. They exhibit intense, homogeneous enhancement after contrast injection (Johnsen et al. 1991).

Intrasellar melanomas are rare entities. These rapidly enlarging tumors appear hyperintense on T_1-weighted sequences and hypointense on T_2-weighted sequences.

Primary lymphoma, histiocytosis X (Fig. 1.20), and sarcoidosis can involve the pituitary gland, the neural stalk, or the floor of the third ventricle. These granulomatous lesions enhance inhomogeneously after contrast injection. There are no specific signs allowing their differentiation. Ganglioneuromas, primary pituitary carcinoma, and pituitary metastases are other rare entities encountered in the sellar region.

1.3.3.11 Tumors of the Skull Base Involving the Sellar Region

Metastases of the skull base and sphenoidal chordomas predominate.

Sphenoidal metastases are rare. As for bone metastases in other skeletal sites, sphenoidal metastases present several classical patterns that depend on the primary neoplasm: sclerotic or mixed metastases of prostate cancer, hypervascular metastases of thyroid or renal cancer, hemorrhagic metastases of melanoma. Prostate, lung, and breast cancers are the most frequent primaries. The lytic, mixed, or sclerotic nature of metastases is well demonstrated by CT. Contiguous spread to adjacent soft tissues is usually visualized as a tissue mass extending on either side of the bone plane that enhances after contrast injection. On MRI, sphenoidal metastases image as hyperintense masses on T_2-weighted sequences; they appear hypointense on T_1-weighted sequences and enhance after contrast injection (Fig. 1.21). MR has a high sensitivity for the detection of lytic lesions. Osteosclerotic metastases have a low signal intensity on both T_1- and T_2-weighted sequences owing to their high calcium content. They may enhance moderately after contrast injection (Feydi et al. 1995).

Chordomas are slow-growing destructive tumors that are histologically benign but locally invasive. One third occur in the spheno-occipital region. The majority are located on the midline. The clivus is the site of predilection, although chordomas can also occur at the petrous apex and the trigeminal cavity (Meyers et al. 1992). On CT, these lytic lesions enhance moderately after contrast injection. Chordomas are isointense on T_1-weighted sequences and

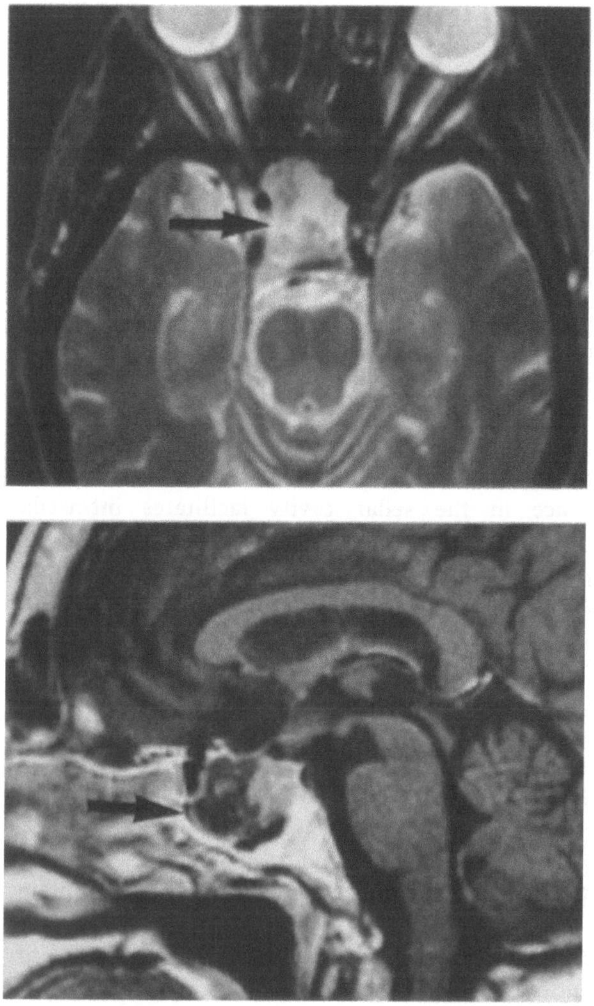

a

b

Fig. 1.21a,b. Sphenoidal metastasis of breast cancer. **a** Axial T_2-weighted sequence. **b** Contrast-enhanced T_1-weighted sequence. Heterogeneous lytic mass invading the sella turcica (*arrows*)

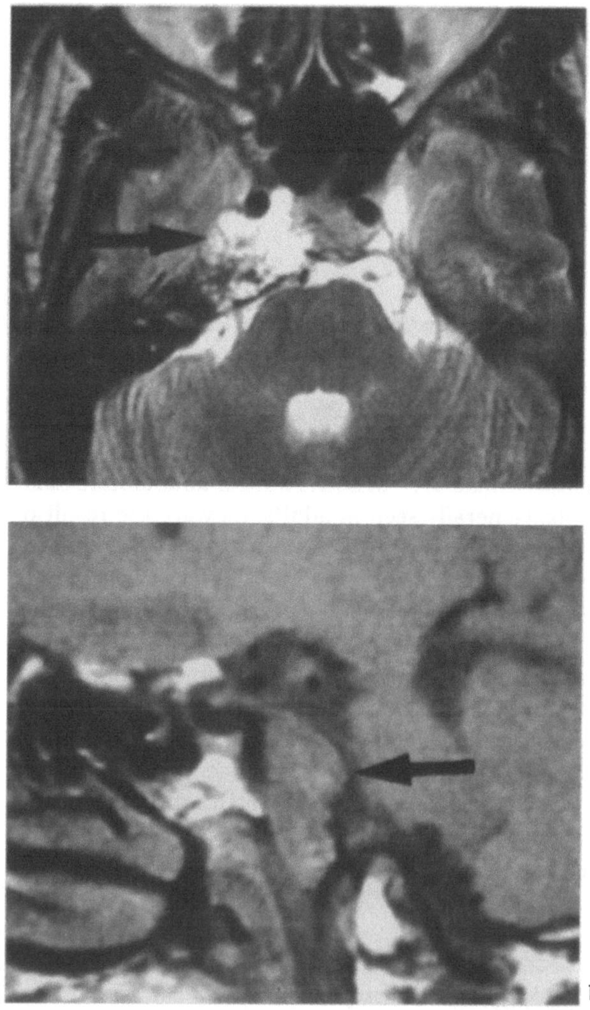

a

b

Fig. 1.22a,b. Chordoma of the petrous apex. **a** Axial T_2-weighted sequence. **b** Sagittal T_1-weighted sequence. This tumor mass invading the clivus and Meckel's cavity (*arrows*) was strongly hyperintense on the T_2-weighted sequence

typically have an extremely high intensity signal on T_2-weighted sequences (Fig. 1.22). They often enhance moderately after contrast injection.

Primary bone tumors of the sellar region are infrequent (chondromas, chondrosarcomas, osteosarcomas). These usually highly destructive tumors tend to have an anarchic calcified matrix that is well analyzed by CT.

1.3.4 Conclusion

MRI is of particular value for examination of tumors of the sellar region due to its high sensitivity and possibilities for tissue characterization. CT can provide complementary information, in particular for bone lesions and calcifications.

1.4 Empty Sella

M.Y. Mourou and G. Michelozzi

1.4.1 Introduction

CT and especially MRI have greatly increased the frequency of detection of normal-sized and slightly enlarged sellae filled primarily by CSF of the suprasellar cisterns that compresses the normal pituitary gland. In the absence of any specific symptoms, such empty sellae are considered normal anatomic variants. Generally seen in adults, they are the result of involution of the pituitary tissue associated with incompetence of the diaphragm of sella turcica.

Symptomatic patients presenting with headache, pituitary endocrine dysfunction, or occasionally visual impairment and/or CSF rhinorrhea often have a more or less enlarged sella occupied primarily by intrasellar herniation of the suprasellar cisterns; marked reduction in the volume of the pituitary gland is accompanied by stretching of the neural stalk. This true pathologic entity is referred to as empty sella syndrome.

1.4.2 Etiology and Pathogenesis

In the absence of any previous pituitary pathology, an empty sella is termed "primary". It is impossible to determine the congenital or acquired causes in such cases. By contrast, an empty sella in a patient with a history of pituitary disease is referred to as "secondary."

1.4.2.1 Primary Empty Sella

Three major pathogenic factors have been implicated in the development of an empty sella: incompetence of the diaphragm of sella turcica, reduction in the volume of the normal pituitary gland, and increased CSF pressure in the suprasellar cisterns. In most cases, a combination of these factors is incriminated.

The diaphragm of sella turcica is a ring-shaped fold of dura mater pierced by an opening, the foramen diaphragmatis sellae, that accommodates the neural stalk and separates the suprasellar chiasmatic compartment (cisterns and optic tracts) from the intrasellar compartment (anterior pituitary and posterior pituitary) and prevents herniation of the suprasellar structures consecutive to CSF pressure.

In their respective autopsy studies, Bush (1951) and Bjerre (1990) found an abnormally large foramen diaphragmatis sellae in at least 20% of normal individuals. The diaphragm of sella turcica in such cases may be no more than a thin peripheral ring or may even be absent, resulting in direct exposure of the pituitary gland.

A normal physiologic reduction in pituitary volume occurs during the postpartum period, after menopause, and in the elderly; the resultant empty space in the sellar cavity facilitates intrasellar herniation of the suprasellar cisterns. Increased CSF pressure (especially when chronic) in the opto-chiasmatic cisterns or on the floor of the third ventricle may lead to intrasellar herniation of the suprasellar cisterns or even the third ventricle.

1.4.2.2 Secondary Empty Sella

An empty sella is referred to as secondary when it is the consequence of a recognized pituitary pathology. The multiple causes include all of the pathologies that can lead to a reduction in the volume of the pituitary gland, e.g., necrotic and hemorrhagic degeneration of space-occupying pituitary lesions (especially adenomas) (Robinson and Michaels 1992; Yokoyama et al. 1992; Le Nestour et al. 1994; Bonneville et al. 1986), ischemic pituitary lesions and infectious or autoimmune hypophysitis (Montalban et al. 1991; Barbaro et al. 1993; Nishiyama et al. 1993; Tollin and Seely 1994), the sequelae of trauma. The major iatrogenic causes are treatment of neoplastic sellar lesions (surgery, medical treatment, and radiotherapy), pharmacologic treatment of peripheral endocrine pathologies, and long-term corticosteroid therapy (Kawano et al. 1994).

Secondary empty sella may also result from an alteration in CSF dynamics, as seen in chronic intracranial hypertension, including pseudotumor cerebri (Silbergleit et al. 1989; Gibby et al. 1993).

Intrasellar invagination of the suprasellar cisterns, sometimes accompanied by herniation of the third ventricle, is seen in patients with intracranial hypertension and individuals who have been treated for a pituitary adenoma (especially by surgery).

The distinction between completely and partially empty sellae is based on the percentage of CSF and residual pituitary tissue in the sellar cavity. Wolpert et al. 1984) devised a scheme based on the amount of residual pituitary parenchyma. In their classification, a completely empty sella corresponds to residual pituitary tissue no more than 2mm thick associated with an arachnoidocele of the suprasellar cisterns that occupies nearly the entire sellar cavity. A partial empty sella corresponds to residual pituitary tissue thicker than 2 mm. GIBBY et al. (1993) proposed a classification based on the percentage of CSF in the sella: grade I, less than 50%; grade II, 50%–75%; grade III, more than 75%.

1.4.3 Empty Sella Syndrome

Symptomatic empty sellae are characterized by clinical manifestations that vary with age.

1.4.3.1 Adults

An asymptomatic primary empty sella is discovered incidentally in at least 20% of the normal adult population (BERGLAND et al. 1968; FORESTI et al. 1991). In patients with a primary empty sella, empty sella syndrome is more frequent in females (approximately 80%–90% of cases), especially in multiparous women and hypertensives. Most cases are diagnosed in adulthood and in the elderly. A higher incidence has been reported in North Africans (FORESTI et al. 1991). Familial cases are exceptional (COLLIOT et al. 1990).

The most common symptom of primary empty sella in adults is headache, followed by endocrine manifestations and visual disorders. CSF rhinorrhea occurs infrequently (SCOTT and REDMAN 1989; GIONAKIS et al. 1992). Headaches, especially associated with papilledema, nausea, vomiting, memory loss, or alterations in mental state, are more frequent in patients with intracranial hypertension, even when benign (pseudotumor cerebri).

Endocrine manifestations due to hypothalamopituitary hypo- or hypersecretion are fairly frequent, as are obesity and hirsutism. Primary empty sella is associated in 20% of cases with a functional or nonfunctional microadenoma. In the absence of a microadenoma responsible for hormone disorders, other potential causal factors include pituitary involution, stretching of the neural stalk, and alterations in CSF dynamics.

GH, FSH, and LH secretion are usually altered less often than PRL (HUNG and FITZ 1992); implication of TSH and ACTH is even rarer (NEELON et al. 1973; RADFAR et al. 1985; MANCINI et al. 1990; SERPICO et al. 1992). Empty sella is exceptionally associated with diabetes insipidus.

Deformation and stretching of the suprasellar optic tracts usually causes visual field defects, papilledema, and optic nerve atrophy. However, these symptoms may also occur in the absence of optic tract distortion (FORESTI et al. 1990).

1.4.3.2 Children

Empty sella syndrome is rare in childhood (RAPAPORT and LOGRONO 1991; CACCIARI et al. 1994; AKCURIN et al. 1995; ZUCCHINI et al. 1995). The main clinical manifestations are hormonal disorders of the hypothalamic–pituitary unit (SHULMAN et al. 1986; RAPAPORT and LOGRONO 1991; CACCIARI et al. 1994; ZUCCHINI et al. 1995). Neuroendocrine disorders are observed in 10.9%–17.9% of children with an empty sella (SOLIMAN et al. 1995,1996). The other features typically found in adults are rare.

Hypopituitarism (especially anterior pituitary deficiency) and disorders in pubertal development are the most typical manifestations. Multiple pituitary hormone deficiency (CACCIARI et al. 1994) and GH deficiency (RAPAPORT and LOGRONO 1991; CACCIARI et al. 1994; AKCURIN et al. 1995; FRANCOIS et al. 1997) are the most frequent manifestations of endocrine dysfunction.

GH deficiency, responsible for pituitary dwarfism (hypophyseal infantilism), may be associated with central precocious puberty (RAPAPORT and LOGRONO 1991; YOKOYAMA et al. 1992; CACCIARI et al. 1994; AKCURIN et al. 1995) or delayed puberty (CACCIARI et al. 1994; ZUCCHINI et al. 1995). Associations have also been reported with duplication of the long arm of the X chromosome (YOKOYAMA et al. 1992), diabetes insipidus, diabetes mellitus, optic atrophy, sensorineural deafness (DIDMOAD) syndrome (SOLIMAN et al. 1995), and 18P monosomy (SCHEBER et al. 1995).

Hypothalamic hypogonadotropic hypogonadism (CACCIARI et al. 1994; AKCURIN et al. 1995) is another manifestation of empty sella in pediatric patients seen in Bardet-Biedl syndrome (SOLIMAN et al. 1996) and Kallmann's syndrome (ZUCCHINI et al. 1995).

Pituitary disorders due to hypersecretion are less frequent (Cacciari et al. 1994). Coexistence of empty sella and septo-optic dysplasia is possible (Kouhiainen and Tirasvirta 1989). Children with multiple hormone deficiencies generally have a completely empty sella (Zucchini et al. 1995). In pituitary dwarfism, empty sella is merely one manifestation of more complex alterations of the hypothalamic-pituitary unit (Root et al. 1989; Mariani et al. 1992). Diabetes insipidus (Hung and Fitz 1992; Lambert et al. 1992; Cacciari et al. 1994) and hypothyroidism due to TSH deficiency are very rare clinical manifestations of empty sella syndrome.

1.4.4 Neuroradiology

MRI is the modality of choice for examination of the pituitary region in general, and empty sellae in particular. Thanks to direct demonstration of the characteristic components of an empty sella, MRI optimizes diagnosis and is more sensitive than CT for identification of the origin of the empty sella (Sacco Vinci et al. 1990; Hardjasudarma et al. 1994).

Conventional skull X-rays may remain helpful to guide the diagnosis. In contrast, arteriography of the circle of Willis and phlebography of the cavernous sinuses are no longer indicated for evaluation of an empty sella.

Despite its overall diagnostic value, CT (even helical CT) is currently reserved for evaluation of bone erosion, in particular of the sellar floor, and the search for microcalcifications as a complement to MRI (Bonneville et al. 1986). Intrathecal injection of an iodinated contrast agent is indicated solely for evaluation of fluid fistulae and differential diagnosis of intrasellar cystic lesions.

The MRI protocol for evaluation of the sellar region consists in T_1- and T_2-weighted SE sequences and two-echo fast SE sequences, preferably with a large matrix and thin slices (1–3 mm). Coronal and sagittal views may be completed by axial scans. Dynamic MRI during gadolinium administration can provide supplementary diagnostic information about space-occupying lesions associated with an empty sella. Vascular and CSF flow analysis techniques and fat-suppression sequences are required occasionally.

Workup of primary empty sella requires evaluation of supra- and infratentorial anatomy. MRI allows detailed analysis of the different structures involved in primary empty sella, and especially secondary empty sella: the sellar cavity, posterior pituitary, anterior pituitary, neural stalk, diaphragm of sella turcica, chiasmatic cisterns, suprasellar optic tracts, hypothalamus, and the third ventricle.

1.4.4.1 *Sella Turcica*

The size and shape of the sellar cavity depend on the primary or secondary nature of the empty sella.

In primary empty sella, the sella turcica may appear normal or nearly normal (Fig. 1.23). However, over 50% of pediatric cases and at least 70% of cases in adults are associated with more or less extensive enlargement of the sellar cavity. Sellar enlargement is usually symmetrical and generally occurs in the vertical axis following collapse of the floor of the sellae, which is convex downward toward the sphenoidal sinus. The floor of the sella is usually thinned or focally interrupted (Fig. 1.24), but may remain normal (Fig. 1.25).

The dorsum sellae may be thinned and convex posteriorly. The posterior clinoid processes may exhibit signs of erosion. Lysis of the dorsum sellae is infrequent, however. The anterior clinoid processes are generally preserved.

Secondary empty sella not related to prior surgery is usually accompanied by major bone destruction caused by the original pathology. Sellar enlargement is frequently asymmetrical; more or less extensive lysis of the dorsum sellae is more common. Erosion of the anterior clinoid processes is also possible.

In postsurgical secondary empty sella, the appearance of the sellar cavity depends on the pathology treated and the surgical approach (frontal or transsphenoidal).

1.4.4.2 *Pituitary Gland*

The posterior pituitary may be difficult to identify in primary empty sella, but the anterior pituitary is always recognizable. The residual pituitary tissue is visible as a thin smooth layer lying against the bottom of the middle and posterior portions of the sellar cavity. Visualization of the anterior pituitary in a paramedian position or lateralized towards the me-

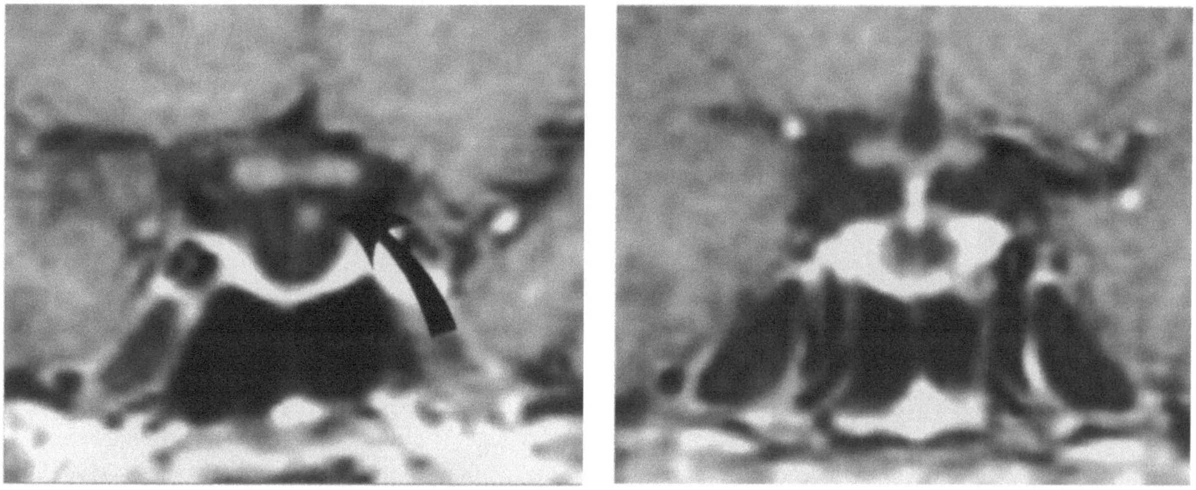

a b

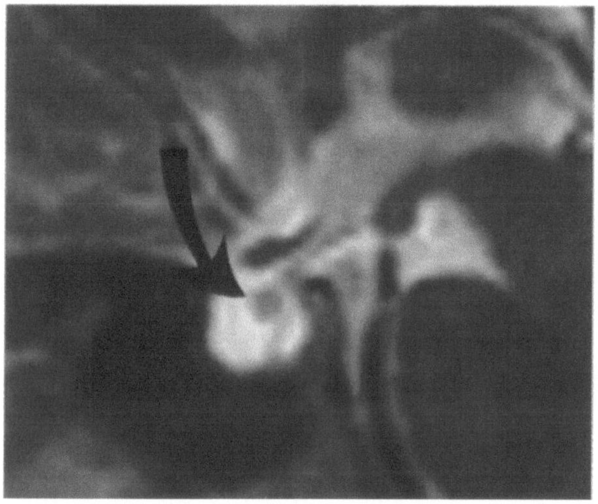

c

Fig. 1.23a–c. Primary empty sella. **a,b** Contrast-enhanced coronal T_1-weighted SE scans. **c** Sagittal T_2-weighted SE scan. Incidental discovery of an empty sella: the sellar cavity is not enlarged, and the volume of the pituitary gland is reduced. Note the intrasellar herniation of the suprasellar cisterns. Presence of a nonspecific micronodular lesion (*arrows*) of intermediate signal intensity lying against the left anterolateral aspect of the neural stalk. This lesion did not enhance after gadolinium injection

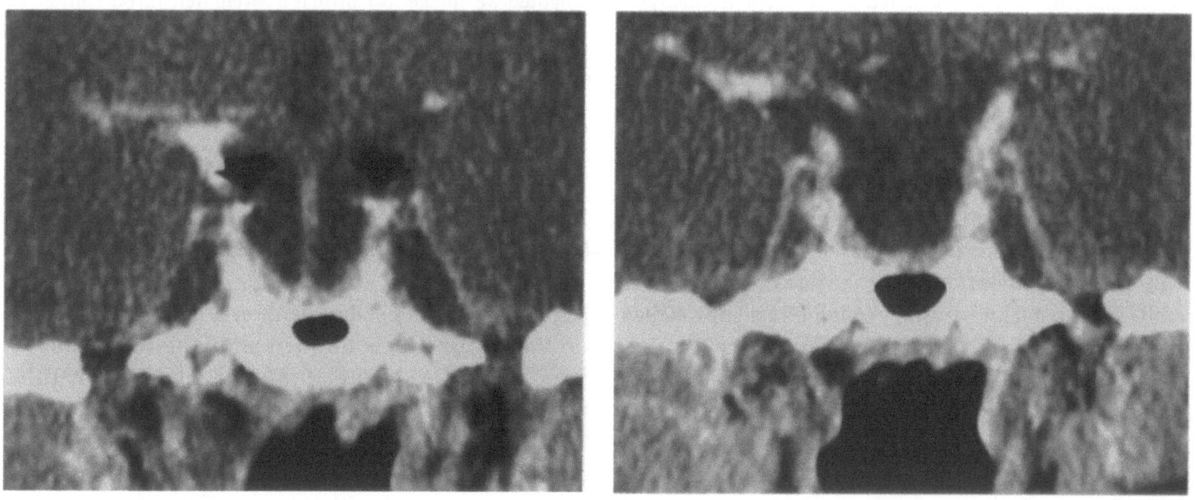

a b

Fig. 1.24a,b. Primary empty sella. Contrast-enhanced coronal CT scans. Enlarged sella turcica with collapse and lysis (*arrowheads*) of the floor of the sella. The sellar cavity is filled essentially by cerebrospinal fluid (CSF) from the suprasellar cisterns that has herniated into the sellar cavity. The pituitary gland is reduced to a thin layer of tissue lying against the sellar floor. The pituitary stalk lies on the midline and is not thinned. The suprasellar optic tracts are in their normal position. The residual diaphragm sella turcica is partially visible

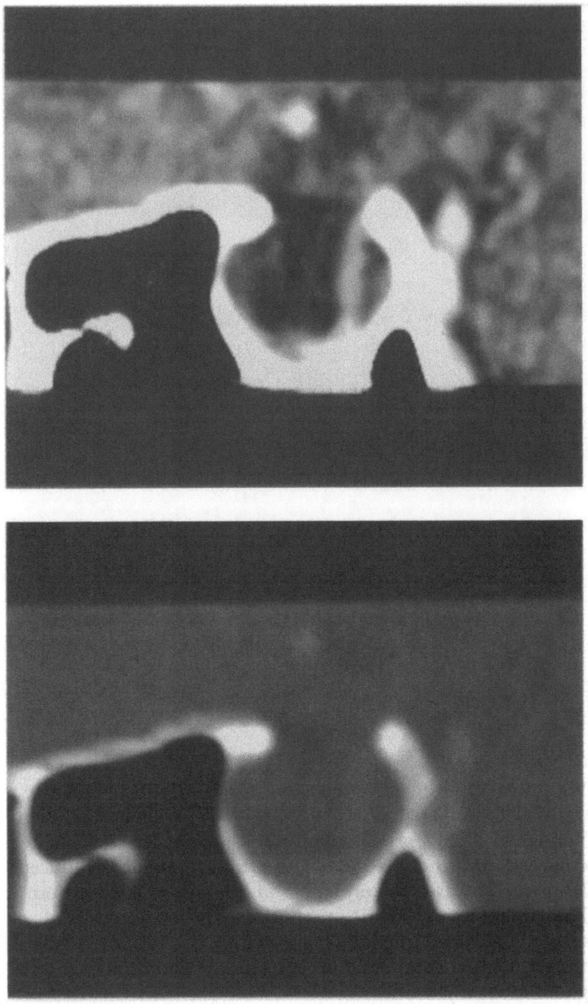

a

b

Fig. 1.25a,b. Primary empty sella. Sagittal CT reconstructions after enhancement by an iodinated contrast agent. Enlarged sellar cavity without signs of thinning of the floor or the dorsum sellae; the superior aspect of the anterior wall appears thinned. The suprasellar cisterns have herniated into the middle and anterior portions of the sellar cavity, anterior to the neural stalk

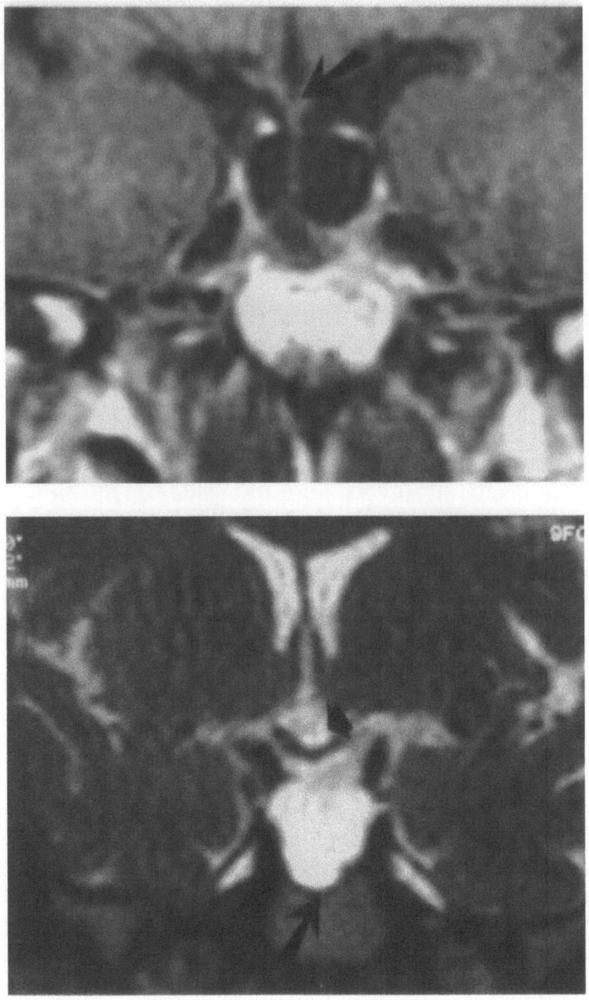

a

b

Fig. 1.26a,b. Primary empty sella. **a** Postcontrast coronal T_1-weighted SE image. **b** Coronal T_2-weighted turbo spin-echo (TSE) sequence. Enlarged sella turcica with collapse of the sellar floor. Presence of a microadenoma (*arrow*) on the bottom of the sellar cavity in a right paramedian location. The midline neural stalk is stretched. Note the deformation of the suprasellar optic tracts (*arrowhead*)

dial wall of a parasellar sinus suggests the existence of an associated microadenoma (Fig. 1.26).

In pituitary dwarfism, the anterior pituitary is small. The posterior pituitary may lie in a suprasellar position rather than within the sellar cavity.

The appearance of the pituitary gland in secondary empty sella obviously depends on the original pathology and subsequent treatment (medical therapy, surgery, or irradiation) (Fig. 1.27). Remnants of pituitary adenomas are common and often show cystic/necrotic degeneration.

1.4.4.3 Neural Stalk – Diaphragm of Sella Turcica

In primary empty sella, the neural stalk typically lies on the midline. It is thinned and lengthened due to traction by the shrunken pituitary lying against the bottom of the usually enlarged sellar cavity. When the stalk courses obliquely rather than being located on the midline (Fig. 1.28), it is usually, although not always, associated with a microadenoma. The MRI signal of the stalk is usually normal on both unenhanced and contrast-enhanced sequences.

In pituitary dwarfism, it may not be possible to clearly identify the stalk because of its small size or

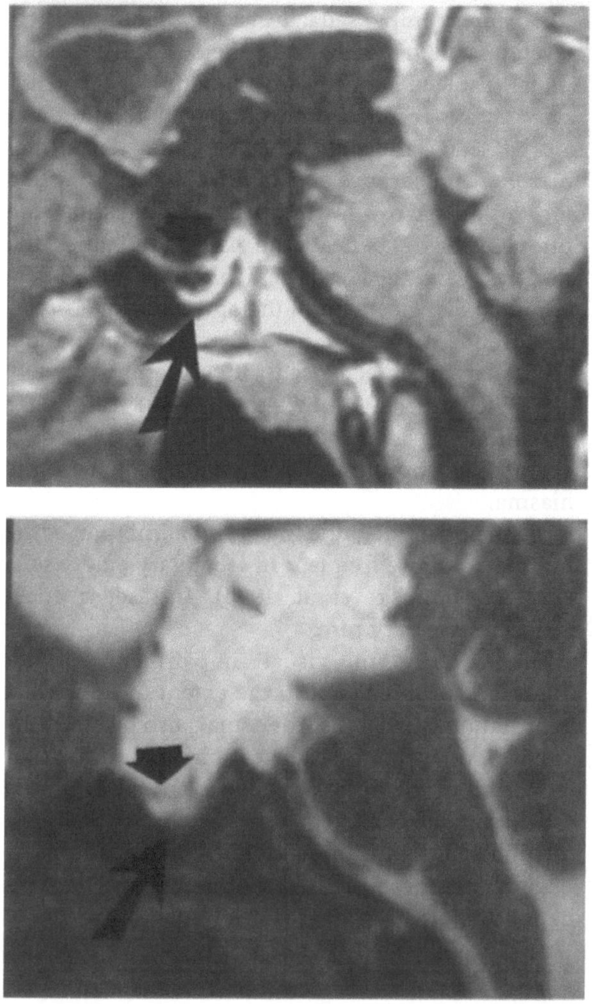

a

b

Fig. 1.27a,b. Empty sella in a patient with hydrocephalus due to tumor stenosis of the cerebral aqueduct (glioma of the tectum mesencephali). **a** Contrast-enhanced sagittal T_1-weighted SE sequence. **b** Sagittal T_2-weighted turbo spin-echo (TSE) sequence. Enlarged and widened sellar cavity with deformation of the dorsum sellae. Intrasellar herniation of the enlarged third ventricle (*arrowhead*) associated with intrasellar herniation of the suprasellar cisterns (*arrow*). The shrunken pituitary gland is compressed against the bottom of the sellar cavity

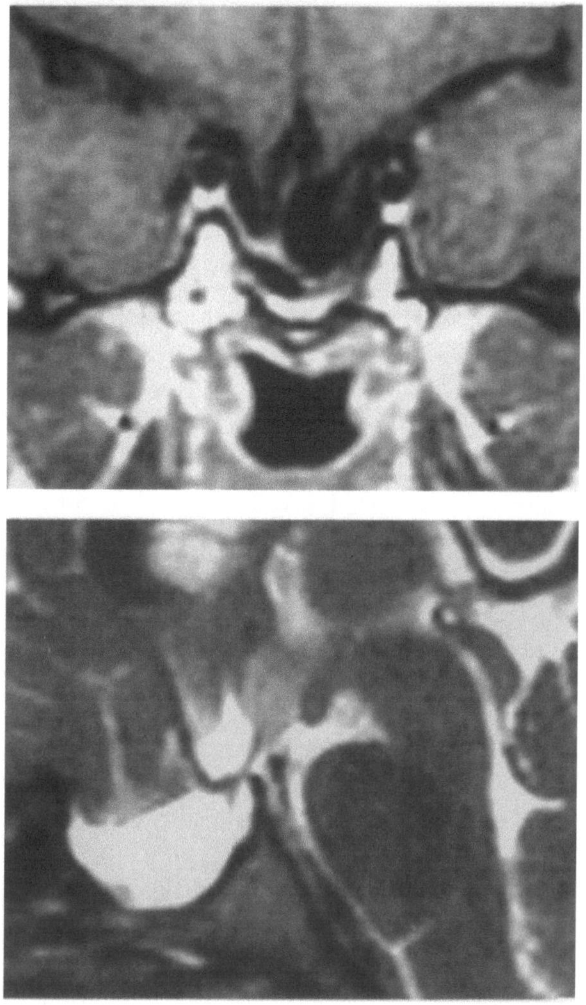

a

b

Fig. 1.28a,b. Primary empty sella. **a** Contrast-enhanced coronal T_1-weighted SE sequence. **b** Sagittal T_2-weighted turbo spin-echo (TSE) sequence. Enlarged sellar cavity with intrasellar herniation of the suprasellar cisterns, the posterior portion of the gyri recti, and the suprasellar optic tracts. Eccentric right-sided position of the pituitary gland and the neural stalk (**a**). Chiari malformation

because it is interrupted. In secondary empty sella, the appearance of the neural stalk may be the same as in primary empty sella. However, it usually presents modifications linked to the original pathology and subsequent treatment.

The diaphragm of sella turcica can almost never be visualized in patients with an empty sella by CT or MRI, not even on T_2-weighted sequences using large matrices.

1.4.4.4 Suprasellar Cisterns

Herniation of the chiasmatic cisterns into the sellar cavity is the characteristic neuroradiological feature of empty sellae. Cisternal CSF occupies the sellar cavity above the residual pituitary tissue.

In primary empty sella, the intrasellar fluid compartment anterior to the neural stalk is usually the largest.

In secondary empty sella in patients with a history of chronic intracranial hypertension and in postsur-

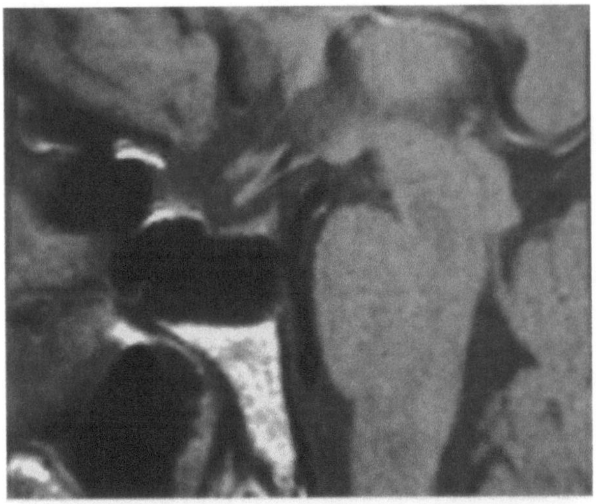

a

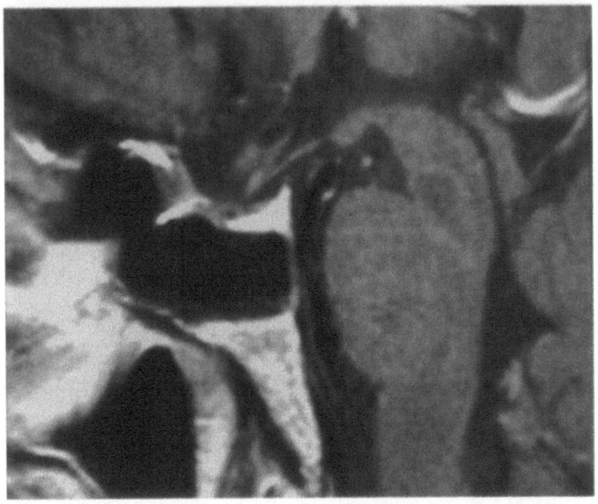

b

Fig. 1.29a,b. Secondary empty sella following surgery for a pituitary macroadenoma. **a** Unenhanced sagittal T_1-weighted SE image. **b** Contrast-enhanced sagittal T_1-weighted SE sequence. Sequelae of nonrecent transsphenoidal surgery are visible at the level of the sellar floor. No sign of tumor recurrence. Intrasellar herniation of the optic chiasma

gical secondary empty sella, the third ventricle may be displaced downward toward the roof of the sellar cavity and may even herniate directly into it. In such cases, the CSF in the sellar cavity is both cisternal and ventricular.

1.4.4.5 Optic Tracts

The optic chiasma and adjacent intracranial portions of the optic nerves and roots of the optic tract lie within the suprasellar cisterns. The chiasma is the most mobile portion of the optic tracts.

In primary empty sella, the suprasellar optic tracts may retain their normal morphology and location. Caudal displacement toward the entry of the sellar cavity always results in morphologic alteration. On coronal scans, the optic chiasma loses its normal horizontal appearance and appears V-shaped, with a more or less narrow lower tip. On sagittal scans, the optic chiasma lies beneath the plane that reunites the optic tracts and the lateral geniculate bodies. Moderate caudal displacement of the optic chiasma is relatively frequent, but true intrasellar herniation of the suprasellar optic tracts occurs in only approximately 12.5% of cases (Kaufman et al. 1989). Intrasellar herniation of the third ventricle is always accompanied by intrasellar herniation of the optic chiasma.

Distortion of the optic tracts and herniation of the chiasma are more frequent in secondary empty sella (Fig. 1.29; Foresti et al. 1990). Intrasellar encephaloceles are very rare.

The severity of visual impairment is not necessarily proportional to the extent of optic tract deformation. Visual disorders may also occur in the absence of optic tract distortion, and intrasellar herniation of the optic tracts does not always cause visual field defects.

Opticochiasmatic arachnoiditis may complicate secondary empty sella, especially after surgery or radiation therapy, and aggravates visual disorders.

1.4.4.6 Differential Diagnosis

MRI readily demonstrates empty sellae, particularly those of primary origin. Differential diagnosis usually involves no problems, except occasionally for differentiation from fluid or semifluid intrasellar space-occupying lesions such as cystic adenomas, cystic craniopharyngiomas, Rathke cleft cysts, arachnoid cysts, epidermoid cysts, and pituitary abscesses. However, expanding lesions exert mass effect, especially on the neural stalk and the optic chiasma, which is absent in empty sellae. Demonstration of the superior wall of a space-occupying cystic lesion facilitates differential diagnosis.

Cisternography, though rarely indicated, can demonstrate passage of contrast agent into an empty sella.

1.4.4.7
Magnetic Resonance Imaging Follow-Up

No follow-up is required for asymptomatic empty sellae. MRI remains the modality of choice for post-therapy follow-up. Normalization of sellar contents is possible (Zanardo et al. 1996).

Primary empty sella in patients with empty sella syndrome should be followed up by MRI, even if symptoms are mild. This is particularly true for patients with visual field defects. Follow-up is indispensable for secondary empty sella. Particular attention must be paid to evaluation of neoplastic remnants and chiasmatic herniation of the suprasellar optic tracts.

Aggravation of symptoms in empty sella syndrome, especially visual field defects, intracranial hypertension refractory to antiedema therapy, and CSF rhinorrhea are the main indications for surgery (Gallardo et al. 1992), which may consist in chiasmapexy, ventricular bypass, or intrasellar balloon inflation (Cybulski et al. 1989).

1.5
Conclusions

The spatial resolution and multiplanar imaging capacities of MRI have made it the technique of choice for all sellar and parasellar pathologies. Thanks to accurate evaluation of the components of an empty sella, MRI permits easy diagnosis and facilitates follow-up. Although CT can usually diagnose an empty sella, it is now reserved for second-line use as a complement to MRI. CT cisternography has been virtually abandoned.

References

Ahmadi J, North CM, Segal HD et al (1985) Cavernous invasion by pituitary adenomas. AJNR 6:893–898

Ahmadi J, Meyers GS, Segall HD et al (1995) Lymphocytic adenohypophysitis: contrast-enhanced MR imaging in five cases. Radiology 195:30–34

Akcurin S, Ocal Ahmadi H, Larsson EM, Jinkins JR (1990) Normal pituitary gland: coronal MR imaging of infundibular tilt. Radiology 177:389–392

Akcurin S, Ocal G, Berberoglu M, Memioglu N (1995) Association of empty sella and neuroendocrine disorders in childhood. Acta Paediatr Jpn 37:347–351

Amadi J, Destian S, Apuzzo MLJ et al (1992) Cystic fluid in craniopharyngiomas: MR imaging and quantitative analysis. Radiology 182:783–785

Anderson DF, Afshar F (1993) Pituitary apoplexy presenting as multiple ocular nerve palsies of sudden onset. Br J Neurosurg 7:443–445

Arita K, Uozumi T, Yano T et al (1993) MRI visualization of complete bilateral optic nerve involvement by pituitary adenoma: A case report. Neuroradiology 35:549–550

Baleriaux D, Jacquemin C, Lemort M (1990) Magnetic resonance imaging of the pituitary gland and the sella turcica region. Normal and pathological aspect. Ann Endocrinol (Paris) 51:173–180

Barbaro D, Boldrin M, Repeti M et al (1993) L'ipofisite autoimmune. Rassegna della letteratura. Minerva Med 84:637–640

Barkovich AJ, Atlas SW (1988) Magnetic resonance imaging of intracranial hemorrhage. Radiol Clin North Am 26:801–820

Barrou Z, Abecassis JP, Guilhaume B et al (1997) Magnetic resonance imaging in Cushing disease. Prediction of surgical results. Presse Med 26:7–11

Bartinsky WS, Lin L (1997) Dynamic and conventional spin-echo MR of pituitary microlesions. AJNR 18:965–972

Baskin DS, Townsend JJ, Wilson CB (1982) Lymphocytic adenohypophysitis of pregnancy simulating a pituitary adenoma: a distinct pathological entity. J Neurosurg 56:148–153

Benesch H, Felber SR, Finkenstedt G et al (1995) MR volumetry for monitoring intramuscular bromocriptine treatment in macroprolactinomas. J Comput Assist Tomogr 19:866–870

Berger SA, Edberg SC, David G (1986) Infectious disease in the sella turcica. Rev Infect Dis 8:747–755

Bergland RM, Ray BS, Torack RM (1968) Anatomical variations in the pituitary gland and adjacent structures in 225 human autopsy cases. J Neurosurg 28:93–99

Bessac L, Bachelot I, Vasdev A et al (1992) Le cathétérisme des sinus pétreux inférieurs. Sa place dans le diagnostic du syndrome de Cushing. Expérience de 23 explorations. Ann Endocrinol 53:16–27

Bevan JS, Webster J, Burke CW (1992) Dopamine agonists and pituitary tumour shrinkage. Endocr Rev 13:220–240

Bjerre P (1990) The empty sella: a reappraisal of etiology and pathogenesis. Acta Neurol Scand 82 (suppl 130):7–23

Bonneville JF, Cattin F, Dietmann JL (1986) Computed tomography of pituitary gland. Springer, Berlin Heidelberg New York

Bonneville JF, Cattin F, Gorczyca W et al (1993) Pituitary microadenomas: early enhancement with dynamic CT-implications of arterial blood supply and potential importance. Radiology 187:857–861

Boyko OB, Curnes JT, Oakes WJ, Burger PC (1991) Hamartomas of the tuber cinereum: CT, MR, and pathologic findings. AJR 12:309–314

Brechtelsbauer D, Klisch J, Urbach H (1996) Radiologic diagnosis of hypophyseal adenomas. Aktuelle Radiol 6:301–307

Brooks BS, Gammal TE, Allison JD et al (1989) Frequency and variation of posterior pituitary bright signal on MR images. AJNR 10:943–948

Buchfelder M, Nistor R, Fahlbusch R et al (1993) The accuracy of CT and MR evaluation of the sella turcica for detection of adrenocorticotropic hormone-secreting adenomas in Cushing disease. AJNR 14:1183–1190

Bush W (1951) Die Morphologie der sella turcica und ihre Beziehungen zur Hypopyse. Virchows Arch Pat Anat 320:437–458

Cacciari E, Zucchini S, Arnbrosetto P et al (1994) Empty sella in children and adolescents with possible hypothalamic-pituitary disorders. J Clin Endrocrinol Metab 78:767–771

Chacko AG, Chandy MJ (1992) Incidental pituitary macroadenomas. Br J Neurosurg 6:233–236

Chanson P, Timsit J, Harris AG (1993) Octreotide, analog of somatostatin. Pharmacological properties and therapeutic

applications in pituitary endocrine tumours. Presse Med 22:2009–2016
Chong BW, Kucharczyk W, Singer W et al (1994) Pituitary gland MR: a comparative study of healthy volunteers and patients with microadenomas. AJNR 15:675–679
Clarke H, Clarke V, Gill J et al (1992) Painful ophtalmoplegia secondary to a mucocele involving the sella turcica, superior orbital fissure and sphenoid sinus. J Natl Med Assoc 84:279–280
Colliot S, Heim M, Vincentelli JM, Jacquet P, Simonin R (1990) Familial primary empty sella turcica. A propos of a family with 3 cases. Ann Endocrinol (Paris) 51:39–42
Colombo N, Berry I, Kucharczyk J et al (1987) Posterior pituitary gland: appearance on MR images in normal and pathologic states. Radiology 165:481–485
Colombo N, Loli P, Vignati F et al (1994) MR of corticotropin-secreting pituitary microadenomas. AJNR 15:1591–1595
Cremonini N, Graziano E, Chiarini V et al (1992) Atypical McCune-Albright syndrome associated with growth hormone-prolactin pituitary adenoma: natural history, long-term follow-up, and SMS 201-995-bromocriptine combined treatment results. J Clin Endocrinol Metab 75:1166–1169
Cybulski Gr, Stone JL, Geremia G (1989) Intrasellar balloon inflation for treatment of symptomatic empty sella syndrome. Neurosurgery 24:105–108
Daita G, Yonemasu Y, Nakai H et al (1995) Cavernous sinus invasion by pituitary adenomas-relationship between magnetic resonance imaging findings and histologically verified dural invasion. Neurol Med Chir (Tokyo) 35:17–21
Daniel DL, Pech P, Mark L et al (1985) Magnetic resonance imaging of cavernous sinus. AJNR 6:187–192
Daniel DL, Czervionke LF, Bonneville JF et al (1988) MR imaging of cavernous sinus: value of spin-echo and gradient recalled echo images. AJNR 9:947–952
Davis PC, Hoffman JC Jr, Spencer T et al (1987a) MR imaging of pituitary adenoma: CT, clinical and surgical correlation. AJNR 8:107–112
Davis PC, Hoffman JC Jr, Malko JA et al (1987b) Gadolinium-DTPA and MR imaging of pituitary adenoma: a preliminary report. AJNR 8:817–823
Davis PC, Gokhale KA, Joseph GJ et al (1991) Pituitary adenoma: correlation of half-dose Gadolinium-enhanced MR imaging with surgical findings in 26 patients. Neuroradiology 180:779–784
Davis WL, Lee JN, King BD et al (1994) Dynamic contrast-enhanced MR imaging of the pituitary gland with fast spin-echo technique. J Magn Reson Imaging 4:509–511
De Bruin TW, Kwekkeboom DJ, Van't Verlaat JW et al (1992) Clinically non functioning pitutary adenoma and octreotide response to long term high dose treatment, and studies in vitro. J Clin Endocrinol Metab 75:1310–1317
De Herder WW, Uitterlinden P, Pieterman H et al (1994) Pituitary tumour localization in patients with Cushing's disease by magnetic resonance imaging. Is there a place for petrosal sinus sampling? Clin Endocrinol (Oxf) 40:87–92
Delgrange E, Maiter D, Donckier J (1996) Effects of the dopamine agonist carbegoline in patients with prolactinoma intolerant or resistant to bromocriptine. Eur J Endocrinol 134:454–456
Dietemann JL, Cromero C, Tajahmady T et al (1992) Scanographie et IRM des lésions suprâ-sellaires. J Neuroradiol 19:1–22
Dina TS, Feaster SH, Laws ER (1993) MR of the pituitary gland postsurgery: serial MR studies following transsphenoidal resection. AJNR 14:763–769
Doppman JL, Oldfield EH, Krudy AG et al (1984) Petrosal sinus sampling for Cushing's syndrome: anatomical and technical considerations. Radiology 150:99–103
Doppman JL, Miller DL, Patronas NJ et al (1990) The diagnosis of acromegaly: value of inferior petrosal sinus sampling. AJR 154:1075–1077
Doppman JL, Ram Z, Shawker TH et al (1994) Intraoperative US of the pituitary gland, work in progress. Radiology 192:111–115
Edal AL, Skjodt K, Nepper-Rasmussen HJ (1997) SIPAP: a new MR classification for pituitary adenomas. Suprasellar, infrasellar, parasellar, anterior and posterior. Acta Radiol 38:30–36
Elster AD (1993a) Modern imaging of the pituitary. Radiology 187:1–14
Elster AD (1993b) Imaging of the sella: Anatomy and pathology. Semin Ultrasound CT MR 14:182–194
Elster AD (1994) High-resolution, dynamic pituitary MR imaging: standard of care or academic pastime? AJR 163:680–682
Elster AD, Chen MYM, Williams III DW et al (1990) Pituitary gland: MR imaging of physiologic hypertrophy in adolescence. Radiology 174:681–685
Elster AD, Sanders TG, Frederick SV et al (1991) Size and shape of the pituitary gland during pregnancy and post partum: measurement with MR imaging. Radiology 181:531–535
Ezzat S, Horvath E, Harris AG (1994) Morphological effects of octreotide on growth hormone-producing pituitary adenomas. J Clin Endocrinol Metab 79:113–118
Fagel WJ, Hekster REM, Smith SJ et al (1986) Transient intrasellar collection of air during bromocriptine treatment of a prolactinoma. Neuroradiology 28:364–366
Fassbender WJ, Stracke H, Bachmann G et al (1992) Disappearance of a pituitary tumour after 15 months of treatment with CV205–502, a new dopamine agonist. Clin Invest 70:444–446
Feydi A, Carlier R, Vallée C et al (1995) Imagerie des métastases ostéocondensantes. J Radiol 76:561–572
Findling JW, Tyrell JB (1986) Occult secretion of corticotropin. Arch Intern Med 146:929–933
Finelli DA, Kaufman B (1993) Varied microcirculation of pituitary adenomas at rapid, dynamic, contrast-enhanced MR imaging. Radiology 189:205–210
Fisher BJ, Gaspar LE, Noone B (1993) Radiation therapy of pituitary adenoma: delayed sequelae. Radiology 187:843–846
Fisher BJ, Gaspar LE, Stitt LW et al (1994) Pituitary adenoma in adolescents: a biologically more agressive disease? Radiology 192:869–872
Foresti M, Guidali A, Susanna P (1990) Ernia del chiasma in sella vuota secondaria: immagini di risonanza magnetica in paziente asintomatico. Radiol Med 80:93–97
Foresti M, Guidali A, Susanna P (1991) Sella vuota primitiva: frequenza in 500 soggetti asintomatici esanainati con rizonanza magnetica. Radiol Med 81:803–807
Francois I, Casteels I, Silberstein J, Casaer P, De Zegher F (1997) Empty sella, growth hormone deficiency and pseudotumour cerebri: effect of initiation, withdrawal and resumption of growth hormone therapy. Eur J Pediatr 156:69–70
Gallardo E, Schachter D, Caceres E et al (1992) The empty sella: results of treatment in 76 successive cases and high frequency of endocrine and neuroradiological disturbances. Clin Endocrinol (Oxf) 37:529–533
Gancel A, Vuillermet P, Legrand A et al (1994) Effects of a slow-release formulation of the new somaotostatin ana-

logue lanreotide in TSH-secreting pituitary adenomas. Clin Endocrinol (Oxf) 40:421–428
Gibby WA, Cohen MS, Goldberg HI (1993) Pseudotumor cerebri: findings and correlation with vision loss. AJR 160:143–146
Girard N, Brue T, Chabert-Orsini V et al (1994) 3D-FT thin sections MRI of prolactin-secreting pituitary microadenomas. Neuroradiology 36:376–379
Gòniakis M, Segas J, Kontou FK et al (1992) Empty sella syndrome, diagnosed as allergic rhinitis. ORL J 54:91–94
Guy RL, Benn JJ, Ayers AB et al (1991) A comparison of CT and MRI in the assessment of the pituitary and parasellar region. Clin Radiol 43:156–161
Hald JK, Nakstad PH, Kollevold T et al (1992) MR imaging of pituitary microadenomas before and after transphenoidal surgery. Acta Radiol 33:396–399
Hall WA, Luciano MG, Doppman JL et al (1994) Pituitary magnetic resonance imaging in normal human volunteers: occult adenomas in the general population. Ann Intern Med 120:817–820
Hamon-Kerautret M, Leclerc X, Dewailly D et al (1994) Pituitary microadenomas: experience with Gd-DOTA-enhanced MR imaging at 0.5 Tesla. Eur J Radiol 18:185–190
Hardjasudarma M, White KE, Nandy I (1994) Sellar emptiness on routine magnetic resonance imaging. South Med J 87:340–343
Hirohata T, Uozumi T, Mukada K et al (1992) Microprolactinoma invading the cavernous sinus-report of three cases. Neurol Med Chir (Tokyo) 32:10–12
Hirsh WL, Frank GH (1988) Comparison of MR imaging, CT and angiography in the evaluation of the enlarged cavernous sinus. AJNR 9:907–915
Holland BA, Kucharczyk W, Brandt-Zawadzki M et al (1985) MR imaging of calcified intracranial lesions. Radiology 157:353–356
Howlet TA, Drury PL, Perry L et al (1986) Diagnosis and management of ACTH-dependent Cushing's syndrome: comparison of the features in ectopic and pituitary ACTH production. Clin Endocrinol 24:699–713
Hung W, Fitz CR (1992) The primary empty sella syndrome and diabetes insipidus in a child. Acta Paediatr 81:459–461
Jack PC, Krecke KN, Luetmer PH et al (1994) Diagnosis of mesial temporal sclerosis with conventional versus fast spin echo MR imaging. Radiology 192:123–127
Johnsen DE, Woodruff WW, Allen IS et al (1991) MR imaging of the sellar and juxtasellar regions. Radiographics 11:727–758
Johnson MR, Hoare RD, Cox T et al (1992) The evaluation of patients with a suspected pituitary microadenoma: computed tomography compared to magnetic resonance imaging. Clin Endocrinol (Oxf) 36:335–338
Kaufman B, Tomsak RL, Kaufman BA et al (1989) Herniation of the suprasellar visual system and third ventricle into empty sella: morphologic and clinical considerations. AJR 152:597–608
Kawano T, Kobayashi S, Ebizuka T et al (1994) Hypopituitarism associated with empty sella after steroid pulse therapy. Ryumamachi 34:54–58
Kayath MJ, Lenggyel AM, Nogueira R et al (1991) Giant aneurism of the sellar region simulating pituitary adenomas: a diagnosis to be considered. J Endocrinol Invest 14:975–979
Kaye TB, Crapo L (1990) The Cushing's syndrome: an update on diagnostic tests. Ann Intern Med 112:434–444
Kobayashi S, Ikeda H, Yashimoto T (1994) A clinical and histopathological study of factors affecting MRI signal intensities of pituitary adenomas. Neuroradiology 36:298–302
Kouhiainen H, Tirasvirta M (1989) Coexistence of empty sella syndrome and low tension glaucoma. Acta Ophthalmo (Copenh) 67:367–370
Kovacs K, Horovath E, Asa SL (1995) Classification and pathology of pituitary tumours. In: Wilkins RH, Rengachary SS (eds) Neurosurgery. McGraw-Hill, New York, pp 834–842
Kreft B, Peters A, Kerner W (1996) The therapy of a macroprolactinoma with the intramuscular application of a long-acting bromocriptine preparation. Dtsch Med Wochenschr 121:865–868
Kremer P, Forsting M, Hamer J et al (1996) MR imaging of residual tumour tissue after transsphenoidal surgery of hormone-inactive pituitary macroadenomas: a prospective study. Acta Neurochir Suppl (Wien) 65:27–30
Kucharczyk W, Bishop JE, Plewes DB et al (1994a) Detection of pituitary microadenomas: comparison of dynamic keyhole fast spin-echo, unenhanced, and conventional contrast-enhanced MR imaging. AJR 163:671–679
Kucharczyk W, David DO, Kelly WM et al (1994b) Pituitary adenomas: high resolution MR imaging at 1.5T. Radiology 161:761–765
Kulkarni MV, Lee KF, McArdle CB et al (1988) 1.5T MR imaging of pituitary microadenomas: technical considerations and CT correlation. AJNR 9:5–11
Lambert M, Gaillard RC, Vallotton MB et al (1992) Emtpy sella syndrome associated with diabetes insipidus: case report and review of the literature. J Endocrinol Invest 12:433–437
Landolt AM, Valavanis A, Girard J et al (1986) Corticotropin-release factor-test used with bilateral simultaneous inferior petrosal sinus blood sampling for the diagnosis of pituitary-dependent Cushing's disease. Clin Endocrinol 25:687–696
Lazaro CM, Guo WY, Sami et al (1994) Haemorrhagic pituitary tumours. Neuroradiology 36:111–114
Le Nestour E, Abecassis JP, Bertagna X et al (1994) Silent necrosis of a pituitary corticotroph adenoma revealed by timely magnetic resonance imaging. Eur J Endrocrinol 130:469–471
Loes DJ, Barloon TJ, Yuh WTC et al (1991) MR anatomy and pathology of the hypothalamus. AJR 156:579–585
Lundin P, Bergstrom K (1992) Gd-DTPA-enhanced MR imaging of pituitary macroadenomas. Acta Radiol 33:323–332
Lundin P, Bergstrom K, Thuomas KA et al (1991) Comparison of MR imaging and CT in pituitary macroadenomas. Acta Radiol 32:189–196
Lundin P, Pedersen F (1992) Volume of pituitary macroadenomas: assessment by MRI. J Comput Assist Tomogr 16:519–528
Lundin P, Bergstrom K, Nyman R et al (1992a) Macroprolactinomas: serial MR imaging in long-term bromocriptine therapy. AJNR 13:1279–1291
Lundin P, Nyman R, Burman P et al (1992b) MRI of pituitary macroadenomas with reference to hormonal activity. Neuroradiology 34:45–51
Mampalam TJ, Tyrell JB, Wilson CB (1988) Transsphenoidal microsurgery for Cushing's disease. A report of 216 cases. Ann Intern Med 109:487–493
Mancini A, Calabro F, Lagonigro C et al (1990) Cushing's syndrome: new variants and association with empty sella syndrome. J Nucl Med Allied Sci 34:59–66
Mariani M, Coussement A, Berard E et al (1992) Apport de l'IRM dans les diverses variétés de déficit idiopathique en hormone de croissance. Arch Fr Pediatr 49:345–350
Mariuzzi GM, Cavazzini L, Morosini PP (1987) Sistema diencefalo-ipofiario. In: Lanza G (ed) Anatomia patologica sistemica, 2nd edn, vol 1. Piccin, Padua, pp 1047–1065

Mark L, Pech P, Daniels D et al (1984) The pituitary fossa: a correlative anatomic and MR study. Radiology 153:453–457
Mark LP, Haughton VM, Hendrix LE et al (1991) High-intensity signals within the posterior pituitary fossa: a study with fat-suppression MR techniques. AJNR 12:529–532
Meyers SP, Hirsch WL Jr, Curtin HD et al (1992) Chordomas of the skull base: MR features. AJNR 13:1627–1636
Michael AS, Paige ML (1988) MR imaging of intrasellar meningiomas simulating pituitary adenomas. J Comput Assist Tomogr 12:946–949
Miki Y, Matsuo M, Sadahiko N et al (1990) Pituitary adenomas and normal pituitary tissue: enhancement patterns on gadopentate-enhanced MR imaging. Radiology 177:35–38
Miyanohara O, Kusumoto K, Asakura T et al (1993) Juvenile male prolactinoma: a case report. No Shinkei Geka 21:361–366
Moberg E, Trampe E, Wersall J et al (1991) Long-term effects of radiotherapy and bromocriptine treatment in patients with previous surgery for macroprolactinomas. Neurosurgery 29:200–204
Montalban J, Simo R, Sumalla J et al (1991) Pituitary apoplexy and empty sella. Med Clin (Barc) 97:107–109
Mortiyama T, Shigemori M, Hirohata Y et al (1992) Multiple intracranial aneurysms following radiation therapy for pituitary adenoma: a case report. No Shinkei Geka 20:487–492
Mukherji SK, Tart RP, Fitzsimmons J et al (1994) Fat-suppressed MR of the orbit and cavernous sinus: comparison of fast spin-echo and conventional spin-echo. AJNR 15:1707–1714
Nakamura T, Schorner W, Bittner RC et al (1988) The value of paramagnetic contrast agent gadolinium-DTPA in the diagnosis of pituitary adenomas. Neuroradiology 30:481–486
Neelon FA, Gorfe JA, Lebovitz HE (1973) The primary empty sella: clinical and radiographic characteristics and endocrine function. Medicine 52:79–83
Nemoto Y, Inoue Y, Fukuda T et al (1988) MR appearance of Rathke's cleft cysts. Neuroradiology 30:155–159
Newton DR, Dillon WP, Norman D et al (1989) Gd-DTPA-enhanced MR imaging of pituitary adenomas. AJNR 10:949–954
Nishiyama S, Takano T, Hidaka Y et al (1993) A case of postpartum hypopituitarism associated with empty sella: possible relation to postpartum autoimmune hypophysitis. Endrocr J 40:431–438
Nomura M, Tachbana O, Hasegawa M et al (1996) Contrast-enhanced MRI of intrasellar arachnoid cysts: relationship between the pituitary gland and cyst. Neuroradiology 38:566–568
Oldfield EH, Doppman JL, Lynnette K et al (1991) Petrosal sinus sampling with and without corticoprotin-releasing hormone for the differential diagnosis of Cushing's syndrome. N Engl J Med 325:897–905
Ostrov SG, Quencer RM, Hoffman JC et al (1989) Hemorrhage within pituitary adenomas: how often associated with pituitary apoplexy syndrome? AJNR 10:503–510
Paoletti AM, Cagnacci A, Mais V et al (1994) Shrinkage of pituitary adenoma after short-term treatment with bromocriptine long-acting repeatable injections. Clin Exp Obstet Gynecol 21:124–128
Parent AD, Bebin J, Smith RR (1981) Incidental pituitary adenomas. J Neurosurgery 54:228–231
Pascal-Vigneron V, Weryha G, Braun M et al (1994) Rhinorrhea and otorrhea: rare complications of the medical treatment in invasive prolactinomas. Ann Endocrinol (Paris) 54:347–351
Peck WW, Dillon WP, Norman D et al (1988) High-resolution MR imaging of microadenomas at 1.5T: experience with Cushing disease. AJNR 9:1085–1091
Plockinger U, Reichel M, Fett U et al (1994) Preoperative octreotide treatment of growth hormone secreting and clinically nonfunctioning pituitary macroadenomas: effect on tumour volume and lack of correlation with immunohistochemistry and somatostatin receptor scintigraphy. J Clin Endocrinol Metab 79:1416–1423
Pojunas KW, Daniels DL, Williams AL et al (1986) MR imaging of prolactin secreting microadenomas. AJNR 7:209–213
Radfar N, Raji N, Dastur KJ, Drash A (1985) Hypopituitarism in children with primary empty sella syndrome. Pediatr Res 19:191
Rapaport R, Logrono R (1991) Primary empty sella syndrome in childhood: assocation with precocious puberty. Clin Pediatr (Phila) 30:466–471
Reul J, Weis J, Spetzger U et al (1995) Differential diagnosis of truly suprasellar space occupying masses: synopsis of clinical findings, CT and MRI. Eur Radiol 5:224–237
Robinson DB, Michaels RD (1992) Empty sella resulting from the spontaneous resolution of a pituitary macroadenoma. Arch Intern Med 152:1920–1923
Rolih CA, Ober KP (1993) Pituitary apoplexy. Endocrinol Metab Clin North Am 22:291–302
Root AW, Martinez CR, Muroff LR (1989) Subhypothalamic high-intensity signals identified by magnetic resonance imaging in children with idiopathic anterior hypopituitarism. Evidence suggestive of an ectopic posterior pituitary gland. Am J Dis Child 143:366–367
Rossitch EJ, Carrazana EJ, Black PM (1992) Isolated oculomotor nerve palsy following apoplexy of a pituitary adenoma. J Neurosurg Sci 36:103–105
Sacco Vinci V, Majoli A, Citro G et al (1990) La sindrome della sella vuota: studio clinico e neuroradiologico. Medicina 10:273–277
Sadoul JL, Thyss A, Freychet P (1992) Invasive mixed growth hormone/prolactin secreting pituitary tumour: complete shrinking by octreotide and bromocriptine, and lack of tumour growth relapse 20 months after octreotide withdrawal. Acta Endocrinol (Copenh) 126:179–183
Sautner D, Saeger W, Ludecke DK (1993) Tumours of the sellar region mimicking pituitary adenomas. Exp Clin Endocrinol 101:283–289
Scheber E, Scheibenreiter S, Frisch H (1995) 18 P monosomy with GH deficiency and empty sella: good response to GH treatment. Clin Genet 47:254–256
Scheithauer BW, Horvath E, Kovacs K et al (1986a) Plurihormonal pituitary adenomas. Semin Diagn Pathol 3:69–82
Scheithauer BW, Kovacs KT, Laws ER et al (1986b) Pathology of invasive pituitary tumours with special reference to functional classification. J Neurosurg 65:733–744
Schwarzstein D, Garcia-Patterson A, Gimenez G et al (1993) Dopaminergic resistance in a case of invasive macroprolactinoma. J Endocrinol Invest 16:443–447
Scott RJ, Redmon MJ (1989) Nontraumatic cerebrospinal-fluid rhinorrhea in cases of primary empty sella syndrome. Med J Aust 150:458–461
Scotti G, Yuh CY, Dillon WP et al (1988) MRI of the cavernous sinus involvement by pituitary adenomas. AJR 151:799–806
Sener RN, Jinkins JR (1991) CT of intrasellar colloid cyst. J Comput Assist Tomogr 15:671–672
Serpico PC, Freeman JS, Marks B (1992) Empty sella syndrome associated with parital hypopituitarism visualized on MRI scan. J Am Osteopath Assoc 92:1172–1174

Shulman DI, Martinez CR, Bercu BB et al (1986) Hypothalamic-pituitary dysfunction in primary empty sella syndrome in childhood. J Pediatr 108:500–504

Silbergleit R, Junck L, Gebarski SS (1989) Idiopathic intracranial hypertension (pseudotumor cerebri). MR imaging. Radiology 170:207–209

Smith MV, Laws ER Jr (1994) Magnetic resonance imaging measurements of pituitary stalk compression and deviation in patients with non-prolactin-secreting intrasellar and parasellar tumours: lack of correlation with serum prolactin levels. Neurosurgery 34:834--839

Snow RB, Patterson RH Jr, Horwith M et al (1988) Usefulness of preoperative inferior petrosal vein sampling in Cushing's disease. Surg Neurol 29:17–21

Snow RB, Johnson CE, Morgello S et al (1990) Is magnetic resonance imaging useful in guiding the operative approach to large pituitary tumours? Neurosurgery 26:801–803

Soliman AT, Bappal B, Darwisch A, Rajab A, Asfour M (1995) Growth hormone deficiency and empty sella in DIDMOAD syndrome: an endocrine study. Arch Dis Child 73:251–253

Soliman AT, Rajab A, Alsalmi I, Asfour MG (1996) Empty sella impaired testosterone secretion, and defective hypothalamic-pituitary growth and gonadal axes in children with Bardet-Bield syndrome. Metabolism 45:1230–1234

Stadnik T, Stevenaert A, Beckers A et al (1992) Contrast behavior between microadenoma and normal pituitary gland after gadolinium injection as a function of time at 1.5T. Neuroradiology 34:184–189

Stadnik T, D'Haens J, Luypaert R et al (1994a) The value of three-dimensional turbo-FLASH and spin-echo sequences in the detection of pituitary microadenomas following gadolinium administration. Neuroradiology 36:598–601

Stadnik T, Spruyt D, van Binst A et al (1994b) Pituitary microadenomas: diagnosis with dynamic serial CT, conventional CT and T1-weighted MR imaging before and after injection of gadolinium. Eur J Radiol 18:191–198

Steiner E, Imhof H, Knosp E (1989) Gd-DTPA enhanced high resolution MR imaging of pituitary adenomas. Radiographics 9:587–598

Steiner E, Knosp E, Herold CJ et al (1992) Pituitary adenomas: findings of postoperative MR imaging. Radiology 185:521–527

Steiner E, Math G, Knosp E et al (1994) MR appearance of the pituitary gland before and after resection of pituitary macroadenomas. Clin Radiol 49:524–530

Sumida M, Uozumi T, Mukada K et al (1994a) MRI of pituitary adenomas: the position of the normal pituitary gland. Neuroradiology 36:295–297

Sumida M, Uozumi T, Yamanaka M et al (1994b) Displacement of the normal pituitary gland by sellar and juxtasellar tumours: surgical-MRI correlation and use in differential diagnosis. Neuroradiology 36:372–375

Sy RA, Bernstein R, Chynn KY (1992) Reduction in size of a thyrotropin- and gonadotropin-secreting pituitary adenoma treated with octreotide acetate (somatostatin analogue). J Clin Endocrinol Metab 74:690–694

Tabarin A, Greselle JF, San-Galli F et al (1991) Usefulness of the corticotropin-releasing hormone test during bilateral inferior petrosal sinus sampling for the diagnosis of Cushing's disease. J Clin Endocrinol Metab 73:53–59

Tamaki N, Yonezawa K (1993) Prolactin producing adenoma. Nippon Rinsho 51:2685–2690

Tamura M, Misumi S, Kurosaki et al (1992) Anaplastic astrocytoma 14 years after radiotherapy for pituitary adenoma. No Shinkei Geka 20:493–497

Teramoto A, Hirakawa K, Sanno N et al (1994) Incidental pituitary lesions in 1,000 unselected autopsy specimens. Radiology 193:161–164

Thorner MO, Vance ML, Horovath E et al (1992) The anterior pituitary. In: Wilson JD, Foster DW (eds) Williams textbook of endocrinology, 8th edn. Saunders, Philadelphia, pp 221–310

Tollin SR, Seely EW (1994) Case report: postpartum hypopituitarism in a patient with sickle cell trait. Am J Med Sci 308:35–37

Trandafir T, Sipot C, Froicu P (1990) On a possible neural ridge origin of the adenohypophysis. Endocrinologie 28:67–72

Tsang RW, Brierley JD, Panzarella T et al (1994) Radiation therapy for pituitary adenoma: treatment outcome and prognostic factors. Int J Rad Oncol Biol Phys 30:557–565

Ur E, Mather SJ, Bomanji J et al (1992) Pituitary imaging using a labelled somatostatin analogue in acromegaly. Clin Endocrinol 36:147–150

Van Effenterre R, Boch AL (1993) Radionecrosis of the optic chiasma. A clinical and radiological study of three cases. Neurochirurgie 39:75–84

Van Royen EA, Verheff NP, Meylaerts SA et al (1996) Indium-111-DTPA-octreotide uptake measured in normal and abnormal pituitary glands. J Nucl Med 36:1449–1451

Van'T Verlaat JW, Croughs RJ, Hendriks MJ et al (1990) Results of primary treatment with bromocriptine of prolactinomas with extrasellar extension. Can J Neurol Sci 17:71–73

Verhoeff NP, Bemelman FJ, Wiersinga WM et al (1993) Imaging of dopamine D2 and somatostatin receptors in vivo using single-photon emission tomography in a patient with a TSH/PRL-producing pituitary macroadenoma. Eur J Nucl Med 20:555–561

Warnet A (1992) The role of octreotide (Sandostatin) in non-growth hormone, non-thyroid-stimulating hormone, and non-prolacting-secreting adenomas. Metabolism 41 [Suppl 2]:59–61

Webb SM, Ruscalleda J, Schwarzstein D et al (1992) Computerized tomography versus magnetic resonance imaging: a comparative study in hypothalamic-pituitary and parasellar pathology. Clin Endocrinol (Oxf) 36:459–465

Webster J, Peters JR, John R et al (1994) Pituitary stone: two cases of densely calcified thyrotrophin-secreting pituitary adenomas. Clin Endocrinol (Oxf) 40:137–143

Weissbuch SS (1986) Explanation and implications of MR signal changes within pituitary adenomas after bromocriptine therapy. AJNR 7:214–216

Wiener SN, Rzeszotarski MS, Droege RT et al (1985) Measurement of pituitary gland height with MR imaging. AJNR 6:717–722

Wolansky LJ, Leavitt GD, Elias BJ et al (1996) MRI of pituitary hyperplasia in hypothyroidism. Neuroradiology 38:50–52

Wolpert SM, Molitch ME, Goldman JA et al (1984) Size, shape and appearance of the normal female pituitary gland. AJR 143:377–381

Wu W, Thoumas KA (1995) Pituitary microadenoma: MR appearance and correlation with CT. Acta Radiol 36:529–535

Yokoyama Y, Narahara K, Tsuyi K et al (1992) Growth hormone deficiency and empty sella syndrome in a boy with Dup (X). Am J Med Genet 42:660–664

Yu YQ, Jiang XX, Gao YJ (1995) MRI of a pituitary cryptococcoma simulating an adenoma. Neuroradiology 37:449–450

Yuh WT, Wright DC, Barlan TJ et al (1988) MR imaging of primary tumor of trigeminal nerve and Meckel's cave. AJNR 9:665–670

Yuh WT, Fisher DJ, Nguyen HD et al (1994) Sequential MR enhancement pattern in normal pituitary gland and in pituitary adenoma. AJNR 15:101–108

Yusem DM, Arrington JA, Zinreich SJ et al (1989) Pituitary adenomas: possible role of bromocriptine in intratumoural hemorrhage. Radiology 185:239–249

Zanardo MT, Cail WS, Kelman SE, Rothman I (1996) Reversible empty sella in idiopathic intracranial hypertension: an indicator of successful therapy? AJNR 17:1953–1956

Zaugg M, Adaman O, Pescia R et al (1995) External irradiation of macroinvasive pituitary adenomas with telecobalt: a retrospective study with long-term follow-up in patients irradiated with doses mostly between 40–45Gy. Int J Rad Oncol Biol Phys 32:671–680

Zucchini S, Ambrosetto P, Carla G, Tani G, Franzoni E, Cacciari E (1995) Primary empty sella: differences and similarities between children and adults. Acta Pediatr 83:1382–1385

2 Ultrasonography of the Normal Female Reproductive Tract

B. BENOIT

CONTENTS

2.1 Examination Techniques

2.1.1 Transabdominal Ultrasound

The transabdominal approach was for many years the sole technique available for pelvic ultrasonography. The patient is examined with a full bladder. Transabdominal sonography using 3.5- to 5-MHz transducers is still considered the imaging modality of choice for initial examination of the female pelvis, but is insufficient for detailed characterization of the pelvic organs.

2.1.2 Transvaginal Ultrasound

Transvaginal sonography (TVS) is currently the ideal technique for sonographic analysis of the pelvis. Both mechanical (rotating or pendulous) and electronic endovaginal probes are available. Examination is usually performed at frequencies of 3.5–10 MHz. The higher the frequency, the better the resolution, but the lower the depth of penetration of the ultrasound beam (PRICE and FLEISCHER 1995). The field of view is usually in the axis of the ultrasound beam. The angle of insonation varies between 75° and 240°, depending on the ultrasound unit.

Transvaginal ultrasound must be performed with the empty-bladder technique. The tip of the transducer is introduced into a vaginal cul-de-sac (anterior fornix for an anteverted uterus, posterior fornix for a retroverted uterus). High-resolution images are obtained for structures located within 4–5 cm of the tip of the transducer. The region of interest can be brought closer to the probe by simultaneous external compression on the abdomen.

Owing to the limited depth of ultrasound beam penetration, rapid transabdominal scanning must be performed first in order to localize and analyze any pelvic mass that might escape endovaginal detection owing to its size or high location.

2.1.3 Transperineal Ultrasound

Transperineal sonography is an infrequently used alternative when the endovaginal approach is not feasible.

2.2 Sonographic Techniques

2.2.1 Doppler Techniques

Ultrasound machines have conventional pulsed black and white or color Doppler imaging capability allowing analysis of endometrial vascularity.

Pulsed Doppler allows spectral analysis of endometrial blood flow and measurement of flow indices. The most commonly used indices are the

B. BENOIT, Service de Gynécologie et d'Obstétrique, Hôpital de l'Archet, 151 chemin de Saint-Antoine Ginestière, 06200 Nice, France pulsatility index [PI=(*S*–*D*)/*M*] and the resistive index [RI=(*S*–*D*)/*S*], where *S* is the peak systolic velocity, *D* is the end diastolic velocity, and *M* is the mean velocity.

Color Doppler (CD) permits visualization of endometrial blood flow. This technique depends on the angle between the path of the ultrasound beam and the direction of the vessel. No color signal is obtained for flow perpendicular to the ultrasound beam.

Power Doppler (PD) analyzes the energy retrodiffused by structures in movement (erythrocytes). The angle with the path of the ultrasound beam has little influence, and this technique is five times more sensitive than CD. PD can detect low-impedance blood flow and allows vascular mapping of organs.

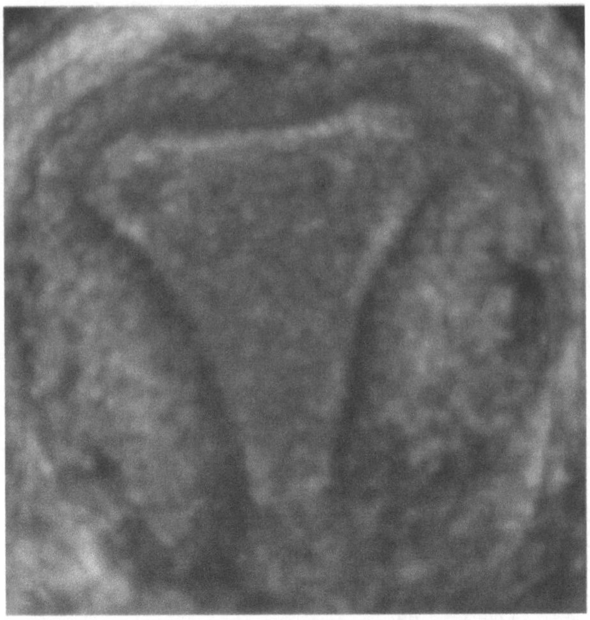

Fig. 2.2. Uterus: coronal scan

2.2.2 Three-Dimensional Ultrasound

Rather than the planar images obtained with two-dimensional sonography, three-dimensional ultrasound provides volume data (Baba and Okai 1997). As volume acquisition is obtained by stacking a series of contiguous scans, multiplanar exploration of the volume matrix is easy (Fig. 2.1). Coronal scans of the uterus (Fig. 2.2) are the most helpful for evaluation of the shape of the uterine cavity, particularly in case of malformations (Steiner et al. 1994; Jurkovic et al. 1995) (Fig.2.3).

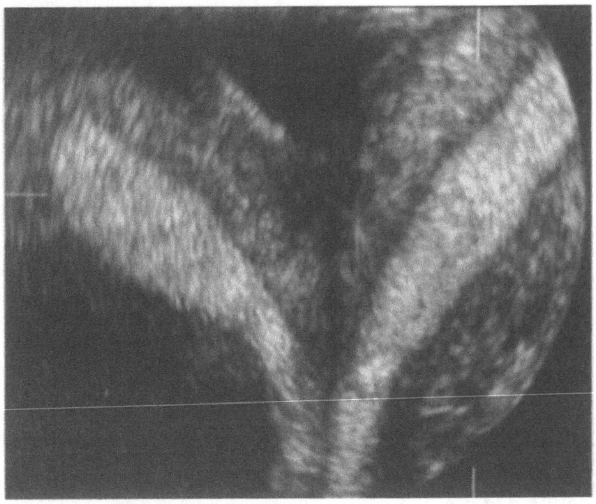

Fig. 2.3. Bicornuate uterus: coronal scan

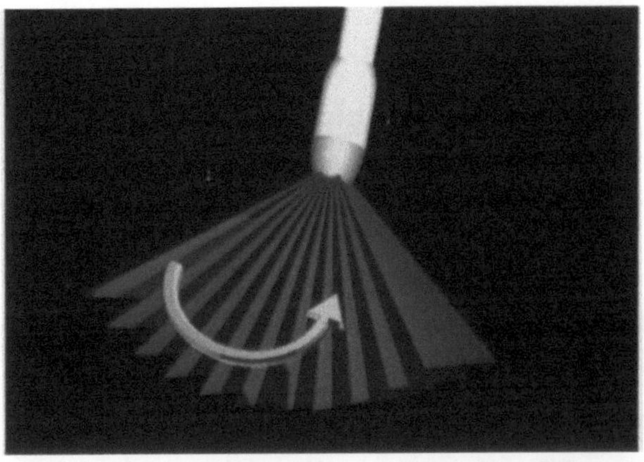

Fig. 2.1. Endovaginal probe for three-dimensional ultrasound

2.2.3 Endouterine Ultrasound

Endouterine sonography can be performed using the very thin 10- to 20-MHz transducers developed for vascular studies. The probe is introduced into the uterine cavity and placed directly in contact with the endometrium. This technique reportedly allows better evaluation of myometrial invasion in patients with endometrial cancer, but the high cost of these disposable transducers limits more widespread use.

2.3 Uterus

The prepubescent uterus is cylindrical; the body and cervix are the same length. On sagittal views, the uterus (cervix plus corpus) measures 20–30 mm, and the diameter ranges from 5 to 10 mm. The endometrium is thin and linear. PD of the uterine arteries demonstrates a weak diastolic component (PI, >3) reflecting the absence of estrogen secretion.

At puberty, the corpus lengthens, ultimately reaching twice the length of the cervix. Uterine dimensions are highly variable and depend on age, the phase of the menstrual cycle, and parity. The sagittal axis may measure anywhere from 60 to 100 mm. Resistances decrease in the uterine arteries (PI, 1.5–2) and vary with the degree of estrogenic stimulation.

The endometrium undergoes changes in thickness and echotexture during the menstrual cycle (Constant and Besson 1989). Interpretation of endometrial status requires knowledge of the period of the cycle to affirm proper synchronization of images with follicular development.

As the mucosa breaks down and is shed during the menstrual phase, endometrial bleeding occurs. Together with the mucosal debris, this constitutes the menstrual flow. Sonographically, the uterine cavity contains echogenic zones (mucosal debris) surrounded by anechoic areas (blood) (Fig. 2.4). Immediately after the phase of desquamation (day 3/4), the endometrium images as an unmeasurably thin echogenic line (Fig. 2.5).

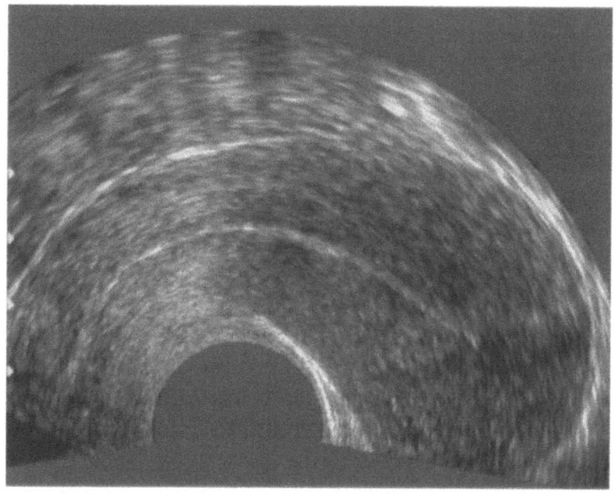
Fig. 2.5. Thin endometrium

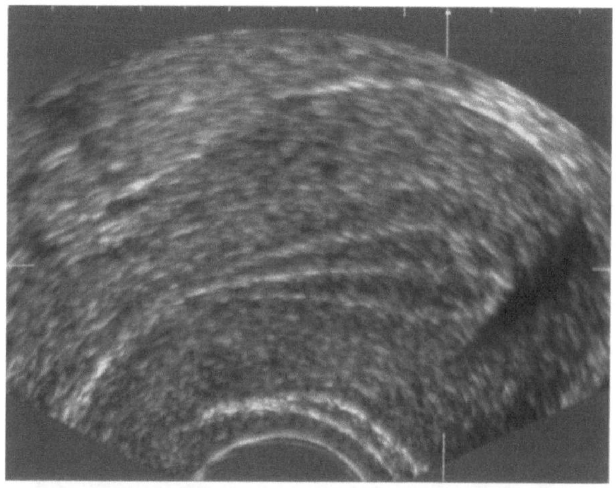
Fig. 2.6. Endometrium: proliferative phase

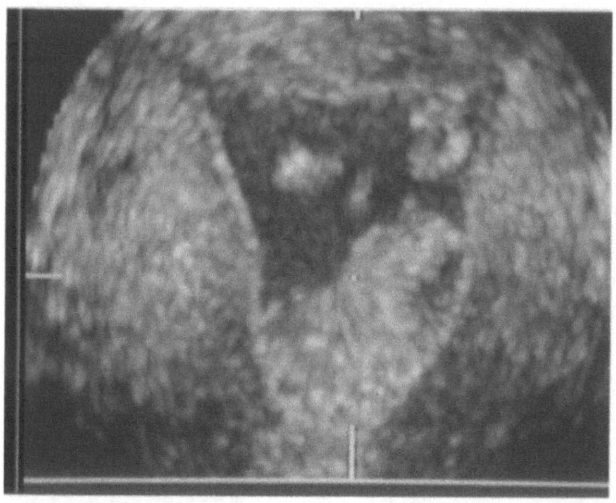
Fig. 2.4. Endometrium (day 3 of the menstrual phase): coronal scan

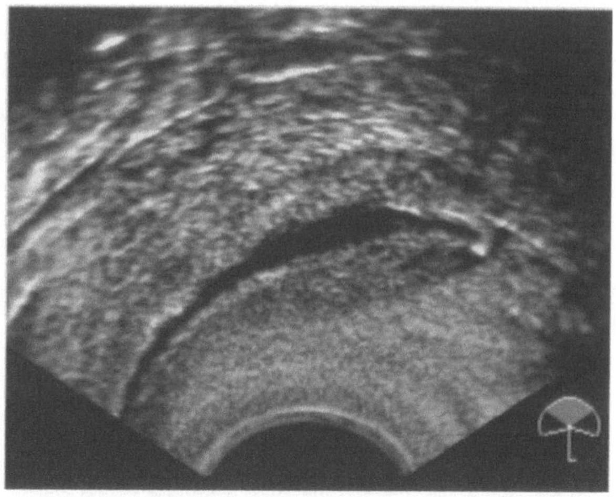
Fig. 2.7. Cervical canal containing cervical mucus

During the proliferative (follicular) phase, the endometrium progressively thickens until it reaches an average of 10mm (total anteroposterior thickness of the double layer). The echotexture is hypoechoic. The endometrial–myometrial interface and the two closely apposed layers of the endometrium are outlined by a hyperechoic line that creates a "coffee bean" appearance (Fig. 2.6). At this point in the cycle, the endocervical mucosa is thick, and the cervical canal contains a small amount of fluid corresponding to cervical mucus (Fig. 2.7).

In contrast to the myometrium and the endocervical mucosa, the normal endometrium does not present any internal vascularity detectable by CD.

During the second phase of the cycle (glandular transformation and secretory activity), the echogenic stripe outlining the contours of the endometrium thickens. The endometrium gradually becomes hyperchoic (Fig. 2.8), and the linear central separation between the two layers is no longer visible.

After menopause, the uterus undergoes involution. It measures less than 70 mm in length and is less than 30 mm thick. The endometrium atrophies progressively. When the two surfaces of the uterine cavity are apposed, a thin, unmeasurable echoic stripe is seen. This stripe is often surrounded by a hypoechoic halo.

The uterine cavity may contain a small amount of fluid (Fig. 2.9). Such endometrial fluid collections, often due to cervical stenosis, are not necessarily indicative of malignancy. Intracavitary fluid facilitates assessment of the endometrial lining of the uterine cavity, as does instillation of fluid into the uterus during sonohysterography.

Doppler analysis of the uterine arteries reveals a considerable decrease in the diastolic component (PI, >3).

The endometrium thickens in response to hormone treatment, but should not exceed the cutoff of 8mm (Gull et al. 1996). Doppler ultrasound reveals a drop in the PI, but this parameter should remain over 1.5.

2.4 Ovaries

The ovaries are usually imaged medial to the iliac vessels (Fig. 2.10).

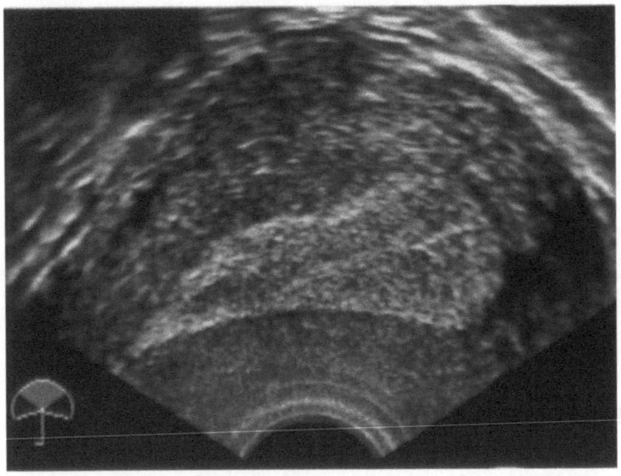

Fig. 2.8. Endometrium: glandular phase

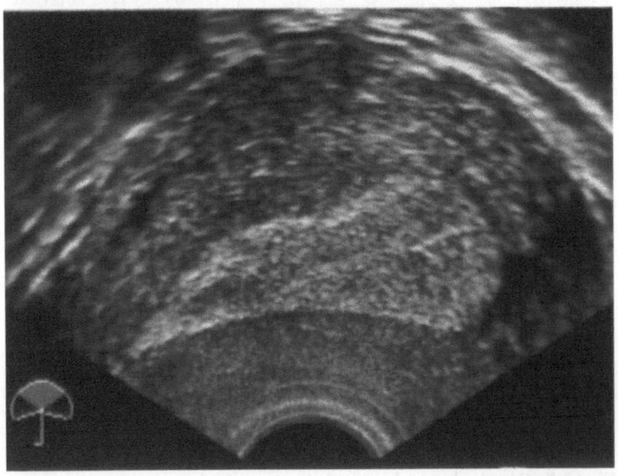

Fig. 2.9. Intracavitary fluid collection

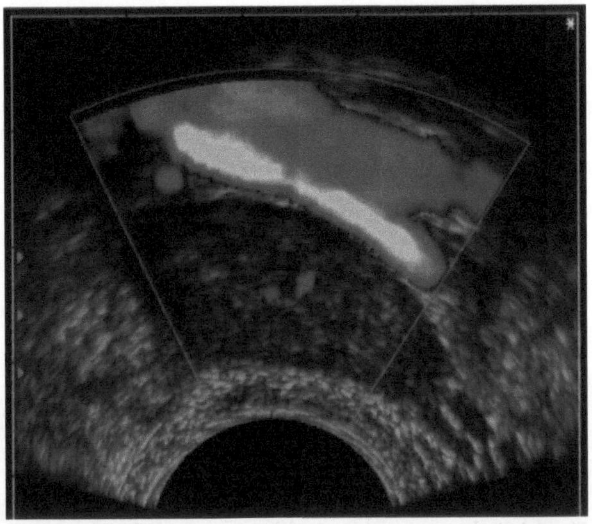

Fig. 2.10. Ovary

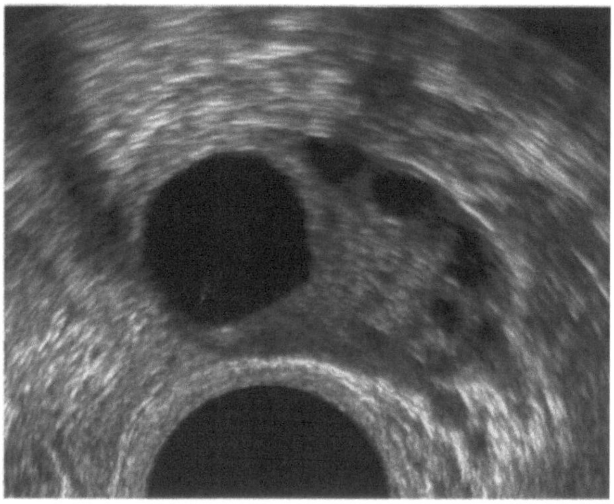

Fig. 2.11. Dominant follicle

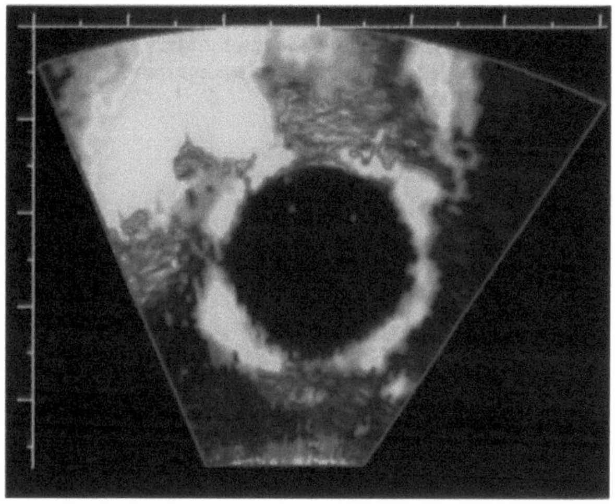

Fig. 2.13. Corpus luteum: color Doppler

The prepubescent ovaries are small (under 15 mm). They are often difficult to visualize, especially because transvaginal ultrasound is not feasible.

During the childbearing years, the size of the normal ovary, like that of the uterus, varies as a function of age and the stage of the cycle. An ovary containing a mature follicle may be twice as large as the contralateral ovary without a follicle.

The normal ovary measures 20–30 mm in length; at its widest portion, the surface area is less than 6 cm^2. These oval structures have an echogenic center. The external portion containing the follicles is hypoechoic.

Typically, only one dominant follicle grows during each menstrual cycle, reaching 20–22 mm in diameter (Fig. 2.11). During this preovulatory follicular stage, the ovarian cumulus is occasionally seen as a small focus of intraparietal thickening. CD demonstration of peripheral vascularity is a good criterion of follicle maturation.

Following ovulation, the follicle transforms into a corpus luteum. Smaller than a follicle, and with much thicker walls (Fig. 2.12), the corpus luteum is characterized by dense vascularity with low blood flow. CD demonstrates a characteristic "annular" appearance (Fig. 2.13). Follicular fluid surrounds the ovary and then collects in the pouch of Douglas.

Postmenopausally, the ovaries atrophy (15–20 mm in long axis) and become homogeneous. Follicles are no longer imaged, and no vascularity is detectable by CD. Postmenopausal ovaries are thus particularly difficult to visualize.

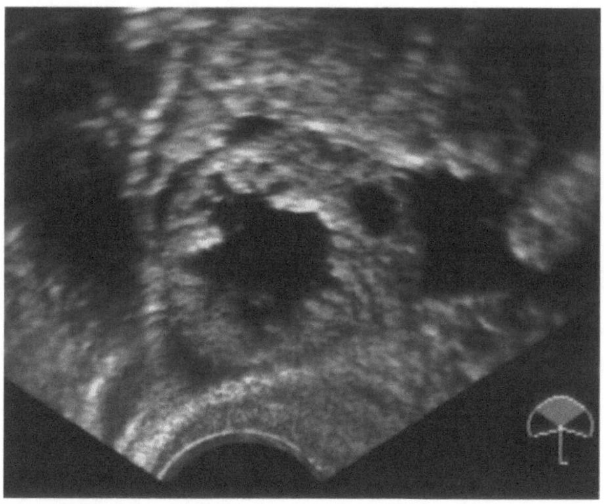

Fig. 2.12. Corpus luteum

References

Baba K, Okai T (1997) Basis and principles of three-dimensional ultrasound. In: Baba K, Jurkovic D (eds) Three-dimensional ultrasound in obstetrics and gynecology. Parthenon, London, pp 1–19

Constant M, Besson P (1989) Echographie endocavitaire en gynécologie. Vigot, Paris

Gull B, Karlsson B, Milsom I, Wiklans M, Granberg S (1996) Transvaginal sonography of the endometrium in a representative sample of postmenopausal women. Ultrasound Obstet Gynecol 7:322–327

Jurkovic D, Geipel A, Gruboek K, Jauniaux E, Natucci M, Campbell S (1995) Three-dimensional ultrasound for the assessment of uterine anatomy and detection of congenital anomalies: a comparison with hysterosalpingography and two-dimensional sonography. Ultrasound Obstet Gynecol 5:233–237

Price R, Fleischer AC (1995) Instrumentation used in transvaginal and transrectal sonography. In: Fleischer AC, Kepple DM (eds) Transvaginal sonography. Lippincott, Philadelphia, pp 1–19

Steiner H, Staudach A, Spitzer D, Schaffer H (1994) Three-dimensional ultrasound in obstetrics and gynaecology: technique, possibilities and limitations. Hum Reprod 4:1773–1778

3 Sonohysterography

Y. Robert, N. Rocourt, I. Damarey, and F. Durand

CONTENTS

3.1 Introduction

The female pelvic reproductive tract is characterized by an endocrine function, related to the ovarian activity, and a target organ, the uterus. Ultrasound has gradually become the technique of reference for assessment of ovarian dysfunction and uterine pathologies. Thanks to technological advances (high-frequency intracavitary transducers, Doppler techniques), morphologic analysis of the ovaries, the myometrium, and the endometrium has progressively improved. Despite the efficacy of ultrasound for endometrial studies, detailed examination of the uterine cavity remains one of the indications for hysterography.

With us, the virtual uterine cavity, imaged sonographically as an echoic midline interface, can be analyzed during sonography by instillation of sterile fluid into the uterus. This enhances visualization of the endometrium and especially depiction of its internal contours (Cullinan et al. 1995). Termed sonohysterography, this recent imaging modality is a supplementary diagnostic procedure for pathologies of the endometrium, the normal target of ovarian endocrine activity.

3.2 Technique

Sonohysterography is a component of comprehensive sonographic exploration of the female genital tract. It requires specific material. Along with standard equipment for visualization and preparation of the cervix, sonohysterography requires that special attention be paid to selection of the catheter and contrast agent.

3.2.1 Catheters

Three types of catheters, each with advantages and drawbacks, can be used to instill the contrast medium (Fig. 3.1): a flexible, small (5F or 7F) dedicated sonohysterography catheter, with a hole at its distal tip, equipped with a balloon; a pediatric Foley cath-

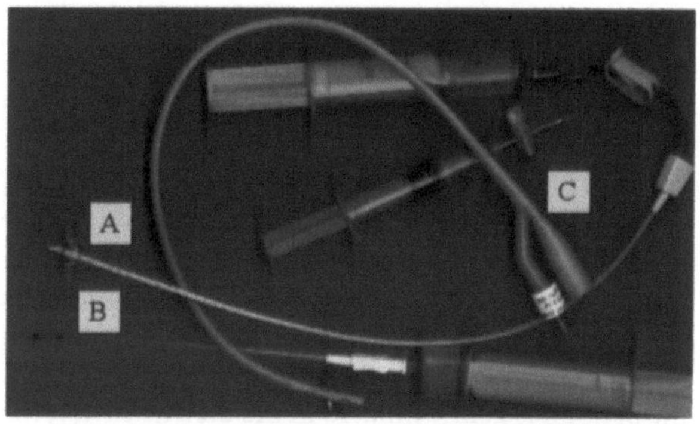

Fig.3.1. Sonohysterography equipment. *A*, sonohysterography catheter (Ackrad Laboratories, Cranford, NJ); *B*, intrauterine insemination catheter (Frydman type); *C*, Foley catheter

Y. Robert, N. Rocourt, I. Damarey, F. Durand, Service de Radiologie et d'Imagerie Médicale, Hôpital Jeanne de Flandre, 2 avenue Oscar Lambert, 59037 Lille, France eter (MITRI et al. 1991); and an intrauterine insemination (IUI) catheter.

Dedicated sonohysterography catheters are easy to insert thanks to a rigid sheath that is positioned against the external os. Its distal tip permits easy air evacuation, eliminating any air bubbles. Proper balloon inflation prevents leakage and ensures satisfactory filling of the uterine cavity. The drawback of these instruments is their cost.

Pediatric Foley catheters are also equipped with a balloon. Although inexpensive, the flexibility of these catheters can complicate insertion into the cervical canal. Furthermore, side holes at the tip prevent complete air evacuation, and introduction of air into the uterine cavity can interfere with sonography.

IUI catheters (Frydman type) are also inexpensive. In addition to a rigid sheath, these catheters have a thin, flexible distal segment that facilitates passage through the cervix with minimal trauma. Their major drawback is absence of a balloon. In certain cases, reflux of the contrast agent precludes adequate distention of the uterine cavity.

3.2.2 Contrast Media

Two types of contrast agents can be used to visualize the uterine cavity:

- A negative contrast agent: sterile saline serum is an inexpensive and readily available anechoic fluid.
- A positive sonographic contrast agent (fluid rendered echoic by the presence of microbubbles in suspension). Although more expensive, such products allow easier and reliable passage of the contrast agent into the fallopian tubes.

3.2.3 Method

Following standard transabdominal and transvaginal ultrasound evaluation of the pelvic cavity, sonohysterography is performed in a similar manner to hysterography. A speculum is located into the vagina, then the cervix is cleansed, and the catheter is threaded through the cervical canal and advanced into the uterine cavity. If a balloon catheter is used, the balloon is gently inflated in the uterine cavity; the patient is requested to signal any discomfort or pain as the balloon is filled with water. The balloon is then pulled back against the internal cervical os to prevent outflow of the contrast agent (CULLINAN et al. 1995).

The contrast agent is instilled into the uterine cavity under ultrasound observation, care being taken to avoid excessive and thus painful distention. The entire uterine cavity is scanned from right to left in the sagittal plane, and from bottom to top in a transverse orientation.

Analysis of the lower uterus requires advancement of the balloon all the way to the fundus.

Tubal status can be assessed by identification of contrast medium in the interstitial portions of the fallopian tubes and in the peritoneal cavity around the ovaries. Fallopian tube studies are facilitated by the use of positive ultrasound contrast agents, which occasionally allow identification of the isthmic portion of the fallopian tube.

The cervical canal is imaged at the end of the procedure, during evacuation of the contrast agent.

As for hysterography, examination should be performed during the first half of the cycle, preferably in the absence of active vaginal bleeding. Pelvic infection and pregnancy contraindicate the procedure.

3.3 Results

3.3.1 Normal Uterine Cavity and Fallopian Tubes

Complete filling of the uterine cavity usually requires 10–30 ml contrast medium. Distention is facilitated by occluding the cervical os with a catheter balloon. The entire uterine cavity can be assessed, in particular its contents and regular contours. During the first half of the cycle, the uterine cavity is lined by a regular hypoechoic endometrium 2–4 mm thick (Fig. 3.2).

Transverse scans through the uterine fundus may depict two small linear images with an echoic rim corresponding to the interstitial portions of the fallopian tubes (Fig. 3.3). The fallopian tubes are usually not visualized beyond this point unless a positive contrast agent is used. Passage of the agent into the isthmic portion is visualized as progressive displacement of the echogenic line as filling progresses. Similarly, dynamic appearance of the contrast agent around the ovary can be identified by B-mode scanning or color Doppler.

On scans during evacuation, the cervical canal appears more or less regular, sometimes with small outpouchings corresponding to the normal mucosal

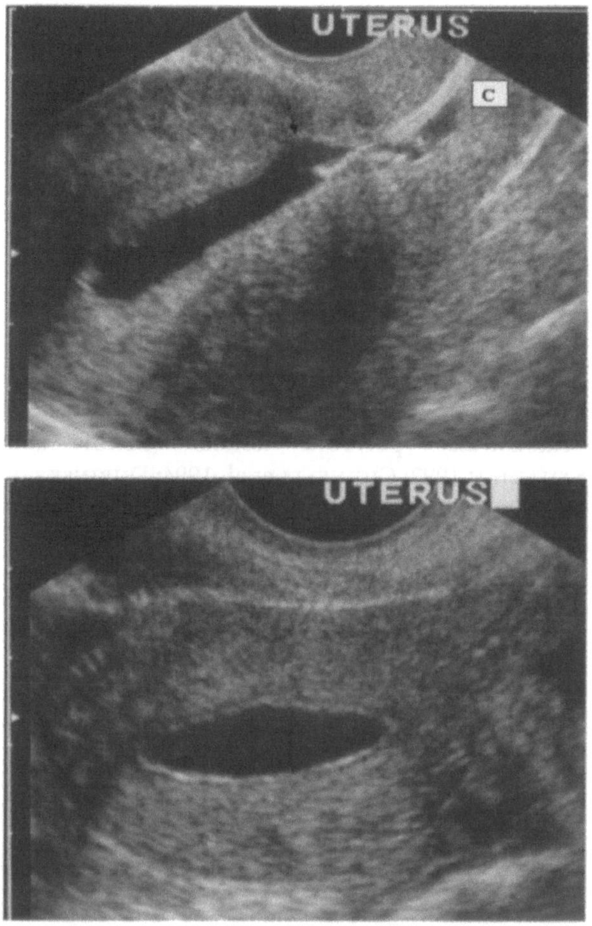

a

b

Fig. 3.2a,b. Sonohysterogram of the normal uterine cavity. **a** Sagittal view of the uterus: the endometrium is thin with regular contours. The catheter (*C*) is visible in the lower uterus. The anterior notch at the cervicouterine junction (*arrow*) corresponds to a cesarean delivery scar. **b** Transverse view through the upper uterine cavity in another patient. The regular contours of the thin endometrium (fine hypoechoic stripe) are outlined by a thin echoic rim

folds. In women who have undergone cesarean delivery, an anterior lobulation corresponding to the scar is sometimes seen (Fig. 3.2a).

3.3.2 Endometrial Hyperplasia

On B-mode ultrasound, the upper normal limits of endometrial thickening are 5 mm in postmenopausal women, 5–8mm in postmenopausal women on hormone replacement therapy, and 15 mm in women of reproductive age. Endometrial thickening may be homogeneously hyperechoic or heterogeneous with multiple cystic spaces. Suggestive of

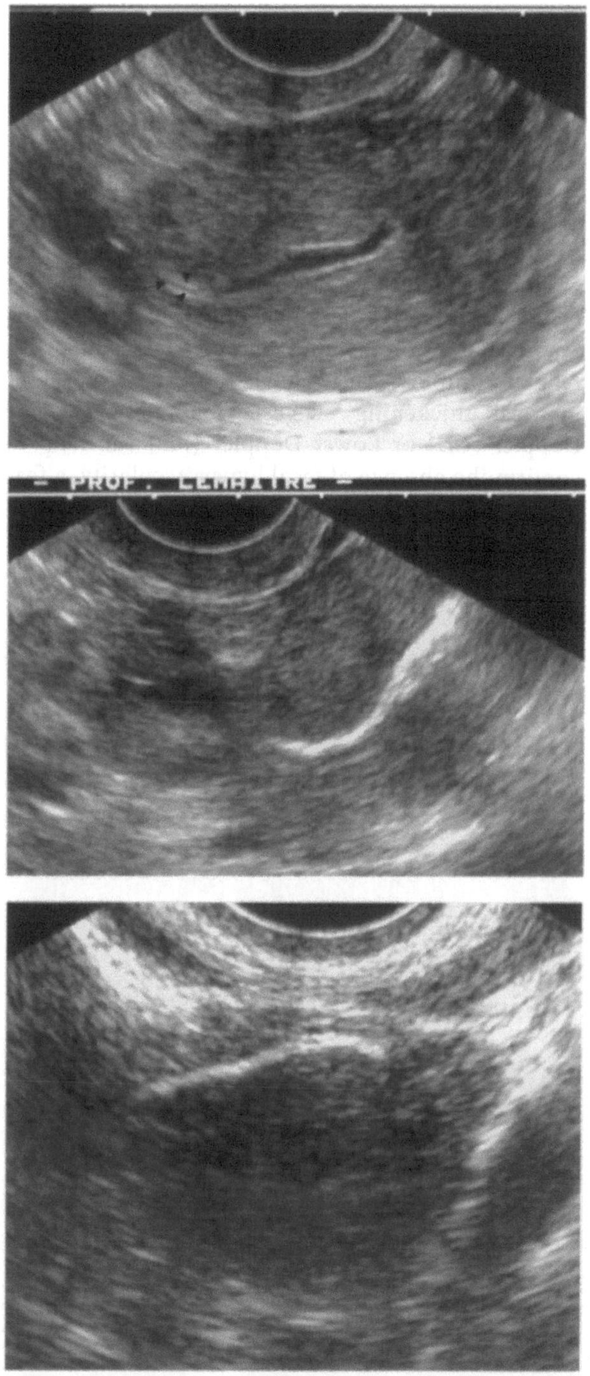

a

b

c

Fig. 3.3a–c. Sonohysterography of the normal interstitial portion of the fallopian tubes. **a** Transverse scan: passage of the saline solution (*arrow*) into the fallopian tubes separates the walls (*arrowheads*) of the interstitial portion of the tube. **b** Use of a positive contrast agent allows visualization of the initial portion of the fallopian tubes and, advantage over saline. depiction of contrast progression into the isthmic portion (**c**) and passage into the peritoneal cavity (see Fig.3.12) mucosal hypertrophy, this latter pattern may correspond to endometrial hyperplasia. However, it may also correspond to a large polyp obliterating the uterine cavity or to endometrial carcinoma (PARSONS and LENSE 1993; COHEN et al. 1994).

Because it allows detailled assessment of the entire endometrial surface, sonohysterography can accurately differentiate between these different pathological entities. Endometrial hyperplasia is depicted as diffuse regular thickening (Fig. 3.4). Polyps are imaged as focal, round endometrial lesions with regular contours. An irregular focal mass or asymmetrical thickening suggests malignancy. Color Doppler (CD) or power Doppler (PD) can help to confirm the absence of focal hypervascularity, a feature suggestive of a neoplastic process.

3.3.3 Endometrial Polyps

Although variable in size, mucosal polyps are typically under 15–20mm. Diagnosis is easiest during the first part of the cycle, when a round hyperechoic mass (Fig. 3.5) is seen distorting or disrupting the echoic midline interface of endometrium (Fig. 3.6). Recognition of small polyps can be difficult, however. Large polyps may occupy the entire uterine cavity and mimic mucosal hypertrophy (homogeneous or with cystic spaces), as seen in endometrial hyperplasia. Sonohysterography readily demonstrates polypoid lesions (SYROP and SAHAKIAN 1992; CICINELLI et al. 1994; DUBINSKY et al. 1995). Small (<5 mm) polyps image as round

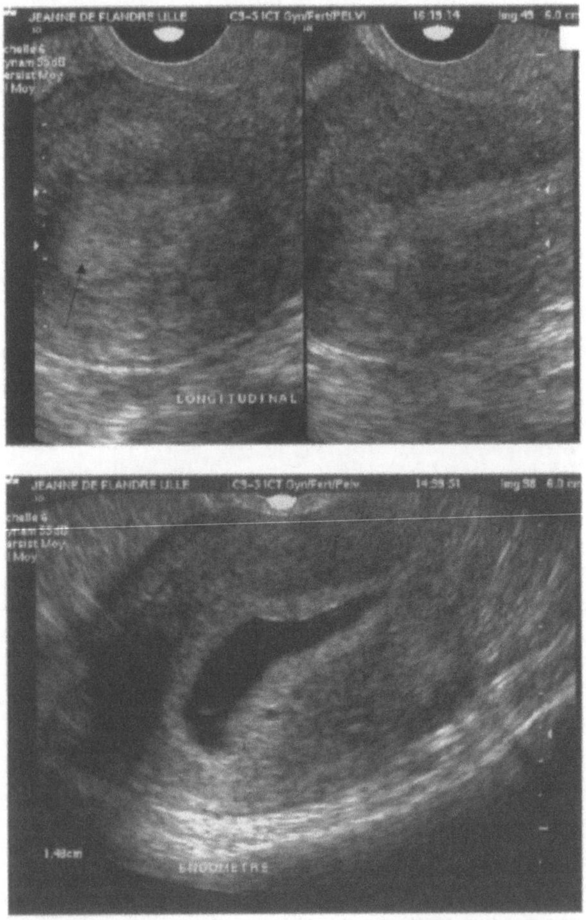

a

b

Fig. 3.4a,b. Endometrial hyperplasia. **a** B-mode scanning depicts the thickened endometrium containing an echoic area suggestive of a mucosal polyp (*arrow*). **b** After distention of the uterine cavity, visualization of diffuse and moderate regular thickening of the hyperechoic endometrium rules out a polyp (14.8mm between the two *crosses*). Endometrial thickening is merely slightly more marked on the upper posterior surface of the uterine cavity

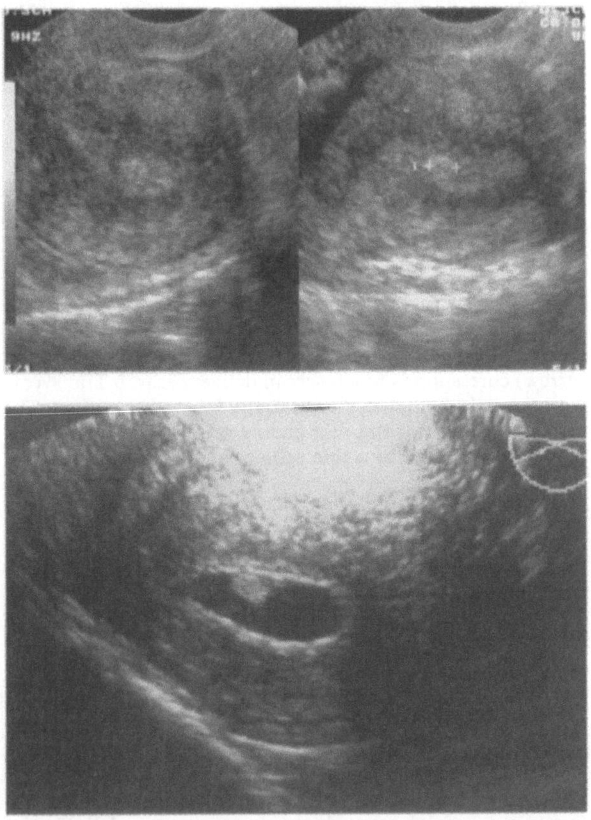

a

b

Fig. 3.5a,b. Uterine polyp. **a** B-mode ultrasound: a small echoic mass (5mm between the two *crosses*) can be suspected in the hypoechoic endometrium. **b** Sonohysterogram: the polyp is readily identified as a round echogenic mass protruding from the thin, regular endometrium

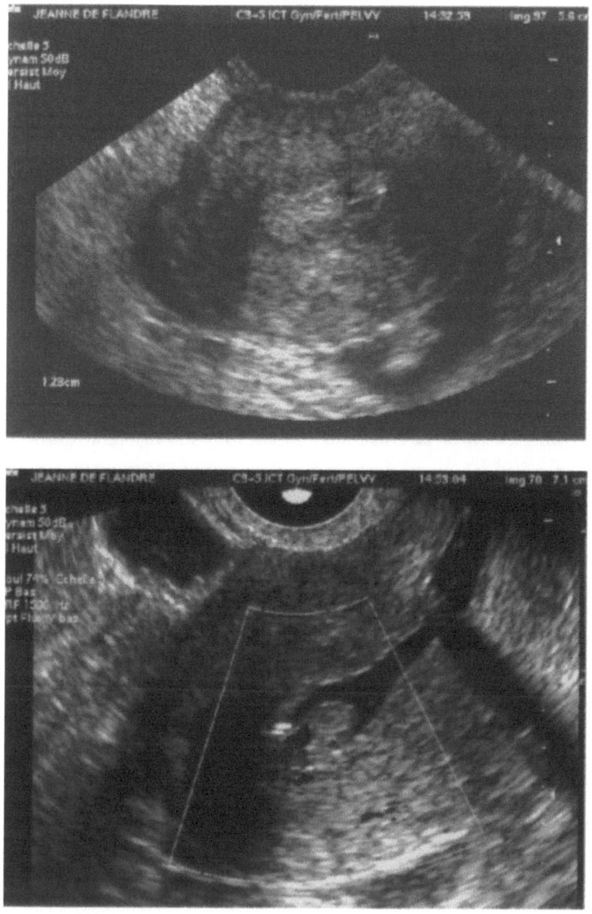

a

b

Fig. 3.6a,b. Uterine polyp. a Presence of a central echoic image (12.8mm between the two *crosses*). b The margins and location of the polyp are readily evaluated by sonohysterography; adjunction of color Doppler (CD) permits visualization of the vascular pedicle

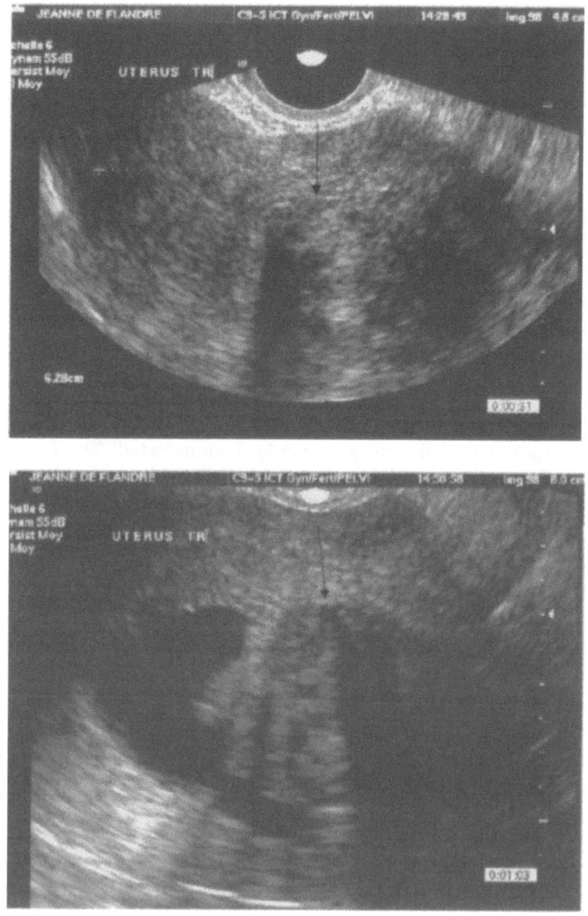

a

b

Fig. 3.7a,b. Submucosal fibroid. a The fibroid (*arrow*) is easily identifiable on B-mode scanning (transverse diameter of the uterus, 6.28cm between the two *crosses*). b Sonohysterography allows excellent assessment of the fibroid's relations with the uterine cavity and reveals its small intracavitary component

masses arising from the surface of the endometrium. Larger polyps are seen as round echogenic masses that project into the endometrial cavity and are surrounded by contrast agent; this allows localization of their fibrovascular stalk. CD may demonstrate vascularity within the pedicle, especially in large polyps.

3.3.4 Submucosal Fibroids

Diagnosis is generally made by B-mode scanning because fibroids tend to be hypoechoic and discretely inhomogeneous. Diagnosis and demonstration of their relations with the uterine cavity are facilitated when the examination is performed during the second half of the cycle, when contrast between the hypoechoic fibroid and the hyperechoic endometrium is greatest.

Sonohysterography facilitates diagnosis during the first half of the cycle, and particularly allows evaluation of the fibroid's intracavitary component (Fukuda et al. 1993; Cicinelli et al. 1995). Pedunculated fibroids that protrude into the uterine cavity may be amenable to hysteroscopic resection (Figs. 3.7, 3.8). Sonohysterography coupled with Doppler allows evaluation of fibroid vascularity.

3.3.5 Endometrial Carcinoma

Endometrial carcinoma is most prevalent in women over 40years of age, particularly after the meno-

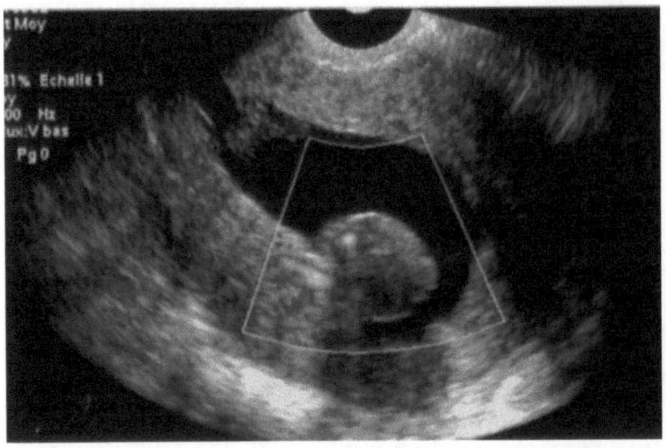

Fig. 3.8. The contours of this hypoechoic, discretely attenuating submucosal fibroid are readily demonstrated. The large intracavitary component makes this fibroid amenable to treatment by hysteroscopic resection

pause. Patients with menometrorrhagia and especially those with postmenopausal bleeding are at particular risk (Goldstein et al. 1990; Goldstein 1994; Emanuel et al. 1995). Whereas endometrial carcinoma may image as diffuse thickening on B-mode scanning, sonohysterography can demonstrate focal thickening or diffuse but asymmetrical thickening suggesting endometrial malignancy (Hoetzinger 1991; Lin et al. 1991; Sheth et al. 1993; Shiply et al. 1994). The following ultrasound and Doppler signs suggest the diagnosis and should prompt directed biopsy (preferably by hysteroscopy) rather than blind endometrial sampling: irregular endometrial contours, hypervascularity of the lesion and/or the area of tumor implantation (Fig. 3.9). The improved contrast resolution of the structures observed with sonohysterography also facilitates tumor localization and evaluation of the depth of invasion, although this last feature is probably best determined by magnetic resonance imaging (MRI).

3.3.6 Endometrial Changes in Response to Tamoxifen Therapy

Tamoxifen therapy, generally prescribed for the treatment of breast cancer, requires particular vigilance (see Chap.12). The slightest clinical symptom should prompt assessment of the endometrium, because endometrial carcinoma may occur in association with this drug (Bourne et al. 1994; Achiron et al. 1995; Bonnier et al. 1995). Tamoxifen-induced endometrial thickening may correspond to true hyperplasia or endometrial carcinoma. Pseudohyper-

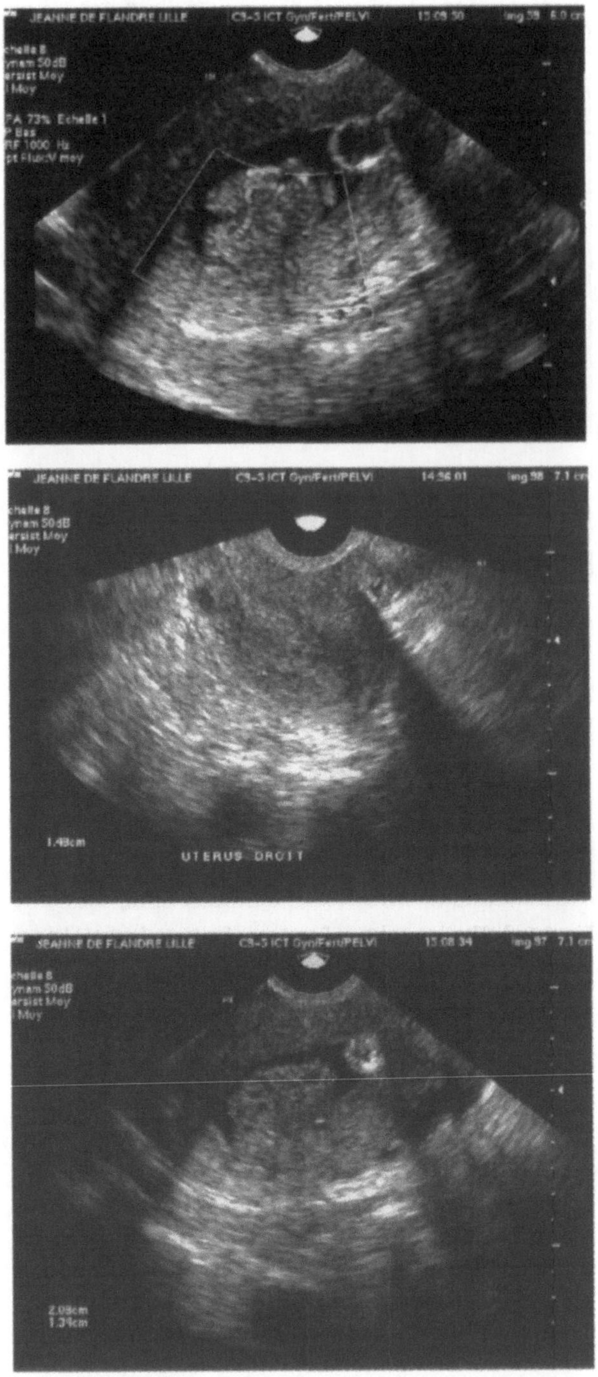

a

b

c

Fig. 3.9a–c. Endometrial carcinoma. **a** B-mode imaging: the thickened endometrium (14.9mm between the two *crosses*) is hyperechoic and discretely inhomogeneous. **b** Sonohysterogram: accurate delineation of this broad-based focal echoic lesion (20.9+13.4mm) rules out endometrial hyperplasia. **c** Sonohysterogram with power Doppler (PD, sagittal view) reveals marked vascularity of the focal lesion, even in the distal portion, and irregular contours, suggesting malignancy trophy, corresponding histologically to endometrial atrophy, frequently images as endometrial thickening with multiple small cystic spaces.

In view of these patterns of endometrial thickening (homogeneous or inhomogeneous with cystic spaces), sonohysterography facilitates differentiation of "hyperplasia" (diffuse, regular thickening of the endometrium) from polyps (round focal mass) or cystic pseudothickening suggestive of tamoxifen-induced cystic atrophy (cysts separated from the uterine cavity by a regular echoic line or discrete distortion of the endometrium by subendometrial cysts). Focal thickening should prompt a search for endometrial carcinoma.

3.3.7 Infertility

Infertility may be an indication for ultrasound and sonohysterography (Mitri et al. 1991; Deichert et al. 1992; Campbell et al. 1994). Although fibromyomata and polyps are not in themselves proven causes of infertility, they merit diagnosis and treatment before fertility management is pursued. By improving the quality of the examination, sonohysterography can aid in the diagnosis and management of these lesions (Fig. 3.7 and 3.8).

Diagnosis of uterine synechiae is difficult with B-mode scanning. Interruption of the echoic midline endometrial stripe by a hypoechoic linear image suggests a uterine adhesion, but this feature is not always easy to distinguish from the normal surrounding tissues. Sonohysterography may prove useful for patients with a history of curettage (Romano et al. 1994; Dijkhuizen et al. 1996). The diagnosis of an adhesion is suggested when the uterine cavity is only slightly distended, the patient experiences pain, and one or more echogenic structures are visualized adherent to the endometrial walls (Fig. 3.10).

Malformations are usually easy to diagnose using a combination of physical examination and ultrasound. However, differentiation of bicornuate uteri and septate uteri can prove difficult. Endovaginal ultrasound during the second part of the cycle usually allows satisfactory identification of both endometrial cavities. In unicervical bicornuate uteri, the two hyperechoic endometrial cavities are surrounded by myometrium with its own vascularity. Associated modifications in uterine contours are frequent. The bladder may "mold" to a notch on the uterine fundus, giving the classical bladder "V" sign

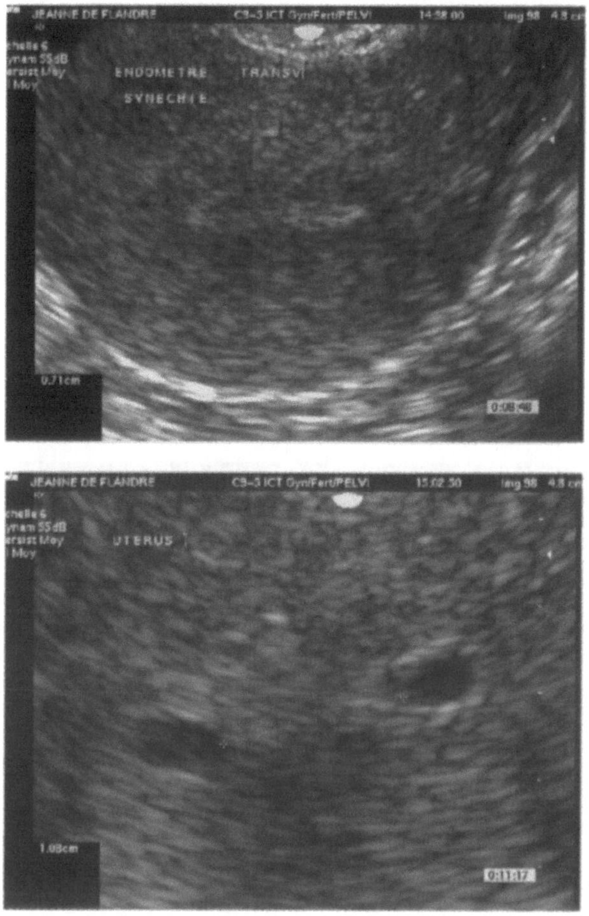

Fig. 3.10a,b. Uterine synechia. **a** B-mode scanning suggests disruption of the endometrium (7.1mm between the two *crosses*). **b** Sonohysterography demonstrated the adhesion between the adherence of the walls of the uterine cavity, which appears double (10.8mm between the two *crosses*)

on transabdominal scans. In contrast, septate uteri have a single myometrium with regular contours; their peripheral vascularity does not extend between the two endometrial cavities.

Sonohysterography may facilitate recognition of the two uterine cavities and the septum that separates them (Van Roessel et al. 1987). Adjunction of CD reveals the presence or absence of vascularity. The divergence of the uterine cavities is also easily evaluated by this technique. Simultaneous opacification of both cavities can be problematic; if the catheter is advanced too far, for example, only one of the cavities may be opacified, with the risk of a false-negative result. Two catheters may prove necessary to opacify both cavities (Fig.3.11).

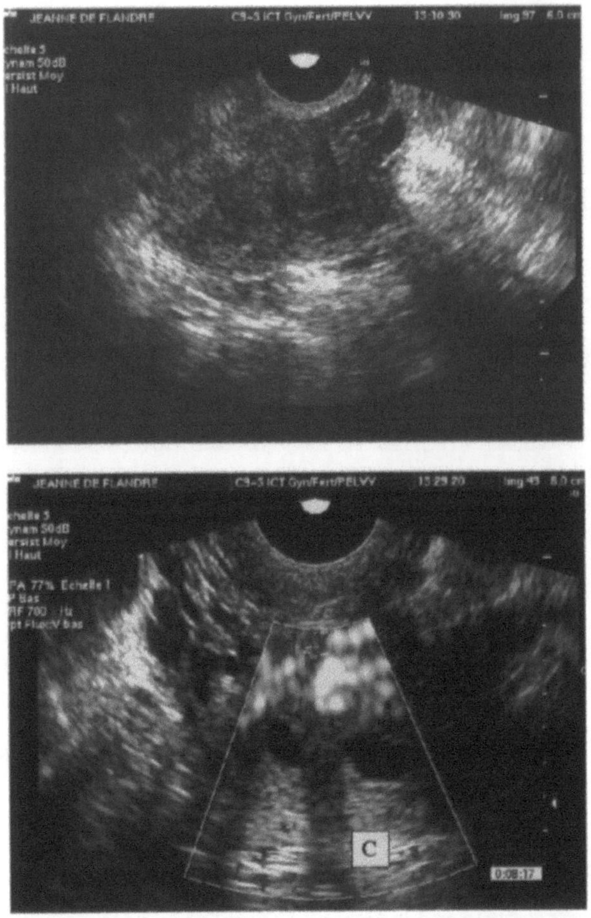

Fig. 3.11a,b. Septate uterus. **a** The septum is difficult to discern with B-mode scanning. **b** Opacification of the uterine cavities may allow identification of the septum (*C*), which is avascular on power Doppler (PD). Insertion of two catheters was necessary because the septum extended into the cervix

3.3.8 Tubal Patency

Tubal status can be reliably assessed using either saline solution or, even better, an ultrasound contrast agent. Passage of the contrast medium from the ampullary portion into the peritoneal cavity around the ovary reflects patency (Deichert et al. 1992; Tufekci et al. 1992; Campbell et al. 1994; Heikkinen et al. 1995). When sterile saline is used, increased free fluid around the ovary indicates passage of the contrast agent. When an ultrasound contrast agent is used, documentation of a sonographic "blush" corresponds to free spill of the contrast agent into the peritoneal cavity (Fig. 3.12).

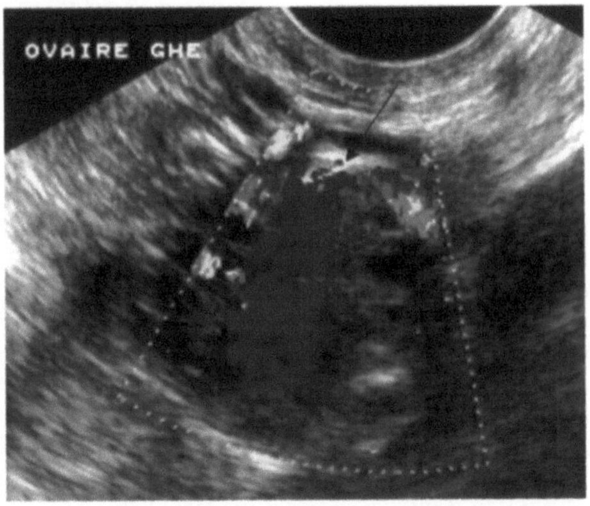

Fig. 3.12. Assessment of tubal patency. Distal tubal spill of the echogenic contrast medium around the ovary (*arrow*) can be depicted by B-mode scanning alone or combined with color Doppler (CD)

3.4 Limitations

False-negative results may be caused by small lesions and suboptimal examination technique with inadequate distention of the uterine cavity. Blood clots, distortions of the mucosal surface, and irregularities in endometrial thickness are sometimes merely normal physiological occurrences and can explain false-positive results for "lesions" that are not found at hysteroscopy. Introduction of air bubbles into the uterus during placement of an insufficiently purged catheter can create artifacts, but they are easily identified and transient.

The cervical canal is not always easy to evaluate during evacuation of the contrast medium.

Catheterization of the endocervical canal may fail because of cervical stenosis. Large myomata can hinder assessment of the uterine cavity by preventing complete distention.

Pain can easily be avoided by progressive and nonexcessive distention of the cavity. The potential risk of infection requires standard precautions, in particular antibiotic prophylaxis, especially for patients with a history of infection and infertility patients.

Finally, while sonohysterography can evaluate tubal patency by demonstrating passage of the contrast medium, the technique does not allow detailed assessment of fallopian tube morphology.

3.5 Conclusion

Sonohysterography has enriched the diagnostic capabilities of ultrasound, just as transvaginal scanning, CD, and PD previously complemented transabdominal B-mode scanning. According to Gaucherand et al. (1995), sonohysterography has improved the sensitivity of ultrasound while retaining satisfactory specificity. These authors consider the technique more sensitive than hysterosalpingography. Similar observations were made by Saidi et al. (1997) for the evaluation of abnormal uterine bleeding, although in their study the major improvement was in specificity rather than sensitivity.

Sonohysterography has also been used to assess tubal patency (Randolf et al. 1986; Schlief and Deichert 1991). Results are reportedly similar to those obtained with hysterosalpingography. Nevertheless, demonstration of the passage of contrast medium, which merely reflects tubal patency, must not be confused with the detailed morphologic analysis of the fallopian tubes provided by hysterosalpingography.

Sonohysterography has broad indications: in addition to workup of clinical symptoms such as metrorrhagia (especially postmenopausal), it is helpful whenever conventional diagnostic ultrasound is equivocal and better visualization of the uterine cavity is required. Therapeutic management is also facilitated because improved imaging allows those patients who do not require any further investigations to be distinguished from those who merit complementary studies.

References

Achiron R, Lipitz S, Sivan E, Goldenberg M, Mashiach S (1995) Sonohysterography for ultrasonographic evaluation of tamoxifen-associated cystic thickened endometrium. J Ultrasound Med 14:685–688

Bonnier P, Romain S, Giacalone PL, Laffargue F, Martin PM, Piana L (1995) Clinical and biological prognostic factor in breast cancer diagnosed during postmenopausal hormone replacement therapy. Obstet Gynecol 85:11–17

Bourne TH, Lawton F, Leather A et al (1994) Use of intracavity saline instillation and transvaginal ultrasonography to detect tamoxifen-associated endometrial polyps. Ultrasound Obstet Gynecol 4:73–75

Campbell S, Bourne TH, Collins WP (1994) Hysterosalpingo-contrast sonography (HyCoSy) and its future role within the investigation of infertility in Europe. Ultrasound Obstet Gynecol 4:245

Cicinelli E, Romano F, Anastasio PS, Blasi N, Parisi C (1994) Sonohysterography versus hysteroscopy in the diagnosis of endouterine polyps. Gynecol Obstet Invest 38:266–271

Cicinelli E, Romano F, Anastasio PS, Blasi N, Parisi C, Galantino P (1995) Transabdominal sonohysterography, transvaginal sonography, and hysteroscopy in the evaluation of submucous myomas. Obstet Gynecol 85:42–47

Cohen JR, Luxman D, Sagi J et al (1994) Sonohysterography for distinguishing endometrial thickening from endometrial polyps in post-menopausal bleeding. Ultrasound Obstet Gynecol 4:227–230

Cullinan JA, Fleischer AC, Kepple DM, Arnold AL (1995) Sonohysterography: a technique for endometrial evaluation. Radiographics 15:501–514

Deichert U, Schlief R, Van de Sandt M, Daume E (1992) Transvaginal hysterosalpingo-contrast sonography for the assessment of tubal patency with gray scale imaging and additional use of pulsed wave Doppler. Fertil Steril 57:62–67

Dijkhuizen PFHI, Brolmann HA, Potters AE et al (1996) The accuracy of transvaginal ultrasonography in the diagnosis of endometrial abnormalities. Obstet Gynecol 87:345–349

Dubinsky TJ, Parvey HR, Gormaz G, Maklad N (1995) Transvaginal hysterosonography in the evaluation of small endoluminal masses. J Ultrasound Med 14:1–6

Emanuel MH, Verdel MJ, Wamsteker K, Lammes FB (1995) A prospective comparison of transvaginal ultrasonography and diagnostic hysteroscopy in the evaluation of patients with abnormal uterine bleeding: clinical implications. Am J Obstet Gynecol 172:547–552

Fukuda M, Shimizu T, Fukuda K, Yomura W, Shimizu S (1993) Transvaginal hysterosonography for differential diagnosis between submucous and intramural myoma. Gynecol Obstet Invest 35:236–239

Gaucherand P, Piacenza JM, Salle B, Rudigoz RC (1995) Sonohysterography of uterine cavity: preliminary investigations. J Clin Ultrasound 23:339–348

Goldstein SR (1994) Use of ultrasonography for triage of perimenopausal patients with unexplained uterine bleeding. Am J Obstet Gynecol 170:565–570

Goldstein SR, Nachtigall M, Snyder JR et al (1990) Endometrial assessment by vaginal ultrasonography before endometrial sampling in patients with postmenopausal bleeding. Am J Obstet Gynecol 163:119–123

Heikkinen H, Tekay A, Volpi E et al (1995) Transvaginal salpingosonography for the assessment of tubal patency in infertile women: methodological and clinical experiences. Fertil Steril 64:293–298

Hoetzinger H (1993) Hysterosonography and hysterography in benign and malignant diseases of the uterus. A comparative in vitro study. J Ultrasound Med 10:259–263

Lin MC, Gosink BB, Wolf SI, Feldesman MR et al (1991) Endometrial thickness after menopause: effect of hormone replacement. Radiology 180:427–432

Mitri FF, Andronikou AD, Perpinyal SM et al (1991) A clinical comparison of sonographic hydrotubation and hysterosalpingography. Br J Obstet Gynecol 98:1031–1036

Parsons AK, Lense JJ (1993) Sonohysterography for endometrial abnormalities: preliminary results. J Clin Ultrasound 21:87–95

Randolf JR, Ying YK, Main DB, Schmidt CL, Riddick DH (1986) Comparison of real time ultrasonography, hysterosalpingography, and laparoscopy/hysteroscopy in the evaluation of uterine abnormalities and tubal patency. Fertil Steril 46:828–832

Romano F, Cicinelli E, Anastasio PS, Epifani S, Fanelli F, Galantino P (1994) Sonohysterography versus hysteroscopy for diagnosing endouterine abnormalities in fertile women. Int J Gynecol Obstet 45:253–260

Saidi MH, Sadler RK, Theis VD, Akright BD, Farhart SA, Villanueva GR (1997) Comparison of sonohysterography and hysteroscopy for evaluation of abnormal uterine bleeding. J Ultrasound Med 16:587–591
Schlief R, Deichert U (1991) Hysterosalpingo-contrast sonography of the uterus and fallopian tubes: results of a clinical trial of a new contrast medium in 120 patients. Radiology 178:213–215
Sheth S, Hamper UM, Kurman RJ (1993) Thickened endometrium in the postmenopausal woman: sonographic-pathologic correlation. Radiology 187:135–139
Shiply CF, Simmons CL, Nelson GH (1994) Comparison of transvaginal sonography with endometrial biopsy in asymtomatic postmenopausal women. J Ultrasound Med 13:99–104
Syrop CH, Sahakian V (1992) Tranvaginal sonographic detection of endometrial polyps with fluid contrast augmentation. Obstet Gynecol 79:1041–1043
Tufekci EC, Girit S, Bayirli E (1992) Evaluation of tubal patency by transvaginal sonosalpingography. Fertil Steril 57:336–340
Van Roessel J, Wamsteker K, Exalto N (1987) Sonographic investigation of the uterus during artifical uterine cavity distension. J Clin Ultrasound 15:439–450

4 Normal Anatomy of the Female Pelvis

C. Roy

Contents

4.1 Introduction

Although based on totally different principles, computed tomography (CT) and magnetic resonance imaging (MRI) are both capable of providing contiguous or noncontiguous scans of variable thickness. The density observed on CT scans and the signal intensity obtained by MRI correspond to the mean of all tissues located in the imaging plane. Such "partial volume averaging" results in degradation of the image of anatomic structures that are not perpendicular to the imaging plane and poor evaluation of visceral contours. Analysis of small masses requires thin slices. This is easy on CT, where the use of thin slices (1–3mm) improves image quality. In contrast, thin slices considerably degrade the quality of MR images. The presence of a sufficient quantity of fat between organs facilitates interpretation.

C. Roy, Service de Radiologie B, Hôpital Civil, 1 place de l'Hôpital, 67091 Strasbourg, France

4.2 Computed Tomography

4.2.1 Technique

Satisfactory CT examination requires adequate opacification of the small bowel, a partially distended bladder at the start of the procedure, without the need to urinate, and insertion of a venous catheter. Contiguous sections 5 mm thick are obtained before and after intravenous administration of an iodinated contrast agent. The best results are obtained with helical data acquisition in the arterial and parenchymal phases, as this allows two-dimensional reconstructions.

4.2.2 Uterus

The uterus and the ovaries have the particularity of being highly mobile. There are no precise anatomic landmarks allowing localization (Roy et al. 1993). On CT scans, the shape of the body of the uterus is influenced by its position in the pelvic cavity (Figs.4.1–4.4). Although most commonly anteverted and anteflexed, the uterus may be deviated to the right or left, retroverted, or even vertical when the bladder is full. Size and shape vary considerably depending on the period of genital activity and parity; they also depend on uterine position in the pelvic cavity because of partial volume averaging. A uterus that assumes a vertical position due to a full bladder appears oval with a transverse long axis. A horizontal uterus imaged when the bladder is empty appears oval, with an anteroposterior long axis. It is thus impossible to give numerical values for normal dimensions. On CT, uterine contours may be sharp; however, extensive partial volume averaging can result in slightly blurry images. The isthmus cannot be accurately localized. Anteversion of the uterine body

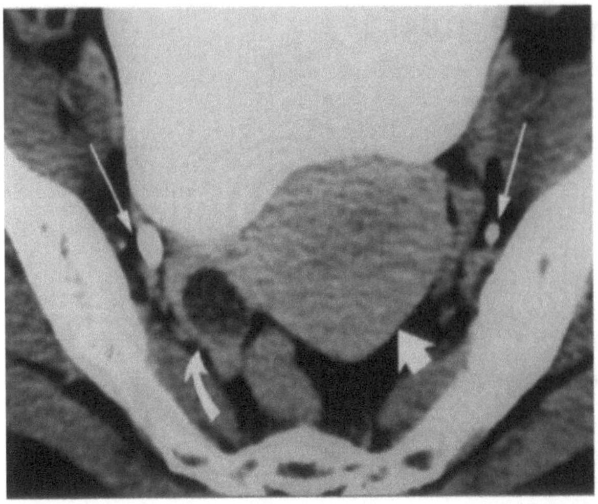

Fig. 4.1. Contrast-enhanced CT of the uterus (bladder distended). The uterus is vertical and contains an ill-defined hypodense central area (*large arrow*). A dominant follicle is present in the right ovary (*curved arrow*). Opacified ureters (*thin arrows*)

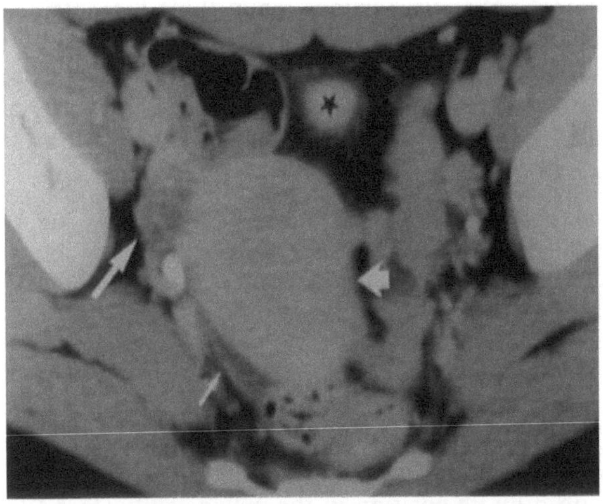

Fig. 4.2. Contrast-enhanced CT of the uterus (bladder empty). This anteverted uterus, deviated to the right, has a homogeneous density (*long arrow*). A small effusion is present in the Douglas cul-de-sac (*small arrow*). Readily identified behind the external iliac pedicle, the right ovary contains several follicles (*short arrow*). *Asterisk*, bladder

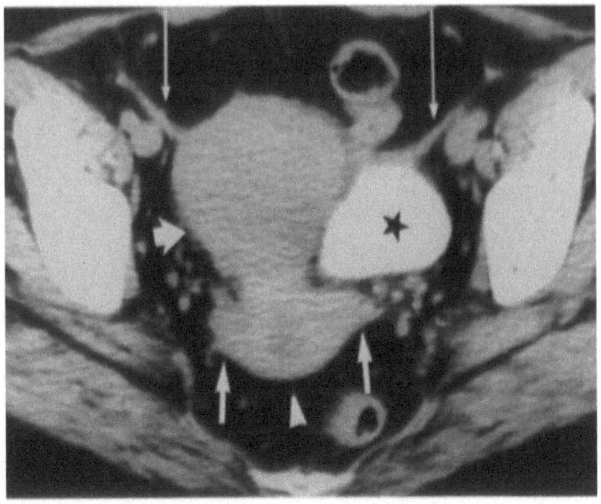

Fig. 4.3. Contrast-enhanced CT of the uterus (bladder partially full). The uterus is anteverted and deviated to the right (*large arrow*). The cervix is distinct, with a hypodense center (*arrowhead*). The parametrial tissues are inhomogeneous and asymmetrical (*small arrows*). Characteristic appearance of the round ligaments (*thin arrows*). *Asterisk*, bladder

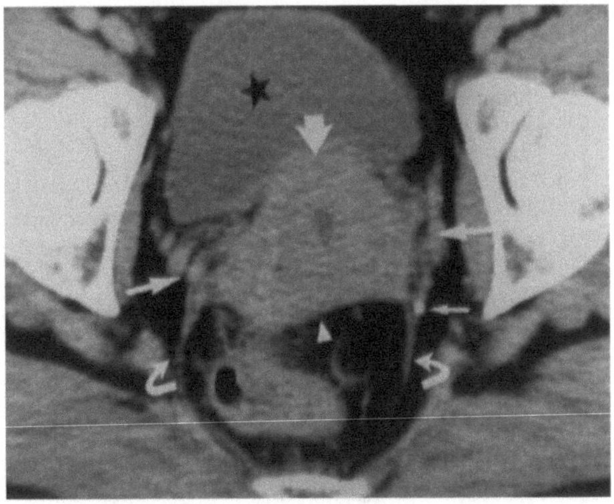

Fig. 4.4. Helical CT of the cervix (bladder full). The cervix is easily identified with its low signal intensity center (*large arrow*). The dense posterior band represents the posterior vaginal cul-de-sac (*arrowhead*). Heterogeneous appearance of the parametrial tissues (*arrows*). The uterosacral ligament is well delineated (*curved arrows*). Note the presence of a pelvic phlebolith (*small arrow*). *Asterisk*, bladder

can lead to suboptimal definition of the anterior uterine wall and the posterior bladder wall. The retroverted uterus images as a round retrovesical mass in the pouch of Douglas and must be distinguished from an abnormal tumoral process. The uterine horns and the fallopian tubes are inconsistently seen, and even then only in a segmental manner. Intrauterine devices (IUD) are readily depicted as a dense structure that appears elongated, punctate, or T-shaped, depending on the type and orientation relative to the imaging plane.

The cervix is seen as a smaller (approximately 3 cm) round or oval mass. It can be identified either due to its location, just above the change in caliber from the vagina, or by the presence of air in the posterior vaginal fornix. The cervix is isodense or slightly hyperdense relative to the corpus. The cervical cavity is sometimes visible; it appears hypodense relative to the cervical stroma because of endocervical secretions. The anterior cervix is difficult to discern from the posterior bladder wall. The posterior aspect of the cervix is clearly separated from the rectum by the perirectal fat planes. No modifications occur during the menstrual cycle.

The corpus and the cervix are both homogeneous before injection (approximately 40–50 HU). They enhance intensely after injection, when their density can reach 80–120HU. Slight changes occur during the menstrual cycle. During the first phase of the cycle, the corpus is homogeneous. During the second phase of the cycle, the endometrium is identified as a linear structure 0.5–1 cm thick that is hyperdense relative to the myometrium. It contains a central hypodense zone corresponding to secretions in the uterine cavity. The uterine cavity is visible on very early scans. During the prepubescent and postmenopausal periods, the uterus is atrophic and displays homogeneous density.

Overall, CT is of limited value for assessment of the uterus because of its low contrast resolution and the poor orientation of CT imaging planes, even with spiral data acquisition. Two-dimensional CT reconstructions, for example, have much lower spatial resolution than MRI.

4.2.3 Parametrial Tissues

The broad ligaments are transverse folds of peritoneum reflected onto the uterus and the adnexa (Figs. 4.3, 4.4). They extend to the lateral walls of the pelvic cavity while delimiting two layers. The parametrium, consisting of fat and fibrous tissue, is located on either side of the uterus, between the two layers of the broad ligament; it contains the uterine vessels and the ureter. The broad base of the parametrium (called the mesometrium) lies at the level of the cervix. There are no precise CT limits. When fat is abundant and the cervix is vertical, the parametrium is easily recognized as a paracervical fat pad containing multiple punctate structures of vascular origin (uterine veins and artery) and the terminal portion of the ureter. The ureter crosses the lateral surface of the cervix and then passes in front of the vaginal vault before entering the base of the bladder. After coursing posterolaterally to the ureter, the uterine artery penetrates the parametrium, curves round in front of the ureter, and curves upward, forming a curved horizontal portion called the cross of the uterine artery. The abundance of vessels (especially veins) is always underestimated compared to anatomic reality. Calcifications of the uterine artery are frequent in elderly women, particularly at the cross of the uterine artery.

After injection of iodinated contrast medium, the ureter is easily identified as a small dense punctate or oval mass, depending on its orientation in the imaging plane. The course of the ureter can be followed up to the ureterovesical pouch; this allows localization of the supravaginal cervical region and the base of the broad ligament. Demonstration of the parametrial tissues is more difficult in thin women and when the long axis of the cervix lies in a transverse position.

4.2.4 Ligaments

The round ligaments of the uterus (Fig.4.3) are frequently visualized, although usually only on one side. Attached proximally to the uterine horns, these dense fibrous bands course anteroinferiorly beneath the two layers of the broad ligament towards the inguinal canals. The round ligaments measure several centimeters in length. They are 2–3 mm thick at their origin but narrow as they approach the inguinal canal. They are unchanged after menopause.

The bilateral uterosacral ligaments (Fig. 4.4) extend from the posterolateral surface of the cervix (at the level of the cervicoisthmic junction) to the front of the sacrum (S2 or S3). These fibromuscular bands are related to the superior aspect of the perirectal fascia that they reinforce. The semicircular uterosacral ligaments form a "horseshoe" that surrounds the rectum. A fold of these ligaments delimits the pouch of Douglas. These ligaments may reach 1–2 mm in thickness.

The ovarian ligament is a small fibromuscular band connecting the ovary to the uterus, below and posterior to the attachment of the fallopian tubes and the round ligaments. It is rarely identified.

4.2.5 Vagina

The vagina is surrounded by the vesicovaginal and rectovaginal septa (Fig. 4.5). Lying anteroinferiorly in an oblique direction, the vagina is ovoid, with a transverse long axis on axial views. The vagina is bounded laterally by the levator ani muscles, anteriorly by the posterior aspect of the bladder, then the

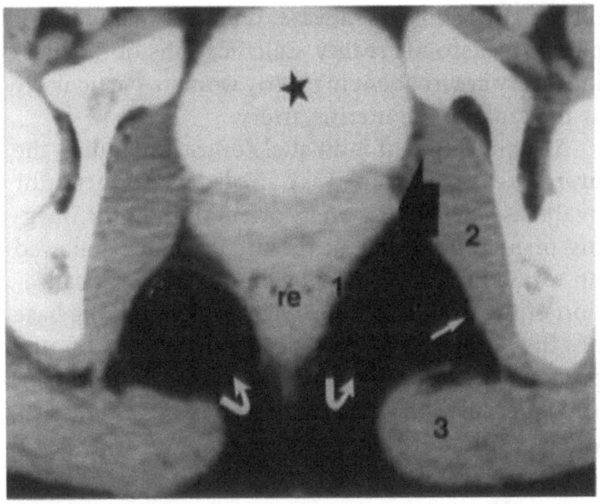

Fig.4.5. Contrast-enhanced CT of the vagina (bladder distended). The vaginal walls are distinct from the hypodense virtual cavity (*large black arrow*). The ischiorectal excavation (*curved arrows*) is bounded medially by the levator ani muscles (*1*) in contact with the pelvic viscera, laterally by the internal obturator muscle (*2*), and posteriorly by the gluteus maximus muscle (*3*). *Small arrow*, internal pudendal vessels; *asterisk*, bladder; *re*, rectum

urethra, and posteriorly by the anterior aspect of the rectum. The vagina is separated from these structures by a thin plane of fat and extensive venous plexuses. Enhancement of the vaginal wall after contrast injection sometimes allows identification of several layers. The central portion remains hypodense because of secretions. The presence of a small quantity of intraluminal air is common, occurring in an estimated 11% of cases, and can be observed on one or two scans. By contrast, visualization of a large amount of air at all scan levels is pathologic and suggests a fistula with the digestive tract.

At the external cervical os, the urethra, the vagina, and the anal canal cannot be distinguished from the contents of the deep and superficial perineal spaces.

4.2.6 Ovaries

The ovaries are consistently visualized with state-of-the art CT scanners in women of childbearing age. The ovary images as an oval tissue-density mass (Figs. 4.1, 4.2). It may be homogeneous, but is usually heterogeneous, with small cystic masses corresponding to follicles. The presence of a follicle (+1cm) facilitates localization. The ovaries may lie in a variety of positions: against the pelvic wall, around the internal iliac vessels, or under the iliac bifurcation in contact with the ureter. They are sometimes found closer to the uterus or in the pouch of Douglas. The variability of ovarian positions can lead to difficulties for localization and possible confusion with a poorly opacified loop of small bowel.

4.2.7 Perineum and Peritoneum

The peritoneal folds are not visible except in the presence of ascites (Fig. 4.6). The pouch of Douglas terminates at the level of the posterior aspect of the cervix or the posterior vaginal cul-de-sac. The rectovaginal and vesicovaginal fasciae cannot be visualized.

The external genital organs and the muscles of the anterior urogenital region (superficial and deep spaces) cannot be differentiated. Only the posterior anal region is well visualized. It is composed of the wedge-shaped ischioanal fossa, which is bounded laterally by the internal obturator muscle, medially by the levator ani muscle, and posteriorly by the gluteus maximus muscle. This area contains abundant fat and the internal pudendal canal, lying close to the obturator muscle in the canal of Alcock, a fibrous canal formed by the splitting of the obturator fascia.

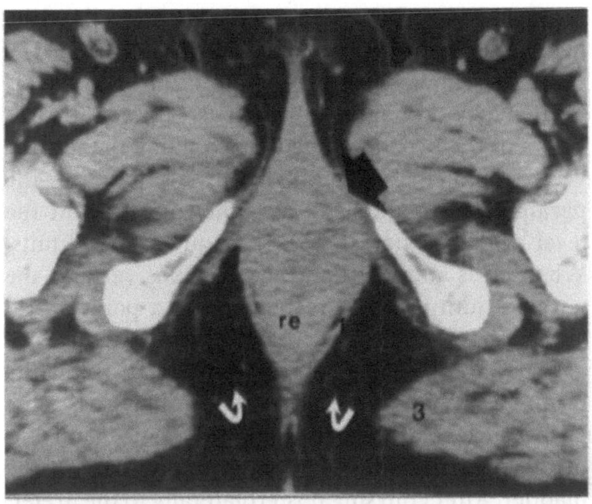

Fig.4.6. Postcontrast CT of the perineum. The muscles of the anterior perineum and the external genital organs are indistinguishable (*large black arrow*). Inferior portion of the ischiorectal excavation (*curved arrows*) with the levator ani muscle (*1*) and the gluteus maximus muscle (*3*). *re*, rectum

4.3 Magnetic Resonance Imaging

MRI is more useful than CT for assessment of female pelvic anatomy because MRI planes (sagittal, coronal, coronal oblique) are better suited to the anatomy of the genital organs and because of the high contrast resolution achieved with T_2-weighted sequences. Phased-array multicoils offer excellent spatial resolution. Endocavitary coils are under development and will probably prove useful for cervical examination.

Presence of an IUD does not contraindicate MRI. Several studies have shown that IUDs do not move, heat up, or cause artifacts. IUDs are imaged as an area of signal void whose size and shape depend on the type and uterine position in the imaging plane (Mark and Hricak 1987).

As detailed hereafter, the normal MR appearance of the female genital organs varies with the phase of the menstrual cycle and drug administration (Bartoli et al. 1991; Lin et al. 1991; Moulin et al. 1991; Scoutt et al. 1991).

4.3.1 Technique

The degree of bladder distention is not important. It is thus preferable to start the examination with the bladder empty or only half-full, but without the need to urinate owing to the risk of motion artifacts. Insertion of a venous catheter for intravenous administration of contrast agent (gadolinium) is indicated for certain pathologies.

Several associated techniques have been proposed, but they usually only complicate the examination:

- Rectal insufflation of air appears justified solely for certain situations (assessment of the anterior rectum and the posterior vaginal cul-de-sac). The patient must remain in ventral decubitus position to maintain the air in the rectum, and this position is not well tolerated.
- Injection of glucagon to reduce intestinal peristalsis is unnecessary, because artifacts due to digestive tract motion cause little degradation of pelvic images.
- Injection of ferrite-based products for localization of gastrointestinal structures also has few indications (evaluation of the node-bearing areas in thin patients in whom the digestive organs are in direct contact with the vessels).

MRI examination is begun with fast gradient-echo sequences for localization purposes. Spin-echo (SE) sequences are then obtained. T_1-weighted SE sequences provide excellent delineation of anatomy and characterization of pelvic fluids. T_2-weighted SE images are particularly suited for demonstration of the internal architecture of the genital organs. Fast SE techniques are advisable because they offer excellent T_2-weighted imaging with a short acquisition time (ranging from several seconds, which allows suspended respiration in case of a small acquisition matrix, to 23min with maximal resolution). Fat-saturation sequences associated with intravenous gadolinium injection improve the diagnostic efficacy of MRI for ovarian masses.

Artifacts are constant in numerous circumstances:

- Nonferromagnetic metal implants distort the magnetic field around them in proportion to their size. An area of signal void is seen at the level of the implant itself. There is no risk of displacement of pelvic surgical clips if care is taken to wait 2–3weeks after surgery so that fibrous tissue can form. The artifact is minimal in such cases and does not hinder interpretation. The focal artifact caused by metal hip prostheses does not interfere with analysis of the uterine cavity and has little influence on pelvic floor images.
- Chemical shift artifacts constantly occur at fat–soft tissue interfaces. This characteristic artifact manifests as a dark band on one side of the interface (hypersignal) and a light band on the opposite side (hyposignal). These artifacts are present on all images, proportional to the intensity of the magnetic field, but are especially conspicuous on T_2-weighted sequences. Such artifacts must not be confused with a pseudocapsule, wall thickening, or a focal fluid effusion (Figs. 4.7, 4.8).
- Flow artifacts are extremely variable and complex. Schematically, vessels with high flows do not have any signal, except on the first or the last scan of a series. Vessels with a lower flow have an intermediate- to high-intensity signal, dependent on numerous factors. Presaturation bands can reduce flow artifacts.

The imaging planes must be adapted to the region of interest. Sagittal views allow accurate assessment of the entire uterus and its relations with the bladder anteriorly and the rectum posteriorly. If the uterus is considerably deviated to the right or left, sagittal

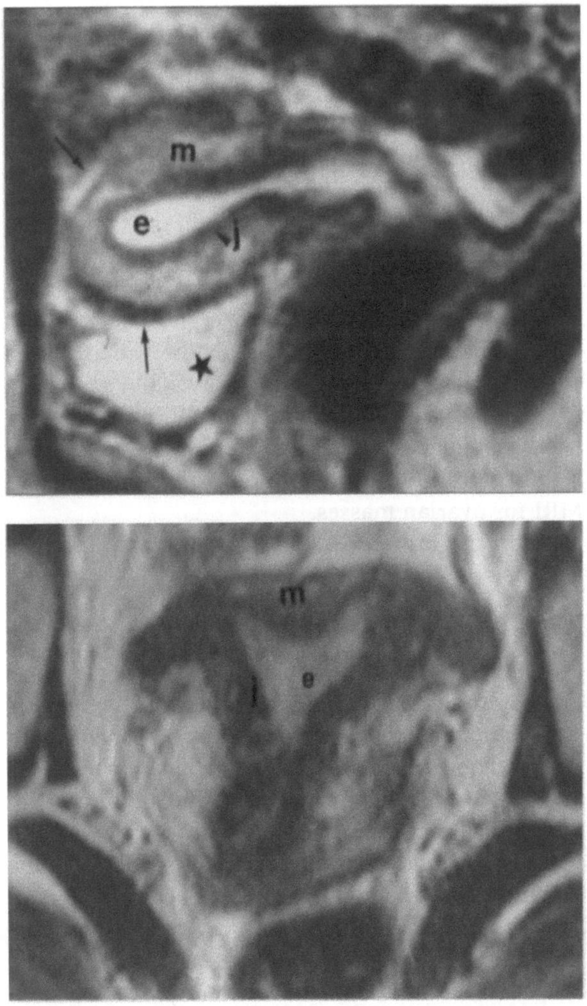

a

b

Fig. 4.7a,b. T_2-weighted SE sequence of the uterus (second phase of the menstrual cycle). **a** Sagittal scan. Hyperintense endometrium (*e*); hypointense junctional zone (*j*); the remainder of the myometrium (*m*) has an inhomogeneous intermediate intensity signal. The chemical shift phenomenon produces a hyperintense rim on one side and a hypointense rim on the other side (*arrows*). Hyperintense urine (*arrowhead*). **b** Axial oblique scan through the long axis of the uterus

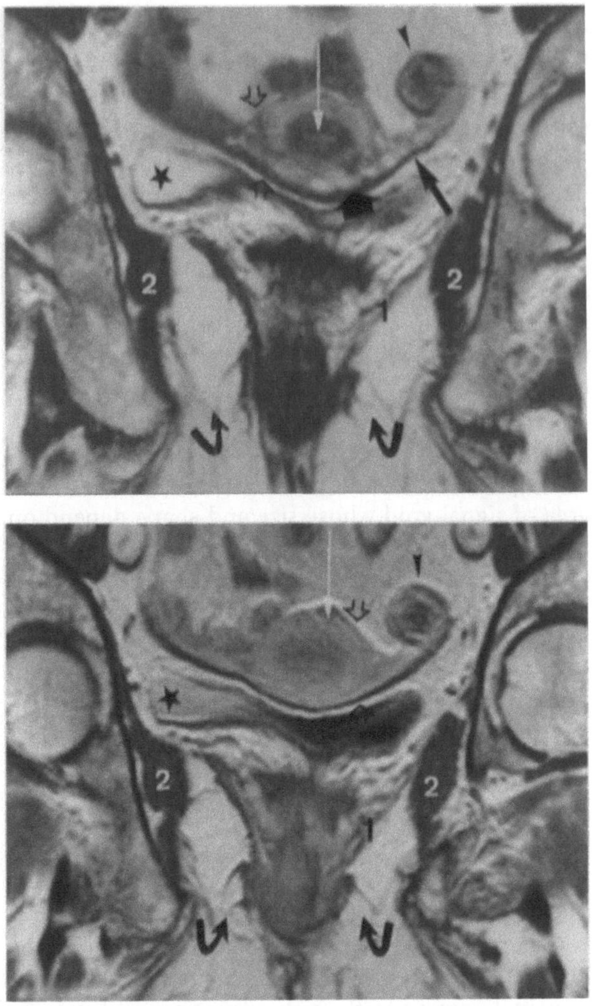

a

b

Fig. 4.8a,b. Coronal oblique MRI scan of the uterus perpendicular to the long axis (first phase of the menstrual cycle) **a** T_2-weighted SE sequence. The endometrium is atrophic (*thin white arrow*). The hyperintense zones in the outer myometrium correspond to the uterine arcuate vessels (*thick arrow*). The right fallopian tube is visible (*arrow*) with the ovary at its superoexternal extremity (*arrowhead*). It has a low signal intensity on the periphery and an intermediate intensity in the center; no follicles are visible on this scan. The large ischiorectal excavation (*curved arrows*) is bounded medially by the levator ani muscle (*1*) and laterally by the internal obturator muscle (*2*). *Asterisk*, bladder. The chemical shift phenomenon is well visible (*open arrows*) and is responsible for the asymmetrical appearance of the levator ani muscles. **b** T_1-weighted SE sequence with contrast enhancement; same imaging plane. The uterus appears more homogeneous (*arrow*); peripheral enhancement of the ovary (*arrowhead*)

oblique views can depict the long axis of the uterus. Axial views are best suited for evaluation of the cervix, which is usually vertical. However, as on CT, relations with the neighboring organs are poorly depicted due to partial volume averaging. Axial views are also useful for evaluation of the parametrial tissues, the vagina, and the ovaries. Coronal scans are indicated for depiction of the cervix and ovaries, evaluation of disease spread to the perineal region, and demonstration of the lateral aspects of the uterus. Coronal oblique scans along the craniocaudal long axis of the uterus permit assessment of the endometrium and the uterine cavity. In practice, T_1- and T_2-weighted sequences are performed in perpendicular planes.

4.3.2 Uterus

4.3.2.1 *Body of the Uterus*

Childbearing Years. The length of the uterine body in women of a childbearing age (Figs.4.7, 4.8) ranges from 6 to 8cm and varies little during the menstrual cycle. On T_1-weighted MR sequences, the uterus is homogeneous and has a low-to-intermediate intensity signal that is usually slightly hyperintense relative to the pelvic muscles. The signal intensity remains constant throughout the cycle. In 40 % of cases, the uterus contains a central band of higher signal intensity corresponding to the endometrium. T_2-weighted images reveal the zonal anatomy of the uterus containing several distinct layers:

- The central endometrial zone can be identified due to its high vascularity and glandular nature as a homogeneous band of intermediate to very high signal intensity (in the latter case equivalent to urine). Endometrial thickness varies from 2.5 to 10mm and includes the two apposed endometrial layers and secretions in the cavity. The endometrium is very thin after menstruation and in the early proliferative phase (1–3 mm). It then thickens progressively, reaching 7–10 mm in the late secretory phase. Accurate measurement of the thickness of the cavity is difficult because the endometrial mucosa is indistinguishable from endometrial secretions. During menstruation, the signal pattern becomes heterogeneous due to blood clots.
- The junctional zone between the endometrium and the myometrium images as a low-intensity line around the endometrial cavity. The nature of the junctional zone remains controversial; histopathologically, it corresponds to the basal layer of the myometrium. Its appearance has been attributed to reduced water content in the extracellular spaces and an increase in the number and size of the nuclei compared to the rest of the myometrium. The junctional zone may reach 10mm in thickness; it is thinnest during the first phase of the menstrual cycle and thickens thereafter.
- The remainder of the myometrium displays an intermediate-to-high signal intensity. On T_2-weighted sequences, the MR signal is increased in the second part of the cycle, whereas it decreases during the first part. The intermediate- to high-intensity signal observed during the proliferative phase is due to the presence of myometrial edema with vasodilatation, proportional to estrogen stimulation. The outer third of the myometrium is often punctuated by hypersignals corresponding to venous lakes or branches of the arcuate arteries. The combined width of the external myometrium and the junctional zone ranges from 14 to 21mm. The thickness of the myometrium increases during the second phase of the cycle. The difference in the signal intensity between the two portions of the myometrium decreases during the secretory phase.

The endometrium and the myometrium both enhance after gadolinium injection, but the junctional zone remains hypointense. The zonal anatomy is seen in only 50% of cases, however. Identification of the three zones permits distinction of the isthmus and the cervix.

Postmenopausal Period. The postmenopausal uterus is ≤4cm in length. On T_1-weighted sequences, the signal is identical to that during the reproductive years. On T_2-weighted images, the endometrium is very thin or absent. The junctional zone is visible in nearly half of all cases, and the signal of the myometrium is decreased. In postmenopausal women on hormone replacement therapy (HRT), the appearance is identical to that during the childbearing years. Endometrial thickness may reach 0.8–1 cm. Higher values are suggestive of endometrial hyperplasia or malignancy. There is no correlation between endometrial thickness, age, and the duration of HRT.

Women on Combination Oral Contraceptives. Predominantly estrogenic regimens cause marked endometrial atrophy. The thickness of the myometrium increases and its signal intensity also increases on T_2-weighted sequences, regardless of the phase of the cycle. The junctional zone is thin or absent. It is sometimes impossible to discern the myometrium from the endometrium. The size of the uterine body decreases in the case of prolonged drug use. Under progestogen therapy, the entire uterus undergoes involution.

Normal Prepubescent Uterus. The uterus is small. The signal is intermediate to high on T_2-weighted sequences and is homogeneous.

4.3.2.2
Cervix and Parametrial Tissues

Although variable in length and position, the cervix is usually better visualized on axial views than on coronal scans (Figs. 4.9, 4.10). On T_1-weighted sequences, the cervix appears isointense or slightly hypointense relative to the corpus. A peripheral band of very low signal intensity is sometimes identified. T_2-weighted sequences reveal a "target" pattern. A maximum of four closely apposed layers can be distinguished, from innermost outward:

- A central zone of high signal intensity corresponding to the endocervical mucosa and mucus.
- An irregular, fringed structure representing the palmate folds (seen inconsistently).
- An intermediate, annular peripheral layer of low signal intensity, isointense to the junctional zone. Histologically, this layer represents the cervical stroma and is distinct from the junctional zone. It consists of a muscular coat rich in connective tissue and elastin fibers.
- An outer layer, isointense to the external layer of the myometrium, is distinguished in 15% of

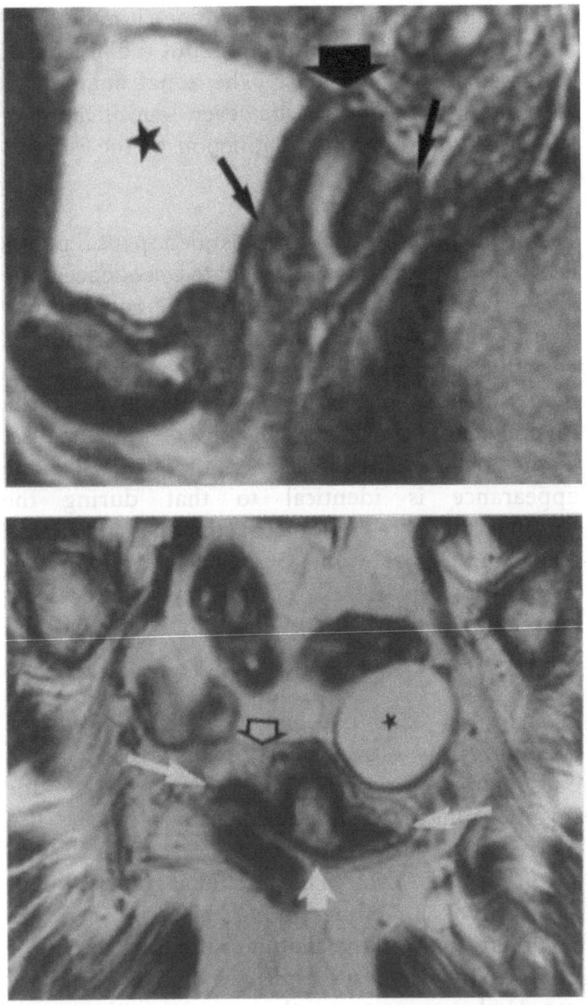

Fig. 4.9a,b. T_2-weighted SE images of the cervix. **a** Sagittal plane. The four cervical layers can be identified along with the central hyperintense cervical cavity (*thick arrow*). The posterior and anterior cul-de-sacs (*small arrows*) are visible. *Asterisk*, bladder. **b** Coronal scan. The lateral vaginal fornices appear hypointense (*small arrows*). Only three cervical layers are visible (*thick arrow*). The heterogeneous parametrium displays an intermediate intensity signal (*open arrow*). Presence of a large right ovarian follicle (*asterisk*)

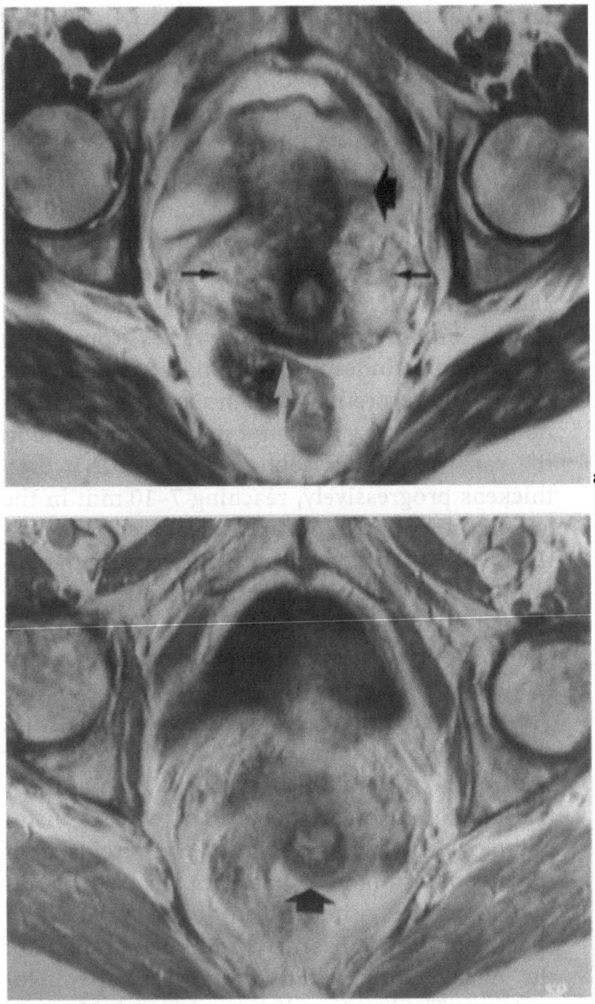

Fig. 4.10a,b. Axial MRI of the parametrial tissues. **a** T_2-weighted SE sequence. Characteristic appearance of the cervix and the heterogeneous parametrial tissues (*small arrows*). Posterior vaginal cul-de-sac (*white arrow*). The posterior bladder wall is not visible because of partial volume averaging with the anteverted uterine body (*large arrow*). **b** Contrast-enhanced T_1-weighted SE sequence (1cm higher). The zonal anatomy is readily visible, and the cervical mucosa is distinct from the cavity (*arrow*). The parametrial vessels are enhanced

cases. Like the external layer of the myometrium, this outer layer changes in appearance as a function of the menstrual cycle. This layer corresponds to bundles of smooth muscle fibers that predominate at the periphery of the cervix.

The parametrium is easily distinguished from the stroma. It has a high T_1 signal intensity and is punctuated by multiple round or oval hypointense zones corresponding to vessels. The parametrium has an intermediate to high intensity signal on T_2-weighted sequences. Hyperintense zones correspond to slow blood flow in the parametrial vessels.

Few changes occur as a function of the menstrual cycle. The appearance of the cervix does not change after the menopause.

After gadolinium injection, the paracervical space and the epithelium of the internal mucosa appear hyperintense, whereas the stroma remains hypointense. The zonal anatomy is well delineated on contrast-enhanced T_1-weighted sequences.

4.3.2.3
Fallopian Tubes

The fallopian tubes are occasionally visible on coronal scans.

4.3.3
Vagina

Anatomically, the vagina can be divided into three portions, which are easily identified on axial views (Hricak et al. 1988). The upper third corresponds to the lateral fornices, the middle third lies at the level of the base of the bladder, and the lower third is located opposite the urethra (Fig.4.11).

Women of Reproductive Age. Regardless of the imaging plane, it is difficult to differentiate the vaginal wall from the posterior aspect of the bladder and the rectal wall on T_1-weighted images. The vagina has a homogeneous, low-intensity signal and sometimes presents a central zone of slightly higher signal intensity.

On T_2-weighted sequences, the vagina is easily distinguished from other structures. Sagittal views permit accurate evaluation of the vaginal fornices (especially the posterior fornix) and the anterior and posterior vaginal walls and relations with the other organs. The rectovaginal and vesicovaginal septa

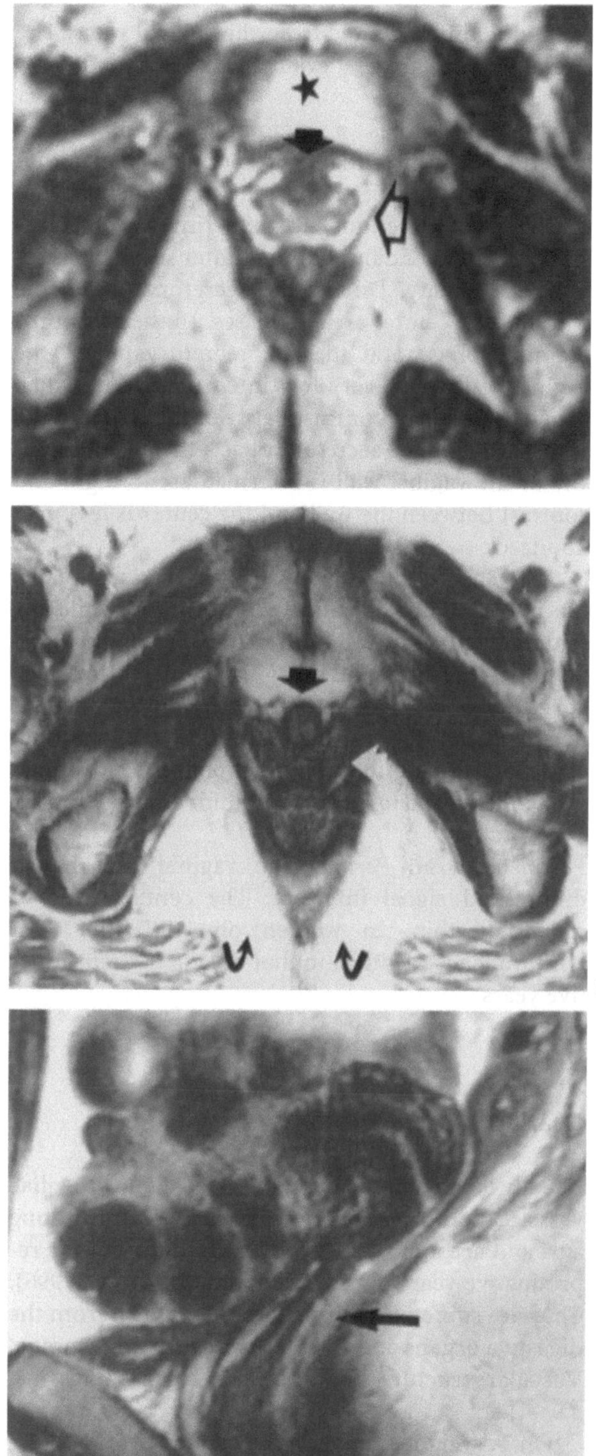

Fig. 4.11a–c. Axial MRI of the vagina. **a** Axial T_2-weighted SE image. The vaginal wall appears hypointense (*white arrow*). Ischiorectal excavation (*curved arrows*). Urethra (*black arrow*). **b** Axial T_2-weighted SE image. The abundance of hyperintense perivaginal venous plexuses is due to slow flow (*open arrow*). *Asterisk*, bladder; *black arrow*, urethra. **c** Sagittal T_2-weighted SE image. The hypointense wall is surrounded by venous plexuses (*arrow*). The scant vaginal contents are hyperintense

cannot be differentiated from the vaginal walls. The lateral fornices are best evaluated by axial and coronal scans.

The vagina has a hypointense wall and a hyperintense center that corresponds to the epithelium and mucus. The endovaginal signal depends on the extent of secretions; it is hyperintense when secretions are abundant, but hypointense when secretions are scanty. During the secretory phase, the width of the central area increases. In the early proliferative phase and the late secretory phase, the vaginal wall has a very low intensity signal, which provides excellent contrast between the wall and the center. During the secretory phase, the signal intensity of the vaginal wall is intermediate to high, and contrast between the wall and the center is less pronounced.

The shape of the vagina varies in the axial plane; the upper vagina is concave posteriorly, while the middle vagina is oval, with a transverse long axis. Opposite the ureter, the vagina is curves forward. Large peripheral vascular structures with a high-intensity signal due to slow blood flow are common, especially during the secretory phase. The vaginal wall enhances following gadolinium administration.

Postmenopausal Period. The vaginal wall has a diminished signal intensity. The central zone of mucus is thin. In women on HRT, the MRI appearance is identical to that during the reproductive years.

4.3.4 Ovaries

Usually located in the ovarian fossa, against the iliac vessels, the normal ovaries measure 2–3cm in long axis and are almost always visualized during the reproductive years (OUTWATER and MITCHELL 1996). They are sometimes difficult to distinguish from the digestive organs and the uterus in very thin women. Vascular structures are the best landmarks (Figs. 4.8, 4.9, 4.12).

On T_1-weighted images, the ovarian stroma has a low to intermediate signal intensity identical to that of the myometrium. On T_2-weighted sequences, the ovaries typically exhibit a zonal anatomy; the cortex appears hypointense relative to the medulla. The medulla is isointense relative to the myometrium; on rare occasions, it is hyperintense.

Multiple cyst-like follicles are often visualized. They vary in number from two to nine per ovary; size ranges from 1 to 2 cm, although they occasionally reach 5 cm. Follicles have a low signal intensity on T_1-weighted images and a high signal intensity on T_2-weighted sequences. Only 5% have a high T_1 signal, reflecting intracystic hemorrhage. The thin wall of follicles may not be apparent or may be depicted on T_2-weighted sequences as a hypointense rim. A hypervascular corpus luteum with a thick wall and irregular internal contours may also be observed. The presence of a dominant follicle facilitates localization of the ovaries.

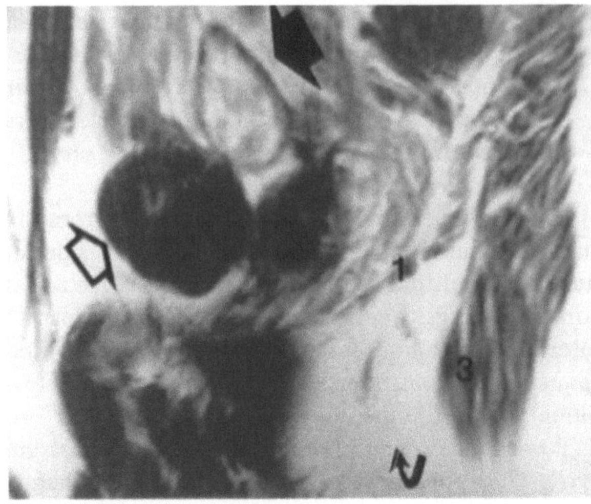

Fig. 4.12. Sagittal T_2-weighted MRI. The ovarian cortex appears hypointense; the intermediate signal intensity medulla contains hyperintense follicles (*large arrow*). Uterine fibromyoma (*open arrow*). The ischiorectal excavation (*curved arrow*) is bounded superiorly by the levator ani (*1*) and posteriorly by the gluteus maximus (*3*)

Following administration of gadolinium, the ovarian stroma enhances less than the myometrium in 75% of individuals and to the same extent as the myometrium in 25%, in particular in elderly patients. The cortex and the medulla appear isointense on gadolinium-enhanced images. Cyst walls enhance discretely, except for corpus luteum cysts, which enhance strongly and have irregular internal margins.

In postmenopausal women who are not on HRT, visualization of the ovaries is not constant. The zonal anatomy of the ovary is rarely observed. The signal intensity on T_2-weighted images is diminished and homogeneous due to replacement of the medulla by fibrous cells and the absence of small follicles. Enhancement after contrast administration is homogeneous and identical to that of the myometrium. Cysts are not infrequent but are small (≤1cm) and not very numerous.

4.3.5
Ligaments and Fasciae

The round ligament is frequently visualized (approximately 50% of cases) as a low-intensity signal on both T_1- and T_2-weighted sequences. The uterosacral ligament is hypointense on T_2-weighted images.

4.3.6
Bladder

Well-demarcated by the hyperintense urine, the bladder wall displays intermediate signal intensity on T_1-weighted sequences and low signal intensity on T_2-weighted sequences.

4.3.7
Perineum and Peritoneum

The muscles of the anterior perineum or urogenital diaphragm appear hypointense on T_2-weighted sequences. The deep perineal pouch contains the deep transverse muscle of perineum and the fibers of the external sphincter muscle of the urethra. The superficial perineal space contains the bulbospongiosus and ischiocavernous muscles and the sphincter muscle of the anus. These structures are particularly well seen on coronal scans. The posterior perineum includes the ischiorectal excavation. Bounded superiorly by the levator ani muscles, this bilateral and symmetrical space contains abundant fat and is readily visualized on all imaging planes.

References

Bartoli JM, Moulin G, Delannoy l, Changaud C, Kasbarian M (1991) The normal uterus on magnetic resonance imaging and variations associated with the hormonal state. Surg Radiol Anat 13:213–220

Hricak H, Chang YC, Thurner S (1988) Vagina: Evaluation with MR imaging. I. Normal anatomy and congenital anomalies. Radiology 169:169–174

Lin MC, Gosink BB, Wolf SI, Feldesman MR, Stuenkel CA, Braly PS, Pretorius DH (1991) Endometrial thickness after menopause: effect of hormone replacement. Radiology 180:427–432

Mark AS, Hricak H (1987) Intrauterine contraceptive devices: MR imaging. Radiology 162:311-314

Moulin G, Bartoli JN, Gaubert JY, Bayle O, Distefano-Louineau D, Kasbarian M (1991) IRM de l'utérus - aspects normaux et pathologiques. Feuillets Radiol 31:222–235

Outwater EK, Mitchell DG (1996) Normal ovaries and functional cysts: MR appearance. Radiology 198:397–402

Roy C, Bourjat P, Beaujeux R (1993) Tomodensitométrie et imagerie par résonance magnétique. In: Buthiau D, Dargent D (eds) Imagerie clinique en gynécologie. Vigot, Paris, pp 39–48

Scoutt LM, Flynn SD, Luthringer DJ, McCauley TR, McCarthy SM (1991) Junctional zone of the uterus: correlation of MR imaging and histologic examination of hysterectomy specimens. Radiology 179:304–407

5 Puberty: Normal and Pathologic Imaging

A. Geoffray, E. Baechler Sadoul, and A. Daneman

CONTENTS

5.1 Normal Puberty

Normal puberty can be adequately evaluated in both sexes solely by clinical signs. In girls, pelvic sonography is a useful complement to physical examination (Andre and Le Bihan 1982; Haber and Mayer 1994) to assess maturation of the internal genital organs.

During the prepubescent period, the ovaries image sonographically as small, homogeneous oval nodules ranging in size from several millimeters to 1cm. The ovaries may also appear microfollicular and contain hypoechoic follicles measuring 2–4 mm. The ovaries are not always visible between the ages of 1 and 3 years. Ovarian cysts are frequent in young prepubertal girls (Cohen et al. 1992), but are not pathologic. They usually measure under 10mm, but macrocysts larger than 9mm are seen occasionally.

The teardrop-shaped uterus measures 3±0.5cm in length (Fig. 5.1). The cervix is larger than the body, which is thin. The isthmus and the cervix represent two thirds of the total uterine volume.

A. Geoffray, Service de Radiologie, Fondation Lenval, 57 avenue de la Californie, 06200 Nice, France
E. Baechler Sadoul, Service de Pédiatrie, Fondation Lenval, 57 avenue de la Californie, 06200 Nice, France
A. Daneman, Department of Radiology, Hospital for Sick Children, 555 University Avenue, Toronto, Ontario M5G1X8, Canada

At puberty, the ovaries enlarge and take on a heterogeneous ultrasound pattern. They measure 2.5–3 cm in the long axis and contain numerous follicles. Measurements should be reported in three dimensions so that the pediatrician can evaluate ovarian volume. According to Colle et al. (1993), Doppler sonography of the ovarian arteries allows assessment of the stage of puberty. Color Doppler (CD) allows visualization of the ovarian arteries, even when small, and permits spectral analysis. Before puberty, the systolic peak is high and there is no diastolic flow; the pulsatility index (PI) is high (over 4). Once puberty begins, diastolic flow appears and the PI decreases. Doppler analysis can thus help to diagnose the onset of puberty (Figs. 5.2, 5.3).

The uterus also undergoes changes at puberty. The corpus enlarges and becomes pear-shaped. On sonograms, the uterine cavity becomes visible as a dense midline echo. Angulation of the isthmus is common (Fig. 5.4). The uterus measures 5–8 cm in length, and the corpus is 2–4 cm thick. Determination of uterine volume is essential because it is the

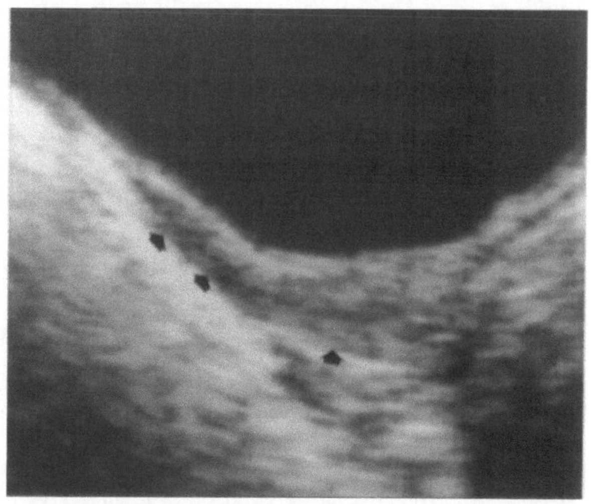

Fig. 5.1. Eight-year-old girl. Midline longitudinal pelvic sonogram revealing the typical infantile morphology of the uterus. The body (*double arrow*) is markedly narrower than the isthmus (*single arrow*)

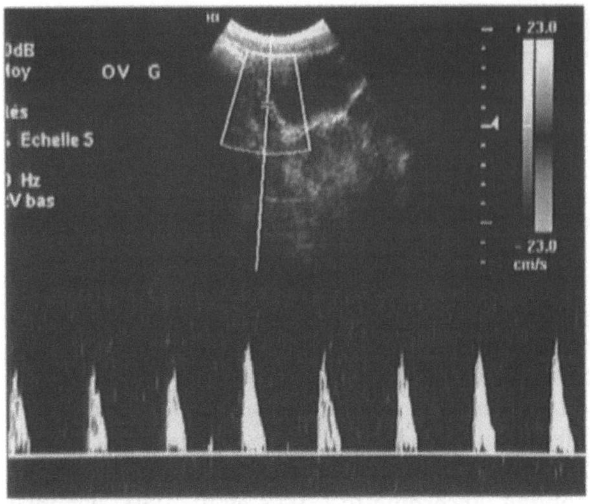

Fig. 5.2. Nine-year-old girl. Left parasagittal pelvic sonogram. Doppler analysis of the ovary reveals the absence of diastolic flow: prepubertal stage

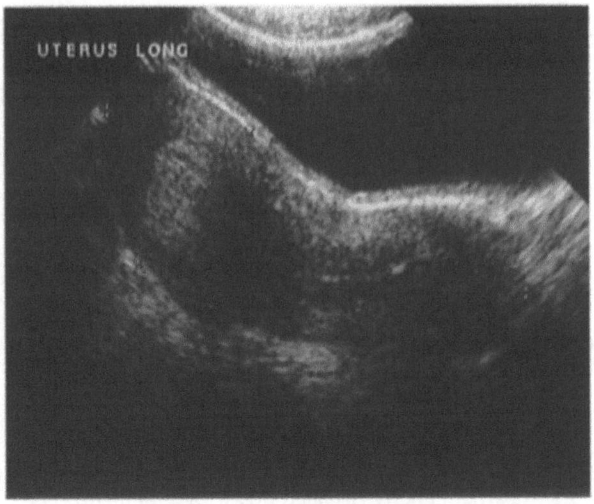

Fig. 5.4. Ten-year-old girl. Midline sagittal pelvic sonogram showing the characteristic pubertal morphology of the uterus; the endometrium is visible

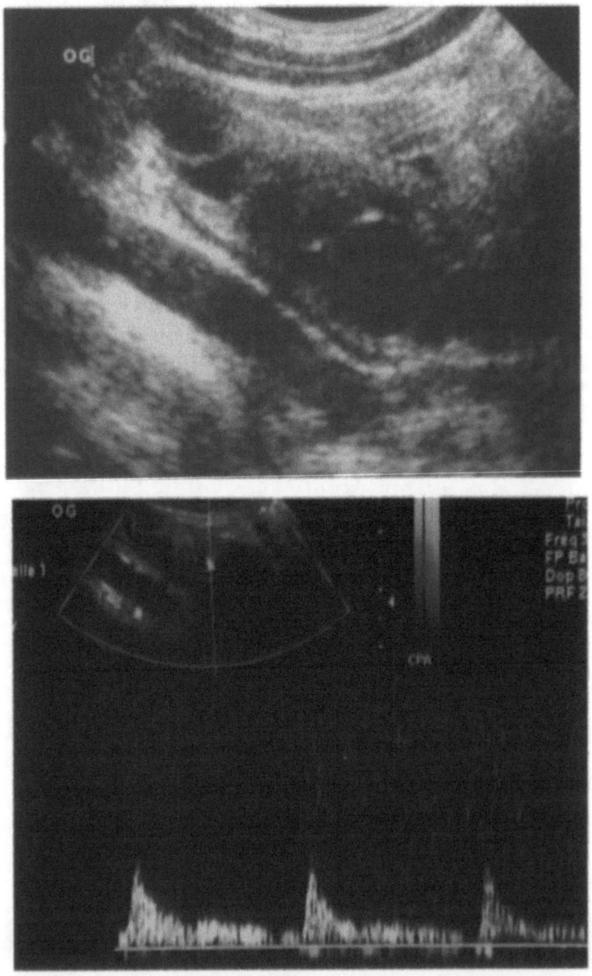

Fig. 5.3 a,b. Eight-year-old girl with breast development. **a** Left parasagittal pelvic sonogram: ovary containing several follicles (at least one is larger than 1cm). **b** Ovarian Doppler reveals diastolic flow suggestive of the onset of puberty

parameter best correlated with the stage of puberty (Haber and Mayer 1994). After puberty, cyclic variations are observed as in adults; endometrial hyperplasia occurs at the end of the menstrual cycle, and a small nonpathologic fluid collection is often noted in the pouch of Douglas during the ovulatory phase.

5.2 Precocious Puberty

Precocious puberty is defined as the onset of sexual maturation before 8years of age in girls and before 10years of age in boys. It is important to distinguish between the following:

- True precocious puberty due to premature activation of the hypothalamus–pituitary–gonadal axis (central precocious puberty)
- Pseudoprecocious puberty due to secretion of sex hormones by the adrenal glands or gonads (peripheral precocious puberty)
- Partial precocious puberty characterized by isolated appearance of a single secondary sexual characteristic (pubic hair, breast development, menstruation)

Diagnosis of precocious puberty is made by physical examination. Pubertal development is evaluated using the Tanner stages. Height–weight growth curves are established to detect any acceleration in growth rate. The onset of the first signs of puberty is recorded and a personal and family history is taken. An alteration in general condition, cutaneous patches of pigmentation, an increase in arterial blood pressure, an abdominal mass, or an abnormal neurologic examination can all help to guide the diagnosis (PERELMAN 1990).

5.2.1
True Precocious Puberty

True precocious puberty affects girls three times as often as boys. Idiopathic cases (80% in girls, 30%–50% in boys) are much more common than those due to secondary causes (20% in girls, 50%–70% in boys) (BRAUNER and RAPPAPORT 1989). Clinically, the onset of puberty is characterized by breast development in girls and testicular enlargement in boys. An acceleration in the growth rate and an advance in bone age should be looked for. The diagnosis is confirmed by sex steroid assays (estradiol in girls and testosterone in boys) and follicle-stimulating hormone (FSH) and luteinizing hormone (LH) concentrations after luteinizing hormone-releasing hormone (LHRH) stimulation.

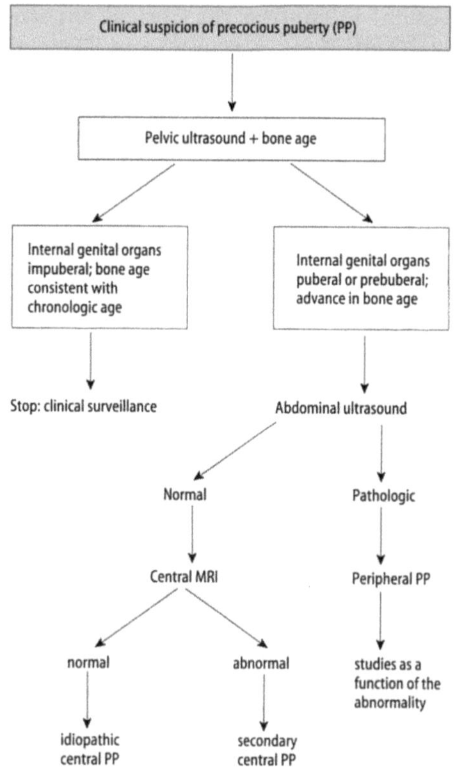

Fig. 5.5. Precocious puberty in girls: algorithm for imaging studies

5.2.1.1
Imaging

Once the clinical diagnosis of pubertal advance has been confirmed by laboratory tests, imaging studies are performed to visualize the internal genital organs, determine their size, and search for a lesion that could explain the symptoms (HEDLUND et al. 1994; Fig.5.5).

Abdominal-pelvic ultrasound is the initial imaging modality in girls (BRAUNER et al. 1986). In true precocious puberty of central origin, abdominal sonograms are normal. Ultrasound confirms pubertal development of the internal genital organs and permits measurement of the uterus and the ovaries (the latter contain follicles but not cysts). The uterus and the ovaries are significantly enlarged in girls with precocious puberty (HABER and MAYER 1994). Enlargement of the uterus precedes that of the ovaries (Table5.1).

Determination of skeletal (bone) age is indispensable. This requires radiography of the left hand and wrist (anteroposterior views) and the left elbow (anteroposterior and lateral views). In children with precocious puberty, skeletal age is greater than chronologic age.

Magnetic resonance imaging (MRI) of the brain is performed systematically because it is the best means to demonstrate an intracranial organic cause (KORNREICH 1995).

The normal appearance of the pituitary gland during puberty, or physiological hypertrophy, must not be confused with a tumor. The height of the pituitary gland typically increases at puberty; the upper aspect of the pituitary gland appears convex at the start and during puberty due to hormone activation (ARGYROPOLOU et al. 1991; KAO et al. 1992; SHARAFUDDIN et al. 1994).

In boys, abdominal-pelvic ultrasound is performed to search for a tumoral origin especially hepatic and adrenal tumors. Scrotal sonography may

Table 5.1. Volume of the uterus and ovaries as a function of the pubertal stage (after Haber 1994)

Tanner stage	Uterine volume (ml)	Ovarian volume (ml)
P0	0.9±0.3	0.6±0.2
P1, S1–S2	3.8±2.0	2.2±1.3
P2–P3, S3–S4	8.0±4.4	2.6±3.1

prove useful to confirm the normal appearance of the testes and allow measurements. Skeletal age is determined, as in girls. MRI is indispensable, especially because tumors are more common in boys than in girls. True precocious puberty may occur secondary to a central nervous system (CNS) tumor, a nontumoral neurogenic cause, or a non-neurogenic cause. True precocious puberty is refered to as idiopathic if no CNS abnormality is identified.

5.2.1.2 Central Nervous System Tumors

Brain tumors are the most frequent neurogenic cause of true precocious puberty, particularly in boys.

Hypothalamic hamartomas are masses of normal-appearing nerve tissue at the base of the hypothalamus. These expansive lesions of the floor of the third ventricle protrude into the interpeduncular space. They are often detected only by MRI because they cause no clinical manifestations other than precocious puberty. These homogeneous lesions are isointense to the cerebral parenchyma, but are readily depicted on sagittal MR views (Fig. 5.6). CT is less useful as it can only provide axial views (Barral et al. 1988). Neuroradiologic evaluation of children with precocious puberty should thus be performed by MRI rather than CT. Hypothalamic hamartomas are usually small and are diagnosed solely by imaging studies. Biopsy is contraindicated owing to the localization. Hypothalamic hamartomas appear stable on subsequent examinations (Turjman et al. 1996) and do not require surgical resection. MRI has increased the frequency of detection of hamartomas in children who would often previously have been misdiagnosed as having idiopathic precocious puberty, especially young childen and those with rapidly evolving manifestations of puberty (Colaco et al. 1993; Kornreich et al. 1995).

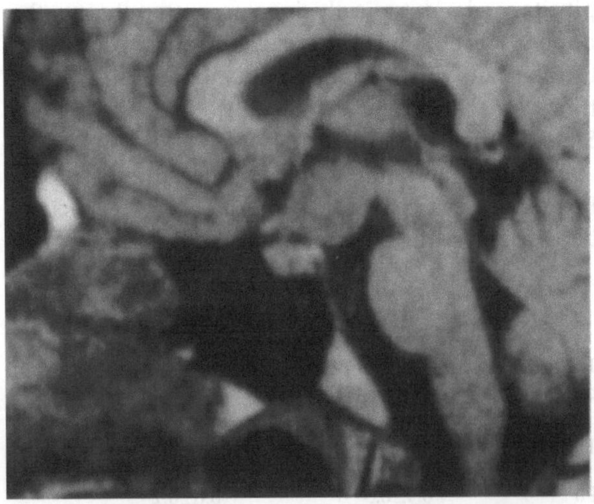

Fig. 5.6. Midline sagittal T_1-weighted MRI: hypothalamic hamartoma. (Courtesy of Prof. F. Brunelle, Hôpital des Enfants Malades, Paris)

Optic tract gliomas are frequent in children with neurofibromatosis. Coexistence of visual or neurologic disorders and precocious puberty may suggest the diagnosis. Precocious puberty may be the initial manifestation of glioma or may occur after treatment of the tumor. MRI demonstrates widening of the optic chiasm and optic nerves (cranial nerve II), which enhance with a contrast agent. MRI can also be used to assess tumor size and its impact on the ventricular system.

Pineal tumors (teratomas, gliomas, or pinealomas) responsible for precocious puberty are most common in boys. The cardinal clinical symptom of these rare entities (Chang et al. 1996) is Parinaud's ophthalmoplegia (conjugate paralysis of upward gaze). Diagnosis is made histologically. Exeresis is often incomplete.

Suprasellar arachnoid cysts, another potential cause of precocious puberty, usually have already been diagnosed at the onset of precocious puberty (Fig. 5.7).

5.2.1.3 Nontumoral Neurogenic Causes

Regardless of the etiology, shunted or stabilized hydrocephalus can cause pubertal advance. This is especially true for myelomeningoceles (Trollman et al. 1996). Increased gonadotropin secretion, probably secondary to abnormal variations in intracranial pressure, is the putative mechanism (Klauschie and Rose 1996; Lopponen et al. 1996). Precocious puberty has also been reported in children with craniostenosis or microcephaly.

Precocious puberty may also have an infectious origin, e.g., as a sequela of meningitis (Desai et al. 1993) or encephalitis. Skull trauma, irradiation (Olgivy-Stuart et al. 1994), meningeal hemorrhage, and encephalopathy are other possible causes.

a

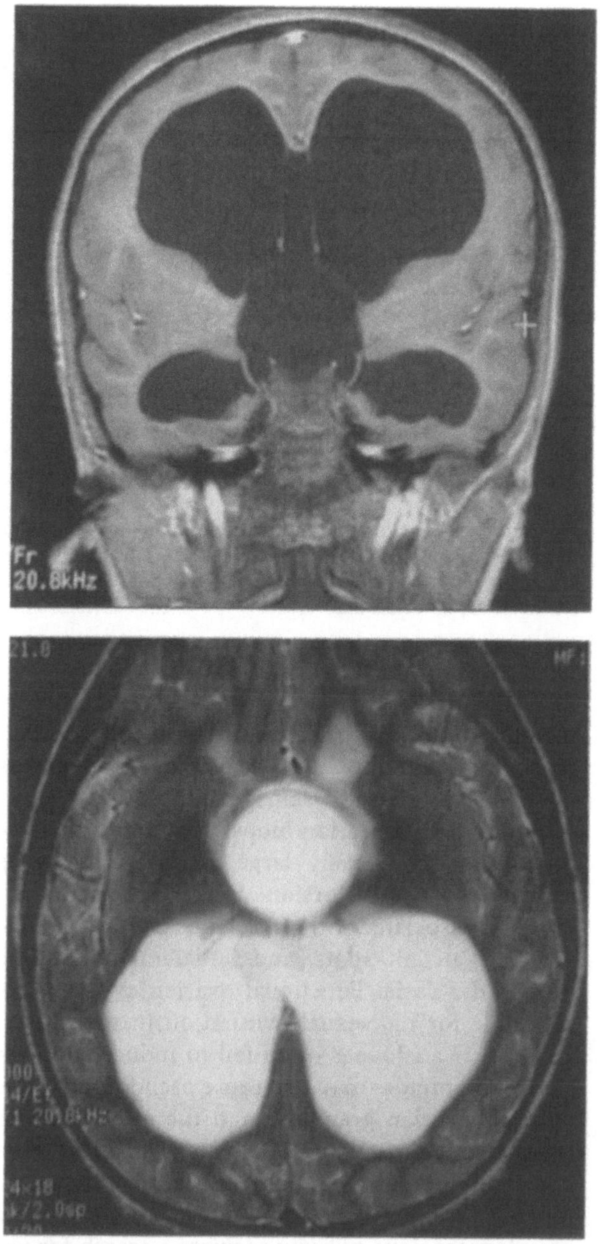

b

Fig. 5.7a,b. Ten-year-old boy presenting with headaches and signs of puberty. MRI revealed a suprasellar arachnoid cyst responsible for hydrocephalus. a Coronal T_1-weighted MRI. b Axial T_2-weighted MRI

5.2.1.4
Non-neurogenic Causes

Non-neurogenic causes of precocious puberty have usually already been recognized before the onset of manifestations.

A number of systemic pathologies are associated with precocious puberty:

- Phakomatosis: Recklinghausen's disease (neurofibromatosis), even in the absence of a chiasmic tumor, tuberous sclerosis (Bourneville's phakomatosis). Cutaneous patches should thus be sought during physical examination.
- Silver-Russell syndrome: intrauterine growth retardation, limb asymmetry, and triangular facies.
- McCune-Albright syndrome (Albright's disease): this entity is discussed in Sect. 5.2.2.2 as it causes pseudoprecocious puberty.

Endocrinologic disorders can cause secondary precocious puberty, because a peripheral endocrine deficiency (hypothyroidism, congenital adrenal hyperplasia) may result in excessive pituitary gonadotropin secretion.

A thorough medical history is necessary to rule out an exogenous source of hormones (lotion or ointment containing estrogen, anabolic steroids).

Treatment of true precocious puberty is rarely that of the underlying cause and always consists in suppressive therapy using LHRH analogues. Ultrasound is effective for surveillance and measurement of the volume of the uterus and ovaries, which decrease in size in response to therapy (Ambrosino et al. 1994; Bridges et al. 1995). Sonographically visible ovarian cysts at the start of treatment may regress after therapy.

5.2.2
Pseudoprecocious Puberty

Pseudoprecocious puberty (peripheral precocious puberty) is usually isosexual; heterosexual cases are exceptional. Abnormal sex hormone secretion by an adrenal or gonadal tumor results in precocious puberty (Figs. 5.8, 5.9). FSH and LH levels are low, and response to stimulation is minimal. Plasma steroid levels are very high.

Abdominal-pelvic sonography is the initial imaging modality of choice for detection of lesions, especially adrenal tumors and ovarian cysts or solid tumors. In boys, scrotal ultrasound can evaluate testicular volume and demonstrate the presence of a tumor. Skeletal age is evaluated just as for patients with true precocious puberty.

Causes of isosexual precocity in boys include congenital adrenal hyperplasia with marked elevation of plasma 17-OH progesterone (usually already diagnosed), adrenal tumors (adenoma, adrenal cortex tumors), testicular tumors (Leydig cell adenomas), nongonadal germ cell tumors secreting human

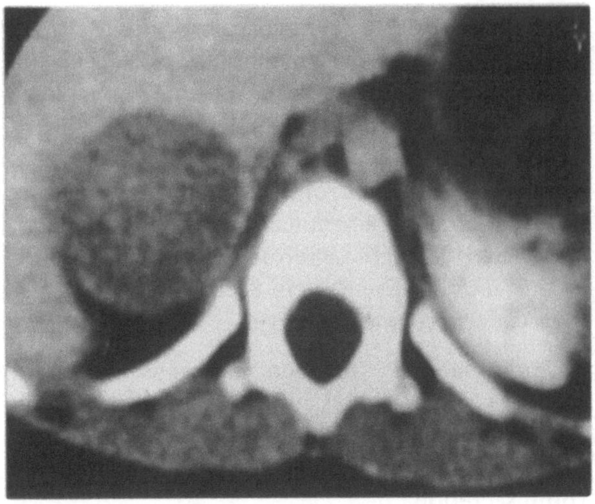

Fig. 5.8. Four-year-old girl with signs of virilization. Contrast-enhanced CT revealed a well-delimited hypodense right adrenal mass: adenoma

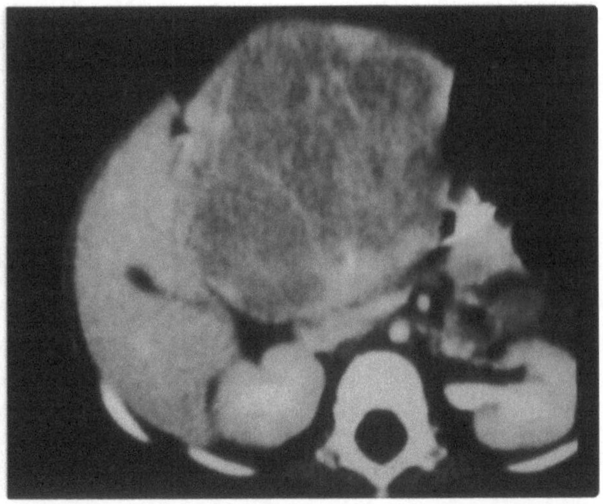

Fig. 5.10. Two-year-old boy with an abdominal mass and signs of precocious puberty. Contrast-enhanced CT of the liver revealed an inhomogeneously enhancing hypodense mass in the left liver: hepatoblastoma

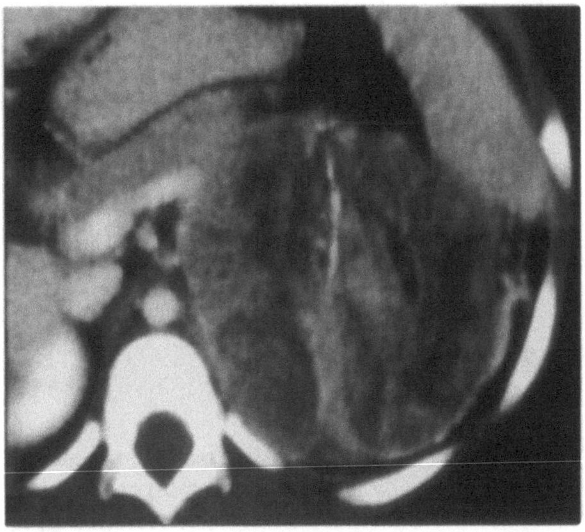

Fig. 5.9. Six-year-old girl with precocious puberty and virilization. Contrast-enhanced CT demonstrated a left adrenal mass invading the upper pole of the kidney: adrenal carcinoma

chorionic gonadotropin (HCG) (mediastinal teratoma, hepatoblastoma), and testitoxicosis (Fig. 5.10). Heterosexual pseudoprecocious puberty is exceptional. Unilateral or bilateral breast development (gynecomastia) is common, occurring during normal puberty in 30% of boys, and must not be mistaken for heterosexual precocity.

In girls, isosexual pseudoprecocious puberty may be related to exogenous estrogens, but follicular ovarian cysts over 2 cm in size (Fig. 5.11) are the most prevalent cause (Wemeau-Jacquemont 1988). Sex steroids are secreted by these cysts, which often evolve in episodes. The severity of clinical manifestations may be correlated with cyst size. Pelvic sonography should thus be performed as soon as the first signs appear. Drainage of the cysts by ultrasound-guided aspiration biopsy may arrest the episode. The occasionally large size of these cysts explains the risk of torsion. McCune-Albright syndrome is associated with precocious puberty, unilateral café au lait spots, and unilateral polyostotic fibrous dysplasia. Functional ovarian cysts are responsible for the sexual maturation in such cases, and LHRH analogues often fail to induce suppression. Solid tumors may also cause pseudoprecocious puberty: ovarian granulosa and thecal cell tumors (Bouffet et al. 1997) predominate (Fig. 5.12), while choriocarcinomas, teratomas, and adrenal cortex tumors are less common. Heterosexual pseudoprecocious puberty requires a search for use of exogenous androgens. It may also be secondary to congenital adrenal hyperplasia or, occasionally, an adrenal tumor (adenoma, carcinoma) or an androgen-secreting ovarian tumor (teratoma, arrhenoblastoma). These lesions can be detected by abdominal-pelvic sonography.

5.2.3 Partial Puberty (Isolated Breast Development)

Diagnosis is made by physical examination, but ultrasound is helpful to demonstrate the absence of development of the internal genital organs.

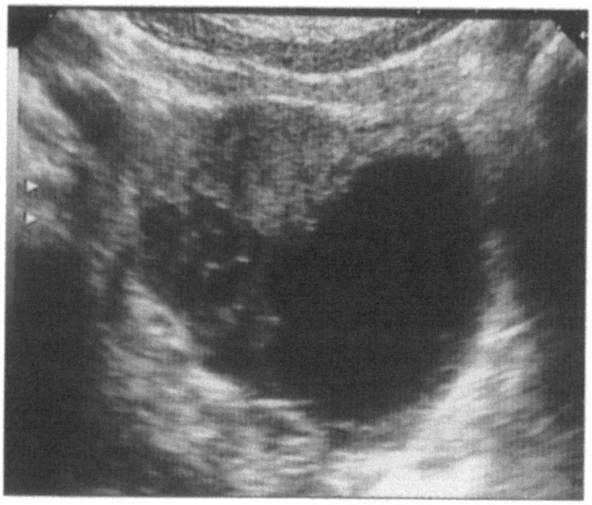

Fig. 5.11. Seven-year-old girl with precocious puberty and metrorrhagia. Transverse pelvic sonogram showing a left ovarian cyst

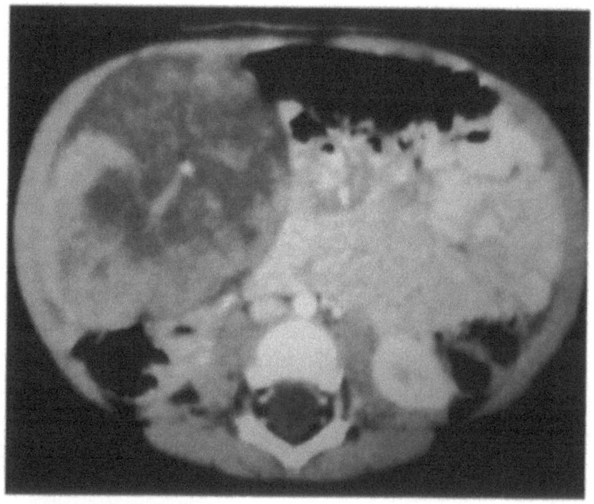

a

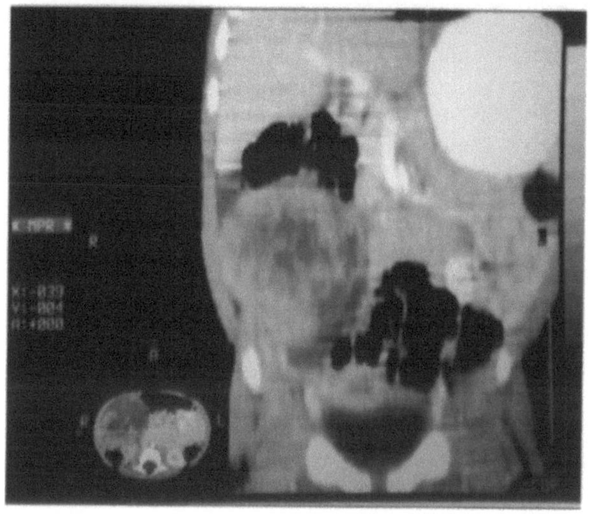

b

Fig. 5.12a,b. Ten-month-old girl with precocious puberty. a Contrast-enhanced CT scan. b Coronal reconstruction. Large heterogeneous mass in the right ovary: granulosa tumor. (Courtesy of Dr. Leroux, Hôpital de l'Archet, Nice)

5.2.4 Summary

In summary, imaging studies have four major purposes in the evaluation of precocious puberty: (1) to confirm the clinical diagnosis by measuring the genital organs, (2) to evaluate bone age, (3) to rule out an organic cause (cerebral or other), and (4) to monitor the efficacy of suppressive therapy (ultrasound, bone age).

5.3 Delayed Puberty

The term "delayed puberty" refers to the lack of appearance of secondary sexual characters at 13years of age in girls and by the age of 15 in boys. Most cases are actually mere delays in sexual maturation. Nine out of ten patients are boys with a history of late growth in their family (constitutional delay). Skeletal age lags behind chronologic age, but the course is spontaneously favorable. Treatment of secondary delayed puberty consists in hormone replacement. Imaging plays a minor role in delayed puberty and is essentially used to confirm the delay in sexual maturation by evaluating bone age.

Secondary pubertal delays are relatively rare. There are three major causes: a chronic illness or condition, hypogonadotropic hypogonadism, and primary gonadal failure.

5.3.1 Chronic Illness or Condition

Delayed puberty may be due to a chronic illness or condition that has generally already been diagnosed (asthma, chronic arthritis, enteropathy, chronic anemia, neurologic affections, glycogen storage disease). In girls, pelvic ultrasound is useful to monitor the progression of puberty; visualization of uterine development reflects the onset of puberty.

a

b

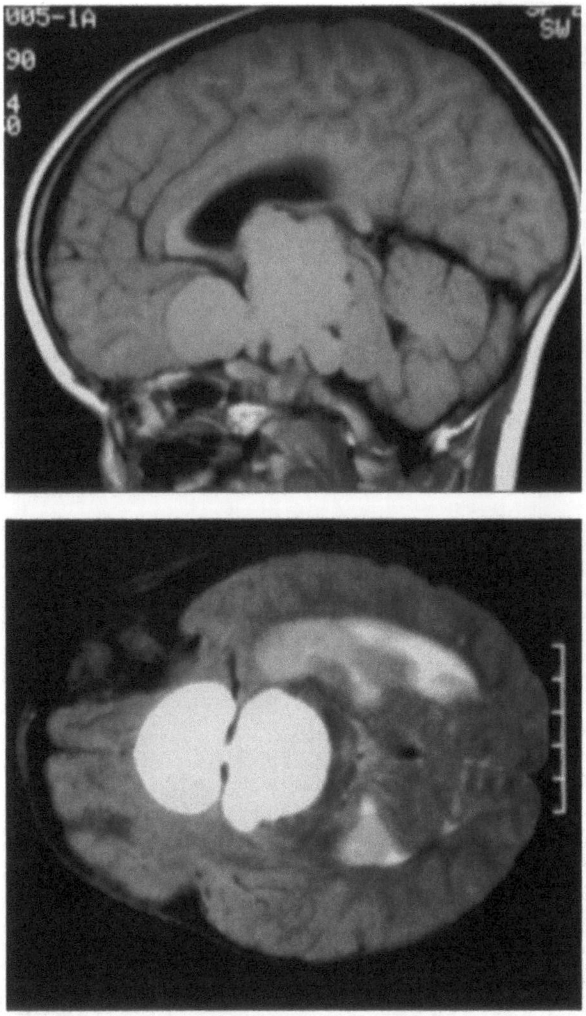

Fig. 5.13a,b. Cystic mass in the hypothalamic region of a 5-year-old girl with below-normal weight gain: craniopharyngioma. a Sagittal T_1-weighted MRI. b Axial T_2-weighted MRI

5.3.2 Hypogonadotropic Hypogonadism

Hypogonadotropic hypogonadism, characterized by a lack of gonadotropic secretion, is caused by absent or weak pituitary stimulation. On pelvic ultrasound, the ovaries appear small, with a homogeneous echotexture. The uterus appears impuberal. Possible causes include the following:

1. Anterior pituitary aplasia, brain tumor (craniopharyngioma), sequelae of irradiation, malformation, idiopathic origin (Fig.5.13)
2. A congenital malformation syndrome:
   - Kallmann syndrome (olfactogenital syndrome): gonadotropic insufficiency and hyposmia or anosmia, sometimes related to development of the rhinencephalon
   - Prader-Willi syndrome: intrauterine and postnatal hypotonia, obesity, short stature, mental deficiency, hypogonadism
   - Laurence-Moon-Biedl syndrome: polydactylia, mental retardation, obesity, pigmentary retinopathy, hypogonadism with cryptochidism in boys

The diagnosis is confirmed by failure of gonadotropin levels to rise in response to LHRH stimulation tests.

5.3.3 Primary Gonadal Failure

Primary gonadal failure is characterized by elevated gonadotropin concentrations and low steroid levels (hypergonadotropic hypogonadism).

Etiologies in boys include the following:

- Gonadal dysgenesis: Noonan syndrome, Klinefelter syndrome (primary testicular dysfunction)
- Abnormal testosterone biosynthesis
- Testicular atrophy due to trauma, exposure to the mumps virus, irradiation, and very occasionally chemotherapy

In girls, primary gonadal failure may be caused by gonadal dysgenesis with chromosomal abnormalities; the most frequent form is Turner syndrome. The ovaries cannot be detected by ultrasound or are mere fibrous gonadal streaks. The uterus is tiny, flattened, and totally impuberal.

References

Ambrosino MM, Heernanz-Schulman M, Genieser NB, Sklar CA, Fefferman NR, David R (1994) Monitoring of girls undergoing medical therapy for isosexual precocious puberty. J Ultrasound Med 13:501–508

André C, Le Bihan B (1982) Echographie pédiatrique. Vigot, Paris, pp 241–267

Argyropoulou M, Perignon F, Brunelle F, Brauner R, Rappaport R (1991) Height of normal pituitary gland as a function of age evaluated by magnetic resonance imaging in children. Pediatr Radiol 21:247–249

Barral V, Brunelle F, Brauner R, Rappaport R, Lallemand D (1988) MRI of hypothalamic hamartomas in children. Pediatr Radiol 18:449–452

Bouffet E, Basset T, Chetail N et al. (1997) Juvenile granulosa tumor of the ovary in infants: a clinicopathologic study of three cases and review of the literature. J Pediatr Surg 32:762–765

Brauner R, Rappaport R (1989) Pubertés précoces centrales. Ann Pediatr (Paris) 36:653–658

Brauner R, Hauschild MC, Pariente D, Thibaud E, Rappaport R (1986) Place de l'échographie dans le diagnostic, les indications thérapeutiques et la surveillance des pubertés précoces centrales. Arch Fr Pediatr 43:601–606

Brauner R, Rappaport R, Nicod C et al. (1987) Pubertés précoces vraies au cours de l'hydrocéphalie non tumorale. Arch Fr Pediatr 44:433–436

Bridges NA, Cooke A, Healy MJ, Hindmarsh PC, Brook CG (1995) Ovaries in sexual precocity. Clin Endocrinol (Oxf) 42:135–140

Chang YL, Lin SZ, Chiang YH, Liu MY, Lee WH (1996) Pineal ganglioglioma with premature thelarche. Report of a case and review of the literature. Childs Nerv Syst 12:103–106

Cohen HL, Eisenberg P, Mandel FS, Maller JO (1992) Ovarian cysts are common in premenarchal girls: a sonographic study of 101 children 2–12 years old. AJR 159:89–91

Colaco MP, Desai MP, Choksi CS, Shah KN, Mehta RU (1993) Hypothalamic hamartomas and precocious puberty. Ind J Pediatr 60:445–450

Colle M, Broussin B, Auzerie J (1993) Doppler des artères ovariennes: une aide à la détermination de l'entrée en puberté chez la fille? Ref Gynecol Obstet 1:259–264

Desai MP, Colaco MP, Choksi CS, Ambadkar MC, Vaz FE, Gupte C (1993) Isosexual precocity: the clinical and etiologic profile. Ind Pediatr 30:607–623

Haber HP, Mayer EL (1994) Ultrasound evaluation of uterine and ovarian size from birth to puberty. Pediatr Radiol 24:11–13

Hedlund GL, Royal SA, Parker KL (1994) Disorders of puberty: a practical imaging approach. Semin Ultrasound CT MR 15:49–77

Kao SCS, Cook JS, Hansen JR, Simonson TM (1992) MR imaging of the pituitary gland in central precocious puberty. Pediatr Radiol 22:481–484

Klauschie J, Rose SR (1996) Incidence of short stature in children with hydrocephalus. J Pediatr Endrocinol Metab 9:181–187

Kornreich L, Horev G, Blaser S, Denman D, Kauli R, Grunebaum M (1995) Central precocious puberty: evaluation by neuroimaging. Pediatr Radiol 25:7–11

Lopponen T, Saukkonen AL, Serlo W, Tapanainen P, Ruokonen A, Knip M (1996) Accelerated pubertal development in patients with shunted hydrocephalus. Arch Dis Child 74:490–496

Ogilvy-Stuart AL, Clayton PE, Shalet SM (1994) Cranial irradiation and early puberty. J Clin Endocrinol Metab 78:1282–1286

Perelman R (1990) Comment s'orienter devant une précocité isosexuelle? Med Infant 2:158–161

Sharafuddin MJA, Luisiri A, Garibaldi (1994) MR imaging diagnosis of central precocious puberty: importance of changes in the shape and size of the pituitary gland. AJR 162:1167–1173

Trollmann R, Dorr HG, Strehl E, Katalinic A, Beyer R, Wenzel D (1996) Growth and pubertal development in patients with meningomyelocele: a retrospective analysis. Acta Paediatr 85:76–80

Turjman F, Xavier JL, Froment JC, Tran-Minh VA, David L, Lapras C (1996) Late MR follow-up of hypothalamic hamartomas. Childs Nerv Syst 12:63–68

Wemeau-Jacquemont C (1988) Pubertés précoces et kystes ovariens folliculaires. Pédiatrie 43:355–360

6 Female Infertility

A. MAUBON and J.P. ROUANET

CONTENTS

6.1 Introduction

Imaging studies for female infertility include a variety of procedures. Indications for the different modalities vary with the clinical presentation of the individual case, but the following questions must always be addressed:

- Is there an abnormality of the female reproductive tract (uterine cavity or fallopian tubes)? This information is generally provided by hysterosalpingography (HSG) and its complement, selective tubal catheterization and recanalization.
- Is there an abnormality near the uterine cavity or the tubes? If so, additional investigations are warranted. Ultrasound and/or magnetic resonance imaging (MRI), when available, usually provide the answer.

A. MAUBON, J.P. ROUANET, Imagerie Médicale, CMC Beau Soleil, 119 avenue de Lodève, 34000 Montpellier, France

6.2 Assessment of the Female Reproductive Tract

6.2.1 Hysterosalpingography

6.2.1.1 Preparation

Examination should preferably be performed during the first part of the cycle (follicular phase), after the menses, but in any case before ovulation. If the tubes are occluded and are to be unblocked by the procedure, it is important that the patient should be able to benefit from the next ovulation and start a pregnancy as soon as possible. In addition, because HSG involves ionizing radiation, it should be avoided later in the cycle owing to the possibility of an early pregnancy of which the patient and the physician are not aware. Depending on the duration of the menses, days 7–11 are optimal.

HSG should be postponed in the case of persistent uterine bleeding owing to the potential risk of endometrial migration and the increased difficulty in interpretation of radiographs; blood clots can easily be mistaken for genuine cavitary lesions.

Wide-spectrum antibiotic prophylaxis is strongly advised 2 days before the procedure and 3 days afterwards. No other premedication is usually required.

6.2.1.2 Contraindications

HSG is contraindicated in the case of acute pelvic infection (chronic pelvic inflammatory disease is a relative contraindication), intolerance to iodinated contrast media, severe coagulation disorders, etc.

6.2.1.3
Technique

The patient is placed in the gynecologic position, with stirrup leg rest, on the fluoroscopy table. The anovulvar region is swabbed with an antiseptic. A sterile drape is placed under the patient and whenever possible on the patient's abdomen and lower extremities. The cervix is exposed with a vaginal speculum. Care must be taken to obtain a "bull's eye" view, with the cervix in the center of the field, in order to facilitate subsequent steps. The cervical canal is then probed with a hysterometer to determine the size of the cavity and to slightly dilate the endocervical canal. Depending on the physician's preference and availability, a vacuum cup, a tenaculum at 12 o'clock position, or a specially designed balloon catheter is applied on the cervix.

Contrast agent is then slowly injected manually into the uterine cavity under fluoroscopic control, as gently as possible. Injection is stopped when the uterine cavity is filled; tubal opacification is obtained with peritoneal spillage of contrast. Most commercially available, water-soluble iodinated contrast agents are adequate. Preference should be given to nonionic, iso-osmolar compounds. Oil-soluble media should no longer be used. Radiographs should include early-filling and late-filling coronal views, left and right oblique views, a lateral view, two views during voiding after removal of the hysterograph, and, if needed, a late view a few minutes after the procedure to assess peritoneal contrast spillage.

Optimal imaging may require traction on the cervical canal to straighten the uterus, especially in patients with a retroverted uterus.

6.2.1.4
Results

The normal uterine cavity is triangular in shape. In addition to interindividual variations, shape depends on parity. Borders should be smooth, without filling defects or lateral outpouchings (Fig. 6.1).

The normal fallopian tube has four segments:

- The interstitial portion within the uterine wall (2 cm long from the tubal ostium).
- The isthmic portion (8 cm long from the outer uterine wall to the ampulla); this sinuous portion is mobile.
- The ampulla, which embraces the ovary (5 cm long). This is the widest part of the tube and presents wide longitudinal folds.

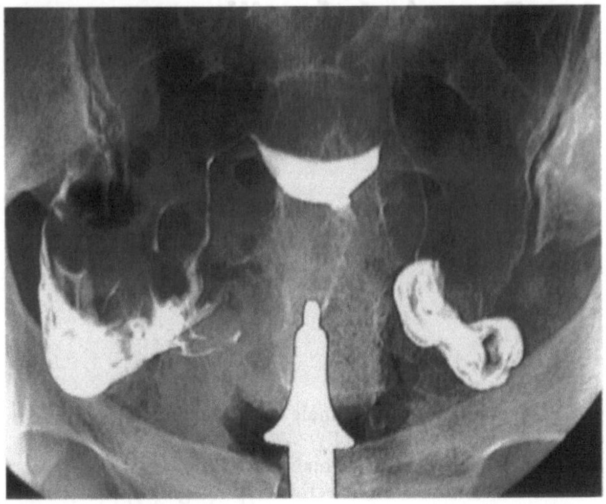

Fig. 6.1. Hysterosalpingography (HSG): the walls of the normal uterine cavity are smooth, with bilateral tubal and peritoneal passage of contrast

- The infundibulum, which is hardly visible. Peritoneal spill of contrast begins in the ovarian peritoneal fossa.

A number of situations are encountered after HSG for assessment of infertility:

- The uterine cavity is normal, the tubes are patent with normal ampullary folds, contrast medium flows freely into the peritoneum, and no tubal or uterine cause of infertility is demonstrated.
- The tubes are patent, but the cavity is abnormal.
- The tubes are patent, but peritoneal spillage is poor or absent, indicating the presence of peritubal and/or periovarian adhesions.
- The tubes are not opacified or only partially opacified. Selective salpingography should be performed in these cases (see Fig. 6.2).

6.2.2
Uterine Cavity Abnormalities

6.2.2.1
Synechiae

Fibrotic scar tissue bridging the anterior and posterior aspects of the uterine mucosa is generally due to endometrial injury during curettage or instrumentation or the sequelae of infections (genital tuberculosis). HSG demonstrates a sharply marginated geographic filling defect that remains unchanged during the course of the procedure (Fig. 6.2). Synechiae may be central or lateral; they may be partial or may oblit-

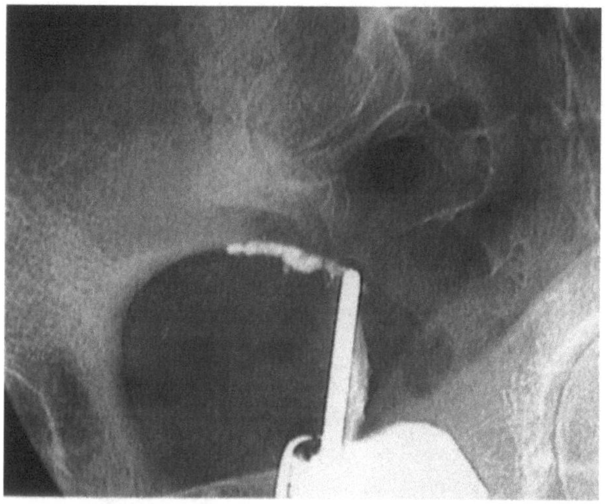

Fig. 6.2. Hysterosalpingography (HSG) oblique view: the uterus was almost completely obliterated by adhesions after endometrial curettage

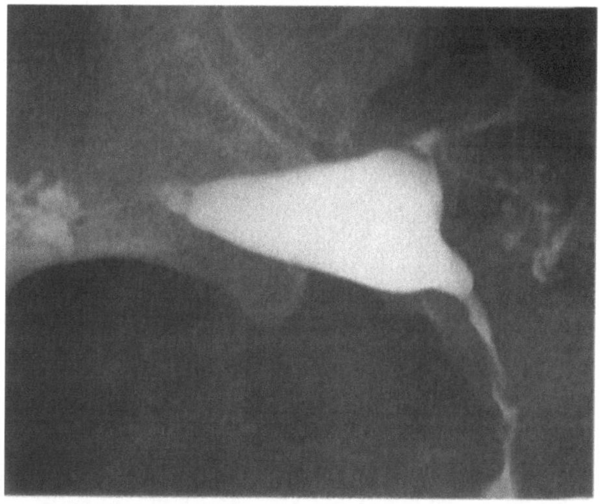

Fig. 6.3. Hysterosalpingography (HSG) oblique view: bilateral tubal endometriosis

erate the entire cavity. In the latter case, only the cervix or isthmus are opacified. Traumatic synechiae sometimes retain the shape of the instrument responsible for the injury (Thurmond 1997).

6.2.2.2 Adenomyosis

Adenomyosis corresponds to invaginations of functional endometrium in the myometrium. HSG typically demonstrates small diverticulae. These lesions appear early during opacification as round images connected with the cavity by a thin channel. Located beyond the ideal mucosal line (Fig. 6.3), they may be scattered throughout the entire uterine cavity or limited to a small portion. Other signs include a rigid uterus that remains fixed despite traction on the tenaculum or the "upright" position of the interstitial portion of the tubes (Thurmond 1997).

6.2.2.3 Uterine Fibroids

Fibroids can be considered responsible for infertility only after several miscarriages and only if they significantly modify the anatomy of the uterine cavity. Submucosal fibroids image as round filling defects with regular borders surrounded by contrast medium. They are best detected on early filling views and on late views after voiding. They tend to be less conspicuous when the uterine cavity is completely filled (Dudiak et al. 1988).

6.2.2.4 Uterine Anomalies

Two types of malformations must be distinguished: müllerian duct anomalies of embryologic origin and malformations caused by exposure to diethylstilbestrol (DES) in utero.

Müllerian Duct Anomalies. Developmental disorders of müllerian ducts are the result of embryologic insult during weeks 8–17 of intrauterine life. These common anomalies cause primary infertility or repeated miscarriages. Malformations commonly detected by HSG include:

- Unicornuate uterus with a characteristic banana-shaped cavity deviated to one side. The fallopian tube arises from the distal end of the hemicavity without angulation (Fig. 6.4). This should be distinguished from partial synechiae with tubal obstruction.
- Bicornuate uterus with two cavities separated by more than 110° and an intercornual distance of over 4 cm. There may be one or two cervices (Fig. 6.5).
- Septate uterus. There is always a single cervix. Angulation between the horns is usually less than 90°. Depending on the length of the septum within the cavity, septate uteri are classified as complete, partial, or arcuate (Fig. 6.6).

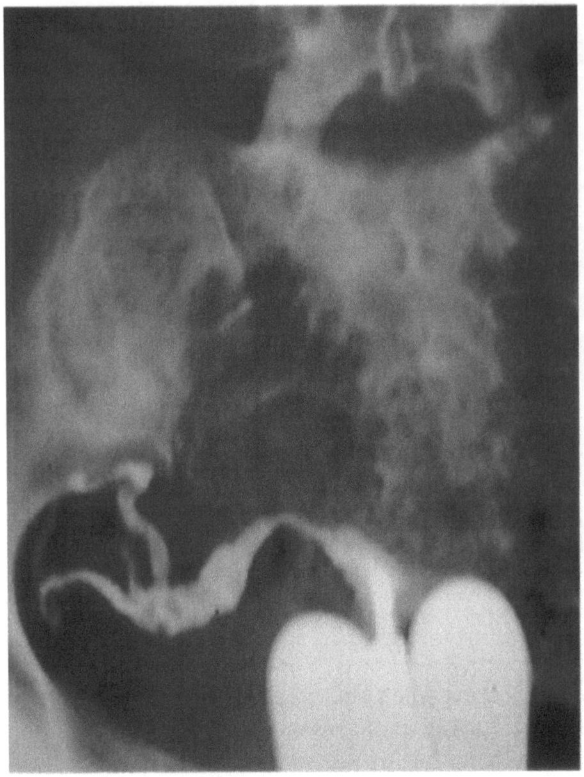

Fig. 6.4. Hysterosalpingography (HSG): right unicornuate uterus. This patient also has a single kidney, on the right

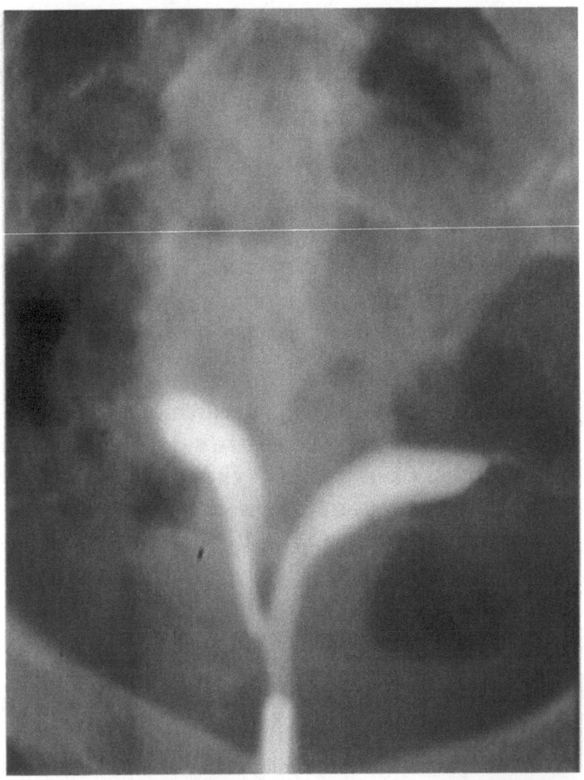

Fig. 6.5. Hysterosalpingography (HSG): unicervical bicornuate uterus

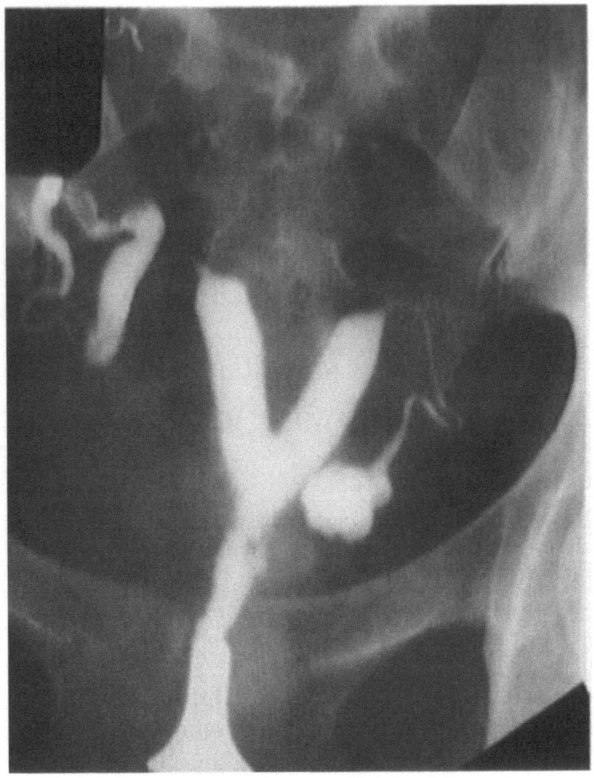

Fig. 6.6. Hysterosalpingography (HSG): septate uterus

Uterine Anomalies Due to DES Exposure In Utero. DES is a synthetic estrogen that was given to prevent miscarriage. The daughters of women treated with this drug may present a variety of uterine malformations that are readily detected by HSG: hypoplasia, T-shaped uterus, "gun barrel" cornua, or cornual strictures (Fig. 6.7; MAUBON et al. 1996).

6.2.3 Tubal Anomalies: Selective Salpingography and Tubal Recanalization

If tubal opacification is not obtained during HSG performed for infertility workup, the injection pressure should be gently increased in an attempt to fill the tubes. If the tubes remain invisible, selective tubal catheterization and recanalization can be performed. First described in 1977 by ROUANET and CHALUT, this technique has both diagnostic and therapeutic goals:

- Visualization of the fallopian tubes and the site of any tubal obstruction
- Determination of the cause of the tubal obstruction

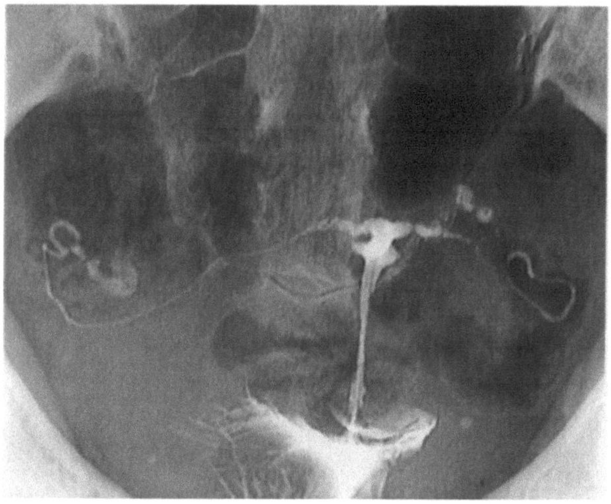

Fig. 6.7. Hysterosalpingography (HSG): typical diethylstilbestrol (DES) uterine malformation associating a hypogenetic uterus and strictures on the uterine horns (a small catheter was required for HSG)

- Elimination of the tubal obstruction to obtain peritoneal passage of contrast, indicative of tubal patency
- Evaluation of the distal fallopian tube and peritoneal spill

6.2.3.1 Indications

All cases of tubal infertility can benefit from selective recanalization (THURMOND 1991). Three conditions must be met to avoid unnecessary examinations and to optimize results:

- Infertility (primary or secondary) after at least 1 year of unprotected intercourse
- A gynecologic examination for evaluation of infertility
- A good-quality, standard hysterogram that shows tubal occlusion or absence of tubal passage of contrast

A new indication has recently appeared: persistent infertility after reversal of a temporary or permanent sterilization procedure (THURMOND et al. 1995a,b). The decision to perform selective recanalization should ideally be made together by the radiology and gynecology teams.

6.2.3.2 Technique

Ideally, selective recanalization should be performed during the same session as sonohysterography, immediately after attempts to demonstrate the tubes fail. Commercially available kits (HOVSEPIAN et al. 1996) allow selective catheterization using the same material as for HSG.

A precurved 5F catheter is passed through the hysterograph, directly laterally towards the uterine orifice. If the position is incorrect, a torque movement is required. It is often easier to advance a smooth J-tipped guidewire into the cornu first.

The catheter is then gently pushed through the tubal ostium (the patient feels a slight abutting sensation), and selective manual injection is performed under fluoroscopic guidance.

In the case of bilateral obstruction, the other tube should be catheterized during the same procedure. The catheter is withdrawn into the uterine cavity and then torqued to direct it into the contralateral cornu.

Three situations may be encountered:

- Opacification of a radiologically normal fallopian tube with peritoneal spill of contrast (Fig. 6.8)
- Tubal obstruction without opacification of the ampulla
- Opacification of a pathologic tube, with or without peritoneal spill

Tubal recanalization should be attempted in the last two situations (Fig. 6.9). As the diameter of the 5F catheter is larger than the tubal lumen, it should not be advanced into the fallopian tube. A precurved or straight, flexible-tipped polyethylene-covered 0.032-inch guidewire or a 0.016-inch steerable guidewire on a 3F catheter is more appropriate. Using a back-and-forth movement, the catheter is gently advanced up to the point of stenosis. Exertion of slight pressure usually allows passage beyond the stricture. Manual injection of contrast material through the 3F catheter allows better control of guidewire progression, may identify any tubal tears, and is mandatory to assess peritoneal spill.

The entire procedure usually takes 10–30 min, depending primarily on the position of the uterus and the extent of tubal lesions. Tubal recanalization can be performed on an outpatient basis. It is usually painless, but discomfort can occur if the uterus has to be tracted to pass through the endocervix or if tubal catheterization is difficult.

a

b

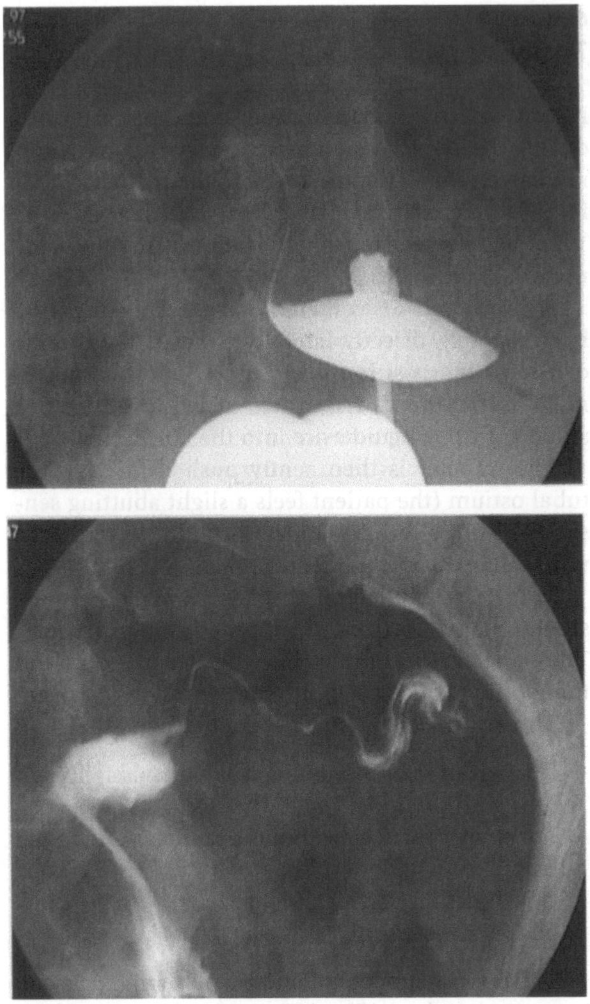

Fig 6.8. **a** Hysterosalpingography (HSG): only the right tube is opacified. **b** Selective salpingography on the left side opacifies a normal tube with normal ampullary folds and peritoneal spillage of contrast

a

b

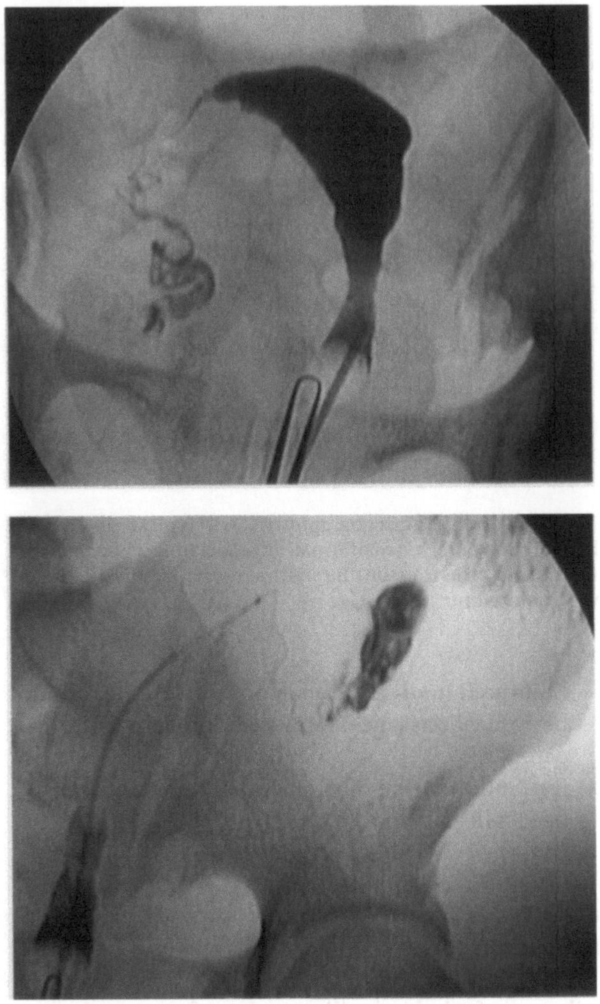

Fig. 6.9. a Hysterosalpingography (HSG): the right fallopian tube is normal, the left tube is not visible. **b** Selective tubal catheterization of the left tube with a microcatheter allows visualization of the entire fallopian tube, with peritoneal spillage of contrast

6.2.3.3 Results

Selective tubal catheterization is usually possible in 90% of cases (bilaterally in 80%, on only one side in 10%). A retrofixed uterus, uterine synechiae, bilateral polyps at the uterotubal junction, or huge fibroids may prevent successful catheterization.

Tubal Opacification Under Pressure. After catheterization, manual injection opacifies the fallopian tube with peritoneal spill in 75% of cases; no peritoneal spill is seen in 25%. In one of our own series, two thirds of patent tubes were considered normal, while one third presented peritubal adhesions or tubal endometriosis (Maubon et al. 1996).

Recanalization. For the 25% of cases in which no peritoneal spill is visualized, recanalization successfully reestablishes tubal patency in approximately half the patients. The main causes of unsuccessful recanalization are hydrosalpinx, peritubal adhesions, and impermeable tubal occlusions of unknown origin.

Pregnancies. Depending on patient recruitment and the series, the pregnancy rate varies from 10% to 55%. On average, approximately 25% of patients achieve pregnancy. The best results are obtained in the 6 months following recanalization. The risk of extrauterine pregnancy appears correlated with tubal status; the risk is lower in cases of interstitial occlusion of a normal tube than in cases of damaged tubes, even if these are patent. The risk of first-term miscarriage also seems to be slightly higher than in "normal" pregnancies, but tends to be lower than after tubal microsurgery.

Complications. No cases of mortality have been reported to date. Small asymptomatic tubal tears are not uncommon during guidewire recanalization. They can be prevented by careful manipulation of the guidewire. Tubal perforation is essentially a theoretical risk. Pelvic or peritoneal infection can be avoided by appropriate prophylaxis. Mild vaginal bleeding can persist for as long as 48 h, especially after difficult catheterization.

6.2.3.4 Comments

In trained hands, selective salpingography is a simple technique with few complications. It restores tubal patency in over 80% of patients in which the fallopian tubes are not seen on conventional hysterograms. It can therefore be proposed as the initial procedure, prior to more invasive methods such as tubal microsurgery or in vitro fertilization (MAUBON et al. 1992). Furthermore, these latter techniques remain feasible if pregnancy is not achieved despite technically successful selective salpingography. These conclusions were confirmed in the *Guidelines for Practice* issued by the American Fertility Society after the 1992 meeting in Birmingham (AMERICAN FERTILITY SOCIETY 1993).

The high percentage (80%) of fallopian tubes opacified merely by contrast injection into the tubal ostium has two explanations. Many tubal "occlusions" are actually simply due to uterine nonopacification during conventional hysterography. Selective injection at a higher pressure often suffices to restore tubal patency. In other cases of tubal occlusion, opacification appears to be blocked in the proximal tube. A slight increase in the injection pressure may suffice to eliminate a "plug" of tubal secretions in the interstitial portion of the tube by pushing it through into the peritoneum (SULAK et al. 1987). These tubes are more likely to reocclude.

Peritoneal spill is also affected by the status of the distal tube. Recanalization of a severely damaged tube may prove useless if the ampulla is not patent. Although technically feasible, aspiration of a hydrosalpinx should not be attempted due to the risk of spread of infection. Peritubal adhesions are easily diagnosed by HSG and selective salpingography. Such patients should be referred back to their gynecologist for laparoscopy and adhesiolysis.

Sonohysterography, coupled when necessary with salpingography, appears advisable as the initial procedure. This approach is much less invasive than laparoscopy and results in a significant number of relatively "easy" pregnancies. If pregnancy is not achieved within a reasonable interval (this depends on the patient's age), laparoscopic evaluation is required before deciding whether to perform tubal microsurgery or in vitro fertilization.

6.3 Infertility Not Directly Related to the Uterine Cavity or the Fallopian Tubes: Ultrasound and Magnetic Resonance Imaging

6.3.1 Techniques

Gynecologic ultrasound requires a 3.5-MHz transducer for transabdominal examination and a 7.5-MHz probe for endovaginal imaging. Color Doppler (CD) capability is a useful adjunct. When available, MRI is the ideal, radiation-free complement to sonography for assessment of extracanalar pathologies. Sagittal and coronal T_1- and T_2-weighted sequences of the pelvis are the minimum requirements in all cases.

6.3.2 Ovarian Pathologies

Although usually temporary, ovarian pathologies are undoubtedly responsible for some cases of infertility.

6.3.2.1 Functional Cysts

Follicular cysts are thin-walled, hypoechoic fluid-like structures. Their diameter is usually less than 5 cm. On MRI, these cysts have a fluid signal (low-intensity T_1-weighted signal, high-intensity T_2-weighted signal). Luteal cysts are sonographically hypoechoic with a thick wall. On MRI, they have a high signal intensity on T_1- and T_2-weighted sequences (OUTWATER and MITCHELL 1996). The best diagnostic criterion is their disappearance after several cycles.

6.3.2.2 *Luteinized Unruptured Follicle Syndrome*

Pathologically, the lesions seen in luteinized unruptured follicle syndrome correspond to an unruptured mature follicle colonized by a corpus luteum. During the luteal phase, these follicles increase to over 4–5 cm in diameter. Ultrasound demonstrates internal echoes indicative of intrafollicular hemorrhage. On MRI, these lesions have a high-intensity signal on both T_1- and T_2-weighted sequences.

6.3.2.3 *Polycystic Ovary Syndrome*

Polycystic ovary disease can be divided into two types on the basis of clinical and anatomic features (MAUBON et al. 1993):

- Micropolycystic ovaries: clinical manifestations in these young patients include obesity, hirsutism, and menstrual disorders. Imaging reveals large ovaries (>5 cm in diameter) containing multiple (more than ten) small peripheral follicles. The hypertrophic ovarian stroma appears hyperechoic.
- Macropolycystic ovaries: these are characterized by the presence of several cysts greater than 15 mm in diameter in one or both ovaries in the absence of medical ovarian stimulation. Clinical symptoms include pelvic pain, sometimes with a history of infections or endometriosis. Ultrasound demonstrates large asymmetrical ovaries containing multiple cysts of different sizes (Fig. 6.10).

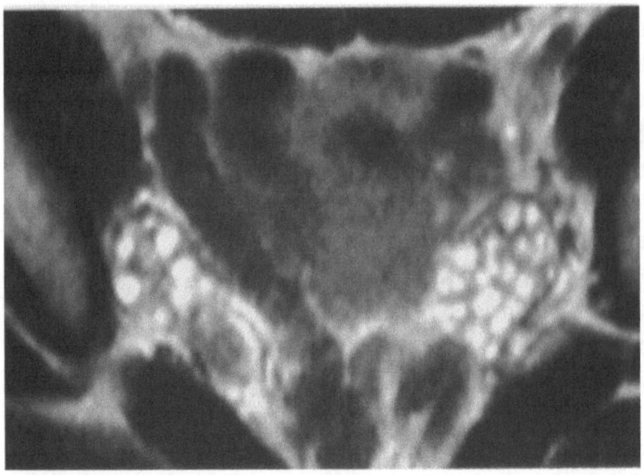

Fig. 6.10. Axial T_2-weighted image: polycystic ovarian disease. More than ten peripheral cysts are visible in these enlarged ovaries with stromal hypertrophy

6.3.3 Endometriosis

Endometriosis is defined as the presence of ectopic foci of endometrial tissue outside of the uterine cavity. These foci are under hormonal stimulation and may cause bleeding during the menstrual period. Endometrial cysts may thus be symptomatic (menstrual pain) or incidental findings (BIS et al. 1997). Sonographically, endometriotic cysts are round or oval masses with punctate hyperechoic foci. MRI demonstrates high signal intensity masses on T_1-sequences. Endometriomas may also have a typical "mirror-like" appearance, with inversion of the signal between cysts of different ages on T_1- and T_2-weighted sequences. The cyst wall is usually thin (2 mm) and hypointense; there are no internal implants. A fluid–fluid level may be present due to the sedimentation of menstrual blood (Fig. 6.11). MRI is the only imaging modality that can detect intraovarian endometriosis, which images on T_1-weighted sequences as hyperintense foci deep within the ovary, without ovarian enlargement (Fig. 6.12). Small extragenital or peritoneal implants can only be detected by laparoscopy.

6.3.4 Adenomyosis

Adenomyosis refers to the presence of ectopic foci of endometrium in the myometrium (REINHOLD et al. 1997). Ultrasound visualizes round, hypoechoic foci deep within the myometrium or poorly defined areas of abnormal echotexture. MRI demonstrates diffuse or focal thickening of the junctional zone (Fig. 6.13).

6.3.5 Uterine Anomalies

Congenital anomalies of the uterus are the result of developmental disorders of the müllerian ducts. These ducts normally give rise to the tubes and fuse medially to create the uterus, cervix, and upper two thirds of the vagina. Müllerian duct anomalies are classified as hypoplasia or agenesis and duplication anomalies (FIELDING 1996; MAUBON et al. 1996).

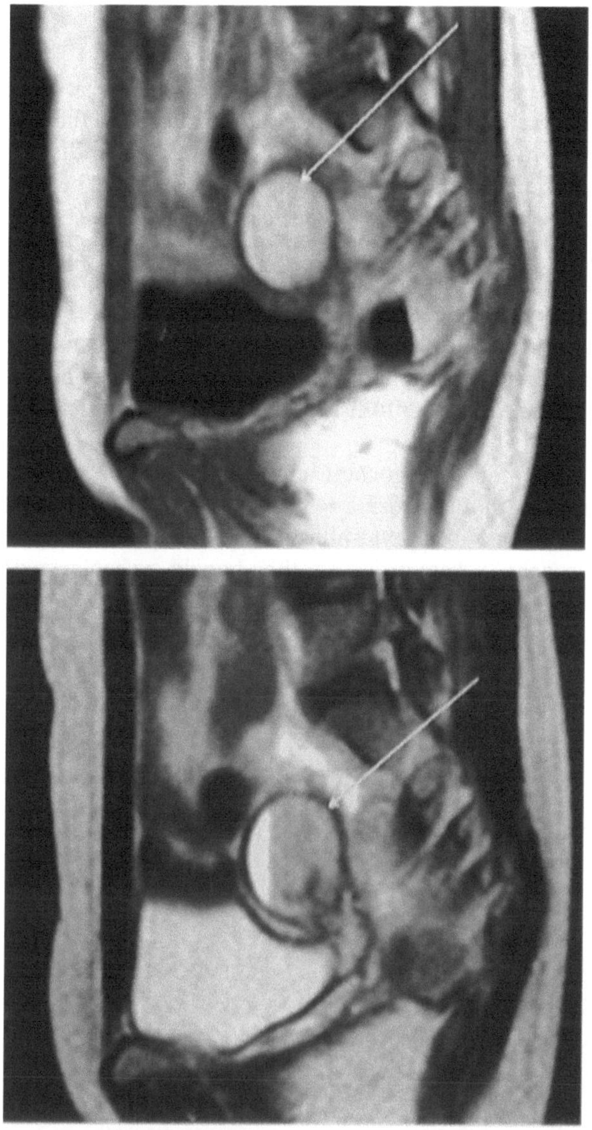

a

b

Fig. 6.11a,b. Parasagittal MRI scans: Ovarian endometrioma with **a** a high T_1 signal and **b** an intermediate T_2 signal. Note the fluid-fluid level (*arrows*)

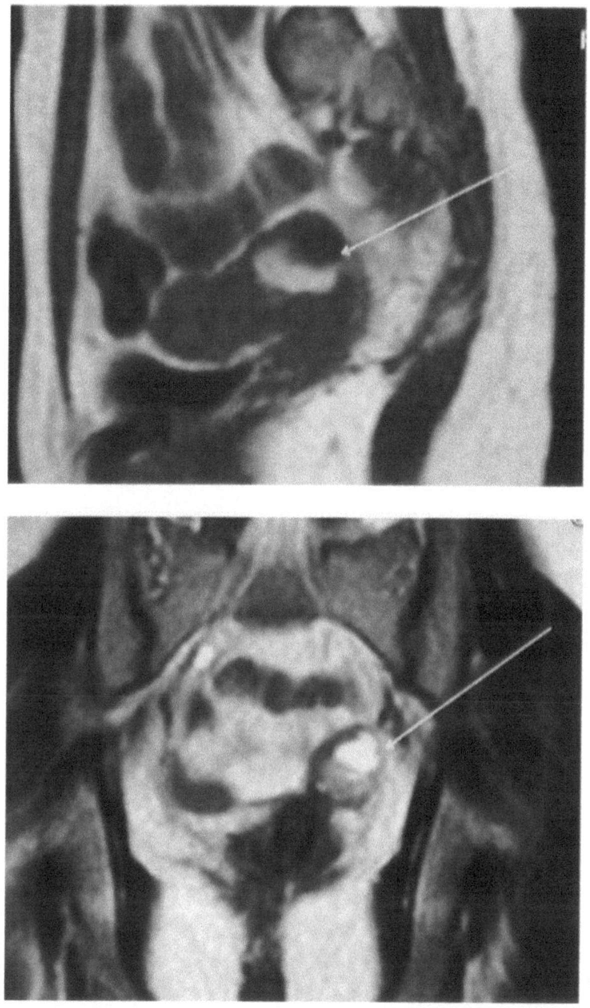

a

b

Fig 6.12a,b. Intraovarian endometriosis with a high-intensity signal on both sequences (*arrows*). **a** Parasagittal plane. **b** Coronal plane

6.3.5.1
Hypoplasia and Agenesis

These patients often present with vaginal agenesis. Clinical features and management depend on the extent of uterine and cervical tissue:

- If endometrium is present, patients usually have hematometra and/or hematocolpos and/or reflux endometriomas, sometimes presenting as a pelvic mass.
- If no functional endometrium is present, patients usually present with primary amenorrhea (Reinhold et al. 1997).

MRI is a useful tool for preoperative workup of these patients for whom suprapubic sonography is often difficult and endovaginal sonography is usually impossible. MRI demonstrates blood collections, the presence and size or the absence of the uterus, cervix, and vagina, the presence of functional endothelium, and the distance between the existing vagina and the uterus in cases of cervical atresia.

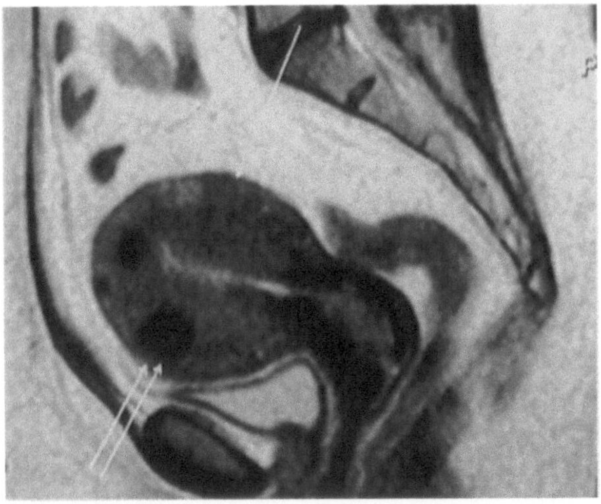

Fig. 6.13. Sagittal T_2-weighted image: diffuse adenomyosis is seen as thickening of the junctional zone (*arrow*); uterine myomata are also present (*double arrow*)

6.3.5.2
Uterine Duplication Anomalies

Uterine duplication anomalies are caused by maldevelopment or fusion of one or both müllerian ducts. Most malformations – unicornuate, didelphic, bicornuate with one or two cervices, septate (Figs. 6.4–6.6), and arcuate uteri – are accurately evaluated by ultrasound and MRI. To various degrees, these uterine anomalies can all cause infertility. Septate uteri are the most common and the most frequent cause of miscarriage, probably because the poor vascularity of the midline septum rapidly proves insufficient to support the fetus.

The most important clinical distinction to be made is that between a septate uterus and a bicornuate uterus. A septate uterus may benefit from hysteroscopic resection of the poorly vascularized

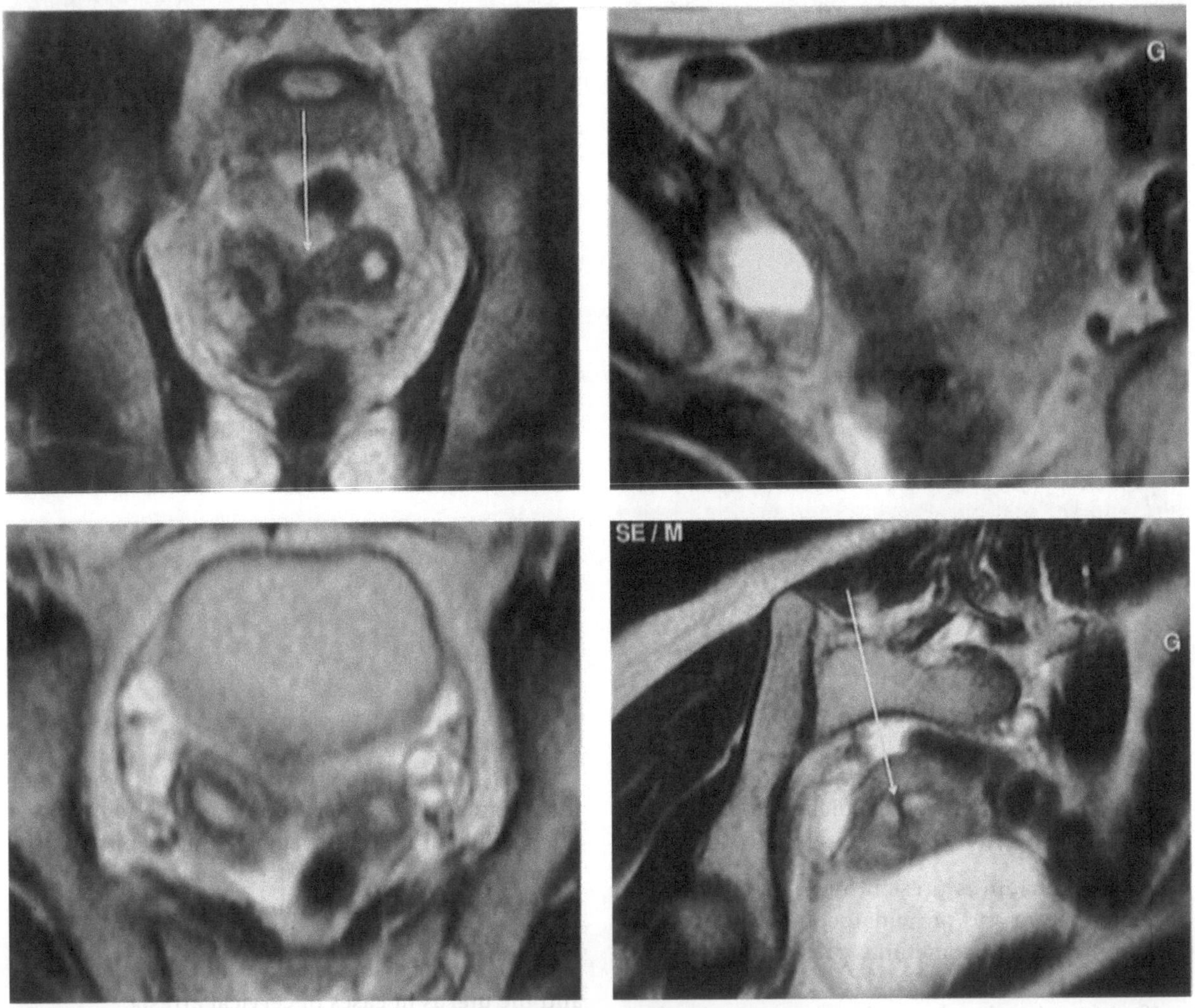

a c b d

Fig. 6.14a–d. MRI comparison of bicornuate and septate uteri. **a** Coronal view and **b** transverse view of a bicornuate uterus: the uterine horns are wide apart and a fundal notch is present (*arrow*). **c** Axial view and **d** oblique coronal view of a septate uterus: the uterine horns appear closer together; the external shape of the cavity is usually normal. Tissue with low signal intensity, corresponding to the septum, separates the two cavities (*arrow*) septum, whereas a bicornuate uterus should not be operated on. Distinction by HSG is possible, but difficult. Ultrasound and MRI reveal a fundal notch in bicornuate uteri, whereas the fundus of septate uteri is flat. On MRI, the midline portion of bicornuate uteri has a high-intensity signal due to the presence of myometrium and vessels. In contrast, the midline portion of septate uteri appears uniformly hypointense on both T_1- and T_2-weighted sequences (Fig. 6.14).

Patients with müllerian duct anomalies require comprehensive examination of the entire genitourinary tract and the spine owing to the frequency of associated renal and vertebral anomalies.

6.4 Conclusion

In conclusion, imaging of infertile patients is a complex matter that requires comprehensive management of the infertile couple. HSG is the baseline examination for the female partner to rule out a uterine or tubal cause. Ultrasound and MRI aid in assessment of the many possible causes of infertility.

References

American Fertility Society (1993) Guidelines for practice: tubal disease. American Fertility Society, Birmingham

Bis KG, Vrachliotis TG, Agrawal R, Shetty AN, Maximovich A, Hricak H (1997) Pelvic endometriosis: MR imaging spectrum with laparoscopic correlation and diagnostic pitfalls. Radiographics 17:639–655

Chen MYM, Zagoria RJ, Fayez JA et al (1995) Comparison of patient reactions and diagnostic quality for hysterosalpingography using ionic and non ionic contrast media. Acad Radiol 2:123

Dudiak CM, Turner DA, Patel SK et al (1988) Uterine leiomyomas in the infertile patient: preoperataive localization with MR imaging versus US and hysterosalpingography. Radiology 167:627–630

Fielding JR (1996) MR imaging of müllerian anomalies: impact on therapy. AJR 167:1491–1495

Hovsepian DM, Thurmond A, Confino E (1996) Recent food and drug administration clearance of a catheter system for selective catheterization of the fallopian tubes. Radiology 201:582–583

Maubon A, Rouanet JP, Cover S et al (1992) Fallopian tube recanalization by selective salpingography, an alternative to more invasive techniques. Hum Reprod 17:1425–1428

7 Parauterine Masses

J.N. Buy, M. Ghossain, and D. Vadrot

CONTENTS

7.1 Introduction

Determination of the benign or malignant nature of an adnexal mass is essential for appropriate therapeutic planning. Functional cysts and uncomplicated cysts smaller than 5 cm in postmenopausal women may merely be kept under surveillance (Levine et al. 1992). Stage I and II endometriosis of the American Fertility Society classification are managed medically, at least initially (American Fertility Society 1985). Certain benign lesions can be resected by celioscopy, whereas malignant and borderline tumors require laparotomy. Due to its excellent capabilities for morphological analysis, transvaginal ultrasound can characterize most ovarian masses smaller than 10 cm. More recently, color Doppler (CD) evaluation of the vascularity of adnexal masses combined with morphologic assessment has improved diagnostic characterization of these lesions (Buy et al. 1996). Adnexal masses larger than 10 cm in diameter and lesions with equivocal sonographic patterns all require further investigation by computed tomography (CT) or magnetic resonance imaging (MRI).

7.2 Imaging Modalities

7.2.1 Ultrasound

Pelvic sonography using a 2- to 4-MHz transducer is complemented by transabdominal ultrasound, with particular attention paid to the right subphrenic region and the kidneys. In the absence of contraindications, transvaginal ultrasound is systematically performed with a wide-band 5- to 9-MHz probe. Examination comprises the following:

- Demonstration of anatomy and morphologic analysis
- CD of any echogenic components of the mass, either in the conventional mode (pulse repetition frequency, 1000–1500, 50- to 100-Hz wall filter, high-priority color setting) or in the energy mode (power Doppler, PD)
- Doppler waveform analysis: measurement of the resistive index (RI), the pulsatility index (PI), and the peak systolic velocity (PSV).

7.2.2 Computed Tomography

Pelvic scans are obtained without contrast enhancement in the helical mode. CT angiography of the region of interest is performed by injecting 60 cc contrast medium at a rate of 6 cc/s. Scans are taken every 10 s for 60 s. Systematic abdominal–pelvic CT is mandatory to search for signs of disease spread and to evaluate contrast diffusion in the adnexal mass on late scans.

J.N. Buy, M. Ghossain, D. Vadrot, Service de Radiologie, Hôtel Dieu, Place du Parvis Notre Dame, 75004 Paris France

7.2.3 Magnetic Resonance Imaging

MRI of adnexal masses requires axial T_2-weighted sequences and T_1-weighted sequences without and with gadolinium enhancement. Complementary projections may be required for optimal evaluation. In particular, T_2-weighted sagittal sequences allow correct examination of the uterus and the pouch of Douglas. If the signal of the mass is isointense to subcutaneous fat on T_1-weighted images, a fat-suppression sequence should also be obtained.

7.3 Results

7.3.1 Ultrasound

7.3.1.1 Conventional Ultrasound

Sonographic criteria associated with borderline or malignant tumors include the following:

- An echogenic structure against the wall of a cyst, suggesting a papillary vegetation
- A large, irregular homogeneous or heterogeneous echogenic structure, suggesting an irregular solid component, with or without degenerative changes
- An irregular, thickened (>3 mm) wall or septum

A mass is considered benign if it does not present any of these signs of malignancy or if it exhibits the typical pattern of a benign ovarian mass (characteristic features are described hereafter for each etiology). Occasionally, it is impossible to determine whether a mass is solid or cystic, or benign or malignant. Although indeterminate, such lesions are considered malignant in statistical analyses.

7.3.1.2 Color Doppler and Morphological Modifications

The presence or absence of color flow is evaluated in the various portions of the mass (wall, septa, large echogenic portion, or small echogenic nodule lying against the cyst wall; Buy et al. 1996):

- In a mass characterized as malignant by conventional ultrasound, demonstration of color flow in the echogenic portion indicates its solid hypervascular nature, and the mass is considered malignant. Absence of color flow in the echogenic portion of a mass suspected to be malignant at ultrasound indicates its cystic or poorly vascularized nature, and the mass is considered benign.
- In a mass characterized as benign by conventional ultrasound, the presence of color flow in a regular wall or septum or a regular solid component is not indicative of malignancy. In the absence of color flow, the tumor is considered benign.
- If a mass is considered indeterminate by conventional ultrasound, the presence of color flow in the echogenic portion indicates its partially solid character, and the mass is considered malignant. In contrast, the absence of color flow in the echogenic portion indicates that the mass is completely cystic and thus benign (e.g., hemorrhagic cyst or cystic teratoma).

7.3.1.3 Spectral Doppler Analysis

Spectral Doppler analysis is of limited interest (Buy et al. 1996). However, a low RI or PI and an elevated PSV are suggestive of malignancy (Fleischer et al. 1992; Levine et al. 1994; Stein et al. 1995; Buy et al. 1996)

7.3.2 Computed Tomography

7.3.2.1 Malignant Tumors

Diagnosis of malignancy is based on three types of findings:

1. Morphological features suggestive of malignancy identical to those defined by conventional ultrasound.
2. Features on CT angiography highly suggestive of malignancy (Buy et al. 1991): hypervascularity consisting of thin irregular vessels on the arterial phase (20 s after the start of injection) that disappear rapidly on the next film and early contrast enhancement on the parenchymal phase (40 s after the start of injection)
3. Signs of extraovarian spread (Buy et al. 1991):
   a) Contiguous spread, namely to the uterus
   b) Peritoneal involvement, especially implants in the pouch of Douglas, the greater omentum, and the right subphrenic region
   c) Nodal metastases, namely involving the para-aortic nodes
   d) Distant metastases, in particular right pleural effusion

7.3.2.2
Benign Lesions

Adnexal masses are considered benign in the absence of any sign of malignancy or if the characteristic pattern of a specific benign tumor is depicted (e.g., cystic teratoma).

7.3.2.3
Indeterminate Tumors

Indeterminate tumors are considered malignant for purposes of analysis unless proven otherwise.

7.3.3
Magnetic Resonance Imaging

7.3.3.1
Malignant Tumors

The morphological features of malignancy on MRI are the same as for conventional ultrasound. On T_1-weighted sequences, solid components usually have a signal intensity similar to that of the pelvic muscles. On postcontrast MRI scans, these morphological abnormalities have a signal intermediate between muscle and fat (Ghossain et al. 1991). On T_2-weighted sequences, solid components have a signal intensity comparable to the pelvic muscles. Cystic components have a signal intensity comparable to urine. Pelvic spread, in particular to the uterus, is suggestive of malignancy.

7.3.3.2
Benign Tumors

A tumor is considered benign in the absence of signs of malignancy or if it presents the typical pattern of a specific benign ovarian mass (e.g., endometriotic cyst).

7.3.3.3
Indeterminate Tumors

Indeterminate tumors are considered malignant for purposes of analysis.

7.4
Non-neoplastic Lesions

7.4.1
Ovarian Adnexal Masses

7.4.1.1
Functional Cysts

On conventional ultrasound, functional cysts are typically unilocular, anechoic masses. These regular structures with thin walls (or sometimes without any visible wall) do not contain papillae and measure under 8 cm (Clement 1987). These criteria are diagnostic for benignancy. However, other benign lesions (benign serous cystadenoma, simple cyst, parovarian cyst) have similar sonographic features. A repeat sonogram performed after the next menstrual cycle or after hormone treatment that shows a decrease in size or resolution of the lesion confirms its functional nature. CD does not yield any diagnostic information.

7.4.1.2
Hemorrhagic Functional Cysts

Diagnosis of hemorrhagic functional cysts is suggested sonographically by demonstration of a central clot that is hyperechoic relative to the myometrium and is connected to the periphery of the cyst by thin bands or echogenic contents with a characteristic "fishnet" appearance (Jain et al. 1993). However, these characteristic patterns were observed in only 46% of cases in one of our own series (Buy et al. 1996). Modification in the cyst's echotexture after an interval of at least 10 days, a reduction in size, or even complete resolution are highly suggestive of the diagnosis.

As ultrasound is usually diagnostic, there are few indications for MRI. Certain investigators consider ultrasound rather than MRI the most suitable modality for characterization of these cysts (Jain et al. 1993). Others have defined certain MRI features characteristic of hemorrhagic functional cysts:

- For Outwater and Dunton (1995), hemorrhagic functional cysts typically have an intermediate- to high-intensity T_1 signal and an intermediate- to high-intensity T_2 signal. The decrease in signal intensity on T_2-weighted images that is characteristic of endometriosis is absent.
- Togashi et al. (1991) described hemorrhagic functional cysts that presented as hyperintense

subacute hematoma with decreased central signal on T_1-weighted sequences.
- A fluid level is considered by certain authors to be specific to hemorrhagic functional cysts (Nyberg et al. 1987). However, this feature is also encountered in endometriosis (Togashi et al. 1991).

7.4.1.3 Benign Serous Cystadenomas

Simple serous cystadenomas have the same features as functional cysts. Serial studies are required to distinguish the two based on differences in their course. CD provides no useful information. CT and MRI have no indications except for those rare masses over 10 cm in diameter.

Complex serous cystadenomas may be multiseptate and contain stromal tissue or papillary vegetations:

- The differential diagnosis for multilocular masses includes mucinous cystadenoma and other multilocular tumors. The loculi may be of different a nature.
- Lesions containing abundant stromal tissue are termed cystadenofibromas. These tumors contain weakly vascular solid material with regular borders, which distinguishes them from malignant lesions. They may undergo calcification.
- Papillae are present in 66% of cases (Buy et al. 1996; Fig. 7.1). These papillary vegetations are not very numerous; they are typically small (1–3 mm) with a regular surface. Unfortunately, there are no morphologic criteria that affirm their benignity, and any tumor containing vegetations must be verified surgically. CD does not demonstrate any flow in these vegetations, even when they are over 10 mm. In contrast, flow is constantly visible in malignant vegetations over 1 cm. Minute vegetations in a small tumor are usually best demonstrated by ultrasound. However, ultrasound is usually not sufficient for diagnosis of complex lesions.

On CT, these papillary vegetations usually appear denser than the cystic contents. They do not exhibit hypervascularity on the arterial phase of CT angiograms or contrast enhancement on the parenchymal phase. Contrast enhancement in these vegetations or solid components is usually seen only on late scans (10 min after injection). Slow diffusion of the contrast agent is characteristic of the vascularity of benign connective tissue.

On MRI, these vegetations typically have a fluid signal on T_1-weighted sequences. On T_2-weighted sequences, their signal is comparable to that of muscle; the cystic contents have a high-intensity signal similar to urine. After gadolinium injection, these vegetations enhance with a signal intermediate between muscle and fat.

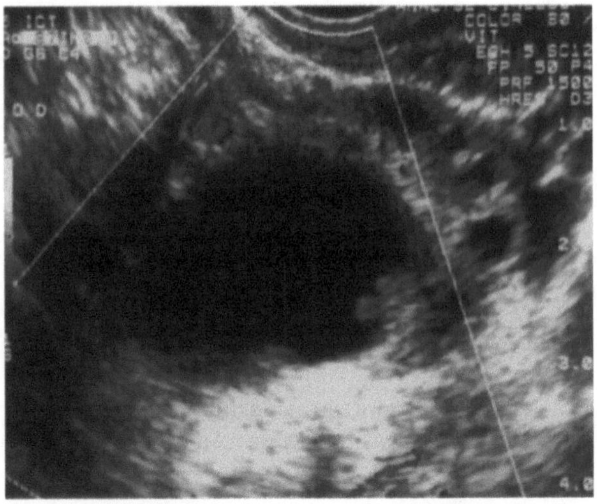

Fig. 7.1. Serous cystadenoma with a papillary projection. The absence of vascularity in the papillary projection on color Doppler makes a malignant vegetation highly unlikely

In these cases, both CT and MRI can demonstrate that the echogenic mass seen in contact with the cyst wall on sonograms is solid in nature and corresponds to a vegetation, despite the absence of vascularity at Doppler analysis.

7.4.1.4 Benign Mucinous Cystadenomas

On conventional ultrasound, benign mucinous cystadenomas are characteristically multilocular cystic masses. The loculations contain fluids of different echogenicities separated by smooth thin walls and septa (although thicker than those of benign serous cystadenoma) without endocystic vegetations (Buy et al. 1991).

CD usually depicts thin regular vessels within the walls or septa. Visualization of such vascularity is not a sign of malignancy. CD is useful primarily to affirm the purely cystic character of the echogenic portions, which can reach a considerable size.

As these tumors are often larger than 10 cm in diameter, CT or MRI is helpful for complete analysis of the tumor to confirm the absence of any morphologic sign of malignancy. CT angiography, in particular, can confirm the cystic nature of the echogenic zones (Buy et al. 1991).

The difference in contrast between the various fluids is more conspicuous on MRI (especially T_2-weighted images) than on sonograms or CT scans (GHOSSAIN et al. 1991; Fig. 7.2). Comparison of pre- and postgadolinium T_1-weighted images allows confirmation of the absence of contrast enhancement throughout the mass.

While the morphologic features of mucinous tumors usually facilitate diagnosis, radiologic affirmation of their benign nature remains difficult: their gross characteristics are similar to those of borderline mucinous tumors and even, in certain cases, to mucinous cystadenocarcinomas.

7.4.1.5
Benign Mature Cystic Teratomas (Dermoid Cysts)

Sonographic findings suggestive of the diagnosis of benign mature cystic teratomas include:

- A hyperechoic mass with an echogenicity greater than that of the myometrium
- A mural nodule containing hyperechoic structures and sharp acoustic shadowing suggesting the presence of dense structures (tooth-like structures, bone, cartilage, calcifications) in a Rokitansky nodule
- A mass containing a structure that is hyperechoic relative to the myometrium, containing lines or dots corresponding to hair, and broad acoustic shadowing (BRONSTEIN et al. 1991)
- A round, well-defined ball that is hyperechoic relative to the myometrium or an echogenic mass floating at the fluid interface (SHETH et al. 1988)

Sonographic depiction of one or more of these features allows diagnosis of dermoid cysts in 60% of patients (BUY et al. 1996). In the remaining patients, nonvisualization of vascularity within these masses with echogenic contents by CD confirms their cystic nature.

CT demonstration of fat (93% of patients according to BUY et al. 1989; Fig. 7.3) and accurate analysis of the components of Rokitansky's protuberance (dense elements, fat, connective tissue, in certain cases a fluid component; 81% of patients) allows def-

a

b

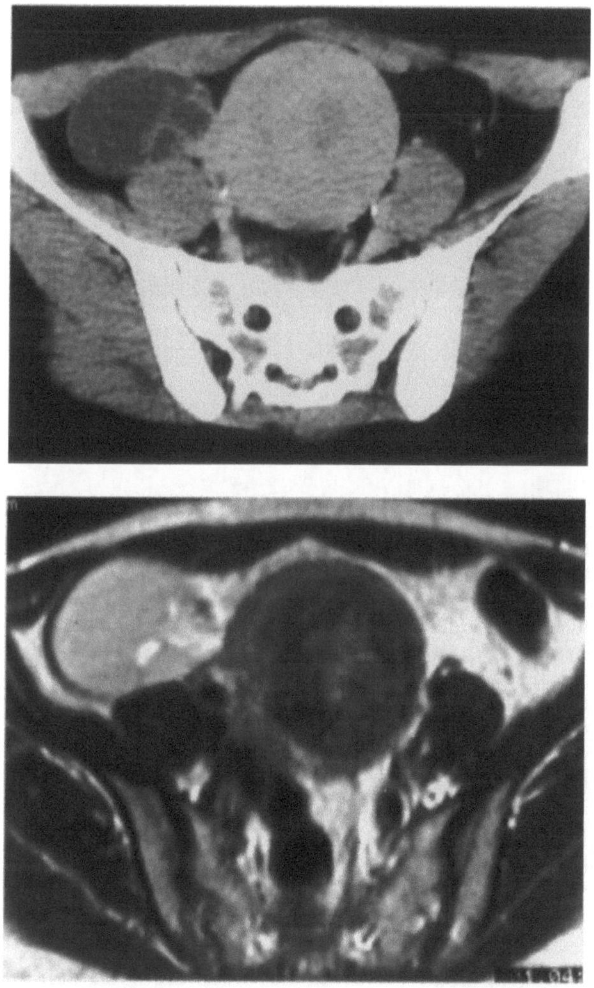

Fig. 7.2a,b. Benign multilocular mucinous cystadenoma in the right ovary. **a** CT failed to reveal any difference in density between the fluids in the various loculi. **b** T_2-weighted MRI demonstrated different signal intensities in the fluids, a pattern characteristic of these tumors

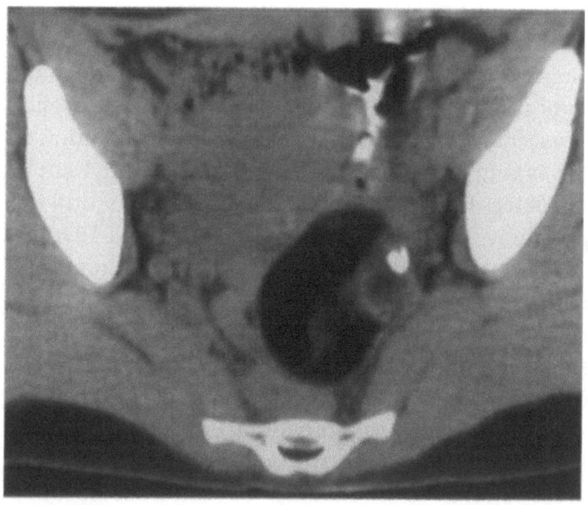

Fig. 7.3. Mature cystic teratoma. The density of the sebaceous content of this left ovarian cystic mass is −115 HU. A Rokitansky protuberance adherent to the cyst wall contains a tooth-like structure and fat. Hair is visible in the sebum

inite diagnosis of cystic mature teratoma in 98% of patients. CT can also accurately depict the following:

- The presence or absence of a mature cystic teratoma in the contralateral ovary (6%–12% of patients; SCULLY 1979).
- Another tumor in the same ovary (especially a mucinous tumor)
- Malignant degeneration in Rokitansky's protuberance, a rare possibility (BUY et al. 1989)

On MRI, the dense elements in Rokitansky's protuberance are less apparent than on CT. The fat component of the cyst has a signal close to that of subcutaneous fat on T_1- and T_2-weighted sequences. Fat-suppression sequences allow characterization of the sebaceous material in these tumors with the same reliability as CT.

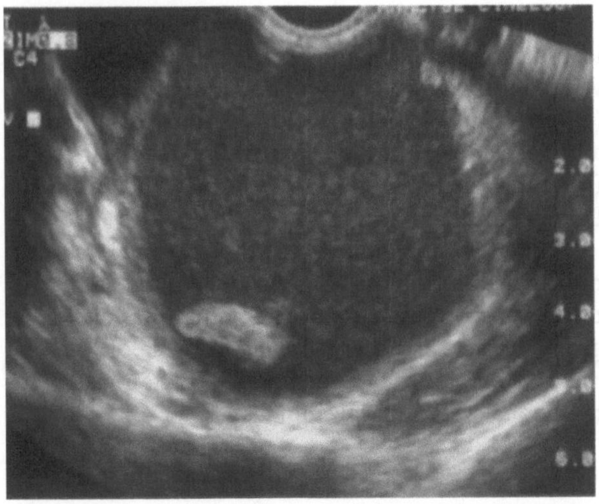

Fig. 7.4. Endometrioma seen as a homogeneously echogenic cystic mass with a more echogenic curvilinear mass against the internal wall corresponding to a blood clot

7.4.1.6
Endometriomas (Endometriotic Cysts)

On conventional ultrasound, endometriomas typically image as a more or less round, homogeneously echogenic structure (hypoechoic relative to the myometrium) containing diffuse, low-level echoes due to clots. Usually located against the inner wall, with or without acoustic shadowing, these blood clots appear more echogenic than the myometrium and are highly suggestive of the diagnosis when curvilinear and slightly separated from the wall (SANDLER and KARO 1978; BUY et al. 1992; Fig. 7.4). Endometriomas may also be visualized as round masses or may resemble papillary projections (LAING 1994), which explains why they may be mistaken for malignant tumors (BUY et al. 1996). CD can confirm the absence of vascularity within these masses. Demonstration of the avascular nature of these structures over 1 cm in diameter adherent to the inner wall rules out the possibility of malignant papillae (BUY et al. 1996).

CT has limited diagnostic value for endometriomas. By contrast, MRI (Fig. 7.5) reveals their hemorrhagic nature by demonstrating a cystic mass with a signal intensity equivalent to fat on T_1-weighted sequences that remains unchanged on fat-suppression sequences. On T_2-weighted images, these cysts may have a variety of signals; some contain hypointense areas referred to as "shading" (TOGASHI et al. 1991). Clots have a characteristic appearance, without any signal on the various sequences (BUY et al. 1992). MRI can also depict peritoneal implants and implants in the bladder or bowel.

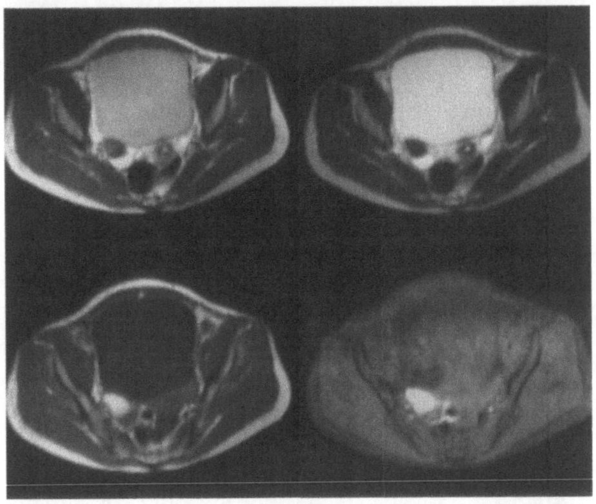

Fig. 7.5. Endometrioma in the right ovary associated with a follicle. *Bottom left*, T_1-weighted MRI: the high signal intensity of this endometrioma is similar to that of subcutaneous fat. A hypointense follicle is visible posterior to the endometrioma. *Bottom right*, fat-suppression sequence: the persistently high signal intensity of this endometrioma confirms its hemorrhagic character and rules out the presence of fat. *Top*, T_2-weighted MRI (*left*, first echo; *right*, second echo): shading is observed in the hypointense endometrioma, whereas the follicle is hyperintense

7.4.1.7
Ovarian Fibromas

Sonographically, ovarian fibromas are solid benign tumors imaging as a round or slightly bosselated mass that is nearly isoechoic relative to the myometrium and contains multiple acoustic shadows without calcification due to fibrous tissue.

Difficulties occur for differential diagnosis of ovarian fibromas from subserosal fibromyomas because these lesions have similar morphologic characteristics. A subserosal fibromyoma is more probable only if the ovary can be discerned on the same side as the myoma or if the mass contains large calcifications. CD consistently depicts vessels within ovarian fibromas and subserosal myomas (Buy et al. 1996), confirming the solid nature of these echogenic masses. Ovarian fibromas and subserosal fibromyomas also have different patterns of vascularity (Laing 1967; Bazot et al. 1993). Subserosal leiomyomas always present a peripheral ring, typical of hypervascularity, more or less associated with central vessels, whereas solid ovarian fibromas contain only a few vessels on the periphery or in the center (Buy et al. 1996).

On CT, ovarian fibromas have a density similar to the myometrium. CT angiography allows differentiation (Bazot et al. 1993). On the arterial phase, hypervascularity is constant in subserosal myomas, whereas it is absent in ovarian fibromas. Intense contrast enhancement or enhancement equivalent to the myometrium on the parenchymal phase is consistently observed for subserosal myomas, whereas it is absent or minimal in ovarian fibromas. On late films (10 min after the start of injection), subserosal myomas enhance to the same extent the myometrium. Ovarian fibromas usually enhance slightly less than the myometrium, and late films are thus necessary to confirm their solid nature.

The differences in vascularity demonstrated by Doppler and CT angiography and the differences in contrast enhancement on CT appear related to the specific vascular characteristics of subserosal myomas and ovarian fibromas. The intense peripheral vascularity of subserosal myomas, for example, is due to the numerous branches of the arcuate arteries arising from the marginal segment of the uterine artery that penetrates the serosa of the myoma. In contrast, the vascularity of ovarian fibromas derives from the ovarian artery and consists of much thinner vessels.

Fibroids and fibrothecomas have a homogeneous, low-intensity signal on T_1-weighted MRI. On T_2-weighted sequences, these lesions are completely or predominantly hypointense. Areas of edema and cystic degeneration appear hyperintense (Troiano et al. 1997).

Enhancement with gadolinium is necessary to establish the tissue character of these masses; this allows differentiation from certain cystic lesions, in particular endometriomas, which can have similar appearances.

7.4.2 Extraovarian Adnexal Masses

7.4.2.1 *Hydrosalpinges*

A hydrosalpinx images as a tubular, fluid-filled mass separate from the normal-appearing ovary. Demonstration of mucosal folds (Jain et al. 1993) or echogenic debris corresponding to pus or blood is highly suggestive of the diagnosis.

7.4.2.2 *Parovarian Cysts*

Parovarian cysts are thin-walled, unilocular cystic masses that display good through transmission and are separate from the normal ipsilateral ovary. Conventional ultrasound suffices for diagnosis. CD provides no complementary information.

7.4.2.3 *Peritoneal Pseudocysts*

Peritoneal pseudocysts typically image as a unilocular or multilocular mass separate from the ovary, with thin or thick septa, that conforms to the shape of the adjacent structures (Outwater and Dunton 1995). A history of pelvic surgery or pelvic inflammatory disease supports the diagnosis. CT can usefully demonstrate the lesion's relations with adjacent structures, particularly the pelvic ureter, because adhesions are constant. MRI is of little value for characterization.

7.5 Malignant and Borderline Tumors

Borderline tumors are defined histopathologically by cytologic criteria of malignancy without invasion of the stroma, in contrast to carcinoma. Borderline tumors are typically unilateral and confined to the ovary, whereas carcinomas are usually bilateral and have generally already invaded the ovary at diagnosis. As borderline tumors cannot be distinguished from their malignant counterparts on the basis of their gross morphology, their radiologic diagnosis is discussed together with malignant neoplasms.

7.5.1 Ultrasound

On conventional ultrasound, "typical" borderline or malignant tumors (Figs. 7.6, 7.7) present one or more of the following morphologic characteristics of malignancy:

- An echogenic component with irregular borders and areas of architectural change.
- One or more echogenic structures in contact with the inner cyst wall, corresponding to papillae. These usually large, broad-based lesions with an irregular surface are generally numerous.
- A thick (>3 mm) and irregular wall
- Thick, irregular septa (>3 mm)

At CD (Figs. 7.6, 7.7), demonstration of hypervascularity within an echogenic component suspected of being malignant confirms its solid nature and establishes the diagnosis of malignancy.

Doppler waveform analysis of arterial vascularity may provide additional diagnostic data if the RI is less than 0.40. However, this relatively specific sign has low sensitivity.

Carcinoma may present as a complex mass containing both echogenic and anechoic components. Diagnosis of a cystic or solid, benign or malignant tumor is difficult in such cases.

Due to its ability to demonstrate the vascular or avascular nature of an echogenic component, CD can distinguish echogenic vascular solid tissue from

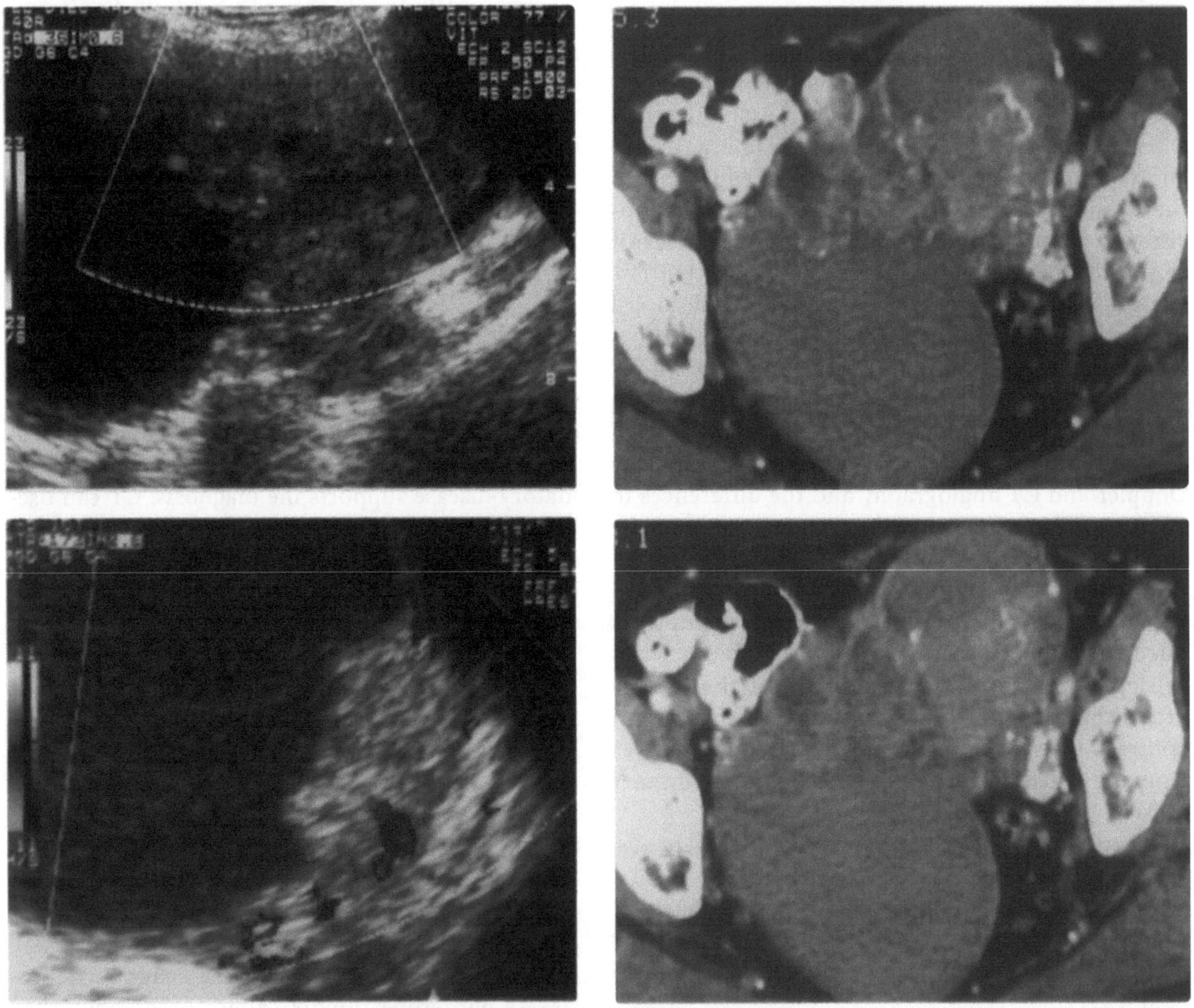

a c b d

Fig. 7.6a–d. Stage I endometroid cystadenocarcinoma of the left ovary. **a** Color Doppler sonogram: complex mass containing an anechoic component and a vascular echogenic component with irregular internal contours. **b** CT angiogram: the precontrast scan reveals a left anterior component containing calcifications and a homogeneous posterior component. **c** Arterial phase: the hypervascularity of the anterior tissue component is composed of thin irregular vessels, which is characteristic of a malignant tumor. **d** Parenchymal phase: contrast uptake is visible in the solid component containing areas of architectural change, whereas the posterior fluid component remains unenhanced

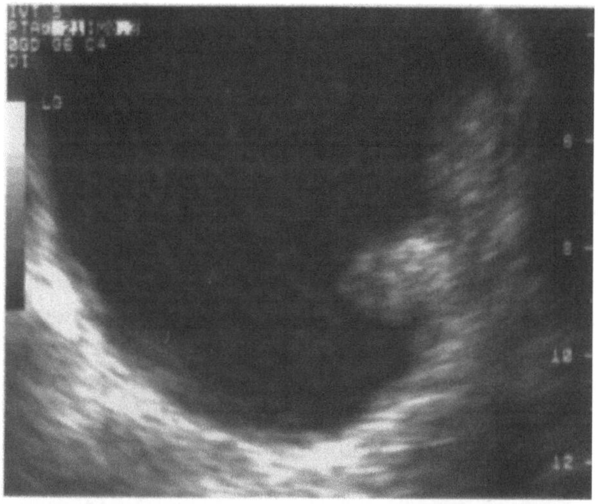

a

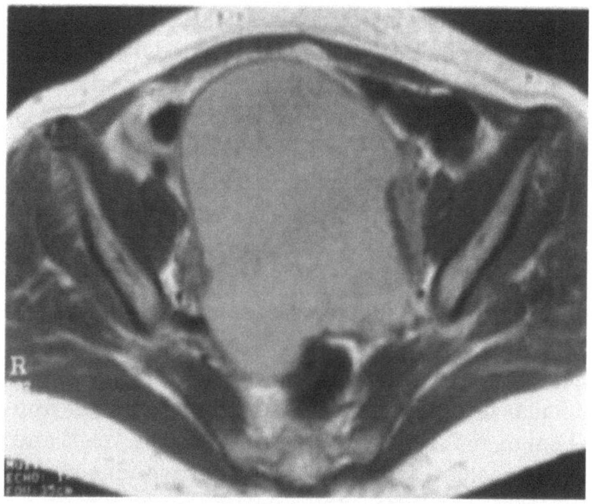

d

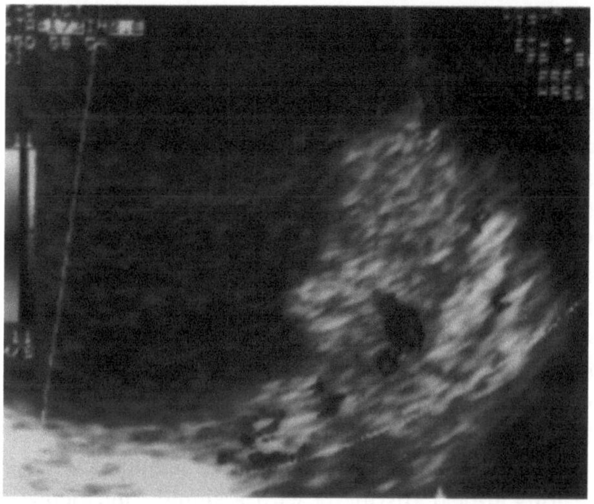

b

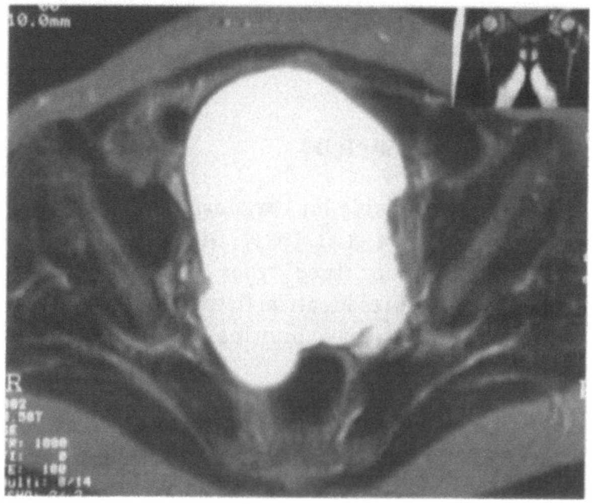

e

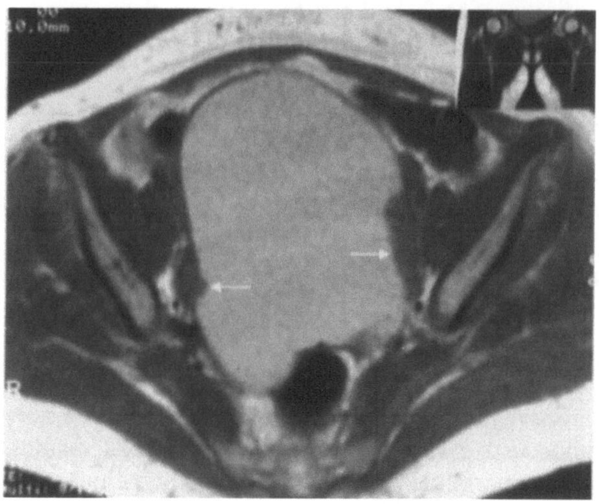

c

Fig. 7.7a–e. Clear cell cystadenocarcinoma of the left ovary. **a** Sonogram revealing a cystic lesion with fine echoes and a more echogenic component against its inner wall. This pattern can correspond to either an endometrioma with blood clots or carcinoma. **b** Color Doppler demonstration of flow in this echogenic mass was consistent with solid tissue and led to a diagnosis of malignancy. **c** T_1-weighted MRI: the cystic mass contains two components adherent to the inner wall (*arrows*) with signal intensities close to that of pelvic muscle. **d** Gadolinium-enhanced MRI showed enhancement of both components, thus confirming that they were papillary projections, a feature consistent with a malignant tumor. **e** T_2-weighted sequence: the papillae have a signal intermediate between muscle and fat echogenic avascular structures (e.g., clots) or elements with flow too weak to be detected by Doppler. Detection of vascularity in the echogenic portion of a complex mass confirms its tissue nature and is highly suggestive of a malignant tumor.

On rare occasions, carcinoma is depicted as a homogeneous echogenic mass. The most common etiologies of these infrequent lesions are lymphomas and metastases.

Borderline mucinous cystadenoma and mucinous cystadenocarcinoma merit special mention owing to their particular macroscopic features. These multilocular tumors can be difficult to differentiate from a benign mucinous tumor. However, the thick and irregular character of the septa, their number, and their location clustered in a portion of the tumor, or even the existence of a solid component, suggest a borderline or malignant nature.

7.5.2 Computed Tomography

CT has proven reliable for diagnosis of benign epithelial tumors (Buy et al. 1991). Diagnosis of carcinoma is based on three types of findings: (1) morphologic features identical to those described for ultrasound, (2) vascular abnormalities, and (3) disease spread.

Vessel abnormalities are analyzed by CT angiography (Fig. 7.6):

1. On the arterial phase (20–30 s after the start of injection), tumor hypervascularity presents certain specific characteristics:
   a) Morphologic features: the vessels are thin and irregular, without any definite origin or termination.
   b) Hemodynamic characteristics: the flow rate is elevated; the vessels appear on scans after 20 s in certain areas, whereas they disappear on the following scan at 30 s. The flow rate varies from one point of the tumor to another.
2. On the parenchymal phase (40–60 s after the start of injection), intense contrast enhancement is seen in the tissue components.
3. Late scans (10 min after the start of injection) often reveal accumulation of the contrast agent in the tissue components.

Evaluation of disease spread is helpful not only for diagnosis, but also for preoperative workup. Dissemination occurs essentially by contiguous spread, peritoneal implants, and lymphatic spread. Contiguous spread to adjacent viscera (uterus, bladder, rectum) can be diagnosed when a mass of the same nature as the tumor invades one of these organs and distorts its contour.

Peritoneal extension can involve the entire cavity, but has a predilection for the pouch of Douglas, the greater omentum, and the right subphrenic region. Nodular or plaque-like lesions occur on the peritoneum, with or without ascites. The difficulty in demonstrating these implants depends less on their size than on their localization (perihepatic implants are much easier to diagnose than implants on the small intestine) and the presence or absence of ascites.

Lymphatic spread occurs to the external and internal iliac nodes and the retroperitoneal nodes.

7.5.3 Magnetic Resonance Imaging

Like CT, MRI permits comprehensive assessment of malignant and borderline lesions. MRI (Fig. 7.7) is also just as effective as CT for morphologic characterization of these tumors (Ghossain et al. 1991). Papillae, solid components, and septa are isointense to pelvic muscle on T_1-weighted sequences. They are not always distinct on these sequences, because their signal is sometimes similar to that of the fluid of epithelial tumors. These tissue components are much more conspicuous on postcontrast scans, as they have a signal intermediate between muscle and subcutaneous fat. On T_2-weighted sequences, these lesions appear distinctly with a signal intermediate between muscle and fat; the fluid in these tumors presents a high-intensity signal greater than or equal to that of urine (Ghossain et al. 1991).

Pelvic extension, especially to the uterus, is accurately depicted by MRI. Tumor spread to the entire abdominal–pelvic cavity is best evaluated by CT (Ghossain et al. 1991).

7.6 Conclusion

Transvaginal ultrasound and CD have considerably improved the characterization of adnexal masses. CD, in particular, offers better specificity and positive predictive value. CT and MRI are systematically indicated for indeterminate lesions and large tumors. Owing to their diagnostic performances, CT is indicated for lesions suspected of being dermoid cysts, while MRI is the most sensitive and most specific modality for the diagnosis of endometriosis.

References

American Fertility Society (1985) Revised American fertility society classification of endometriosis: 1985. Fertil Steril 43:351–352

Bazot M, Ghossain MA, Buy JN et al. (1993) Fibrothecomas of the ovary: CT and US findings. J Comput Assist Tomogr 17:754–579

Bronstein M, Yoffe N, Brandes JM, Blumenfeld Z (1991) Hair as a sonographic marker of ovarian teratomas: improved identification using transvaginal sonography and simulation model. J Clin Ultrasound 19:351–355

Buy JN, Ghossain MA, Moss AA et al (1989) Cystic teratoma of the ovary: CT detection. Radiology 171:697–701

Buy JN, Ghossain MA, Sciot C et al (1991) Epithelial tumors of the ovary: CT findings and correlation with US. Radiology 178:863–870

Buy JN, Ghossain MA, Marks AS et al (1992) Focal hyperdense areas in endometriomas: a characteristic finding on CT. AJR 159:769–771

Buy JN, Ghossain MA, Hugo D et al (1996) Characterization of adnexal masses: combination of color Doppler and conventional sonography compared with spectral Doppler analysis alone and conventional sonography alone. AJR 166:385–393

Clement PB (1987) Nonneoplastic lesions of the ovary. In: Kurman RJ (ed) Blaustein's pathology of the female genital tract. Springer, Berlin Heidelberg New York, pp 471–515

Fleischer AC, Rodgers WH, Kepple DM, Williams LL, Jones HW III, Gross PR (1992) Color Doppler sonography of benign and malignant ovarian masses. Radiographics 12:879–885

Ghossain MA, Buy JN, Lignières C et al (1991) Epithelial tumors of the ovary: CT findings and correlation with US. Radiology 178:811–870

Jain KA, Friedman DL, Pettinger TW, Alagappan R, Jeffrey RB Jr, Sommer FG (1993) Adnexal masses: comparison of specificity of endovaginal US and pelvic MR imaging. Radiology 186:697–704

Laing FC (1994) US analysis of adnexal masses: the art of making the correct diagnosis. Radiology 191:21–22

Lang EK (1967) Arteriography in gynecology. Radiol Clin North Am 5:13–149

Levine D, Gosink BB, Wolf SI, Feldesman MR, Pretorius DH (1992) Simple adnexal cysts: the natural history in postmenopausal women. Radiology 184:653–659

Levine D, Feldstein VA, Babcook CJ, Filly RA (1994) Sonography of ovarian masses: poor sensitivity of resistive index for identifying malignant lesions. AJR 162:1355–1359

Nyberg DA, Porter BA, Olds MO, Olson DO, Andersen R, Wesby GE (1987) MR imaging of hemorrhagic adnexal masses. J Comput Assist Tomogr 11:664–669

Outwater EK, Dunton CJ (1995) Imaging of the ovary and adnexa: clinical issues and applications of MR imaging. Radiology 194:1–18

Sandler MA, Karo JJ (1978) The spectrum of ultrasonic findings in endometriosis. Radiology 127:229–231

Scully RE (1979) Tumors of the ovary and maldeveloped gonads. In: Harman WH (ed) Atlas of tumor pathology. AFIP, Washington, pp 252–268

Sheth S, Fishman EF, Buck JL, Hamper UM, Sanders RC (1988) Hair as a sonographic marker of ovarian teratomas: correlation with CT. AJR 151:331–334

Stein SM, Laifer-Narin S, Johnson MB et al (1995) Differentiation of benign and malignant adnexal masses: relative value of gray-scale, color Doppler, and spectral Doppler sonography. AJR 164:381–386

Togashi K, Nishimura K, Kimura I et al (1991) Endometrial cysts: diagnosis with MR imaging. Radiology 180:73–78

Troiano RB, Lazzarini KM, Scoutt LM, Lange RC, Flynn SD, McCarthy S (1997) Fibroma and fibrothecoma of the ovary: MR imaging findings. Radiology 204:795–798

8 Osteoporosis

P. Brunner, J.M. Cucchi, A. Gangi, O. Louis, M.-Y. Mourou, and M. Osteaux

CONTENTS

8.1 Introduction

M. Osteaux and O. Louis

Numerous techniques are currently available for evaluation of bone mineral status (Faulkner et al. 1991). These modalities are used to assess the risk of osteoporotic fracture at key skeletal sites, classically the spine, hip, or wrist. However, determination of calcium density alone is clearly not always sufficient. Owing to the overlap in bone density values in patients with osteoporotic fractures and in osteoporotic individuals without fracture, research has been directed at development of techniques capable of analyzing cortical and trabecular bone architecture. The following brief description of the various techniques highlights the advantages of each method. Particular attention is paid to those techniques allowing analysis of bone structure.

P. Brunner, M.-Y. Mourou, Service de Radiologie, Centre Hospitalier Princess Grace, avenue Pasteur, 98000 Monaco
J.M. Cucchi, Centre d'Imagerie Médicale, rue du Gabian, 98000 Monaco
A. Gangi, Service de Radiologie, Hôpital de Hautepierre, avenue Molière, 67098 Strasbourg, France
O. Louis, M. Osteaux, Radiologie en Medische Beeldvorming, Academisch Ziekenhuis, Vrije Universiteit Brussels, Laarbeeklaan 101, 1090 Brussels, Belgium

8.2 Bone Densitometry Techniques

A distinction must be made between projection techniques, which cannot provide density values per unit of volume, and methods that provide true volumetric information. The densities measured by projection techniques are expressed in grams per square centimeter. This areal density is influenced by the body height and weight of the individual examined, which can introduce a bias in clinical and epidemiological studies (Ito et al. 1994; Prentice et al. 1994). Three-dimensional techniques, which are all based on computed tomography (CT), express bone density per unit of volume.

8.2.1 Projection Techniques

The corticodiaphyseal index (Barnett and Nordin 1960) was the first radiologic method to evaluate the cortical bone of a metacarpal. This method is now solely of historical interest, having been abandoned in clinical practice because its sensitivity and specificity are insufficient to be of any real predictive value. In addition, the fact that assessment is restricted to a peripheral site constitutes an intrinsic limitation.

Single-photon absorptiometry (SPA) using an iodine-125 source permits evaluation of the bones of the forearm (Cameron and Sorensen 1963). This technique can be considered the first true quantitative method, even though evaluation is limited to a peripheral site. This method has gradually been almost totally superseded by dual-energy X-ray absorptiometry (DXA or DEXA).

Dual-photon absorptiometry (DPA) (REED 1966; MAZESS et al. 1970) was the first method for dual-energy measurement of the axial skeleton. Performed with gadolinium as the radionuclide, DPA has progressively been replaced by DXA, which provides more consistent results along with improved accuracy and specificity.

A modification of DPA, DXA (WAHNER et al. 1988; MAZESS et al. 1989) is characterized by dual-energy X-ray production either by the generator or by filtration of the emitted spectrum. Currently the most widely used method in clinical practice, DXA can measure bone density at various skeletal sites: spine, hip, forearm, whole body. This increasingly used technique has undergone numerous improvements, having evolved from first-generation "pencil beam" units to third-generation scanners featuring "fan beam" geometry (RÜEGSEGGER 1988; SCHNEIDER and BERGER 1988; Fig. 8.1).

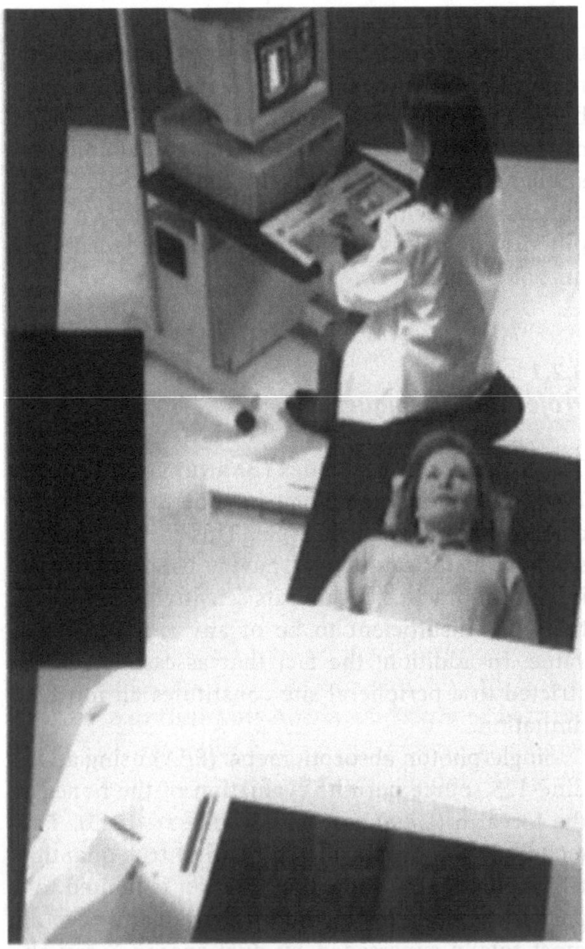

Fig. 8.1. Third-generation dual-energy X-ray absorptiometry (DEXA) unit (fan beam)

8.2.2 Three-Dimensional Techniques

Quantitative CT (QCT) is an application of CT to measurement of bone mineral density (GENANT and BOYD 1977). It is the only true volumetric technique permitting separate assessment of cortical and trabecular bone (Fig. 8.2).

Peripheral QCT (pQCT) performed with small units developed for CT of the wrist allows separate assessment of the cortical and trabecular bone of the radius (RÜEGSEGGER 1988; SCHNEIDER and BERGER 1988; Fig. 8.3).

8.3 Advantages of the Various Techniques

8.3.1 General Comments

The validity and clinical utility of bone densitometry techniques are usually expressed in terms of reproducibility, accuracy, and sensitivity (FAULKNER et al. 1991). Reproducibility, generally expressed as a percentage (CV%), refers to the difference between two measurements made in the same patient or on the same calibration phantom. Good reproducibility is obviously important in clinical practice. Reproducibility is sometimes called "precision," but this can lead to confusion with the notion of accuracy. Accu-

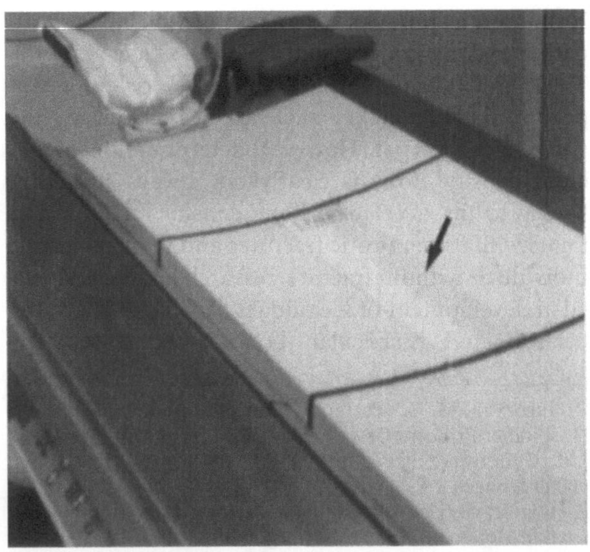

Fig. 8.2. CT unit for measurement of bone mineral density. Note the solid reference phantom (*arrow*) built into the mattress

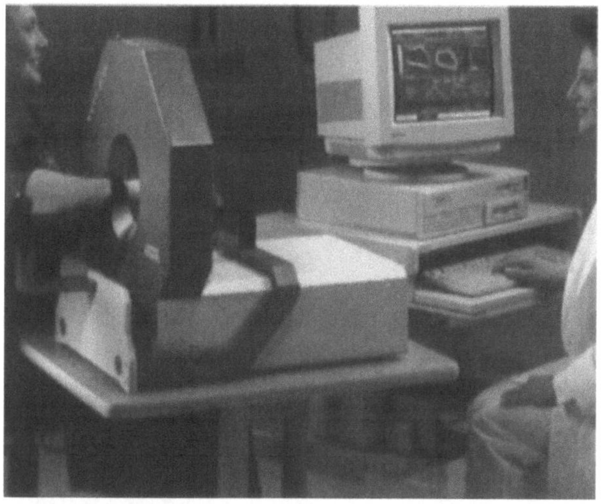

Fig. 8.3. Small dedicated CT unit for quantitative analysis of the extremities

racy reflects the true validity of a technique compared to a physicochemical reference method such as ash density or neutron activation analysis. Sensitivity refers to a technique's ability to discriminate between normal and abnormal situations. A "good" clinical method is one that associates "good" reproducibility with "good" accuracy and "good" sensitivity.

8.3.2 Normal Evolution of Bone Mass

Peak bone mass is usually achieved around 30 years of age in both sexes. Bone mass declines progressively thereafter as part of the normal aging process. The decrease is more abrupt in women after the menopause (SCHOUTENS 1993).

8.3.3 Expression of Results

Bone mass is expressed as the bone mineral content (BMC) in grams or milligrams of calcium hydroxyapatite. Bone mineral density (BMD) is expressed in grams per square centimeter in DXA (areal density) and in milligrams per milliliter (density per unit of volume) in QCT and pQCT. The measured density is then compared to reference values established for a normal population, usually by means of multicenter studies. Several years ago, the present authors participated in a European collaborative study to define normal values for QCT (KALENDER et al. 1990). These studies allowed normal values to be determined (mean±2 SD). Comparison of an individual value with these normal values provides two indices or scores. The Z score is the difference between the measured value and the mean value in an age- and gender-matched population, while the T score is the difference between the measured value and the mean value at 30 years of age (SCHOUTENS 1993).

8.3.4 Comparison of Dual-Energy X-Ray Absorptiometry and Quantitative Computed Tomography

Compared with projection techniques, QCT is the only technique that provides true volumetric BMD (in mg/m^3) thanks to separate assessment of cortical and trabecular bone (Fig. 8.4). As bone metabolism is much more active in trabecular bone, bone mineral changes are more readily detected in trabecular bone. QCT is thus more sensitive than projection techniques (PACIFICI et al. 1990). In addition, QCT eliminates artifacts attributable to degenerative disease, which is common in elderly individuals with osteoarthritis and osteophytes. Compared to projection techniques, QCT requires higher, although moderate, doses of irradiation (KALENDER 1992). This drawback, which has often been exaggerated due to poor familiarity with proper dosimetry processes during CT, represents a relative contraindication for QCT in children.

Correct application of QCT requires specific application software with automated definition of the region of interest (ROI) and the scan level. Manual definition introduces errors that unacceptably affect reproducibility (LOUIS et al. 1988).

Small CT units have been specifically developed (essentially by two European manufacturers) for quantitative measurement of the cortical and trabecular bone of the forearm (RUEGSEGGER 1988; SCHNEIDER and BERGER 1988). Despite encouraging initial results, high-resolution peripheral QCT remains a predominantly experimental technique available only at a limited number of specialized centers (GRAMPP et al. 1996a).

DXA is currently the method of choice for clinical assessment of BMC. This projection technique has excellent accuracy and reproducibility (LOUIS et al. 1992), but its sensitivity is lower than that of QCT despite recent technological advances (replacement of "pencil beam" scanning by "fan beam" geometry;

a

b

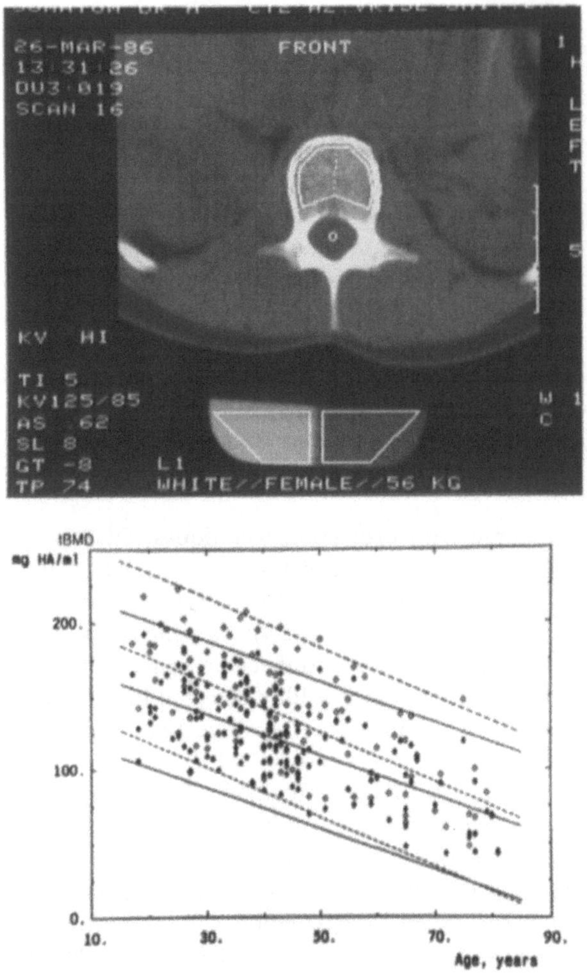

Fig. 8.4. a The CT application software automatically separates the cortical bone from the trabecular bone. The axis of symmetry is used to compare the values of the two hemivertebrae (quality control). **b** The result is then expressed numerically and compared to the database of normal values

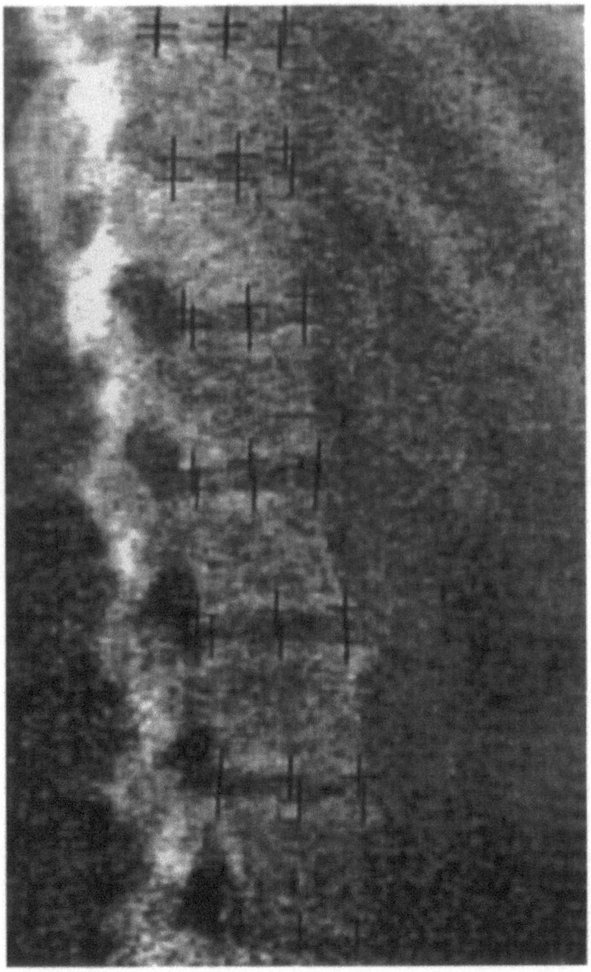

Fig. 8.5. Third-generation dual-energy X-ray absorptiometry (DEXA) units also allow morphometric study, with calculation of the wedge index. Note the excellent image quality (multiple detectors, fan beam technique)

development of entirely automated DXA scanners permitting measurement of the lumbar spine in the lateral projection while the patient remains supine) (Guglielmi et al. 1995; Sabin et al. 1995; Fig. 8.5).

One of the major advantages of DXA is unquestionably the ease of evaluation of sites other than the hip, forearm, and spine (the three primary sites of osteoporotic fracture).

The development of dedicated software has opened the way for application of densitometry techniques to domains other than postmenopausal osteoporosis: diagnosis of the loosening of prostheses in orthopedics (Trevisan et al. 1993), investigation of algodystrophy, and medicolegal appraisals. Whole-body scans (Tothill et al. 1994) are rapidly obtained with the new machines. The rapidity and accuracy with which overall bone mass and soft tissue mass can be determined portends new applications in pediatrics, endocrinology (obesity), sports medicine, etc.

8.4 Techniques Analyzing Bone Structure

8.4.1 Quantitative Magnetic Resonance Imaging

The trabecular architecture of bone has traditionally been evaluated by histomorphometry, usually on a bone biopsy from the iliac crest. In order to study bone architecture in vivo and at more appropriate sites, research has been concentrated on MRI. Two areas are under investigation. The first is based on the existence of two phases in trabecular bone: fat and the bone trabeculae properly so called. Analysis of the inhomogeneity of the magnetic field created by the two phases allows indirect assessment of the trabecular thinning that occurs in osteoporosis (WEHRLI et al. 1995). The second pole of research concerns high-resolution MRI. Initially used for small structures such as the fingers (WEHRLI 1993), high-resolution MR has also been used for the distal radius and the calcaneus (MAJUMDAR and GENANT 1995), but the technique requires very high intensity magnetic fields.

A good correlation has been reported between the trabecular density of the ultradistal radius measured by pQCT and the relaxation time (1/total transverse relaxation [T2*], measured with gradient-echo imaging) (GRAMPP et al.1996b). However, MRI basically remains an experimental technique and is not suitable for large-scale diagnosis of osteoporosis.

8.4.2 Quantitative Ultrasound

Bone ultrasonography is a technique in full expansion. The most commonly used machines analyze the trabecular bone of the calcaneus; others measure the cortical bone of the tibia or the total bone (cortical and trabecular) of the phalanges (VENTURA et al. 1996; Fig. 8.6). Two parameters are measured: attenuation of the ultrasound signal during passage through bone (broadband ultrasound attenuation [BUA], expressed in dB/MHz) and the ultrasound transit velocity through bone (speed of sound [SOS], expressed in m/s). These two parameters are linked to the quantity and the orientation of the trabeculae (FUERST et al. 1995; FUNKE et al. 1995; Fig. 8.7).

The correlation between these parameters and those reflecting BMC (obtained, for example, by DXA of the hip or spine) is generally rather low. By contrast, the correlation between the risk of osteoporotic fracture (especially hip fracture) and ultrasound data is excellent, as demonstrated in a recent prospective study of 1414 women (PORTER et al. 1990; GLUER et al. 1996). Numerous improvements have been made since LANGTON et al. (1984) described the first apparatus. The most noteworthy results have been achieved with ultrasound devices developed for analysis of the calcaneus (LAUGIER et al. 1997), because improvement in the approach to the region of interest has increased reproducibility.

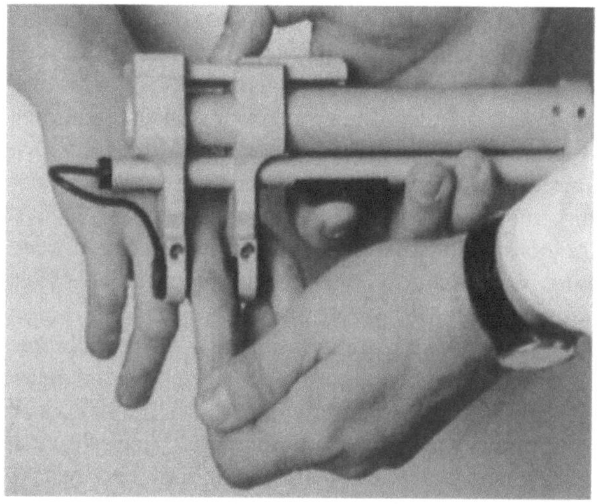

Fig. 8.6. Dedicated quantitative ultrasound unit for assessment of the cortical and trabecular bone of the phalanges

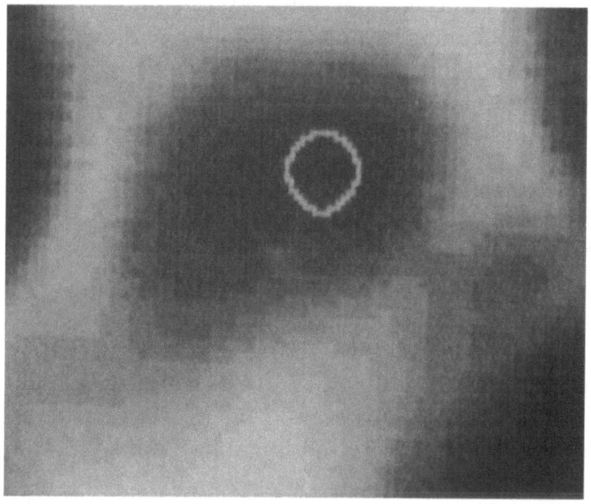

Fig. 8.7. Dedicated ultrasound quantitation: parametric image of the calcaneum

8.5 Percutaneous Vertebroplasty

P. BRUNNER, A. GANGI, J.M. CUCCHI, and M.Y. MOUROU

Percutaneous vertebroplasty is a recent interventional radiology technique consisting in injection of acrylic cement into the body of a vertebra that has been weakened by bone loss due to osteolysis or osteoporosis. In addition to consolidating the vertebra, the technique relieves the related back pain.

Galibert et al. (1987) were the first to describe the results achieved with vertebroplasty. Initially used to treat vertebral bodies damaged by aggressive angiomas, the technique was progressively extended to treatment of osteolytic metastases. Today, hyperalgesic osteoporotic compression fractures refractory to medical management for more than 15 days are increasingly common indications for this procedure (Gangi et al. 1993; Deramond et al. 1996; Cortet et al. 1997).

Osteoporosis is a major public health problem. Although postmenopausal hormone replacement therapy is increasingly frequent, the incidence of compression fractures remains high. These lesions are particularly painful and disabling; bed rest is mandatory, often for prolonged periods, before consolidation and pain sedation can be achieved. The socioeconomic cost of osteoporosis is considerable, as hospitalization alone often exceeds 15 days. Finally, the complications of prolonged immobilization (loss of independent living, bedsores, amyotrophy, thromboembolism) can be life-threatening in the elderly.

8.5.1 Preoperative Workup

Preoperative assessment obviously includes coagulation studies and evaluation of parameters reflecting inflammation; results can serve as reference values should complications occur. MRI is performed systematically to confirm the spinal level involved and to affirm the recent and "active" nature of the fracture (Fig. 8.8).

8.5.2 Technique

With the patient placed in the prone position on the scanner couch, vertebroplasty is performed under local anesthesia (cutaneous, subcutaneous, muscular, posterior articular process, subperiosteal) (Fig. 8.9). The acrylic cement is injected under fluoroscopic control, but concomitant CT guidance now appears mandatory to increase safety and efficacy (Gangi et al. 1994). Attention to asepsis is essential.

Equipment requirements are as follows:

- Size 10 G needles for treatment of lumbar or thoracic vertebrae. Smaller-gauge needles are less suitable owing to the "dough-like" consistency of the cement.

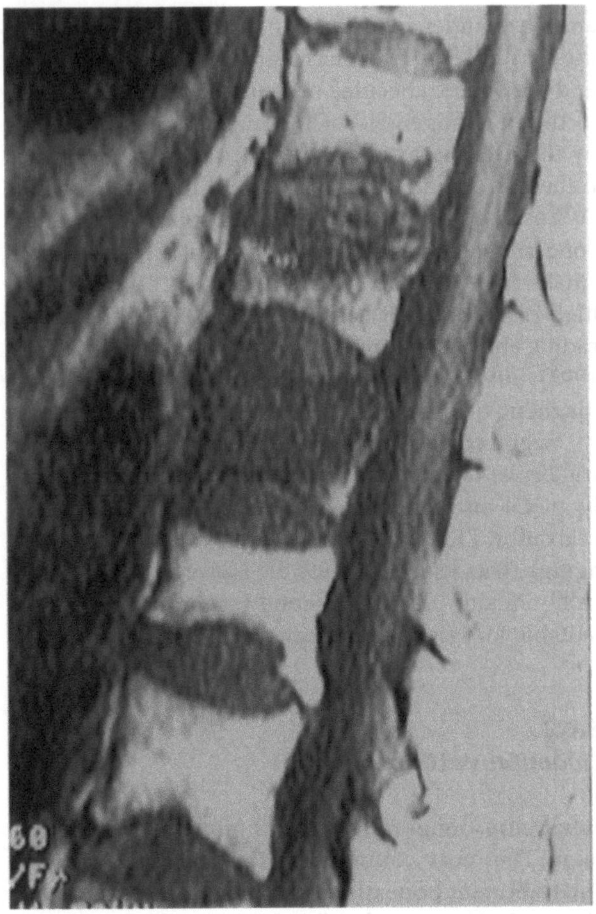

Fig. 8.8. Recent osteoporotic compression fracture of T12 and old compression fracture of T10

- A surgical mallet to facilitate vertebral puncture.
- Luer-Lok syringes (2 cc).
- A sphygmomanometer with an inflatable cuff for regulation of the injection pressure.
- Acrylic cement (methyl methacrylate).
- Tungsten powder to render the cement more opaque and thus facilitate visualization during fluoroscopic control.

Localization of the appropriate point of entry and determination of the ideal needle trajectory are essential for precisional insertion. The weakened vertebral body is punctured under CT guidance to avoid injury to adjacent structures (lung, pleura, spinal canal, spinal nerve roots). Intercostotransverse or transpedicular approaches are indicated for treatment of thoracic vertebrae; for the lumbar spine, transpedicular and posterolateral approaches give equivalent results.

Diffuse bone loss is managed by introducing the tip of the needle at the junction of the anterior third

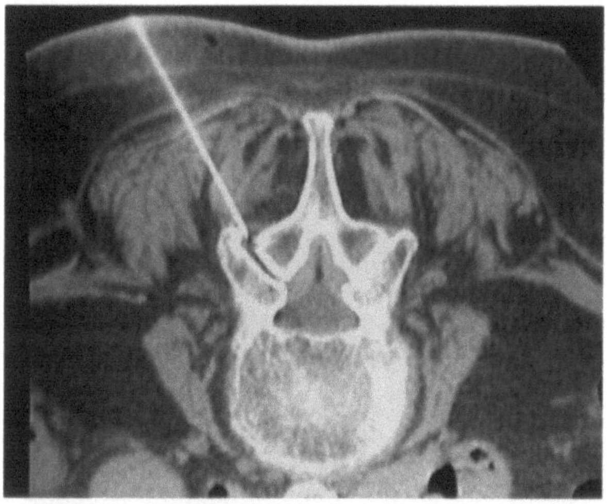
a

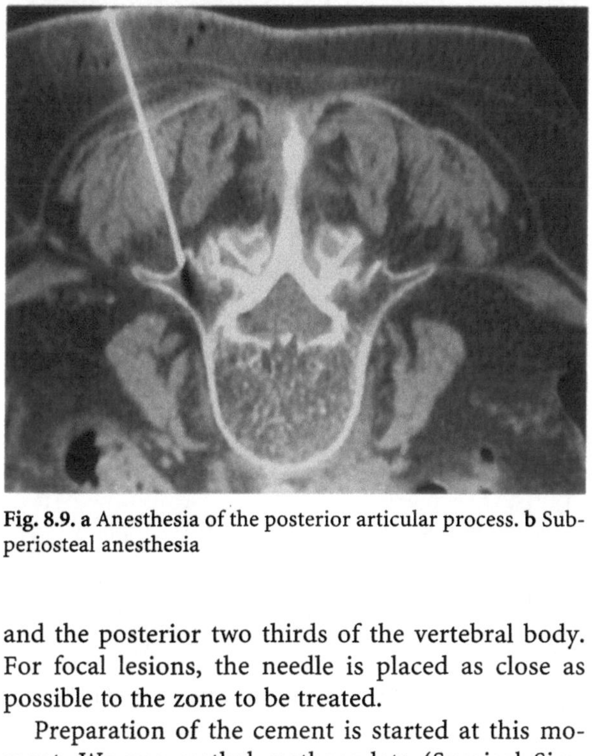
b

Fig. 8.9. a Anesthesia of the posterior articular process. b Subperiosteal anesthesia

and the posterior two thirds of the vertebral body. For focal lesions, the needle is placed as close as possible to the zone to be treated.

Preparation of the cement is started at this moment. We use methyl methacrylate (Surgical Simplex, Howmedica, Limerick, Ireland) to prepare a mixture of 20 volumes of powder, 5 volumes of solvent, and 2 g tungsten. The initially fluid mixture rapidly becomes dough-like as polymerization occurs. The cement is injected solely under fluoroscope control; CT control would waste valuable seconds. The posterior vertebral wall is kept under observation at all times; any leakage of cement into the epidural space requires immediate half of the procedure.

The cement hardens very rapidly (less than 3 min); polymerization prevents any supplementary injection. The amount of cement injected varies from 1 to 7 cc (mean 3 cc). Care must be taken to fill all empty areas; this may require a bilateral approach to the vertebra (Debusshe-Depriester et al. 1991; Cotten et al. 1996). The stylet must be placed back into the needle during withdrawal to prevent leakage into the soft tissues (Fig. 8.10).

Two or three vertebrae may be treated in a single session (Fig. 8.11). The patient is allowed to get up at the end of the day and can be discharged from the hospital the next morning.

8.5.3 Complications

Complications are possible but infrequent (Galibert and Deramond 1990; Gangi et al. 1994, 1996). During injection, cement may leak into the spinal canal. Such leaks may be due to a lesion of the posterior wall or, more often, to injection of excessively fluid cement that passes into a large drainage vein (Brunner et al. 1996; Fig. 8.12). Such incidents usually remain asymptomatic. Radiculalgia may occur, however, and exceptional cases of medullary compression may require neurosurgical decompression. Excessively fluid cement can migrate toward the azygos system or the inferior vena cava system and cause pulmonary embolism. Spondylitis infectiosa, the potential complication in these cases, can be prevented by surgical asepsis.

A drop in arterial pressure may occur during cement delivery. This rare complication has also been encountered by orthopedic surgeons during cement fixation of prostheses. Use of an automatic sphygmomanometer and the assistance of an anesthetist are thus recommended.

Distant compression fractures of fragile supra- or subjacent osteoporotic vertebrae may occur after contact with a very hard, cemented vertebra.

8.5.4 Results

Most reports on percutaneous vertebroplasty have been published by French teams. While the majority concern treatment of osteolytic metastases, the technique also gives spectacular results for osteoporotic fractures. Pain relief is often immediate and complete (Lapras et al. 1989; Galibert and Deramond et al. 1990). Rapid alleviation of pain is essentially due to decreased stimulation of the pain pathway fibers in the periosteum and osteoligamentous apparatus

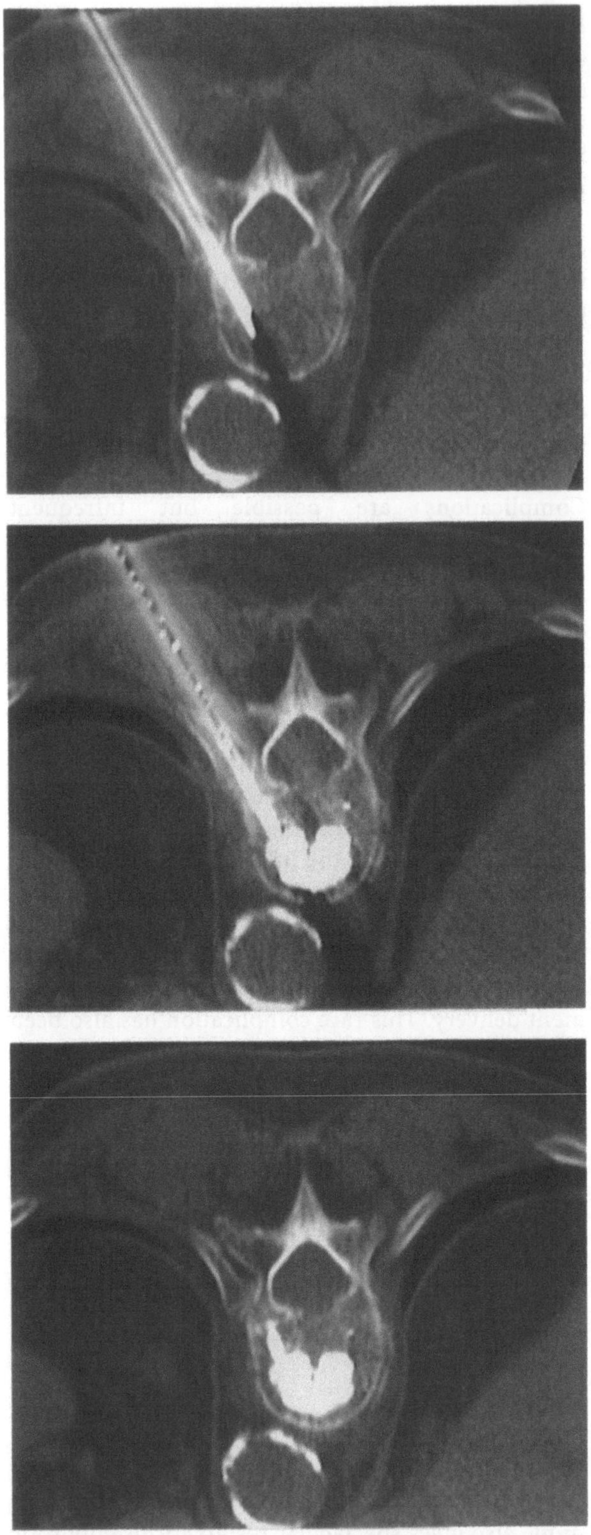

a

b

c

Fig. 8.10. **a** Correct positioning of the 10-G needle. **b** Filling of the vertebra with cement. **c** Final verification

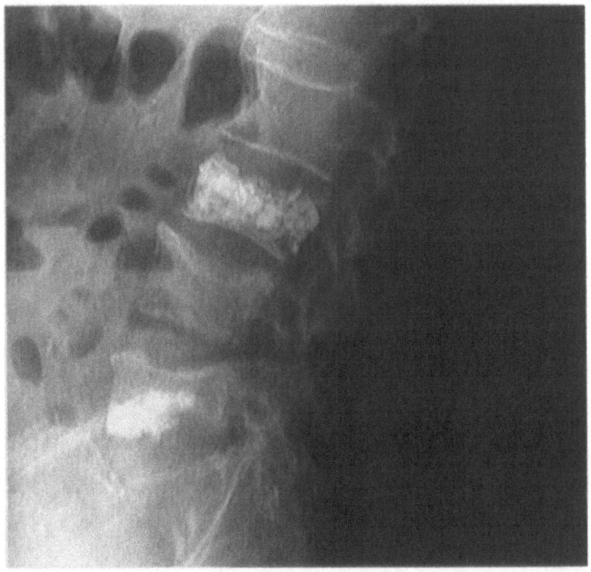

Fig. 8.11. Percutaneous vertebroplasty of L3 and L5

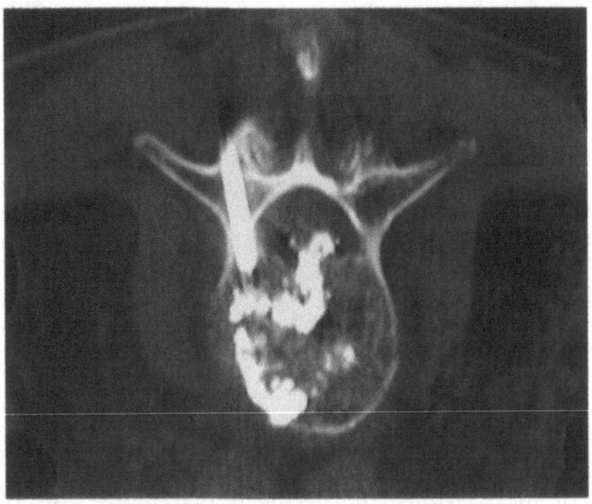

Fig. 8.12. Leakage of cement into the anterior epidural space

following reduction of the forces applied to the initially weak, deformable vertebral body that has been strengthened by the cement (Lapras et al. 1989). Vertebral consolidation is durable; loss of somatic height is stopped.

This technique permits early resumption of weight-bearing. Elevated patient age is thus not a limitation for the indication of the technique; on the contrary, it appears to be a privileged indication.

8.6 Conclusion

Osteoporosis has become a major public health problem in industrialized countries as the twentieth century draws to an end. Thanks to progress in techniques for measurement of bone mass, particularly DXA, the radiologist and the clinician can now take advantage of extremely rapid and reliable machines that provide high-quality images. Current research is[c] focused on the development of apparatus for structural bone measurements, especially those based on ultrasound, a less expensive and nonionizing technique.

Percutaneous vertebroplasty has enlarged our therapeutic arsenal for treatment of vertebral compression fractures, and more widespread use of this treatment alternative appears justified.

References

Barnett E, Nordin BE (1960) The radiological diagnosis of osteoporosis: a new approach. Clin Radiol 11:166–174

Brunner P, Gangi A, Dietmann JL, Mourou MY (1996) Imagerie dans la surveillance de l'ostéoporose sous traitement. In: Bruneton JN, Padovani B (eds) Imagerie en endocrinologie. Masson, Paris, pp 261–266

Cameron JR, Sorensen Y (1963) Measurement of bone mineral in vivo: an improved method. Science 142:230–236

Cortet B, Cotten A, Boutry N et al (1997) Percutaneous vertebroplasty in patients with osteolytic metastases or multiple myeloma. Rev Rhum 64:177–183

Cotten A, Dewatre F, Cortet B et al (1996) Percutaneous vertebroplasty for osteolytic metastases and myeloma: effects of the percentage of lesion filling and the leakage of methyl methacrylate at clinical follow-up. Radiology 200:525–530

Debusshe-Depriester C, Deramond H, Fardelone P et al (1991) Percutaneous vertebroplasty with acrylic cement in the treatment of osteoporosis vertebral crush fracture syndrome. Neuroradiology 33:149–152

Deramond H, Depriester C, Toussaint P (1996) Vertébroplastie et radiologie interventionnelle percutanée dans les métastases osseuses: technique, indications et contre-indications. Bull Cancer Radiother 83:277–282

Faulkner KG, Gluër C, Majumdar S, Lang P, Engelke K, Genant H (1991) Noninvasive measurements of bone mass, structure and strength: current methods and experimental techniques. AJR 157:1229–1237

Fuerst T, Gluër C, Genant HK (1995) Quantitative ultrasound. Eur J Radiol 20:188–192

Funke M, Kopka L, Vosshenrich R et al (1995) Broadband ultrasound attenuation in the diagnosis of osteoporosis: correlation with osteodensitometry and fracture. Radiology 194:77–81

Galibert P, Deramond H (1990) La vertébroplastie acrylique percutanée comme traitement des angiomes vertébraux et des affections dolorigènes et fragilisantes du rachis. Chirurgie 116:326–335

Galibert P, Deramond H, Rosat P et al (1987) Note préliminaire sur le traitement des hémangiomes vertébraux par vertébroplastie acrylique percutanée. Neurochirurgie 33:166–168

Gangi A, Kastler B, Klinkert A, Cejas C, Redondo W, Dietemann JL (1993) Percutaneous vertebroplasty guided by a combination of CT and fluoroscopy: technique and indications. Radiology 189(1):386

Gangi A, Kastler B, Dietemann JL (1994) Percutaneous vertebroplasty guided by a combination of CT and fluoroscopy. AJNR 15:83–86

Gangi A, Dietemann JL, Schultz A, Mortazavi R, Jeung MY, Roy C (1996) Interventional radiologic procedures with CT guidance in cancer pain management. Radiographics 16:1289–1304

Genant HK, Boyd D (1977) Quantitative bone mineral analysis using dual energy computed tomography. Invest Radiol 12:545–551

Gluër C, Cummings S, Bauer D et al (1996) Osteoporosis: association of recent fractures with quantitative US findings. Radiology 199:725–732

Grampp S, Jergas M, Lang P et al (1996a) Quantitative CT assessment of the lumbar spine and radius in patients with osteoporosis. AJR 167:133–140

Grampp S, Majumdar S, Jergas M, Newitt D, Lang P, Genant HK (1996b) Distal radius: in vivo assessment with quantitative MR imaging, peripheral quantitative CT, and dual X-ray absorptiometry. Radiology 198:213–218

Guglielmi G, Grimston S, Fischer K, Pacifici R (1995) Osteoporosis: diagnosis with lateral and posteroanterior dual X-ray absorptiometry compared with quantitative CT. Radiology 192:845–850

Ito M, Hayashi K, Vetani M, Jamada M, Okhi M, Nakamura T (1994) Association between anthropometric measures and spinal bone mineral density. Invest Radiol 29:812–816

Kalender W (1992) Effective dose values in bone mineral measurements by photon absorptiometry and computed tomography. Osteoporos Int 2:82–87

Kalender W, Felsenberg D, Louis O, Klotz E, Osteaux M, Fraga Y (1990) Reference values for trabecular and cortical bone density in single and dual energy QCT. Eur J Radiol 9:75–80

Langton C, Palmer S, Porter R (1984) The measurement of broadband ultrasonic attenuation in cancellous bone. Engl Med 13:89–91

Lapras C, Mottolese C, Deruty R, Lapras, Remond J, Duquesnel J (1989) Injection percutanée de méthyl-métacrylate dans le traitement de l'ostéoporose et ostéolyse vertébrale grave (technique de P.Galibert). Ann Chir 43:371–376

Laugier P, Droin P, Laval-Jeantet AM, Berger C (1997) In vitro assessment of the relationship between acoustic properties and bone mass density of the calcaneus by comparison of ultrasound parametric imaging and quantitative computed tomography. Bone 20:157–165

Louis O, Luypaert R, Kalender W, Osteaux M (1988) Reproducibility of CT bone densitometry: operator versus automated ROI definition. Eur J Radiol 8:82–84

Louis O, Vandenwinkel P, Covens P, Schoutens A, Osteaux M (1992) Dual energy X-ray absorptiometry of lumbar vertebrae: relative contribution of body and posterior elements and accuracy in relation with neutron activation analysis. Bone 13:317–320

Majumdar S, Genant HK (1995) Magnetic resonance imaging in osteoporosis. Eur J Radiol 20:193–197

Mazess RB, Ort M, Judy P (1970) Absorptiometric bone mineral determination using 153 Gd. In: Cameron JR (ed) Proceedings of the Bone Measurement Conference. US Atomic Energy Commission, Washington DC, pp 308–312

Mazess RB, Collie KB, Barden H, Hanson J (1989) Performance evaluation of a dual-energy X-ray bone densitometer. Calcif Tissue Int 44:228–232

Pacifici R, Rupich R, Griggin M, Chines A, Susman N, Avioli LV (1990) Dual energy radiography versus quantitative computer tomography for the diagnosis of osteoporosis. J Clin Endocrinol Metab 70:705–709

Porter RW, Miller CG, Grainger D, Palmer SB (1990) Prediction of hip fracture in elderly women: a prospective study. BMJ 6753:638–641

Prentice A, Parsons Y, Cole T (1994) Uncritical use of bone mineral density in absorptiometry may lead to size-related artefacts in the identification of bone mineral determinants. Am J Clin Nutr 60:837–842

Reed GW (1966) The assessment of bone mineralisation from the relative transmission of 241Am and 137Cs radiations. Phys Med Biol 11:174

Rüegsegger P (1988) Quantitative computed tomography at peripheral measuring sites. Ann Chir Gynecol 77:204–207

Sabin MA, Blake GM, MacLauglin-Black M, Fogelman I (1995) The accuracy of volumetric density measurements in dual X-ray absorptiometry. Calcif Tissue Int 56:210–214

Schneider P, Berger P (1988) Knochendichtebestimmung mit der quantitativ ausgewerten CT und einem Spezialscanner. Nuklearmediziner 11:145–152

Schoutens A (1993) Mesure de la densité minérale de la colonne lombaire: expression des résultats. Rev Med Brux 14:187–189

Tothill P, Avenell A, Reid D (1994) Precision and accuracy of measurement of whole-body bone mineral: comparison between hologic, nuclear and Nordland dual-energy X-ray absorptiometers. Br J Radiol 67:1210–1217

Trevisan C, Bigoni M, Cherubini R, Steiger P, Randelli G, Ortolani S (1993) Dual X-ray absorptiometry for the evaluation of bone density from the proximal femur after total hip arthroplasty: analysis protocols and reproductibility. Calcif Tissue Int 53:158–161

Ventura V, Mauloni M, Mura M, Paltrinieri F, De Aloysio D (1996) Ultrasound velocity changes at the proximal phalanxes of the hand in pre, peri and postmenopausal women. Osteoporos Int 6:368–375

Wahner H, Morin R, Dunn W, Brown M, Riggs B (1988) Dual energy radiography for bone mineral anlaysis of the lumbar spine. J Nucl Med 29:855–858

Wehrli F, Ford Y, Chung H et al (1993) Potential role of nuclear magnetic resonance for the evaluation of trabecular bone quality. Calcif Tissue Int 53:162–169

Wehrli F, Ford J, Haddad J (1995) Osteoporosis: clinical assessment with quantitative MR imaging in diagnosis. Radiology 196:631–641

9 Male Infertility

L. BOYER, A. RAVEL, and J.F. VIALLET

CONTENTS

9.1 Introduction

Infertility is a complex and often multifactorial problem requiring coordinated management by a multidisciplinary team including one or more radiologists. In up to 50% of cases, the problem is partially or totally due to the male partner (Ross 1983; Pontonnier and Bujan. 1993). Semen analysis and the postcoital Huhner test are the initial techniques for assessment of an infertile couple (Belaisch 1987; Nys et al. 1992). If these examinations are abnormal, the cause should be sought in the male partner.

Thorough physical examination and laboratory tests (hormone profile, semen analysis and biochemical assays, spermoculture, urinary microbiology, karyotype) allow several different conditions to be defined:

- Secretory azoospermia: abnormal spermatogenesis may have a peripheral gonadal origin or may be due to hypogonadotropic hypothalamopituitary dysfunction.
- Excretory azoospermia due to impaired sperm transport.
- Oligoasthenoteratospermia, characterized by multiple causes of infertility. Male factors include cytological sperm anomalies, antisperm antibodies, varicocele, inadequate gonadotrophin activity, hyperprolactinemia, primary Sertoli cell or Leydig cell insufficiencies, genetic disorders, chronic genital infections, etc.
- Apparently normal semen, even after the most sophisticated tests.

Imaging studies of the hypothalamopituitary axis and the testes are discussed elsewhere in this book. This chapter is thus limited to imaging of the seminal ducts and diagnostic and interventional radiologic techniques for varicocele.

L. BOYER, A. RAVEL, J.F. VIALLET, Service de Radiologie et d'Imagerie Médicale, Hôpital G. Montpied, 30 place H. Dunant, BP 69, 63003 Clermont-Ferrand, France

9.2 Excretory Infertility

Azoospermia (or severe oligospermia) in a patient with a normal follicle-stimulating hormone (FSH) concentration is suggestive of excretory infertility.

Anejaculation has various origins. Retrograde ejaculation (due to prior prostate resection or pelvic surgery or to neurologic lesions associated with spinal trauma, diabetes, or multiple sclerosis) and psychogenic anejaculation can cause aspermia or hypospermia (ejaculate volume, <2 ml). Postejaculatory urinalysis confirms the absence of sperm.

Ejaculatory duct obstruction can interfere with sperm transit. Diagnosis of obstruction, which is curable in certain cases, relies on the following:

- Physical examination (scrotum, deferent ducts, digital examination of the rectum).
- Determination of the volume of ejaculate. Azoospermia and oligospermia despite a normal ejaculate volume indicate a testicular or scrotal origin. A reduced volume of ejaculate may be due to occlusion of the distal seminal tract or retrograde ejaculation.
- Sperm biochemistry using various markers: carnitine and a-glucosidase for the epididymis, fructose and the pH value for the seminal vesicles, and zinc and citric acid for the prostate.

Ultrasound can effectively explore the entire male genital system except for the deferent ducts and is therefore indicated as the first-line imaging modality. Performed with a high-frequency transducer (5–10 MHz), scrotal ultrasound depicts the normal testis as a homogeneous ovoid structure of intermediate echogenicity and of the same size as the contralateral testis. The normal testis measures 30–50 mm in length and 20–40 mm in transverse diameter. The mediastinum testis may be visible as an echoic eccentric craniocaudal line appearing slightly thicker in its cranial portion. The regular contours are sharply demarcated by the tunica albuginea testis, visualized as a thin echoic rim. The normal epididymis is homogeneous, with an echogenicity similar to that of the testis. The head (1–1.2 cm in diameter) and the tail (0.5 cm) can be discerned, but the body usually cannot be identified.

Transrectal sonography (TRS) allows comprehensive evaluation of the urogenital region; high frequencies permit multiplanar imaging. TRS is often complemented by color Doppler (CD). In addition to the prostate, the following structures are analyzed:

- The seminal vesicles: the echotexture of the normal seminal vesicles is variable, but they are symmetrical in both contents and size. Mean normal dimensions are: height, 19±1.6 mm; transverse length, 7.5±1.3 mm; width (thickness), 2.7±0.45 mm (Carter et al. 1989). Size and appearance vary with the duration of abstinence from sex; awareness of this interval is indispensable for correct image interpretation.
- The ampullae of the deferent ducts: these can be seen on transverse scans along the internal border of the seminal vesicles (3–5 mm in diameter)
- The ejaculatory ducts: these paired structures located in the region of the verumontanum course from the seminal vesicles into the urethra along an oblique sagittal path. These ducts are not always visible; in the normal state, their lumen may measure up to 2 mm in diameter (Kuligowska 1994).

Examination of the lower genitourinary tract must be complemented by renal sonography to search for coexistent anomalies, especially in patients with agenesis, hypoplasia, or a seminal vesicle cyst.

Computed tomography (CT) of the seminal vesicles is generally unsatisfactory because of insufficient tissue contrast. By contrast, magnetic resonance imaging (MRI) is an excellent complement to ultrasound, particularly when performed with an endorectal coil allowing multiplanar imaging. Fast T_2-weighted spin-echo sequences provide excellent contrast of pelvic structures.

Performed by surgical puncture under general anesthesia, vesiculo-deferentography allows direct evaluation of the patency of the deferent duct along its entire course. However, ductal stenosis or occlusion due to secondary fibrosis can complicate the examination.

Transrectal or perineal ultrasound-guided puncture of the seminal vesicles has been proposed for semen aspiration and vesiculography because this method obviates the need for scrototomy (Cornud et al. 1996; Kim and Lipschultz 1996).

9.2.1 Epididymis

Congenital malformations include absence of communication between the rete testis and the epididymis (in which case epididymal markers may be normal) and congenital anomalies of the epididymis itself (fibrous stenosis of the body or agenesis of a segment). Scrotal sonography may demonstrate distention of the upstream canaliculi. Hypertrophy of the globus major epididymis (proximal portion of the head of epididymis) is suggestive of this latter anomaly.

Acquired lesions include the sequelae of epididymitis. Echogenic nodules, sometimes containing calcifications, may be accompanied by upstream dilatation of the seminal vesicle and hypertrophy of the proximal epididymis. Tuberculosis typically causes bipolar nodules, but may also involve the entire epididymis; intravenous pyelography (IVP) is required because of the presence of multifocal urogenital lesions.

In Berry-Perkins-Young syndrome, azoospermia due to progressive distention of the canaliculi of the head of epididymis is a manifestation of a respiratory disorder distinct from cystic fibrosis.

Enlargement of the head of the epididymis may reflect a downstream obstruction. A cystic image may correspond to a true serous cyst or a spermatocele (containing sperm) favored by the obstruction; these entities cannot be differentiated by imaging.

9.2.2 Deferent Ducts

Congenital Lesions. Congenital unilateral agenesis of the deferent ducts is observed in one to seven men per 1000. Congenital bilateral absence of both deferent ducts occurs in 1% of infertile men and accounts for 4%–17% of all cases of azoospermia. This malformation is found in 98% of male patients with cystic fibrosis (CORNUD et al. 1996). Furthermore, 16%–43% of all male patients with bilateral duct agenesis also have renal anomalies such as agenesis (always unilateral) (CORNUD et al. 1996) or ectopia, usually on the left side (KULIGOWSKA 1994). The deferent ducts are not palpable, and the epididymal heads are dilated.

A diagnosis of agenesis should be considered if TRS fails to visualize the ampullae of the deferent ducts or the seminal vesicles, typically associated with dilatation of the tubules of the epididymal head. However, visualization of an atrophic or dilated seminal vesicle does not rule out the diagnosis.

Bilateral agenesis of the deferent ducts may be associated with cystic fibrosis. The diagnosis must be formally established before in vivo fertilization is envisaged (PONTONNIER and BUJAN 1993; CORNUD et al. 1996). Genetic screening of the couple is necessary. Renal sonography is especially important, because demonstration of associated renal agenesis (a developmental anomaly of the mesonephros) probably suffices to rule out cystic fibrosis.

Endorectal MRI is useful whenever the junction between the seminal vesicle and the deferent duct cannot be evaluated by ultrasound.

Acquired Lesions. The patency of the deferent ducts may be altered by the sequelae of infections. In patients with a history of inguinal or scrotal surgery, the possibility of accidental section (BOYER et al. 1990) or adhesions must be entertained. Sonographic depiction of global distention of the epididymis suggests the diagnosis. In cases of long-standing obstruction, rupture of the duct of epididymus due to excessive pressure may result in sclerosis visualized as a focus of hyperechogenicity. Vesiculo-deferentography is required to localize the obstruction.

9.2.3 Seminal Vesicles

Congenital Anomalies (Fig. 9.1). The term "absent seminal vesicle" refers to cases where these structures are not identified or exist solely as minute vestiges. The term "hypoplastic seminal vesicle" refers to structures with a volume 30% below normal (KULIGOWSKA et al. 1992).

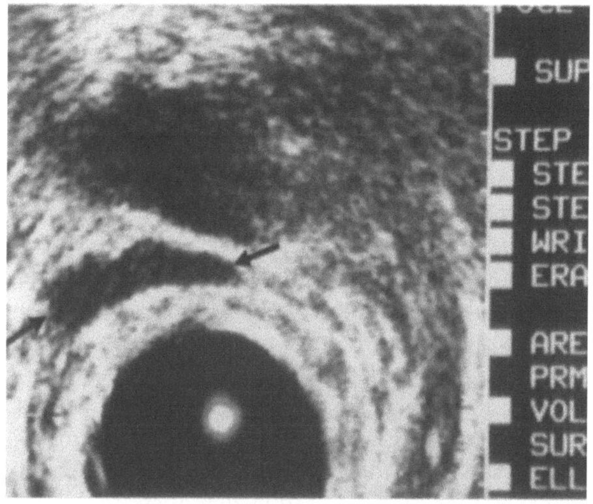

Fig. 9.1. Severe oligospermia. Transverse transrectal sonography (TRS) demonstrates absence of the left seminal vesicle. Right seminal vesicle (*arrows*)

Seminal fluid fructose tests are not always sensitive (BOYER et al. 1994), even though seminal vesicle anomalies are frequent findings. In one of our own series of 91 patients with normal FSH levels examined for oligozoospermia, TRS successfully diagnosed 18 congenital anomalies (no seminal vesicles seen in two patients, only one seminal vesicle seen in eight patients, two atretic seminal vesicles in two patients, one atrophic seminal vesicle in six patients) (BOYER et al. 1994). In a series of 85 patients with azoospermia or severe oligospermia, CARTER et al. (1989) failed to visualize either seminal vesicle in 12 patients. One seminal vesicle was absent in 18 patients, bilateral atrophy was noted in six, and unilateral atrophy was observed in 19.

Congenital seminal vesicle anomalies are frequently associated with malformations of the deferent ducts.

In a group of 40 patients with atresia or agenesis of a deferent duct, TRS demonstrated absence of the seminal vesicles in 21 patients, an atrophic seminal vesicle in eight patients, a thin seminal vesicle in four patients, dilated seminal vesicles in four other patients, and normal seminal vesicles in three patients (CARTER et al. 1989). The seminal vesicles were thin in nine of the 21 patients with an epididymal obstruction. These authors concluded that absence or atrophy of a seminal vesicle associated with failure to visualize a deferent duct is indicative of agenesis, whereas thin or dilated seminal vesicles may be due to a curable obstruction and thus warrant additional investigation by vesiculo-deferentography.

Agenesis of the seminal vesicles and deferent ducts may be accompanied by other sonographically visible developmental anomalies, such as partial agenesis of the epididymis (CARTER et al. 1989; SANDERS 1991) or ipsilateral renal agenesis (PATEL et al. 1987; ABBITT et al. 1991). Agenesis of the ejaculatory ducts is commonly associated with seminal vesicle malformations.

Whether acquired or congenital, seminal vesicle cysts may obstruct the ejaculatory ducts. Congenital seminal vesicle cysts require a search for ipsilateral renal dysgenesis and ectopic ureteral abouchement, which are often associated with such cysts. These cysts may play a role in infertility by reducing the volume of ejaculate (CARVALHO et al. 1986). The origin of small seminal vesicle cysts is readily demonstrated. MRI may prove useful for very large cysts (Fig. 9.2).

Infections. Infection of the seminal vesicles may cause fibrous changes leading to cystic dilatation, obliteration, and/or luminal stenosis. In these cases, the seminal vesicle may image as an inhomogeneous echogenic structure without its typical morphologic features (BOYER et al. 1994; KULIGOWSKA 1994). Infection may also lead to the formation of lithiases in the distal segment of the deferent duct or in the region of the ampulla; these lesions are visible on sonograms as echogenic foci with a posterior shadow.

Chronic inflammatory processes may impair seminal vesicle function, leading to infertility (KULIGOWSKA 1994). Comparison of the volume of the seminal vesicles before and after semen analysis by TRS has been proposed for dynamic evaluation of seminal vesicle drainage (LARDENNOIS et al. 1986).

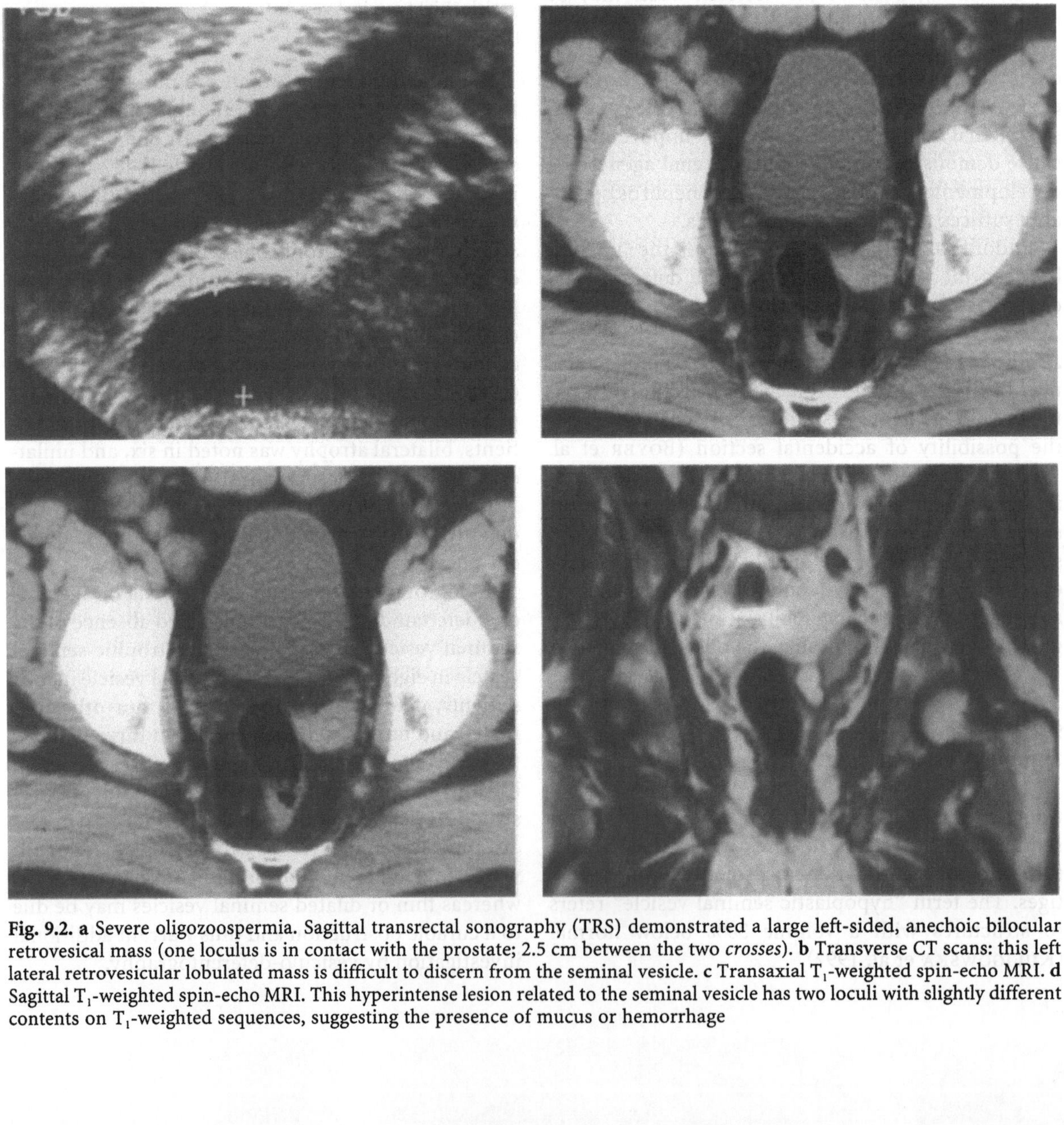

a b c d

Fig. 9.2. **a** Severe oligozoospermia. Sagittal transrectal sonography (TRS) demonstrated a large left-sided, anechoic bilocular retrovesical mass (one loculus is in contact with the prostate; 2.5 cm between the two *crosses*). **b** Transverse CT scans: this left lateral retrovesicular lobulated mass is difficult to discern from the seminal vesicle. **c** Transaxial T_1-weighted spin-echo MRI. **d** Sagittal T_1-weighted spin-echo MRI. This hyperintense lesion related to the seminal vesicle has two loculi with slightly different contents on T_1-weighted sequences, suggesting the presence of mucus or hemorrhage

For COLPI et al. (1987), the presence of anechoic fluid zones within the seminal vesicles reflects poor drainage. Impairment of seminal vesicle contraction has been reported in patients with diabetic neuropathy (PRYOR and HENDRY 1990; CORNUD et al. 1996).

9.2.4 Ejaculatory Ducts

Agenesis is frequently associated with seminal vesicle malformations or dilatation (BOYER et al. 1990). Stenosis may be suggested clinically by azoospermia, a reduced volume of ejaculate with an acid pH that lacks fructose, and a palpable deferent duct.

Dilatation of the ejaculatory ducts is occasionally pseudocystic (MEACHAM et al. 1995); it may be associated with hypotrophy or dilatation of the seminal vesicles. TRS demonstration of dilatation of the ampulla of the deferent duct and the seminal vesicles suggests a distal obstruction (Fig. 9.3). This finding is nonspecific, however, because cystic dilatation of the ejaculatory ducts and the ampulla is occasionally observed in physiological conditions (CORNUD et al. 1993).

Causes of ejaculatory duct obstruction in young infertile men include lithiasis (SANDERS 1991), infection (BOYER et al. 1994), prior surgery (especially correction of a rectal anomaly or ablation of a seminal vesicle cyst in childhood) (PRYOR and HENDRY 1990), and cysts. True seminal vesicle cysts (acquired or congenital), müllerian duct cysts, utricle cysts, and parautricle cysts can all be analyzed by ultrasound-guided fine-needle aspiration (FNA) (SHABSIGH et al. 1989; STASI et al. 1989). Differentiation from prostatic cysts can be difficult.

More frequently than was previously thought, ejaculatory duct obstruction is sometimes amenable to surgical cure, e.g., by TRS-guided endoscopy (MEACHAM et al. 1995; KIM and LIPSCHULTZ 1996).

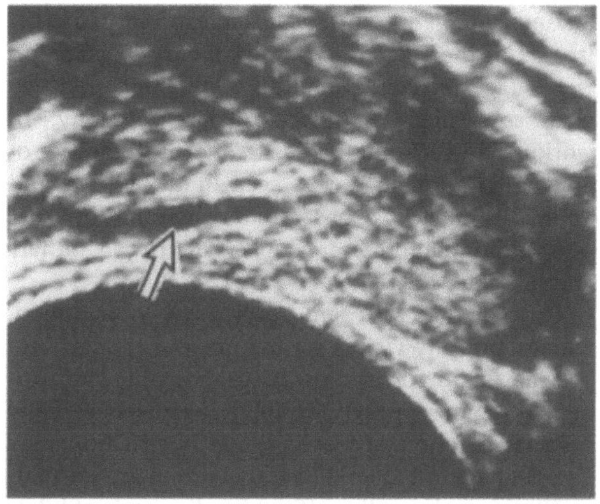

Fig. 9.3. Azoospermia with reduced volume of ejaculate. Sagittal transrectal sonography (TRS) reveals dilatation of the ejaculatory duct (*arrow*) and the seminal vesicles, suggesting a distal obstruction

9.2.5 Prostate

Intraprostatic obstruction can be caused by cysts or scar tissue secondary to infection, sometimes with lithiasis (RIFKIN 1988; KULIGOWSKA 1994). Although ultrasound cannot determine their role in impaired fertility, sonographically visible prostate anomalies are frequently observed during infertility workups. Among 91 patients with clinically suspected excretory infertility, 49 were found to have anomalies on sonograms (eight with solitary calcifications, 25 with solitary or multiple hypoechoic zones, 12 with hyperechoic foci with or without calcifications, and four with prostate enlargement; BOYER et al. 1994).

MRI appears to be much more sensitive than ultrasound for the detection of diffuse or multifocal foci of low signal intensity in the periphery of the prostate in patients with chronic prostatitis (CORNUD et al. 1996).

9.2.6 Indications for Imaging Studies

Excretory infertility has a number of curable causes. As clinical affirmation of the presence or absence of the deferent ducts is difficult, imaging studies efficiently contribute to evaluation of the epididymis and the urogenital region.

TRS and scrotal sonography are first-line imaging modalities that often detect anomalies. In 70 patients with suspected excretory infertility, KULIGOWSKA et al. (1992) observed bilateral absence of the deferent ducts in 26, unilateral absence of the deferent duct associated with a contralateral obstruction in 11, and other obstructive anomalies in 15 patients (bilateral in 13 out of 15 cases); no significant anomaly was found in the remaining 18 patients. CORNUD et al. (1994a) observed suggestive sonographic patterns in the 12 patients with agenesis of the deferent ducts among 25 patients with suspected excretory infertility. Six of the eight stenoses secondary to infection were suggested sonographically, while the other two were confirmed by vesiculo-deferentography. In workups for 91 similar patients, images suggestive of congenital anomalies were seen in 18 patients and anomalies suggestive of seminal vesicle and/or prostate inflammation were observed in 44 others (Boyer et al. 1994).

In patients with an epididymal obstruction, sonographically visible scrotal anomalies may suggest an acquired or congenital anomaly. The urogenital region appears normal in the absence of any associated lesion. An epididymal obstruction may escape diagnosis if epididymal markers are normal.

Ultrasound usually suffices for diagnosis of bilateral agenesis of the seminal vesicles and deferent ducts. In the absence of renal agenesis, the possibility of a genital manifestation of cystic fibrosis must be entertained, and genetic counseling is necessary before in vitro fertilization is attempted (Pontonnier and Bujan 1993; Cornud et al. 1996).

If sonography remains inconclusive for the localization of a distal obstruction, MRI can accurately determine the size of large cystic lesions of the urogenital junction and demonstrate the lesion's anatomic relationships before surgical treatment is attempted (length of the stenosis, distance between the prostatic urethra and the cyst wall) (Cornud et al. 1996). MRI can also better analyze inflammatory changes in the prostate and seminal vesicles.

Today, vesiculo-deferentography should be reserved for those cases where physical examination and noninvasive imaging remain indeterminate (Boyer et al. 1990; Kim and Lipschultz 1996). The technique should be integrated into surgical management. Puncture of the seminal vesicles for sampling of semen and vesiculography has been proposed as an alternative to vesiculo-deferentography.

Although bilateral anomalies may be directly implicated in infertility, unilateral lesions usually do not explain functional anomalies. However, unilateral agenesis of the seminal vesicle and deferent duct may be associated with a contralateral obstruction of another nature (Kuligowska et al. 1992).

9.3 Varicoceles and Infertility

A varicocele is an abnormal dilatation of the veins of the pampiniform plexus that can extend from the internal spermatic vein to its opening in the renal vein and the vena cava. Varicoceles are much more frequent on the left side, but they may be bilateral. Several causes have been identified: an aortomesenteric vascular clip compressing the renal vein, valvular incompetence of the spermatic vein, and an elevated hydrostatic venous pressure in the upright position.

In patients with bilateral varicoceles, certain authors consider the left-sided varicocele the main lesion. Right-sided varicoceles, like varicosities of the deferent ducts, are the consequence of efferent flow owing to the existence of left–right scrotal anastomoses.

Observed in 10%–15% of adult males, varicoceles are commonly associated with complaints of pain, scrotal enlargement, or testicular atrophy, but they are not always symptomatic.

Although a varicocele does not necessarily cause male infertility, these lesions are observed in 20%–40% of infertile men (Demas et al. 1991). A number of possible mechanisms have been implicated in the resultant oligoasthenoteratospermia, e.g., increased scrotal temperature, venous reflux exposing the testicle to adrenal or renal metabolites that interfere with sperm formation, peritesticular venous blood stasis, immunological mechanisms.

9.3.1 Diagnosis

Physical examination in the upright position, before and during a Valsalva maneuver, is usually diagnostic. The potential role of subclinical varicoceles in infertility and the fact that bilateral anomalies are probably underestimated explain the value of imaging techniques for diagnosis and pretherapy workup.

Despite a reported accuracy of 98.4% in 118 patients in whom varicocele is clinically suspected compared with spermatic venography (Hamm et al. 1986), thermography remains controversial and use of this technique has declined considerably.

Color Doppler (CD) is currently the first-line imaging modality. Morphological analysis includes the systematic search for a renal anomaly (tumor), evaluation of the renal veins, and assessment of scrotal contents (especially the size of the testes). Demonstration of a tortuous, often irregular anechoic structure at least 4 mm in diameter that enlarges after initiation of a Valsalva maneuver and persists for the entire duration of the test, but decreases in size as soon as the maneuver is stopped (Fig. 9.4), is suggestive of varicocele (Pascal Suisse et al. 1986).

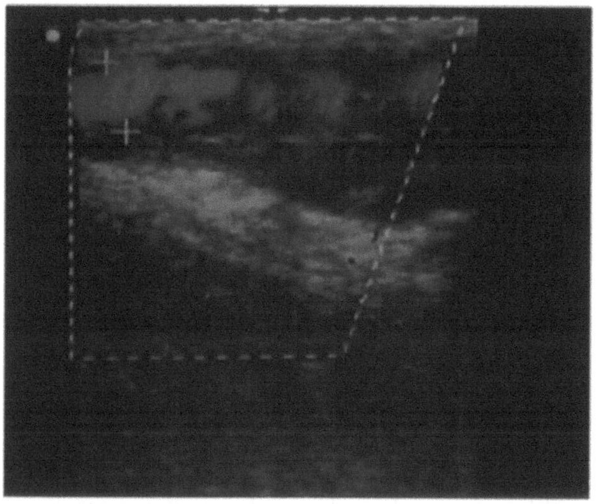

Fig. 9.4. Discomfort during sports in this 12-year-old boy suggested a varicocele: color Doppler (CD) demonstrated persistent venous reflux during a Valsalva maneuver

After localization of the artery, venous reflux is analyzed by examining the patient by duplex Doppler or CD in the dorsal decubitus position during the Valsalva maneuver. Retrograde blood flow (seen as an inversion of the color signal) indicates venous incompetence. CORNUD et al. (1994a) defined three patterns: (1) the probably physiologic transient reflux visible at initiation of the Valsalva maneuver, (2) a decreasing reflux that does not persist during the Valsalva maneuver (the significance of this observation is not univocal; less than half of the cases are associated with venous incompetence on spermatic phlebography, and this pattern can persist during Doppler studies performed after embolization), and (3) permanent reflux that persists during the entire Valsalva maneuver. Permanent reflux is probably the only type that warrants treatment, because it is always associated with venous incompetence, as demonstrated by spermatic venography.

CD is indicated if doubt persists after physical examination. Whenever a left-sided varicocele is incriminated during an infertility workup, it should probably not be treated alone until right-side CD is performed.

Spermatic venography, the current gold standard for diagnosis of varicocele, allows effective pretherapy vascular mapping. This examination is indispensable for evaluation of recurrence after surgical ligation of a varicocele. It may also constitute the initial step in percutaneous embolization.

Performed under local anesthesia, spermatic venography requires transfemoral catheterization (Seldinger's method) of the ostium of the spermatic vein. On the left side, the catheter is introduced into the left renal vein. The orifice of the genital vein is then sought at its anteroinferior border. If this approach fails, an attempt to identify the orifice can be made by opacifying the left renal vein. On the right side, the abouchement of the spermatic vein is sought at the level of the right renal vein (10% of cases). If this approach is not successful, the right anterior border of the infrarenal inferior vena cava is explored. Anatomic variants and the high incidence of valvulation explain the lower success rate on the right than on the left. Two injections of contrast material (10 ml) are then given at a rate of 3–5 ml/s centered first on the lumbar segment and then the pelvic segments of the internal spermatic vein.

An enlarged venous diameter or a varicose or avalvular appearance may be demonstrated. Retrograde flow of contrast material into the spermatic vein is seen only in patients with a varicocele. However, visualization of reflux may not reflect physiological conditions if the catheter is too distal beyond the valvules (DEMAS et al. 1991). SIGMUND et al. (1987b) distinguished two types of varicocele: the stop type, where reflux occurs only in the spermatic vein (subclinical varicoceles are usually of the stop type according to DHABUWALA and PARULKAR 1994), and the shunt type, where retrograde venous blood flow into the internal spermatic vein is followed by anterograde flow into the deferential, cremasteric, or external pudendal veins, which are generally anastomosed (SIGMUND et al. 1989).

Spermatic venograms can also demonstrate anastomoses and collateral venous circulation. In a series of 171 left-sided and 43 right-sided varicoceles, 19% and 17%, respectively, had an aberrant afferent blood supply. Retrograde flow occurred into the internal spermatic vein despite competent valves because of the presence of bypassing anastomoses (MARSMAN 1995).

9.3.2 Interventional Angiography: Percutaneous Sclerotherapy

9.3.2.1 Technique

Percutaneous sclerotherapy is performed under local anesthesia as a prolongation of spermatic venography, either on an outpatient basis or during brief hospitalization. After diagnostic injections, selective distal catheterization is performed up to the pelvic segment of the spermatic vein (Fig. 9.5).

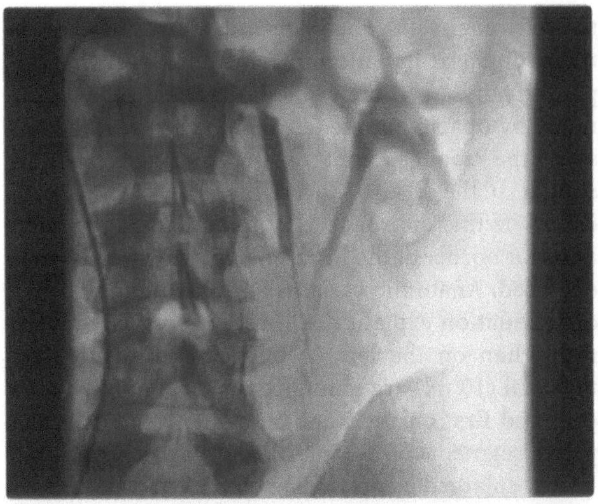

a

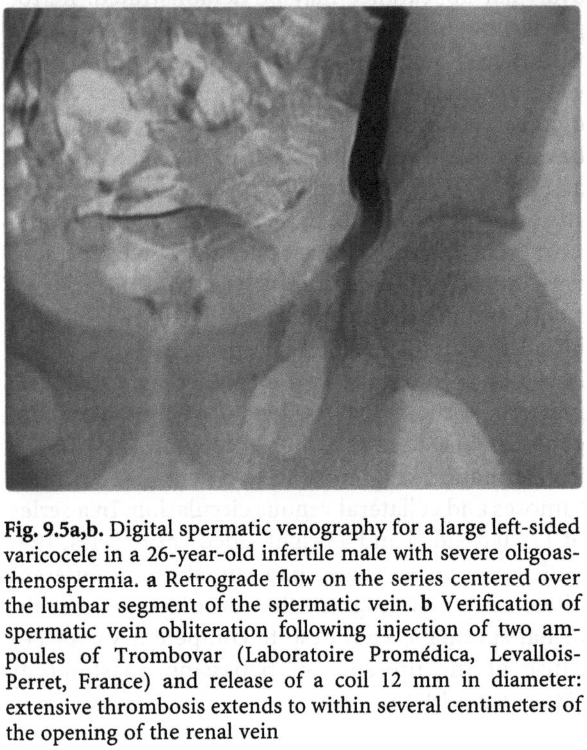

b

Fig. 9.5a,b. Digital spermatic venography for a large left-sided varicocele in a 26-year-old infertile male with severe oligoasthenospermia. **a** Retrograde flow on the series centered over the lumbar segment of the spermatic vein. **b** Verification of spermatic vein obliteration following injection of two ampoules of Trombovar (Laboratoire Promédica, Levallois-Perret, France) and release of a coil 12 mm in diameter: extensive thrombosis extends to within several centimeters of the opening of the renal vein

A variety of embolic agents have been used for spermatic vein obliteration, e.g., hot contrast material, Ivalon (Ingenor, Paris, France), detachable balloons, biologic glue. Numerous authors now use sclerosing agents (e.g., Varicocid, Star, Tampere, Finland; Aethoxysklerol, Dexo, Nanterre, France; Trombovar, Laboratoire Promédica, Levallois-Perret, France), completed when necessary by coil embolization.

Slow injection (several minutes) of one to three ampoules of 3% tetradecyl sodium sulfate (Trombovar) is recommended downstream of the sacroiliac joint. The spermatic vein is compressed at the level of the inguinal canal to prevent intrascrotal reflux. When the spermatic vein is large, coils are released as a supplementary measure.

9.3.2.2
Results

Zuckerman et al. (1994) cited a technical failure rate of only 4.3% in a series of 582 embolizations. Complications are rare, and the postoperative course is usually uneventful. Sigmund et al. (1987a) reported 24 cases of vessel perforation in a series of 717 percutaneous retrograde venographies. Of the 557 patients in this same series who underwent percutaneous sclerotherapy, three experienced acute peroperative inguinoscrotal pain; 43 patients had painless induration of the pampiniform plexus (associated with enlargement of the epididymis in nine patients). Sclerotherapy was impossible in 84 patients because catheterization of the spermatic vein was not selective enough; in 30 other patients, abundant collaterals precluded sclerotherapy. A total of 37 recurrences (9.8%) were found at follow-up 3 months after treatment.

Technical results are the least satisfactory when the main trunk of the spermatic vein has an intact valve but avalvular collaterals cannot be catheterized and establish communication between the spermatic vein and segmental renal or retroperitoneal veins. In a series of 386 patients treated by percutaneous sclerotherapy for idiopathic varicocele, the 73 patients with the Bahren type IVb anatomic variant of spermatic vein accounted for 54% of all failures and 67% of all vessel perforations (Lenz et al. 1996).

Sclerotherapy of the proximal segment of the spermatic vein reportedly involves a greater risk of recurrence owing to the frequency of collateral vessels (Hamm et al. 1986; Fobbe et al. 1987).

Using CD, Cornud et al. (1994) observed persistent permanent reflux after embolization in 6% of patients and anomalies in 20%, including decreasing reflux. Twelve months after percutaneous sclerotherapy for left-sided varicocele in 68 patients, Winkelbauer et al. (1994) demonstrated reflux reflecting a persistent varicocele or recurrence in 29% of cases with Doppler ultrasound. Trombetta et al. (1993) observed a varicocele on scrotal sonograms and Doppler studies in two of 16 patients (12.5%) 6 years after percutaneous sclerotherapy.

Embolization appears effective in alleviating the pain associated with varicoceles. Zuckerman et al.

(1994) embolized ten varicoceles solely because of their painful nature, and eight of the ten patients reported disappearance of this symptom.

Despite the generally admitted benefits of surgical ligation, the factors conditioning success remain controversial. The size of the varicocele does not appear to have any predictive value, whereas early cure in adolescence or young adulthood improves the prognosis.

The efficacy of spermatic embolization for the treatment of infertility remains unclear. Analysis is difficult owing to methodological differences in the various studies published to date, but initial results are encouraging. In 92 patients treated by sclerotherapy, Sigmund et al. (1987b) observed an increased sperm count in 34.8% and increased sperm motility values and sperm morphology in 22.8% and 15.2%, respectively. Marsman (1985) followed up 58 patients after embolization: 14 of the couples (24%) achieved pregnancy. Smith et al. (1988) reported successful conception in 30 couples (40.5%) a minimum of 1 year (mean, 28.5 months) after sclerotherapy for varicocele in 74 infertile men. Nieschlag et al. (1993) observed significant increased sperm count and sperm motility 12 months after embolization in 12 patients, although no modification was seen in sperm morphology, and 11 pregnancies (33%) were achieved. During the 2 years after technically and clinically effective embolization in 79 patients, Ferguson et al. (1995) observed a highly significant increase in sperm motility ($p<0.001$) and a tendency toward an increase in the sperm count ($p<0.1$), but no change in sperm morphology or volume. A pregnancy was achieved by 29 couples (36.7%) in that study.

For 71 of 154 infertile men treated by Zuckerman et al. (1994), embolization of a varicocele constituted the sole therapy for the couple during the study period; 60% of these couples achieved a pregnancy after a mean interval of 11.5 months versus 57% (88 couples) of the entire group of 154 patients after a mean of 17.2 months.

9.3.3 Indications

Establishing a varicocele as the cause of infertility remains highly complex. Surgical ligation was for many years the sole treatment. Percutaneous spermatic vein embolization has become a safe and reliable alternative. Two recent series – Dewire et al. (1994) with 81 patients and Nieschlag et al. (1993) with 71 randomized patients – report equivalent benefits for surgical ligation and percutaneous embolization in terms of restoration of fertility. Embolization offers the advantage of short hospitalization and remains possible even if recurrence occurs after surgical treatment. Numerous authors advocate varicocele repair in adolescence to avoid infertility in adulthood. Only subclinical varicoceles causing permanent reflux require treatment.

References

Abbitt PL, Watson L, Howards S (1991) Abnormalities of the seminal tract causing infertility: diagnosis with endorectal sonography. AJR 157:337–339

Belaisch J (1987) Exploration d'un homme présumé stérile ou hypofertile. In: Arvis G (ed) Andrologie. Maloine, Paris, pp 227

Boyer L, Salicru B, Pujol J, Rouanet JP, Lamarque JL, Viallet JF (1990) Imagerie en andrologie. EMC Paris Gynécologie 760 A10:1–10

Boyer L, Hermabessière J, Boyer-Medeville C, Boissier A, Viallet JF (1994) Place de l'échographie transrectale dans le bilan d'infertilité masculine. A propos de 91 explorations. J Radiol 75:321–326

Carter SS, Shinohara K, Lipshultz LI (1989) Transrectal ultrasonography in disorders of the seminal vesicles and ejaculatory ducts. Urol Clin North Am 16:773–790

Carvalho HA, Paiva JLB, Santos VHV, Andrade M, Galvao-Teles A (1986) Ultrasonic recognition of a cystic seminal vesicle with ipsilateral renal agenesis. J Urol 135:1267–1268

Colpi GM, Casella F, Zanollo A et al (1987) Functional voiding disturbances of the ampullo-vesicular seminal tract a cause of male infertility. Acta Eur Fertil 18:165–179

Cornud F, Belin X, Fromont G (eds) (1993) Imagerie de la prostate. Flammarion, Paris, pp 69–82

Cornud F, Belin X, Delafontaine D et al (1994a) Imagerie de l'infertilité masculine d'origine excrétoire. Rev Imag Med 10:S114

Cornud F, Belin X, Helenon O, Melki P, Moreau JF (1994b) Echo doppler couleur de l'appareil génital masculin. Rev Imag Med 6:S9

Cornud, Belin X, Delafontaine D, Amar J, Helenon O, Moreau JF (1996) Imagerie des azoospermies d'origine excrétoire. Feuillets Radiol 36:374–386

Demas BE, Hricak H, McClure RD (1991) Varicoceles. Radiologic diagnosis and treatment. Radiol Clin North Am 29:619–627

Dewire DM, Thomas AJ, Falk RM, Geisinger MA, Lammert GK (1994) Clinical outcome and cost comparison of percutaneous embolization and surgical ligation of varicocele. J Androl 15 [Suppl]: P 38S–42S

Dhabuwala CB, Parulkar BG (1994) Doppler flow analysis and conventional ultrasonography for evaluation of the infertile male. In: Jaffe R, Pierson RA, Abramowics JS (eds) Imaging in infertility and reproductive endocrinology. Lippincott, Philadelphia, pp 207–216

Ferguson JM, Gillespie IN, Chalmers N, Elton RA, Hargreave TB (1995) Percutaneous varicocele embolization in the treatment of infertility. Br J Radiol 68:700–703

Fobbe F, Hamm B, Sorensen R, Felsenberg D (1987) Percutaneous transluminal treatment of varicoceles: where to occlude the internal spermatic vein. AJR 149:983–987

Hamm B, Fobbe F, Sorensen R, Felsenberg D (1986) Varicoceles: Combined sonography and thermography in diagnosis and post-therapeutic evaluation. Radiology 160:419–424

Kim ED, Lipshultz LI (1996) Role of ultrasound in the assessment of male infertility. J Clin Ultrasound 24:437–453

Kuligowska E (1994) Transrectal ultrasonography in diagnosis and management of male infertility. In: Jaffe R, Pierson RA, Abramowicz JS (eds) Imaging in infertility and reproductive endocrinology. Lippincot, Philadelphia, pp 217–229

Kuligowska E, Baker C, Oates RD (1992) Male infertility: role of transrectal US in diagnosis and management. Radiology 185:653–674

Lardennois B, Lomina D, El Khansa A, Brandt B (1986) Le test de la vidange dynamique des vésicules séminales (VIDYVES). Contrôle du spermogramme en échographie interventionnelle dans l'exploration des stérilités masculines. J Urol 92:239–242

Lenz M, Hof N, Kersting-Sommerhof B, Baultz W (1996) Anatomic variants of the spermatic vein: importance for percutaneous sclerotherapy of idiopathic varicocele. Radiology 198:425–431

Marsman JWP (1985) Clinical versus subclinical varicocele: venographic findings and improvement of fertility after embolization. Radiology 155:635–638

Marsman JWP (1995) The aberrantly fed varicoceles: frequency, venographic appearance and results of transcatheter embolization. AJR 164:649–657

Meacham RB, Townsend R, Drose JA (1995) Ejaculatory obstruction: diagnosis and treatment with transrectal sonography. AJR 165:1463–1466

Nieschlag E, Behre HM, Schlingheider A, Nashan D, Pohl J, Fischedick (1993) Surgical ligation vs angiographic embolization of the vena spermatica: a prospective randomized study for the treatment of varicocele related infertility. Andrologia 25:233–237

Nys P, Merceron RE, Cordray JP, Guillard X (1992) Les stérilités masculines. Concours Med 114:573–579

Pascal Suisse P, Félix F, Laurac J (1986) Echographie des bourses. Vigot, Paris

Patel MR, Dulabon D, Roth R (1987) Case profile: absent seminal vesicle diagnosed by transrectal ultrasound. Urology 39:332

Pontonnier F, Bujan L (1993) Comment reconnaître et classer une infécondité masculine. Rev Prat (Paris) 43:941–948

Pryor JP, Hendry WF (1990) Ejaculatory duct obstruction in subfertiles males: analysis of 87 patients. Fertil Steril 56:725–730

Rifkin MD (1988) Ultrasound of the prostate. Raven, New York

Ross LS (1983) Diagnosis and treatment of infertile men: a clinical perspective. J Urol 130:847–854

Sanders RC (1991) Infertility diagnosis by ultrasound. Urol Radiol 13:41–47

Shabsigh R, Lerner S, Fishman IJ, Kadmon D (1989) The role of transrectal ultra-sonography in diagnosis and management of prostatic and seminal vesicle cysts. J Urol 14:1206–1209

Sigmund G, Bahren W, Gall H, Lenz M, Thon W (1987a) Idiopathic varicoceles: feasibility of percutaneous sclerotherapy. Radiology 164:161–168

Sigmund G, Gall H, Bahren W (1987b) Stop-type and shunt-type varicoceles: venographic findings. Radiology 163:105–110

Sigmund G, Gall H, Bahren W, Wetterauer U (1989) Hemodynamics of varicoceles: venous shunting in grade II and III varicoceles. Ann Radiol 32:24–28

Smith JP, Hunter DW, Cragg AH et al (1988) Spermatic vein embolization with hot contrast material: fertility results. Radiology 168:137–139

Stasi G, Barozzi L, Basunti G et al (1989) L'ecografia operativa delle vescicole seminali nella patologia andrologica. Radiol Med 78:358–362

Trombetta C, Salisci E, Deriu M et al (1993) Echo flowmetric control 6 years after percutaneous treatment of varicocele. Arch Ital Urol Androl 65:367–377

Winkelbauer FN, Amman ME, Karnel F, Lammer J (1994) Doppler sonography of varicocele: long-term follow-up after venography and transcatheter sclerotherapy. J Ultrasound Med 13:953–958

Zuckerman AM, Mitchell SE, Venbru AC et al (1994) Percutaneous varicocele occlusion: long term follow-up. J Vasc Interv Radiol 5:315–319

10 Erectile Dysfunction

V. JUHAN, D. SAMAMA, M. ANDRÉ, and J.M. BARTOLI

CONTENTS

10.1 Introduction

Erectile dysfunction, commonly referred to as impotence, is defined as the failure to initiate or to maintain an erection allowing satisfactory intromission. The causes of erectile dysfunction can be divided into organic and psychogenic causes. Organic impotence can involve vascular, hormonal, and/or neurogenic mechanisms and thus requires a multidisplinary approach for accurate diagnosis. Medical imaging serves essentially to demonstrate or rule out vasculogenic causes of erectile dysfunction.

10.2 Anatomy of the Penis

The penis is composed of three cylindrical fibrous compartments: two lateral corpora cavernosa penis and the central corpus spongiosum (Fig. 10.1). Each of these three erectile bodies is enclosed by a dense fibroelastic sheath (tunica albuginea). The three bodies are collectively surrounded by the deep penile fascia (Buck's fascia). The corpus cavernosum consists of a fibroelastic frame, smooth muscle, and lacunar spaces (sinusoids); the corporal vasculature consists of tortuous arterioles and subtunical venules.

V. JUHAN, D. SAMAMA, M. ANDRÉ, J.M. BARTOLI, Service de Radiologie, Hôpital de la Timone, 264 rue Saint-Pierre, 13385 Marseille, France

10.2.1 Arterial Blood Supply

The penile arterial blood supply is ensured by the internal pudendal artery, which arises from the anterior division of the internal iliac artery. At the root of the penis, the internal pudendal artery divides into two terminal branches: the superficial perineal artery, which supplies the superficial soft tissues of the perineoscrotal region, and the common penile artery, which gives off four branches:

- The artery to the bulb of the corpus spongiosum. This artery is the origin of a blush on arteriograms.
- The bulbourethral artery vascularizes the bulbourethral gland and the walls of the urethra.
- The dorsal penile artery supplies the superficial tissues of the penis, most of the corpus spongiosum, and the glans penis.
- The cavernosal artery (deep artery of penis) is the major vessel involved in erection, as it ensures corporal filling. After piercing the superficial layer of the corpus cavernosum, this slightly eccentric artery runs forward in its center, near the fibrous septum. Along its course, this artery gives off numerous branches (helicine arteries) that radiate out toward the periphery of the corpora cavernosa.

Branches of the dorsal penile artery occasionally communicate with the cavernosal artery. The high frequency of anatomic variations can complicate interpretation of imaging studies.

10.2.2 Venous Drainage

The complex venous anatomy consists of two main drainage systems characterized by considerable variations and numerous communications:

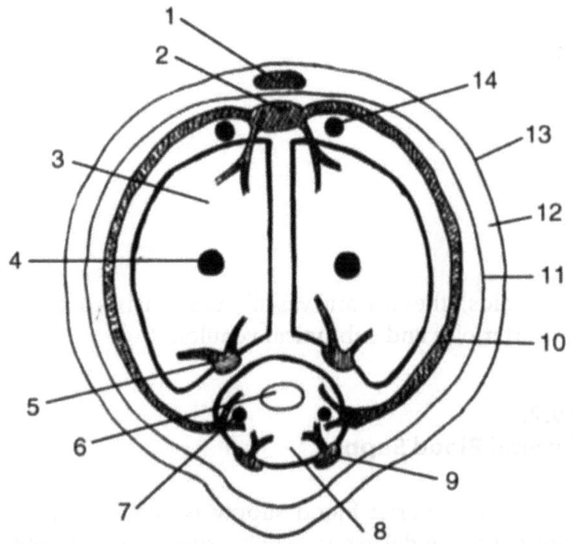

Fig. 10.1. Transverse section through the penis. *1*, superficial dorsal vein; *2*, deep dorsal vein; *3*, corpus cavernosum; *4*, cavernosal artery; *5*, cavernosal vein; *6*, penile urethra; *7*, bulbourethral artery; *8*, corpus spongiosum; *9*, bulbourethral vein; *10*, lateral vein; *11*, deep penile fascia (Buck's fascia); *12*, lacunar space; *13*, skin; *14*, dorsal penile artery. (After Brule et al. 1992)

- The deep venous system ensures nearly all drainage of the erectile bodies through the intermediary of the deep dorsal vein of penis. This single vein, the most important venous structure in the mechanism of erection, arises in small veins around the corona of the glans penis. It lies subfascially between the two dorsal arteries of the penis. The deep dorsal vein drains into the internal pudendal veins and the preprostatic venous plexus (Santorini's venous plexus). The lacunar spaces drain into a network of venules that traverse the tunica albuginea and empty into the circumflex veins. These veins, perpendicular to the long axis of the penis, drain in turn into the deep dorsal vein.
- The superficial venous system consists of an unpaired superficial dorsal vein that runs subcutaneously along the dorsal surface of the penis. This vein, which drains the penile skin, empties into the preprostatic plexus or the external pudendal vein and the internal saphenous vein.
- The posterior venous system is formed by the cavernosal veins that return the blood from the proximal corpora cavernosa directly to the preprostatic venous plexus and/or the internal pudendal veins.

10.3 Physiology of Erection

An erection is a complex cascade of events involving vascular, neurogenic, physiologic, hormonal, and neurologic mechanisms (Lue and Tanagho 1987). Four phases are distinguished:

1. In the flaccid state, the smooth muscle of the corpora cavernosa (walls of the arterioles and sinusoids) is contracted. In this state of high-resistance, low arterial flow, the lacunar spaces are practically empty. The autonomic sympathetic muscle tone is regulated by the secretion of adrenergic and noradrenergic neurotransmitters (norepinephrine). Arterial flow is usually low (10 ml/min). The intracorporal pressure is about 10 mmHg.
2. Tumescence (vascular phase): during induction of penile erection, the release of other neurotransmitters (e.g., acetylcholine, vasoactive intestinal polypeptide) results in a decrease in muscle tone. Smooth muscle relaxation is followed by arterial vasodilation, allowing augmented arterial flow that results in engorgement of the lacunar spaces. The pressure in the corpora cavernosa rises to 50–60 mmHg.
3. In the erect state (rigid erection phase), enlargement of the corpora cavernosa compresses the arteries and veins against the tunica albuginea. The intracavernosal pressure reaches 100–120 mmHg. Conservation of minimal arterial flow prevents priapism.
4. During detumescence, recovery of smooth muscle tone reduces arterial flow and increases venous outflow from the lacunar spaces.

10.4 Pathogenesis of Erectile Dysfunction

Impotence has a psychogenic origin in approximately 25%–30% of patients. Organic causes, which account for 70%–75%, may be purely arteriogenic (5%), purely venogenic (5%), mixed vasculogenic (45%), or neurogenic (15%) (Goldstein et al. 1990). Less frequent organic causes include endocrine disorders and exogenous factors (e.g., drugs, alcohol, tobacco).

Vasculogenic causes can be subdivided into the following:

- Vascular insufficiency due to arterial involvement (atherosclerosis, arteriovenous fistula).

- Impossibility to maintain sufficient intracavernosal pressure due to corporovenous leakage or sinusoidal disease. Mixed etiologies involving both arteriogenic and venogenic factors predominate.

10.5 Evaluation of Erectile Dysfunction

Medical imaging is increasingly used to assess erectile dysfunction. Studies are aimed at diagnosis of vasculogenic causes and determination of their arteriogenic or venogenic nature. Figure 10.2 presents an algorithm for assessment.

10.5.1 Doppler Sonography

Doppler ultrasound is the gold standard for the investigation of organic impotence (LUE et al. 1985). The examination should be performed in a warm and comfortable environment to reduce patient apprehension. Cooperation is improved if the technique and its anticipated benefits are clearly explained.

Exploration of the Iliac Trunk. Examination of the aorta, the common iliac arteries, and the origin of the internal iliac arteries allows demonstration of arterial disease.

Exploration of the Internal Pudendal Arteries. The internal pudendal arteries are accessible to Doppler study in their perineal course. Examination is performed by a perineal approach using a 5- to 7.5-MHz transducer. The patient is examined in the supine position with the legs bent. After external rotation of the lower limb, the transducer is placed on the perineum, midway between the anal margin and the root of the scrotum, medial to the ischial tuberosity localized by palpation. The transducer is angled upward, outward, and forward. The resistive-type tracing is characterized by an elevated systolic peak, a very weak or absent diastole, and occasionally a negative protodiastole. The right and left tracings are symmetrical (Fig. 10.3).

Exploration of the Penile Arteries. The penile arteries are examined with a 7.5- to 10-MHz transducer, first in the flaccid condition and then after intracavernous injection of a smooth muscle relaxant. B-mode scanning is performed prior to Doppler examination.

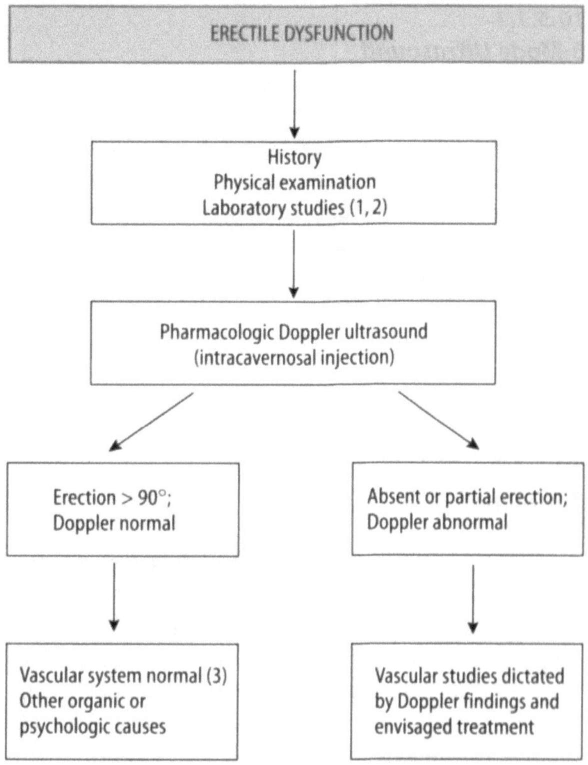

Fig. 10.2. Algorithm for evaluation of erectile dysfunction. *1*, Certain investigators advocate nocturnal penile tumescence (NPT) and/or rigidity tests before Doppler ultrasound because a normal result rules out an organic cause. *2*, Similarly, pharmacologic dynamic infusion testing is sometimes performed without ultrasound based on the assumption that a positive test (full erection) rules out vasculogenic impotence (ROY et al. 1995). *3*, Arteriogenic anomalies may exist despite a positive pharmacological erection test (PESCATORI et al. 1994; CORMIO et al. 1996)

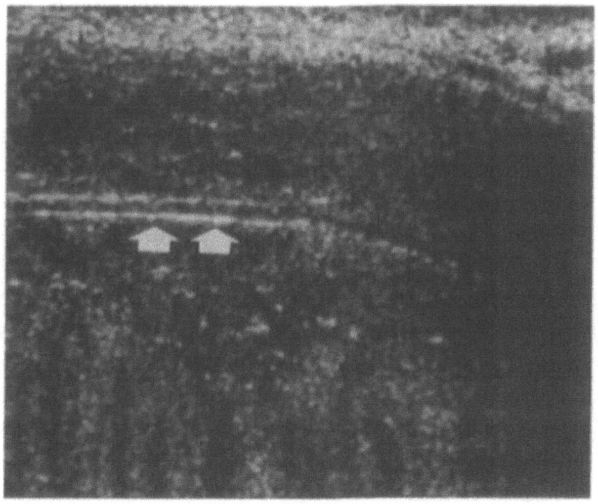

Fig. 10.3. B-mode scan of the corpus cavernosum: localization of the cavernosal artery in the sagittal plane (*arrows*)

10.5.1.1
B-Mode Ultrasound

In the flaccid state, the corpora cavernosa are homogeneously echogenic. During erection, they become hypoechoic; the dilated sinusoids are visible as small anechoic zones. The large dorsal vein is readily visualized, and the dorsal and cavernosal arteries are smaller in diameter. Ultrasound allows evaluation of the corporal architecture. Demonstration of hyperechoic linear images corresponding to fibrous plaques is suggestive of Peyronie's disease.

10.5.1.2
Technique

Accurate assessment of the central cavernosal arteries is dependent on the use of a proper technique. The cavernosal arteries are localized in the sagittal plane, along the ventral aspect of the penis. Recordings are obtained at the root of the penis in the sagittal plane with a Doppler angle of less than 60° relative to the axis of the vessel. The sampling window allows examination of the entire vascular axis with an appropriate pulse repeating frequency (PRF) and wall filter.

Anatomic variations in penile vasculature are common and can result in misinterpretation of Doppler recordings. Most errors are false-positive results in patients without vascular involvement (Jarow et al. 1993; Mancini et al. 1996). The entire penis must thus be carefully examined by means of transverse scans.

10.5.1.3
Results in the Flaccid State

The frequently tortuous cavernosal arteries measure approximately 1.5–2 mm. Peak systolic velocity varies from 10 to 20 cm/s, while diastolic velocity is zero. Absence of a recording has no pathologic significance.

The dorsal arteries are characterized by a resistive spectral waveform. The peak systolic velocity varies from 20 to 25 cm/s, while the diastolic wave may be negative or zero. Doppler ultrasound without intracorporal injection of a pharmacologic agent has little practical value.

10.5.1.4
Intracavernous Injection of Vasoactive Agents

In 1982, Virag reported that injection of papaverine into the corpora cavernosa produces a rigid erection both in healthy males and in men suffering from psychogenic impotence. Papaverine hydrochloride exerts its action essentially by inhibiting the negative effect of noradrenaline, resulting in prolonged blockage of venous return. The potential risk is persistent erection. Papaverine can be used for diagnostic purposes (20–60 mg) or self-injection therapy. An alpha blocker is sometimes given in combination with papaverine.

Prostaglandin is gradually replacing papaverine. A powerful muscle relaxant, prostaglandin is not only more effective but also causes fewer prolonged erections owing to its short half-life (Stackl et al. 1988). A short 26-G needle is used to inject the product into the right or left neck of the glans penis. The injection is made without local anesthesia after careful disinfection of the site, with care being taken to avoid the superficial vessels. Some patients complain of a burning sensation during injection. Manual compression of the puncture site or application of a tourniquet at the base of the penis for 3–5 min slows diffusion of the product into the systemic circulation. Prostaglandin E_1 (PGE_1) is currently the most widely used product (usual dose, 10–40 mg).

Manual genital stimulation after injection reportedly improves the quality of erection in 75% of cases (Donatucci and Lue 1992). Montorsi et al. (1996) advocate a combination of manual genital and audiovisual stimulation after injection of a smooth muscle relaxant; a second injection is given if the erectile response is inadequate.

10.5.1.5
Results After Intracavernous Injection of Vasoactive Agent

Recording is started 5 min after injection and is repeated every 5 min for approximately 30 min. Recordings are not reliable until a full erection has been achieved. Examination of the cavernosal arteries and the dorsal arteries is completed by a search for possible variations in arterial anatomy (Figs. 10.4–10.6).

The following parameters are used:

- Peak flow velocities: the systolic and diastolic velocities are the most commonly used parameters.
- Increase in penile volume: after pharmacologic stimulation, the diameter of the cavernosal artery

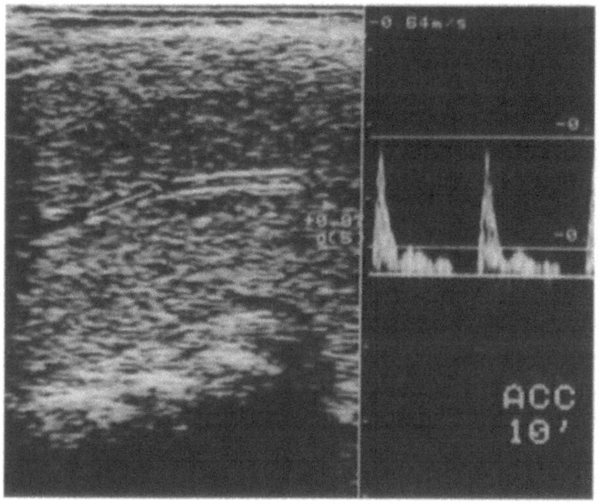

a

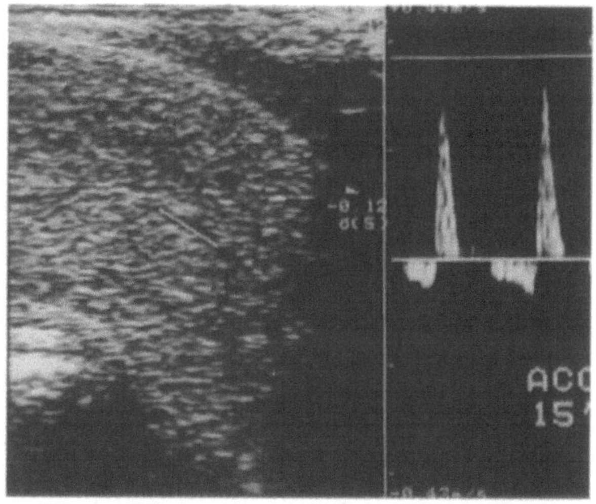
b

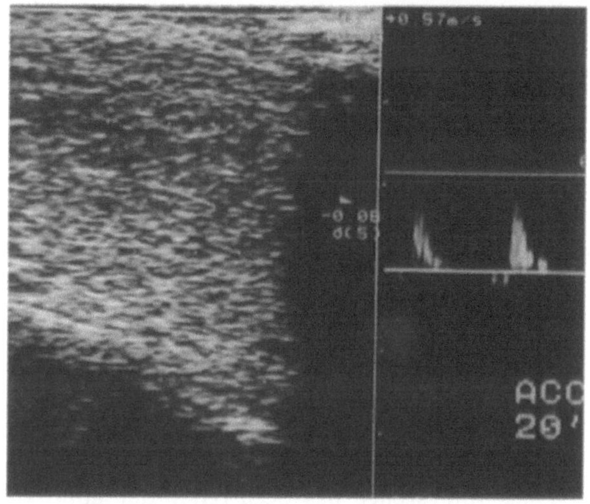
c

Fig. 10.4a–c. Doppler sonogram after intracavernous injection of prostaglandin: normal examination. **a** 10 min after injection: early tumescence. Systolic velocity, >30 cm/s. The diastolic velocity is decreasing (7 cm/s). **b** 15 min after intracavernous injection: rigidity. Elevated systolic peak (37 cm/s in this patient). Inversion of the diastolic flow. **c** 20 min after injection: collapse of the systolic and diastolic peaks

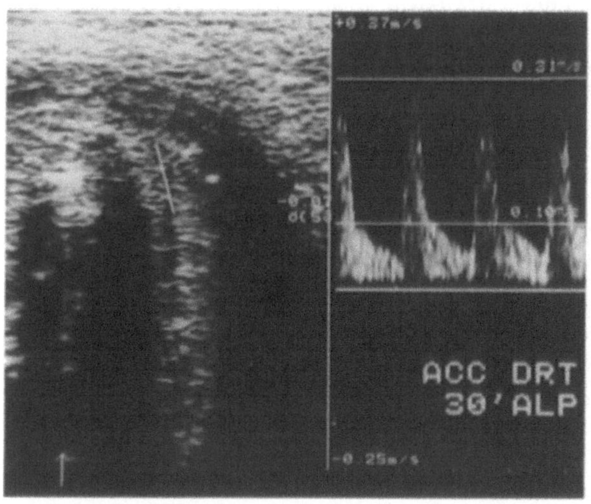

Fig. 10.5. Doppler sonogram 30 min after intracavernous injection of prostaglandin. No erection. Persistence of diastolic flow greater than 5 cm/s reflects corporovenous leakage. Normal systolic velocity

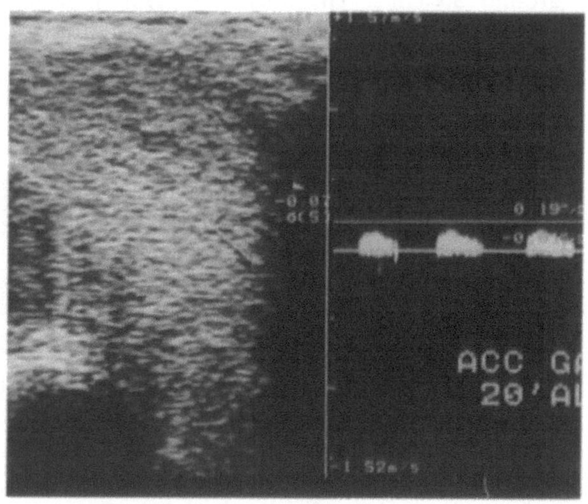

Fig. 10.6. Doppler sonogram 20 min after intracavernous injection of prostaglandin. No erection. The systolic velocity remains very low (<20 cm/s), indicating arterial insufficiency

normally increases (Lue et al. 1985). The maximum diameter is reached 3–5 min after intracavernous injection. Isolated measurement of variations in diameter is not reliable (Meuleman et al. 1992; Benson et al. 1993).
- Systolic acceleration time.
- Systolic acceleration index (i.e., the difference between the maximum systolic velocity and the minimal diastolic velocity divided by systolic acceleration time).
- Pourcelot's resistive index (RI) (i.e., the difference between the mean systolic velocity and the mean diastolic velocity divided by the mean systolic velocity) is of no value for certain authors (Schwartz et al. 1989), whereas others use the RI to evaluate venous drainage (Merckx et al. 1992).
- Penile flow index: this index is considered highly reliable by certain authors (Lopez et al. 1991) because it takes account of the variations in arterial velocity and diameter; however, it is rarely used because the technique is difficult to perform.

The various spectral waveforms reflect the modifications in intracorporal pressure that occur during the different phases of erection (normal values):

- Injection is followed immediately by vasodilation of the cavernosal artery. The systolic velocities rise to 30–40 cm/s (occasionally up to 50 cm/s); a diastolic velocity appears (5–13 cm/s). Velocimetry during this initial phase of tumescence is unreliable.
- Once tumescence has occurred (after approximately 3 min), the systolic velocities stabilize at around 30 cm/s. The normal threshold varies slightly depending on the author. Certain investigators consider the peak systolic velocity normal starting at 25 cm/s (Lue and Tanagho 1987; Jarow et al. 1993), whereas others have cited peak systolic velocities of 30–35 cm/s in normal subjects (Lee et al. 1993; Connolly et al. 1996). These differences can be explained by individual physiologic variations, variations in the angle of the Doppler probe (which must be less than 60°), and differences in the recording site on the penis. The diastole drops during this phase; 5–10 min after injection, it is normally less than 5 cm/s. The intracavernous pressure is greater than 40 mmHg.
- Early rigidity: the peak systolic velocity is only slightly modified. The decrease in the diastolic velocity is accompanied by the appearance of a protodiastolic dicrotic notch.
- Rigidity: the systolic peak becomes very high and narrow. The diastolic velocity is canceled. The intracavernosal pressure is greater than 60 mmHg. When the intracavernosal pressure becomes higher than the diastolic flow (at least 80 mmHg), the diastolic flow is inversed.
- Full erection: collapse of the systolic and diastolic peaks (this phase is inconstant).

The variations in Doppler tracings are summarized in Table 10.1.

Table 10.1. Normal variations in Doppler results after pharmacologic injection

Stage	Systolic velocity	Diastolic velocity
Immediately after injection	>40 cm/s	>5 cm/s
Tumescence	≥30 cm/s	<5 cm/s
Early rigidity	Unchanged	<5 cm/s Protodiastolic dicrotic notch
Rigidity	High narrow systolic peak	Zero
Maximum rigidity	Narrow peak	Inversed diastole

10.5.1.6 Vasculogenic Impotence

Evaluation of Arterial Blood Flow. The systolic velocity reflects arterial blood flow, and a systolic velocity greater than 35 cm/s rules out arterial insufficiency. A peak systolic velocity less than 25 cm/s 20 min after intracavernous injection reflects arterial insufficiency (Shabsigh et al. 1989; Cornud et al. 1992; Vajli and Bookstein 1993) and is an indication for arteriography. For velocities between 25 and 35 cm/s, the decision whether or not to perform arteriography depends on the clinical setting.

In arteriogenic impotence, arterial dilatation is decreased or nonexistent owing to poor arterial compliance or low flow. Most authors have reported little correlation between the percentage of augmentation in vascular diameter and arteriographic images (Rajfer et al. 1990; Chiang et al. 1991; Jarow et al. 1993).

A systolic acceleration time of at least 110 m/s is suggestive of an arterial pathology (Oates et al. 1995). This parameter is increasingly used as a complement to velocimetry.

A systolic acceleration index less than 400 cm/s has been used to assess arterial flow (Vajli and Bookstein 1993). Although sensitive, this parameter is not very specific, and it is rarely used alone.

Penile Doppler sonography has a reported sensitivity of 53%–96% and a specificity of 44%–94% (Mueller et al. 1990; Rajfer et al. 1990; Chiang et al. 1991; Jarow et al. 1993) compared to arteriography, which remains the gold standard.

Evaluation of Venous Drainage. The diastolic velocity is the direct reflection of the intracavernosal pressure and an indirect reflection of venous occlusion (Schwartz et al. 1989). Recordings can only be interpreted in the absence of arterial insufficiency (normal systolic velocity).

If the venocclusive mechanism is impaired, the intracavernous pressure remains less than 40 mmHg and the diastolic velocity remains greater than 5 cm/s 20 min after intracavernous injection (Quam 1989; Fitzgerald et al. 1991; Andresen and Wegner 1997).

If an elevated diastolic flow persists, a second intracavernous injection may demonstrate a late drop in the diastole (Cornud et al. 1992). Color Doppler using this parameter has a reported sensitivity of 94% and a specificity of 69% (Courtheoux et al. 1986; Cornud et al. 1992). However, certain authors have questioned the validity of these parameters (Kropman et al. 1992; Merckx et al. 1992).

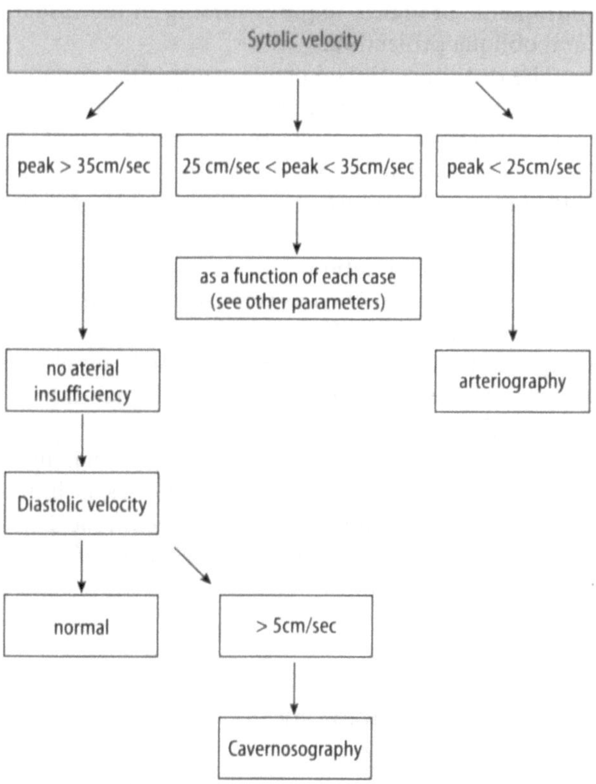

Fig. 10.7. Pharmacological arterial Doppler ultrasound of the penis

The RI has been used by certain investigators to assess venous drainage (Merckx et al. 1992; Nisen et al. 1993). An RI greater than 0.90 20 min after intracavernous injection implies a normal venocclusive mechanism (Fig. 10.7).

10.5.2 Cavernosography

Long considered the examination of reference for confirmation of corporovenous leakage suggested by Doppler ultrasound (Delcour et al. 1986; Malhrotra et al. 1986; Cornud et al. 1992), cavernosography is currently reserved for pretherapy workup (surgery or interventional radiology) (Andresen and Wegner 1997). This technique associates morphologic analysis of the corpora cavernosa and venous drainage with penile blood flow studies (Fig. 10.8).

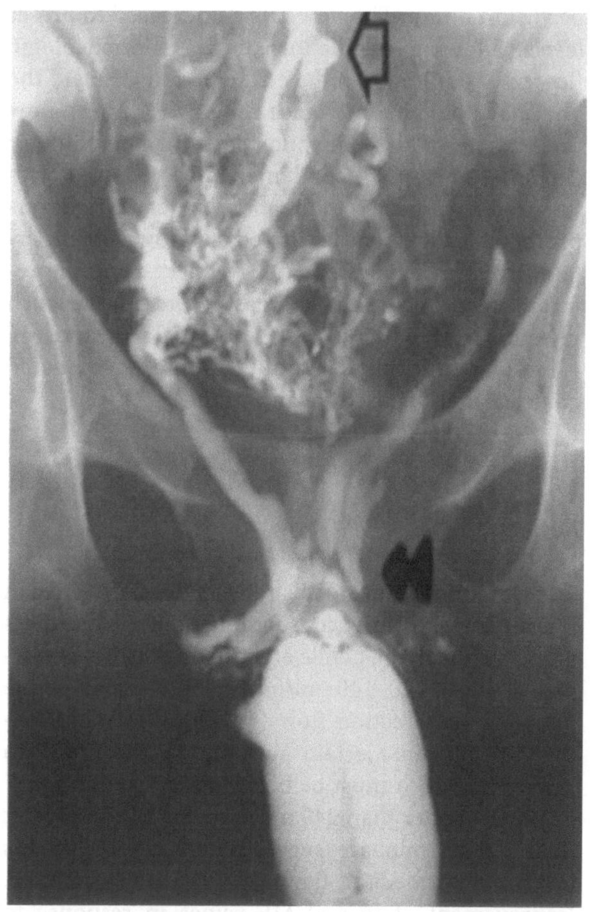

Fig. 10.8. Cavernosography without intracavernous injection of a muscle relaxant. Morphological evaluation of the corpora cavernosa and venous drainage. In this normal variant, drainage occurs preferentially toward the inferior mesenteric vein (*open arrow*). Preprostatic venous plexus (*black arrow*)

10.5.2.1 Technique

The current simplified technique requires contrast injection into a single corpus cavernosum. After disinfection of the injection site, the iodinated medium is injected manually into the neck of the penis with a short Teflonized 19-G or 21-G needle. Manual infusion allows verification of correct needle positioning in the corpus cavernosum and assessment of the architecture of the corpora cavernosa and venous drainage systems. No resistance should be felt during injection, which should be painless. Opacification of the corpora cavernosa is rapid and allows detection of anomalies such as bends or fibrous plaques due to trauma or Peyronie's disease. Analysis of the venous systems allows identification of preferential drainage into the deep or superficial network.

Penile blood flow studies are performed after connection of the needle to an automatic injector or a perfusion pump. The flow rate is increased to preset levels, allowing calculation of the pharmacologic flow rate required to induce an erection (IF) and the pharmacologic maintenance flow (MF). These flow rates can be validated manually or with a manometer (in the latter case, a second injection is required, with the needle connected to the manometer). Numerous protocols have been developed for flowmetry. Certain investigators systematically inject a muscle relaxant intracorporally, whereas others reserve such injections for patients with pathologic IF and MF values. Isotonic saline or a dilute nonionic iodinated contrast agent is used for injection.

10.5.2.2 Results

The variability of protocols reflects the difficulties in interpretation of cavernosographic data. Regardless of the protocol, the penile erection flow (PEF) is normally below 120–140 ml/min. The normal penile maintenance erection flow (PMEF) should not exceed 50 ml/min. Certain authors use the PMEF to PEF ratio, which must be below 40%.

An IF greater than 240 ml/min and an MF greater than 120 ml/min are suggestive of corporovenous leakage; intermediate flow rates are indeterminate. Improvement of IF and MF values in response to intracavernous injection of a muscle relaxant suggests beneficial results if the product is used for self-injection therapy. The main potential complication is prolonged erection, which can progress to priapism; the problem does not always occur immediately, and the patient must be informed of this eventuality. This complication has nearly completely disappeared since the introduction of prostaglandins.

10.5.3 Digital Angiography

Digital angiography is indicated solely for pretherapy workups. Use of this technique has declined markedly due to the efficacy of Doppler ultrasound and the disappointing results of distal arterial penile surgery. The use of a proper technique is crucial to avoid errors in interpretation linked to physiologic or spastic phenomena (Figs. 10.9–10.13).

The examination is performed by a unilateral femoral artery approach, followed by hyperselective contralateral and then ipsilateral catheterization of the ischiopudendal trunk or the internal pudendal artery. Injection of an intra-arterial vasodilator and intracavernous injection of a smooth muscle relaxant are systematically used (Rosen et al. 1990).

The iliac bifurcation is evaluated using a contralateral oblique projection, whereas complete visualization of the internal pudendal artery and its intrapenile branches requires filming in the ipsilateral oblique projection.

The rectilinear dorsal penile artery often communicates with the contralateral artery. The cavernosal artery appears tortuous in the flaccid and in semierect state; it becomes rectilinear only during full erection. Demonstration of an entirely normal arterial tree on one side obviates the need for contralateral catheterization.

Vascular lesions such as stenosis or occlusion are often multiple and diffuse. The most common sites are the ostium or along the trunk of the internal iliac artery, the terminal portion of the internal iliac artery, and along the penile arteries.

Preoperative visualization of the external iliac, common femoral, and epigastric arteries is indispensable for selection of the surgical technique. Digital angiography also allows assessment of distal bypass graft patency.

10.5.4 Interventional Radiology

Embolization of venous leaks by direct injection or, more often, after denudation of the superficial or deep dorsal vein initially raised considerable hopes.

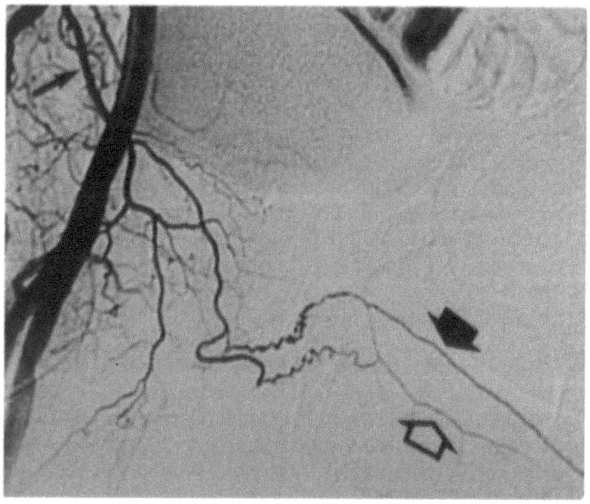

Fig. 10.9. Normal penile arteriogram. Opacification of the right internal pudendal artery (*thin arrow*), the dorsal artery of the penis (*thick solid arrow*), and the cavernosal artery (*open arrow*)

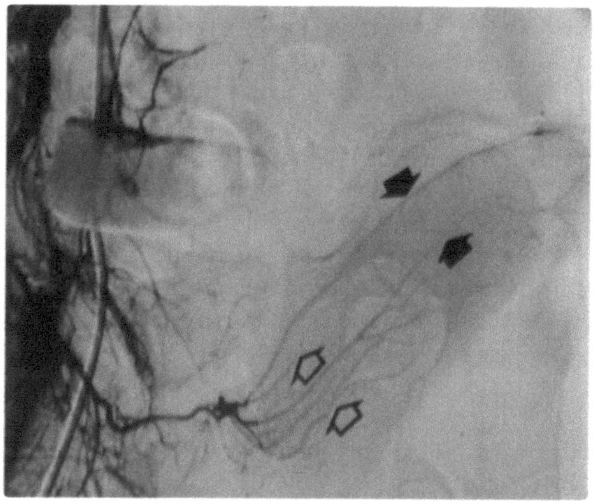

Fig. 10.10. Normal penile arteriogram: anatomic variant. The right internal pudendal artery gives rise to two dorsal penile arteries (*thick solid arrows*) and two cavernosal arteries (*open arrows*)

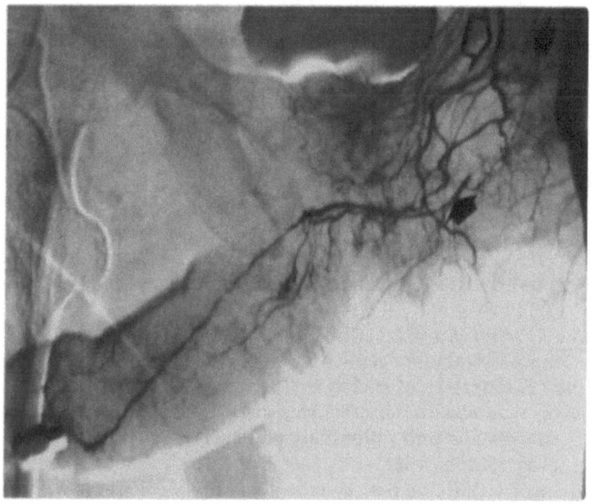

Fig. 10.11. Pathologic penile arteriogram. Thrombosis of the left internal pudendal artery (*solid arrows*) at the level of Alcock's canal. Distal recovery by collateral flow from the obturator artery (*open arrow*)

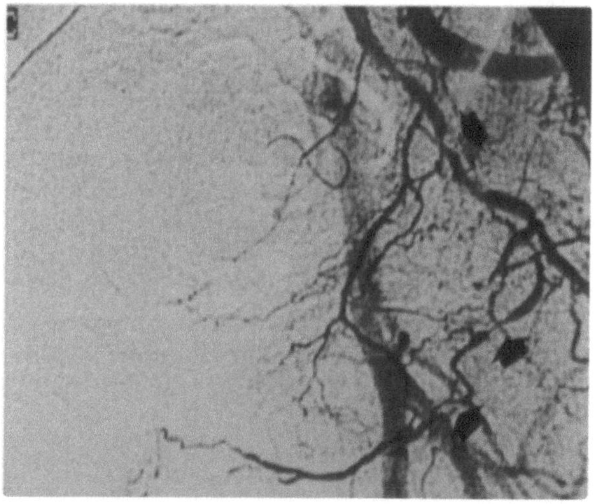

Fig. 10.12. Penile arteriogram revealing multiple sites of stenosis on the left internal pudendal artery (*arrows*)

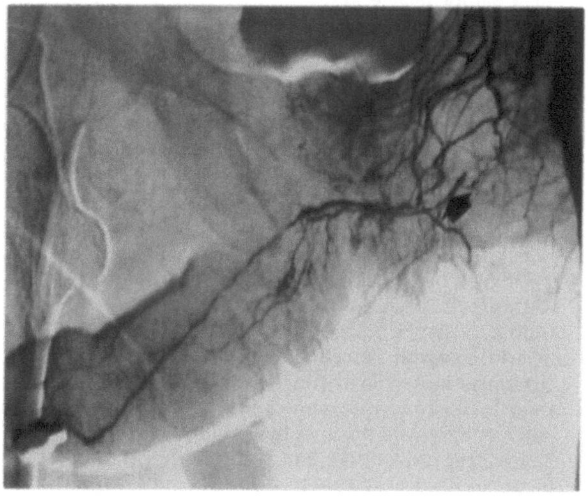

Fig. 10.13. Penile arteriogram. Verification of the patency of a left surgical bypass (*arrows*)

Although early results are often satisfactory, the rapidity and frequency of recurrence has led numerous teams to abandon this therapeutic approach. Despite progress in angioplasty equipment (guide catheters, monorail balloons derived from coronary technology), angioplasty is rarely used to treat arteriogenic lesions in the internal pudendal bed because results remain aleatory. Doppler sonography is effective for surveillance after surgery or embolization to detect recurrence (Keogan et al. 1996).

10.6 Conclusion

Medical imaging plays an important role in the evaluation of erectile dysfunction. Pharmacologic color Doppler is the cornerstone of diagnostic workups; the most frequently used parameters are the systolic and diastolic velocities. Performed increasingly frequently as the initial technique after a thorough medical history and physical examination, pharmacologic color Doppler can be used to diagnose vasculogenic impotence and can suggest its arteriogenic or venogenic nature. This allows identification of those rare patients who merit more sophisticated vascular studies, such as cavernosography or arteriography. Prescribed only after a positive Doppler study, such examinations are reserved for pretherapy workup of candidates for more invasive procedures.

References

Andresen R, Wegner HEH (1997) Assessment of the penile vascular system with color-coded duplex sonography and pharmacocavernosometry and -graphy in impotent men. Acta Radiol 38:303–308

Benson CB, Aruny JE, Vickers MA (1993) Correlation of duplex sonography with arteriography in patients with erectile dysfunction. AJR 160:71–73

Brule JM, Dimitrov Y, Wenger JJ (1992) Diagnostic radiologique de l'impuissance masculine. EMC Paris Urologie-Gynécologie, 34500, A10:12

Chiang PH, Chiang CP, Wu CC et al (1991) Colour duplex sonography in the assessment of impotence. Br J Urol 68:181–186

Connolly JA, Borirakchanyavat S, Lue TF (1996) Ultrasound evaluation of the penis for assessment of impotence. J Clin Ultrasound 24:481–486

Cormio L, Nisen H, Selvaggi FP, Ruutu M (1996) A positive pharmacological erection test does not rule out arteriogenic erectile dysfunction. J Urol 156:1628–1630

Cornud F, Boisrond L, Bonnel D et al (1992) Color Doppler ultrasonograpy in the investigation of vasculogenic impotence. Prog Urol 2:420–426

Courtheoux P, Maiza D, Henriet JP, Vaislic CD, Evrard C, Theron J (1986) Erectile dysfunction caused by venous leakage: treatment with detectable balloons and coils. Radiology 161:807–809

Delcour C, Wespes E, Vandenbosch G, Schulman CC, Struyven J (1986) Impotence: evaluation with cavernosography. Radiology 161:803–806

Donatucci CF, Lue TF (1992) The combined intracavernous injection and stimulation test: diagnostic accuracy. J Urol 148:61–62

Fitzgerald SW, Erickson SJ, Foley WD, Lipchik EO, Lawson TL (1991) Color Doppler sonography in the evaluation of erectile dysfunction: patterns of temporal response to papaverine. AJR 157:331–336

Goldstein I, Krane RJ, Greenfield AJ, Padma-Nathen H (1990) Vascular diseases of the penis: impotence and priapism. In: Pollack HM (ed) Clinical urography, vol 3. Saunders, Philadelphia, pp 2231–2252

Jarow JP, Pugh VW, Routh WD, Dyer RB (1993) Comparison of penile duplex ultrasonography to pudendal arteriography. Invest Radiol 28:806–810

Keogan MT, Kliewer MA, Herzberg BS et al (1996) Doppler sonography in the evaluation of corporo-venous competence after penile vein ligation surgery. J Ultrasound Med 15:227–233

Kropman RF, Schipper J, Oostayen JA, Licklama AAB, Meinhardt W (1992) The value of increased end diastolic velocity during penile duplex sonography in relation to pathological venous leakage in erectile dysfunction. J Urol 148:314–317

Lee B, Sikka SC, Randrup ER et al (1993) Standardization of penile blood flow studies using duplex ultrasonography. J Urol 149:49–52

Lopez JA, Espeland MA, Jarow JP (1991) Interpretation and quantification of penile blood flow studies using duplex ultrasonography. J Urol 146:1271–1275

Lue TF, Tanagho EA (1987) Physiology of erection and pharmacological management of impotence. J Urol 137:829–836

Lue TF, Hricak H, Marich KW, Tanagho EA (1985) Evaluation of vasculogenic impotence with high resolution ultrasonography and pulsed Doppler spectrum analysis. Radiology 155:777–781

Malhrotra CM, Balko A, Wincze JP, Bansal S, Susset JG (1986) Cavernosography in conjunction with arterial erection for evaluation of venous leakage in impotent men. Radiology 161:799–802

Mancini M, Bartolini M, Maggi M, Innocenti P, Forti G (1996) The presence of arterial anatomical variations can affect the results of duplex sonographic evaluation of penile vessels in impotent patients. J Urol 155:1919–1923

Merckx LA, De Bruyne RMG, Goes E, Derde MP, Keuppens F (1992) The value of dynamic color duplex scanning in the diagnosis of venogenic impotence. J Urol 148:318–320

Meuleman EJ, Bemelmans BH, Van Asten WN, Doesburg WH, Skotnicki SH, Debruyne FM (1992) Assessment of penile blood flow by duplex ultrasonography in 44 men with normal erectile potency in different phases of erection. J Urol 147:51–56

Montorsi F, Guazzoni G, Barbieri L et al (1996) The effect of intracorporeal injection plus genital and audiovisual sexual stimulation versus second injection on penile color Doppler sonography parameters. J Urol 155:536–540

Mueller SC, von Wallenberg-Pachaly H, Voges GE, Schild HH (1990) Comparison of selective internal iliac pharmacoangiography, penile brachial index and duplex sonography with pulsed Doppler analysis for the evaluation of vasculogenic impotence. J Urol 143:928–932

Nisen HO, Saarinen O, Ruutu ML, Edgren J (1993) Duplex Doppler scanning with prostaglandin E1 in the diagnosis of cavernous leakage. Acta Radiol 34:335–338

Oates CP, Pickard RS, Powell PH, Murthy LNS, Whittingham TAW (1995) The use of duplex ultrasound in the assessment of arterial supply to the penis in vasculogenic impotence. J Urol 153:354–357

Pescatori ES, Hatzichristou DG, Namburi S, Goldstein I (1994) A positive intracavernous injection test implies normal veno-occlusive but not necessarily normal arterial function: a hemodynamic study. J Urol 151:1209–1216

Quam JP, King BF, James EM et al (1989) Duplex and color Doppler sonographic evaluation of vasculogenic impotence. AJR 153:1141–1147

Rajfer J, Canan V, Dorey FJ, Mehringer CM (1990) Correlation between penile angiography and duplex scanning of cavernous arteries in impotent men. J Urol 143:1128–1130

Rosen MP, Greenfield AJ, Walker TG et al (1990) Arteriogenic impotence: findings in 195 impotent men examined with selective internal pudendal angiography. Radiology 174:1043–1048

Roy C, Brun F, Le Bras F, Leroux E (1995) Imagerie de l'impuissance. Feuillets Radiol 34:440–452

Schwartz A, Wang K, Mack L (1989) Evaluation of normal erectile function with color flow Doppler sonography. AJR 153:1155–1160

Shabsigh R, Fischman IJ, Quesada ET, Seale-Hawkins CK, Dunn JK (1989) Evaluation of vasculogenic erectile impotence using penile duplex ultrasonography. J Urol 142:1469–1474

Stackl W, Hasun R, Marberger M (1988) Intravavernous injection of prostaglandin E1 in impotent men. J Urol 140:66–68

Valji K, Bookstein JJ (1993) Diagnosis of arteriogenic impotence: efficacy of duplex sonography as a screening tool. AJR 160:65–69

Virag R (1982) Intracavernous injection of papaverine for erectile failure. Lancet 8304:938

11 Testicular Tumors

D. JEANBOURQUIN, J. MERRER, and O. BERNARD

CONTENTS

11.1 Introduction

The wide variety of testicular neoplasms is dominated by malignant germ cell tumors, which represent 1% of all malignant tumors in men. Owing to their extreme chemosensitivity, these tumors constitute a nearly unique study model in oncology. Imaging plays an important role because early diagnosis and accurate disease staging are essential for effective management.

11.2 Epidemiology

Although the incidence of primary malignant testicular tumors is relatively well known, less data is available for other testicular tumors (secondary malignancies or benign tumors). Testicular neoplasms are infrequent in France (2–4 per 100,000), where they account for only 0.4% of the general mortality. The incidence is higher in the United States (38 per 100,000 in 1981). Primary testicular tumors have a predilection for young men between 20 and 40 years of age (76%) and are most common in white subjects. Risk factors include congenital causes such as cryptorchidism (which represents an estimated relative risk of 4) and endocrine disorders (excessive estrogen and/or insufficient androgen production), which are often associated with testicular atrophy. The exact role of viral, socioeconomic, thermal, or other factors has not yet been established.

D. JEANBOURQUIN, J. MERRER, O. BERNARD, Service de Radiologie, HIA Percy, 101 avenue Henri Barbusse, BP 406, 92141 Clamart, France

11.3 Histological Classification

It is important to distinguish primary malignant germ cell tumors from other testicular tumors.

11.3.1 Primary Malignant Germ Cell Tumors

Germ cell tumors account for nearly 96% of all testicular tumors (WINTER et al. 1995) and 70%–90% in children (LUKER and SIEGEL 1994, 1996). These lesions are subdivided into pure seminomas, which represent 40% of all germ cell tumors, and nonseminomatous germ cell tumors (NSGCT). NSGCT can be classified histologically into four main types: embryonal cell carcinoma (20%), mature teratoma (5%), choriocarcinoma (1.5%), and mixed tumors (40%).

11.3.2 Non-germ-cell Tumors

11.3.2.1 Secondary Malignant Tumors of the Testis

Testicular localizations of non-Hodgkin lymphoma (NHL), leukemia, or metastases of certain cancers are the most common secondary testicular neoplasms. Malignant lymphoma accounts for 1%–7%

of all testicular tumors (MAZZU et al. 1994), and most of these testicular lesions occur in patients with known lymphoma. Primary lymphoma of the testis is infrequent. Testicular leukemia is most common in children.

Prostate cancer is the origin of most testicular metastases (ROYAL et al. 1994; FORNAGE et al. 1995). Renal and bladder carcinoma may also metastasize to the testis.

11.3.2.2
Stromal Tumors

Leydig cell tumors and Sertoli cell tumors account for approximately 3%–4% of all testicular tumors (DUDIAK et al. 1994). Granulosa tumors are less common.

11.3.2.3
Other Non-germ-cell Tumors

Less frequent benign testicular tumors include epidermoid cyst, carcinoid tumor, adenomatoid tumor, lipoma, fibroma, adrenal rest tumor, and testicular sarcoid (Winter et al. 1995). This list is not exhaustive.

11.4
Germ Cell Tumors

11.4.1
Diagnosis

11.4.1.1
Clinical Diagnosis

Diagnosis of testicular tumors is essentially clinical. Testicular swelling or an enlarged scrotum are highly suggestive. The testis may contain a hard, often craggy mass. However, a normal physical examination does not rule out an occult testicular tumor (SEIDENWURM et al. 1985; VAN DIJK et al. 1994; CORET et al. 1995). In a series of 3019 scrotal ultrasound studies, COMITER et al. (1996) found 15 clinically impalpable intratesticular masses, including five seminomas and six nonseminomas. The first warning sign is occasionally an extratesticular symptom, e.g., gynecomastia, abdominal mass due to nodal enlargement, supraclavicular lymphadenopathy, mediastinopulmonary involvement. Complementary laboratory tests are indicated whenever a testicular tumor is suspected, with particular attention paid to tumor markers.

11.4.1.2
Ultrasound Diagnosis

The patient is examined in the supine position, with the scrotum fixed in position to facilitate exploration. Optimum spatial and contrast resolution are essential; 7.5- or 10-MHz linear phased-array transducers are usually recommended, depending on testicular volume. On occasion, lower frequencies or curved transducers prove helpful. B-mode scanning is usually sufficient for tumor identification, but complementary spectral and color Doppler sonography (CD) is often useful.

As certain germ cell tumors have ultrasound features similar to the normal surrounding tissue, a meticulous examination technique is required. The operator must be familiar with gain settings in order to evaluate subtle differences in echogenicity between normal and pathologic tissue. Image postprocessing is sometimes necessary. A water standoff pad may improve identification of small superficial lesions.

Bilateral examination is mandatory because the contralateral testis is involved in 1%–2.7% of cases (synchronously in 22%) (ROYAL et al. 1994; LENZ et al. 1996).

Localization. The first problem after detection of a testicular mass is extra- or intratesticular localization. Thanks to technological advances, intratesticular sites can now be affirmed in nearly 100% of patients (UCHIYAMA et al. 1994). Bulky tumors may involve problems for topographic diagnosis, but identification of normal testicular tissue either partially or completely surrounding the mass suggests an intratesticular site (UCHIYAMA et al. 1994).

Sonographic Patterns. Most germ cell tumors present as a smoothly contoured focal mass with a hypoechoic echotexture. Some, however, have an inhomogeneous echotexture and contain zones of increased echogenicity. These tissue abnormalities are occasionally associated with hyperechoic masses with shadowing corresponding to calcifications.

CD may be a beneficial complement to B-mode scanning. For HORSTMAN et al. (1992), CD demonstrated hypervascularity in over 95% of tumors larger than 1.6 cm and hypovascularity in 86% of tumors smaller than 1.6 cm.

Although nonspecific, a number of ultrasound patterns have been related to histologic features (GERSCOVICH 1993):

- Seminomas typically have a homogeneous or inhomogeneous hypoechoic echotexture (Fig. 11.1) with more or less well defined contours (GALARDO AGROMAYOR et al. 1996).
- Embryonal cell carcinoma (Fig. 11.2) and choriocarcinoma often present as bulky tumors deforming the contours of the testis; their heterogeneous echotexture combines hypoechoic, hyperechoic, and cystic elements.
- Teratomas are characterized by an inhomogeneous echotexture with calcifications (Fig. 11.3) and cysts (Fig. 11.4)

Following clinical and sonographic detection of such lesions, orchiectomy is indispensable to confirm the diagnosis; it also constitutes the first stage of therapy. Tumor marker assays are also required, in particular human b-chorionic gonadotropin (b-hCG) and α-fetoprotein.

Differential Diagnosis. Once the intratesticular location has been established, differential diagnosis essentially concerns nonprimary malignant intratesticular tumors, benign lesions, and nontumoral pathologies (TESSLER et al. 1996). Other non-germ-cell tumors are dealt with later, and only nontumoral pathologies are included in this discussion on differential diagnosis.

The clinical presentation and medical history provide important diagnostic information. Sonographic demonstration of abnormal intratesticular echotexture in an inflammatory context is suggestive of a pathology such as orchitis. Depiction of testicular

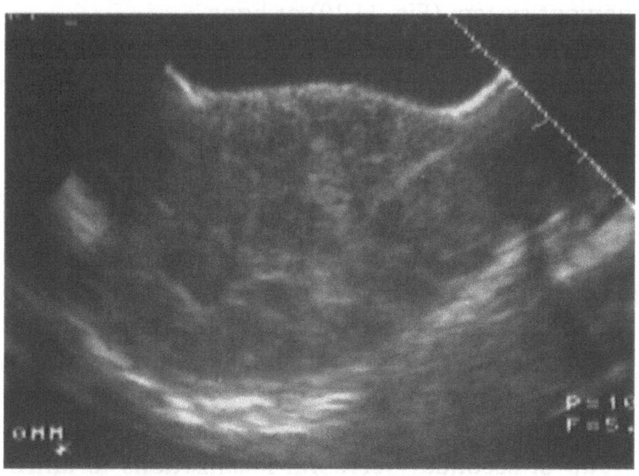

Fig. 11.1. Diffusely enlarged hypoechoic testis with an inhomogeneous echotexture: seminoma

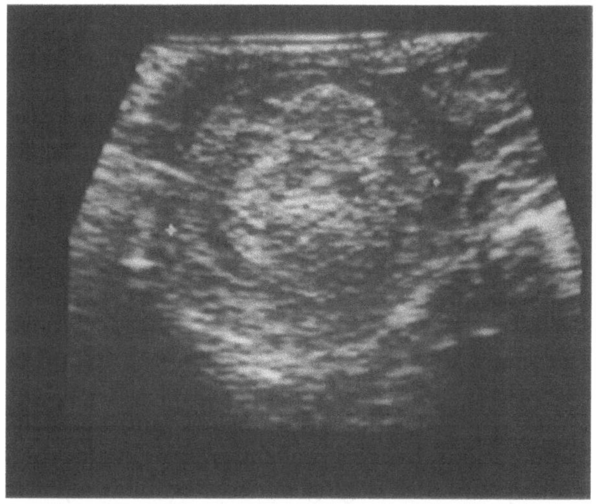

Fig. 11.2. Inhomogeneous tumor with smooth margins distorting the contours of the testis: embryonal cell carcinoma

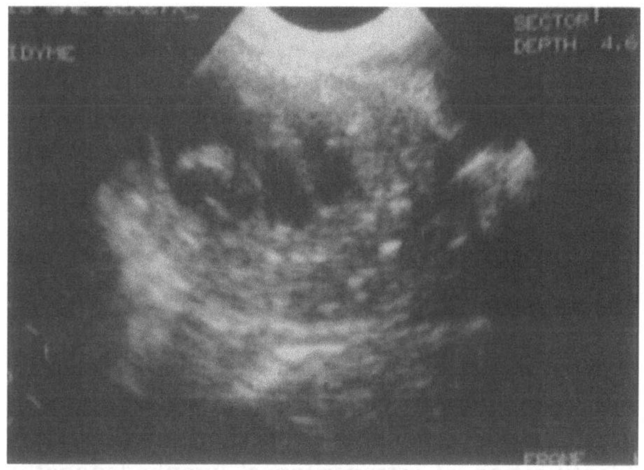

Fig. 11.3. Heterogeneous testicular tumor with cystic zones and microcalcifications: mature teratoma

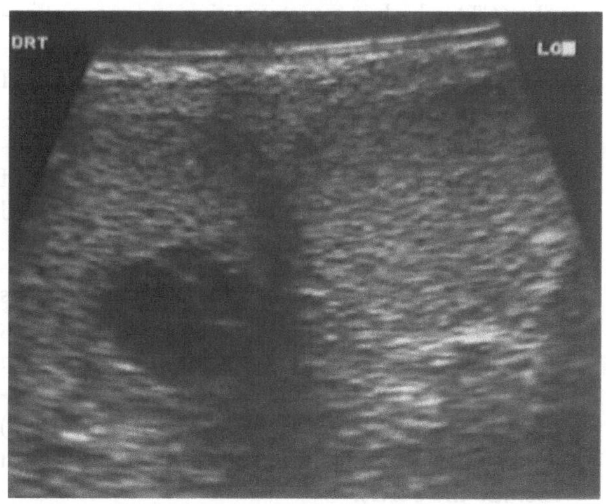

Fig. 11.4. Scrotal sonogram of a tumor with a predominant cystic component: mature teratoma

and epididymal hypervascularity by Doppler examination is also suggestive of an inflammatory process. In contrast, testicular hypervascularity without epididymal hyperhemia is suggestive of a neoplasm (Mazzu et al. 1994). A history of trauma may help differentiate hematoma from a possible tumor.

11.4.2 Disease Staging

Pretherapy disease staging is obligatory following diagnosis because local, locoregional, and distant disease spread determine the prognosis and therapeutic indications. Imaging modalities play a major role, not only for initial staging, but also for follow-up and evaluation of postchemotherapy residual masses.

11.4.2.1 Local Staging

Local disease staging is performed during orchiectomy and may reveal spread to the rete testis, the epididymis, or the spermatic cord. Neoplastic, lymphatic, and vascular emboli may be present.

11.4.2.2 Locoregional Staging

Whenever a suspicious testicular lesion is detected, locoregional disease staging should begin with sonographic evaluation of the retroperitoneum (Fig. 11.5). Identification of retroperitoneal lymphadenopathy corresponding to nodal extension confirms the tumoral nature of the testicular lesion. Locoregional staging is performed primarily by computed tomography (CT), which is more sensitive and more effective for monitoring response to therapy than ultrasound. CT protocols include intravenous injection of a contrast medium and opacification of bowel loops.

The pattern of disease spread to the retroperitoneal nodes is explained by the embryonal origins of the testis and depends on the side involved (Bassoulet et al. 1987; Robson et al. 1996):

- *Left-sided testicular tumors:* nodal spread occurs preferentially to the high left para-aortic nodes, especially at the confluence of the spermatic vein and the left renal vein. Involvement of the primary iliac nodes alone is rare. WHITE et al. (1997) consider abdominal CT sufficient and do not include the pelvis.
- *Right-sided testicular tumors:* nodal spread is to the inter-aorticocaval nodes in nearly half of the patients (Fig. 11.6), but isolated involvement of the precaval or paracaval nodes, right common iliac nodes (Fig. 11.7), and right external iliac nodes or preaortic nodes is not uncommon.

All of the node groups may be involved if massive disease is present; this is particularly true for right-sided testicular tumors owing to extensive right-to-left lymphatic crossover.

CT does, however, have certain limitations. If 2 cm is considered the upper limit for normal nodes, CT has a 20%–30% false-negative rate compared to surgery. Inversely, if a node smaller than 2 cm is considered pathologic at CT, the false-positive rate is 20%–25% compared to surgery (Leibovitch et al. 1995). Interpretation of results must take account of postorchiectomy tumor marker levels: a suspicious node on CT can be considered pathologic if tumor markers are elevated.

11.4.2.3 General Staging

Dissemination occurs by lymphatic and hematogenous spread. General staging also relies greatly on CT and must take into account the modes of extension of these tumors. Lymphatic spread through the diaphragmatic hiatus generally results in left-sided lymphadenopathy of the supraclavicular nodes (Antoine et al. 1995); right-sided lymphadenopathy is much less frequent (10% of patients). Intraperitoneal metastases (Heafield et al. 1994) and extranodal mediastinal involvement (Philips 1994) are rare. Hematogeneous spread through the spermatic vein and the inferior vena cava explains extranodal sites in the lungs (Fig. 11.8) and liver (Fig. 11.9) and occasionally the central nervous system (Fig. 11.10) or bone.

Owing to the benefits of CT, other imaging techniques have limited indications for staging:

- Chest radiography can demonstrate intraparenchymal lung nodules and occasionally mediastinal nodal sites.
- Ultrasound is indicated for detection of hepatic metastases.
- Magnetic resonance imaging (MRI) currently has no role in staging of testicular tumors because it does not provide any supplementary information (Fig. 11.11). The only potential indication is work-up of secondary cerebral localizations to affirm their solitary nature when a local surgical procedure is envisaged.

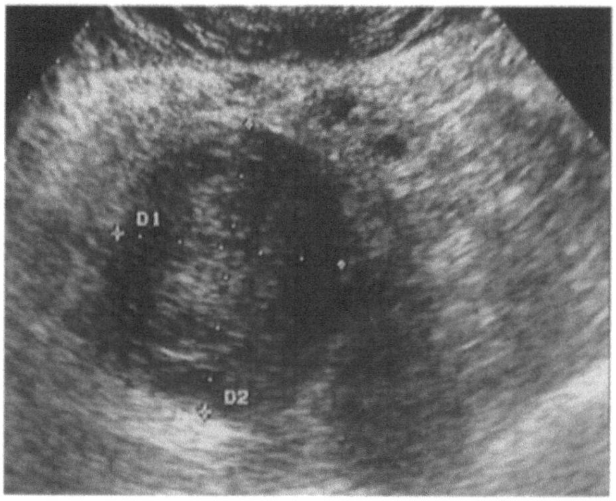

Fig. 11.5. Abdominal sonogram: bulky inhomogeneously hypoechoic inter-aorticocaval nodal mass (same patient as in Fig. 11.2). *D1*, 55 mm between the two *crosses*; *D2*, 56 mm between the two *crosses*

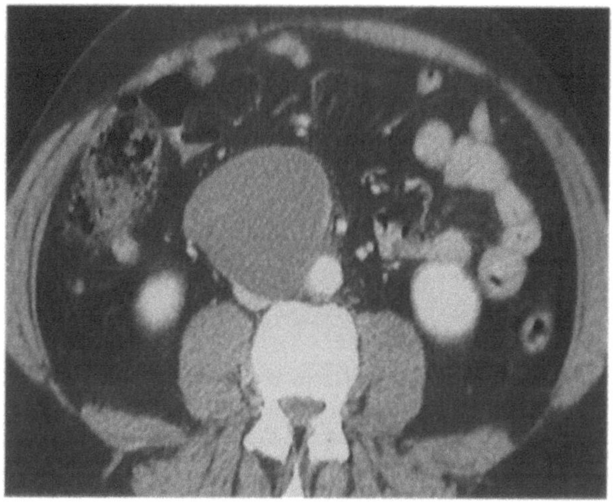

Fig. 11.6. Abdominal CT scan: homogeneous smoothly marginated inter-aorticocaval nodal mass (same patient as in Fig. 11.2)

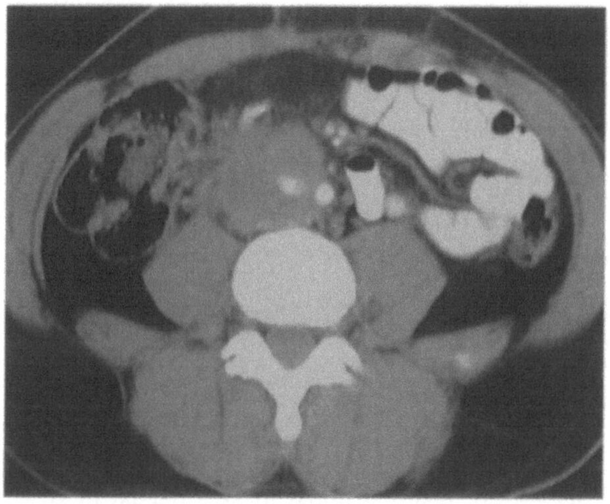

Fig. 11.7. Abdominal CT scan: hypodense right common iliac nodal mass with poorly defined right anterolateral margins encasing the adjacent artery: nodal metastasis of a right mixed germ cell tumor

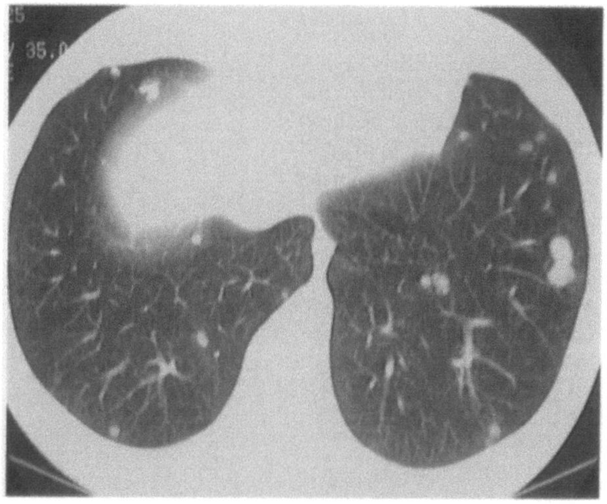

Fig. 11.8. Thoracic CT scan demonstrating multiple bilateral parenchymal lung nodules: metastases of a testicular choriocarcinoma

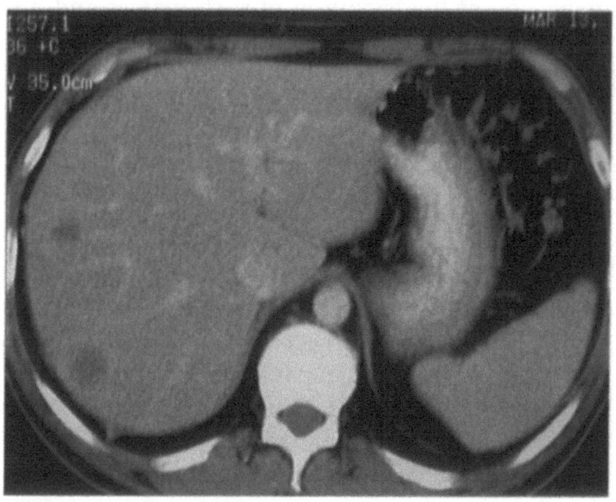

Fig. 11.9. CT scan revealing two hepatic metastases of a testicular embryonal cell carcinoma

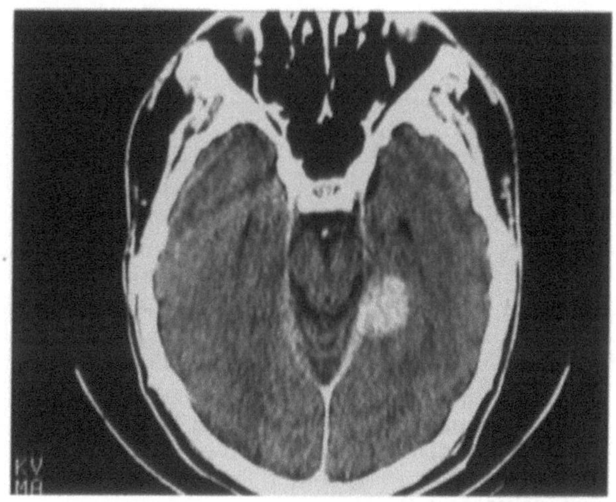

Fig. 11.10. Contrast-enhanced CT brain scan depicting a hyperdense right temporal mass: metastasis of a testicular teratoma

- Fluorodeoxyglucose positron emission tomography (FDG-PET) is reportedly more sensitive and more specific than CT for assessment of nodal involvement (Bender et al. 1997).

Following disease staging, tumors are usually classified according to the Royal Marsden Hospital classification (Tables 11.1, 11.2).

Table 11.1. Royal Marsden Hospital staging classification

Stage	Features
I	*No evidence of metastases*
IM	Rising serum markers with no evidence of metastases
II	*Abdominal node metastases*
IIA	<2 cm in diameter
IIB	2–5 cm in diameter
IIC	>5 cm in diameter
III	*Supradiaphragmatic node metastases*
III0	No abdominal node metastases
IIIA	<2 cm in diameter
IIIB	2–5 cm in diameter
IIIC	>5 cm in diameter
IV	*Extralymphatic metastases*
L1 lung	<3 metastases
L2 lung	>3 metastases, all <2 cm in diameter
L3 lung	>3 metastases, one or more >2 cm in diameter
H+	Liver metastases
Br+	Brain metastases
Bo+	Bone metastases

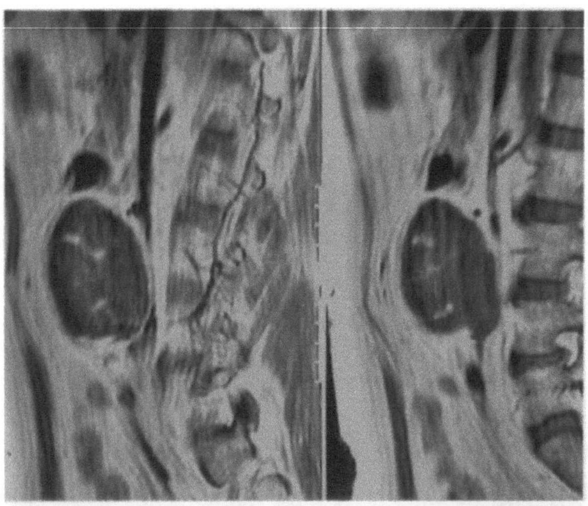

Fig. 11.11. Contrast-enhanced sagittal T_1-weighted MRI of a smoothly contoured, oval retroperitoneal nodal mass with hyperintense central zones exerting mass effect on the inferior vena cava: nodal metastasis of embryonal cell carcinoma (same patient as in Fig. 11.2)

Table 11.2. Royal Marsden Hospital prognostic groups

Stage	Tumor markers	Prognosis
IM, IIA, IIIA, IIIB, IV0ABL1, IV0ABL2, IIC, IIIC, IVCL1, IVCL2	<1000 IU b-hCG/l, <500 IU a-fetoprotein/l	Good
IVL30ABL, IVH+, IIC, IIIC, IVCL1, IVCL2	Elevated	Poor

hCG, human chorionic gonadotropin.

11.4.3 Surveillance Protocols

Pre- and post-therapy surveillance policies rely on the same imaging techniques: chest radiography, abdominal ultrasound, and thoracoabdominal CT. Scanning must always be associated with tumor marker assays. The periodicity of restaging varies with the medical team. Surveillance every 3 months during the first year, every 6 months during the next 2 years, and then once a year for 7 years appears adequate.

11.4.4 Evaluation of Residual Masses

Despite elevated response rates to chemotherapy (70%–90%), residual nodal masses persist in 20%–90% of patients, depending on the series. Evaluation of these masses relies on the same techniques described above (Fig. 11.12). FDG-PET (Fig. 11.13) and gallium scintigraphy appear more effective for documentation of the evolution of such masses and differentiation of active tumor masses from residual fibrosis (Uchiyama 1994). Tumor marker levels must also be taken into consideration.

11.4.4.1 Normalized Tumor Markers

Generally speaking, residual masses consist of one third fibrosis, one third necrotic tissue, and one third active tissue. Imaging, in particular CT, is important because the therapeutic approach depends on their size and location. For stage IIC, II, and IV seminomatous tumors, only residual masses larger than 3 cm require surgery; masses smaller than 3 cm

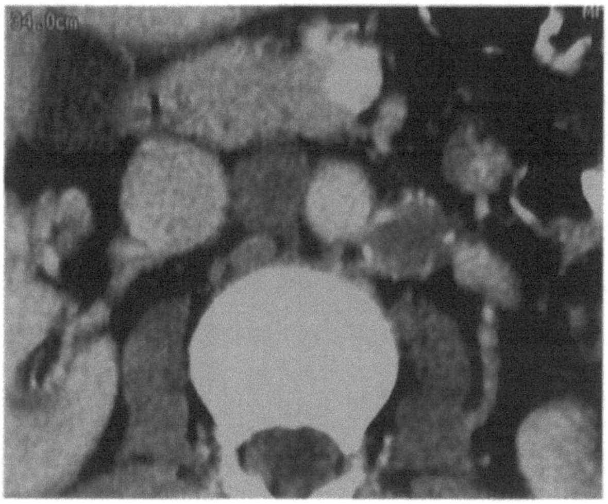

Fig. 11.12. Contrast-enhanced abdominal CT scan of a patient treated for a left testicular germ cell tumor with lymphatic spread, predominantly to the left lateroaortic nodes. Persistence of two residual nodes (inter-aorticocaval and left lateroaortic) after chemotherapy. No active tumor tissue was found on histologic examination of the surgical specimen. Tumor markers were also normal

are merely kept under surveillance. For stage IIA and IIB nonseminomatous germ cell tumors, unilateral lymphadenectomy is performed. For stage IIC, III, and IV tumors, residual nodal and visceral masses require resection.

11.4.4.2
Persistence of Abnormal Tumor Markers

Treatment of residual tumor mass with persistent abnormal tumor markers consists in salvage chemotherapy or an autograft of peripheral stem cells collected after one or two courses of mobilization chemotherapy.

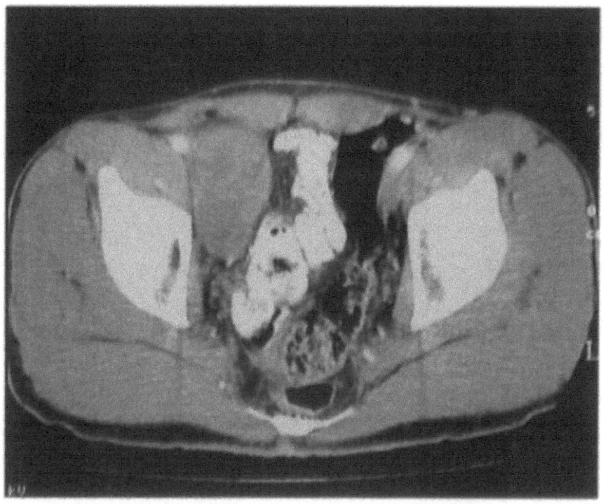

a

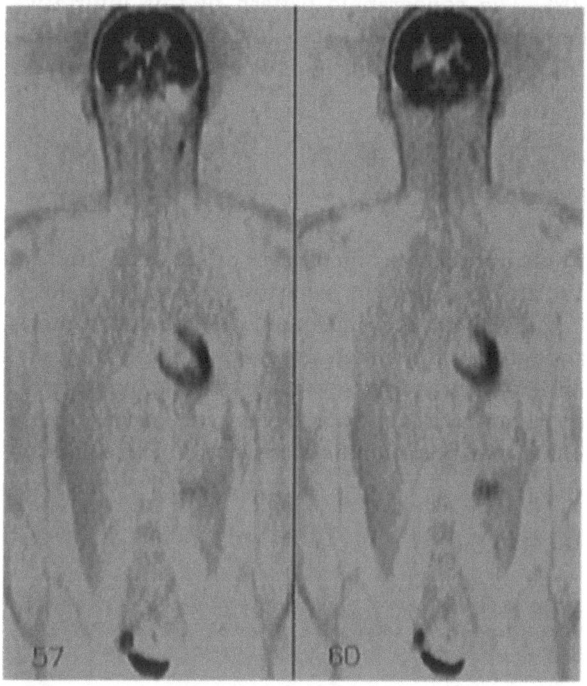

b

Fig. 11.13. **a** Abdominal CT: postchemotherapy right iliac residual nodal mass of a testicular germ cell tumor. **b** Fluorodeoxyglucose positron emission tomography (FDG-PET). High uptake by the right iliac nodal tumor; active tumor tissue was found in the surgical specimen. Tumor markers were also elevated

11.5
Other Non-germ-cell Tumors

11.5.1
Malignant Testicular Tumors

11.5.1.1
Lymphoma

Malignant lymphoma accounts for 1%–7% of all testicular tumors and is one of the most frequent causes of testicular enlargement in men over 50 years of age (Bland et al. 1986; Mazzu et al. 1994). Ultrasound typically demonstrates unilateral or bilateral testicular enlargement; the testes remain ovoid despite the presence of diffuse or focal hypoechoic lesions. Sonographic abnormalities are sometimes subtle

(Fig. 11.14). CD has been advocated as a means of demonstrating hypervascularity that reflects tumor invasion, especially if epididymal vascularity is normal (HORSTMAN et al. 1992)

11.5.1.2
Leukemia

Testicular leukemia is most common in childhood, and testicular involvement is encountered in nearly 8% of all boys with leukemia (MAZZU et al. 1994). According to LUKER and SIEGEL (1994, 1996), testicular involvement is clinically evident in only 5%–30% of patients, whereas it is found at autopsy in 60%. The sonographic pattern of this infiltrative malignancy is similar to that of testicular lymphoma, i.e., diffuse or focal zones of decreased echogenicity.

11.5.1.3
Metastases

Nonlymphomatous metastases of the testis are rare and are dominated by metastases of prostate cancer. Colorectal cancer, malignant neurogenic tumors, and retinoblastoma can also metastasize to the testis. Little information is available on the sonographic appearance of testicular metastases, because these lesions are not sought systematically. Variable echo patterns have been described, e.g., hypoechoic or hyperechoic, inhomogeneous, presence of cystic zones. Prostate cancer is the origin of nearly 75% of all bilateral testicular metastases (FORNAGE et al. 1995).

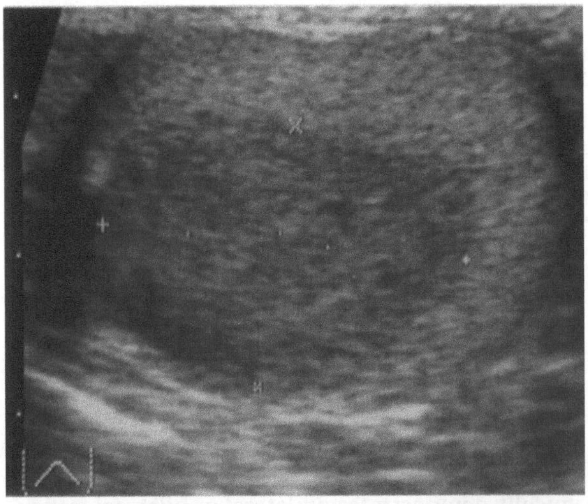

Fig. 11.14. Homogeneously hypoechoic and smoothly marginated intratesticular mass without deformation of testicular contours: testicular site of thoracoabdominal non-Hodgkin lymphoma (NHL)

11.5.2
Stromal Tumors

11.5.2.1
Leydig Cell Tumors

Leydig cell tumors, which account for nearly 3% of all tumors of the testis, are bilateral in 4%–10% of patients (Fig. 11.15). Abnormal sex hormone production by the lesion causes precocious pseudopuberty in boys and gynecomastia, gynecoid obesity, and azoospermia in adults. Between 10% and 15% of these tumors are malignant, and malignancy is encountered particularly frequently in adults. Ultrasound typically demonstrates a hypoechoic tumor, while hyperechoic masses are less common.

11.5.2.2
Sertoli Cell Tumors

Sertoli cell tumors represent 1% of all testicular tumors. Gynecomastia is an accompanying feature in 30% of patients, and features of malignancy are observed in 10%–20%. These hypo- or hyperechoic tumors are usually well circumscribed and smaller than 3 cm. Calcifying Sertoli cell tumors (DUDIAK et al. 1994; GIERKE et al. 1994) may be bilateral and are frequently multifocal (60% of patients). These tumors are associated with various syndromes, e.g., Peutz-Jeghers syndrome, Carney's complex (PREMKUMAR et al. 1997).

11.5.2.3
Granulosa Tumors

Granulosa tumors of the testis are similar to their ovarian counterpart. Half of all patients exhibit feminization. These lesions are encountered in males of all ages and may be associated with congenital urinary tract anomalies.

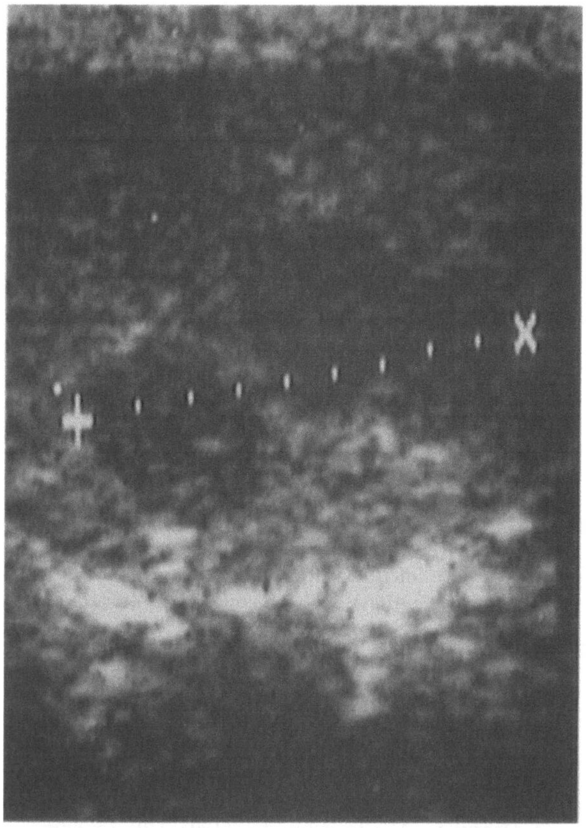

Fig. 11.15. Sonogram of three hypoechoic intratesticular masses without deformation of testicular contours: Leydig cell tumor. 25 mm between the two crosses

11.5.3
Mixed Cell Tumors

Gonadoblastomas are the most common mixed cell tumor; they account for nearly 0.5% of all testicular tumors and are seen in all age-groups. Seminomatous cells are the predominant cell type. Metastases are present in approximately 10% of patients. Other mixed cell tumors are rare and comprise a variety of germ cell lines.

11.5.4
Miscellaneous Tumors

11.5.4.1
Epidermoid Cysts

Epidermoid cysts are benign lesions (1% of all testicular tumors) that consist of a squamous epithelium secreting keratin. They are usually discovered fortuitously. Surgery is required to differentiate them from a potentially malignant mature teratoma.

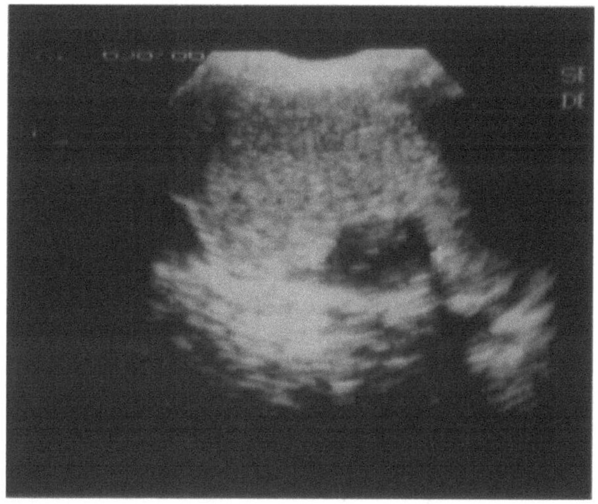

Fig. 11.16. This inhomogeneously hypoechoic intratesticular mass with smooth contours does not distort the contours of the testis

11.5.4.2
Carcinoid Tumors

Testicular carcinoids are divided into three groups: (1) pure primary carcinoid tumors, the most frequent type (Fig. 11.16), (2) pure primary carcinoid tumors with a teratoma, and (3) metastatic carcinoid tumors of the testis.

11.5.4.3
Mesenchymal Tumors

Mesenchymal tumors are rare lesions that may be benign, i.e., leiomyoma, angioma, fibroma, lipoma, adrenal rest tumor (Seidenwurm et al. 1985; Avila et al. 1996), and adenomatoid tumor (Feuer et al. 1996), or malignant, i.e., leiomyosarcoma and rhabdomyosarcoma.

References

Antoine E, Droz JP, Buthiau D (1995) Les tumeurs du testicule. In: Buthiau D, Khayat D (eds) Scanner et IRM en cancérologie. Springer, Berlin Heidelberg New York, pp 325–333

Avila NA, Premkumar A, Shawker TH, Jones JV, Laue L, Cutler GB (1996) Testicular adrenal rest tissue in congenital adrenal hyperplasia: findings at gray scale and color Doppler US. Radiology 198:99–104

Bassoulet J, Pabot du Chatelard P, Timbal Y (1987) Les trois stades du cancer du testicule. Extension, imagerie, marqueurs biologiques. Rev Prat (Paris) 37:1107–1119

Bender H, Schomburg A, Ruhlman J, Biersack HJ (1997) Possible role of FDG-PET in the evaluation of urologic malignancies. Anticancer Res 17:1655–1660

Bland PH, Di Pietro MA, Chenevert TL, Hutchinson RJ, Carson PL (1986) Tissue characterization of the testis using ultrasonic CT. Work in progress. Radiology 159:101–105

Comiter CV, Benson CJ, Capelouto CC et al (1996) Nonpalpable intratesticular masses detected sonographically. Radiology 198:914 (abstr)

Coret A, Leibovitch I, Heyman Z, Goldbasser B, Itschak Y (1995) Ultrasonographic evaluation and clinical correlation of intratesticular lesion: a series of 39 cases. Br J Urol 76:216–219

Dudiak CM, Vade A, Isaac RM (1994) Sonographic demonstration of bilateral large cell calcifying Sertoli cell tumors of the testis. J Ultrasound Med 13:232–235

Feuer A, Dewire DM, Foley WD (1996) Ultrasonographic characteristics of testicular adenomatoid tumors. J Urol 155:174–175

Fornage BD, Logothetis CJ, Swanson DA, Ro JY (1995) Bilateral testicular metastases from prostatic carcinoma: gray-scale and color Doppler sonographic findings. J Ultrasound Med 14:247–249

Galardo Agromayor E, Pena Gomez E, Lopez Rasines G et al (1996) Testicular tumors. Echographic findings. Arch Esp Urol 49:622–626

Gerscovich EO (1993) High resolution ultrasonography in the diagnosis of scrotal pathology. II. Tumors. J Clin Ultrasound 21:375–386

Gierke CL, King BF, Bostwick DG, Choyke PL, Hattery RR (1994) Large cell calcifying cell tumor of the testis: appearance at sonography. AJR 163:373–375

Heafield RJ, Mead GM, Tung KT (1994) Case report: intraperitoneal metastases from testicular germ cell tumor. Br J Radiol 67:501–503

Horstman WG, Melson GL, Middleton WG, Andriole GL (1992) Testicular tumors: findings with Doppler US. Radiology 185:733–737

Leibovitch L, Foster RL, Kopecky KK, Donohue JP (1995) Improved accuracy of computerized tomography-based clinical staging in low stage nonseminomatous germ cell cancer using size criteria of retroperitoneal lymph nodes. J Urol 154:1759–1763

Lenz S, Skakkebaek NE, Hertel NT (1996) Abnormal ultrasonic pattern in controlateral testis in patients with unilateral testicular cancer. World J Urol 14:55–58

Luker GD, Siegel MJ (1994) Pediatric testicular tumors: evaluation with gray-scale and color Doppler US. Radiology 191:561–564

Luker GD, Siegel MJ (1996) Scrotal US in pediatric patients: comparison of power and standard color Doppler US. Radiology 198:381–385

Mazzu D, Jeffrey RB, Ralls PW (1994) Lymphoma and leukemia involving the testicles: findings on gray-scale and color Doppler sonography. AJR 164:645–657

Phillips CJ (1994) Case report: metastatic malignant testicular teratoma of the thymus. Br J Radiol 67:203–204

Premkumar A, Stratakis CA, Shawker TH, Papanicolaou DA, Chrousos GP (1997) Testicular ultrasound in Carney complex: report of three cases. J Clin Ultrasound 25:211–214

Robson AW, Tung K, Mead G (1996) Patterns of supradiaphragmatic metastases in testicular germ cell tumors. Clin Radiol 51:273–276

Royal SA, Joseph DB, Galliani CA (1994) Bilateral testicular teratoma. AJR 163:1130

Seidenwurm D, Smathers RL, Kan P, Hoffman A (1985) Intratesticular adrenal rests diagnosed by ultrasound. Radiology 155:479–481

Tessler FN, Tublin ME, Rifkin MD (1996) Ultrasound assessment of testicular and paratesticular masses. J Clin Ultrasound 24:423–436

Uchiyama M, Kantoff PW, Kaplan WD (1994) Gallium-67-citrate imaging in extragonadal and gonadal seminomas: relationship to radiologic findings. J Nucl Med 35:1624–1630

Van Dijk R, Doesburg WH, Verbeek ALM, Van der Schouw YT, Debruyne FMJ, Rosenbusch G (1994) Ultrasonography versus clinical examination in evaluation of testicular tumors. J Clin Ultrasound 22:179–182

White PM, Howard GC, Best JJ, Wright AR (1997) The role of tomographic examination of the pelvis in the management of testicular germ cell tumor. Clin Radiol 52:124–129

Winter TC, Keener TS, Mack LA (1995) Sonographic appearance of testicular sarcoid. J Ultrasound Med 14:153–156

12 Thyroid Gland

J. N. Bruneton, T. Livraghi, P. Y. Marcy, J. Tramalloni, and F. Tranquart

CONTENTS

12.1 Ultrasonography of Thyroid Nodules

J.N. Bruneton and J. Tramalloni

Evaluation of the thyroid is required in a number of clinical situations (Freitas and Freitas 1994), i.e., clinically solitary thyroid nodule, superior mediastinal mass, hyperthyroidism, diagnosis and postoperative follow-up of thyroid carcinoma, neonatal hypothyroidism, and anomalous thyroid development.

J.N. Bruneton, P.Y. Marcy, Centre Antoine-Lacassagne, 33 avenue de Valombrose, 06189 Nice, France
T. Livraghi, Unita Radiologia, Ospedale Civile, via C. Battisti 23, 20059 Vimercate (MI), Italy
J. Tramalloni, Cabinet de Radiologie, 25 rue du Docteur Paul Bruel, 95380 Louvres, France
F. Tranquart, Médecine Nucléaire et Ultrasons, INSERM U316, CHU Bretonneau, 37044 Tours, France

As the imaging modality of choice for assessment of thyroid morphology, ultrasound (US) can generally determine the number and location of thyroid lesions and rule out nonthyroid pathologies. Sonography facilitates the follow-up of treated patients and is less expensive than other imaging techniques. US also plays an essential role in nodular thyroid disease, in particular in the guidance of fine-needle aspiration (FNA) and the surveillance of nodules not treated surgically.

The dilemma caused by the detection of one or more thyroid nodules is not new. From the very introduction of scintigraphy, the question arose as to whether surgery was indicated for one or more generally palpable nodules. In at least 90% of patients, systematic surgical intervention resulted in excision of a benign nodule; however, a "wait-and-see" attitude involved the risk that a possibly solitary, and thus curable, neoplasm might be overlooked.

Instead of providing the answer, ultrasonography actually tended to complicate the situation, because one or more thyroid nodules are commonly detected at cervical US performed for other purposes. The increased frequency of detection of thyroid nodules can be attributed to better familiarity with their sonographic features and the use of color Doppler (CD), performed either separately or prior to US-guided FNA. US has become indispensable for thyroid examination, with a clearly recognized superiority over physical examination and scintigraphy both in adults (Brander et al. 1992) and in children (Aghini-Lombardi et al. 1997). In addition, although palpation can detect nodules of at least 1 cm, only half of all palpable nodules are truly solitary, as clearly demonstrated by US (Tan et al.1995).

The high prevalence of thyroid nodules was initially a source of controversy between advocates of a wait-and-see attitude and proponents of systematic surgical management. More recently, a consensus has been reached based on the results of US-guided FNA (Cannoni and Demard 1995; Sadoul 1995; Singer et al. 1996).

12.1.1 Nodular Thyroid Disease

12.1.1.1 Frequency of Thyroid Nodules

In a study performed in an adult population using a 13-MHz transducer, one or more thyroid nodules were discovered in 34% of the subjects (BRUNETON et al. 1994a). This figure is much higher than in epidemiological studies, which estimate the frequency of thyroid nodules at only 5% (DANESE and SCHIACCHITANO 1993; RIFAT and RUFFIN 1994). However, the prevalence of thyroid incidentalomas varies greatly in the literature. EZZAT et al. (1994) found one or more thyroid nodules in 67% of patients (physical examination was positive in only 21%), whereas MIKI et al. (1993) discovered a thyroid nodule in less than 21% (physical examination was positive in under 2%). These two series probably represent the extremes concerning the sonographic frequency of thyroid nodules.

Postmortem studies, some of which are quite old, have reported a frequency of benign or malignant thyroid nodules ranging from 8% to 45.6% (VIDONE and SILVERBERG 1966). It should also be remembered that slightly over one third of the general population, in particular women over the age of 40, have one or more thyroid nodules (HORLOCKER et al. 1986).

Thyroid carcinoma is rare. Papillary carcinoma, the main variant, has an indolent course and an excellent prognosis. In light of the anatomic frequency of thyroid nodules, management strategies require an approach that limits the risks of overlooking a carcinoma while also limiting morbidity and the cost of management. The annual rate of detection of clinically significant thyroid cancer in the general population is only 0.004% (GHARIB 1994), and thyroid carcinoma accounts for only 0.5–1.3% of all neoplasms (GANDON and LEDOUX ROBERT 1995). This low clinical frequency contrasts with postmortem rates of up to 38% (ROSS 1991). Most lesions found at autopsy, however, are microcancers. Nevertheless, establishment of guidelines remains difficult because the arguments used to support a wait-and-see attitude also apply to surgical management.

Although thyroid nodules may be fortuitous discoveries at cervical US performed for other reasons (particularly vascular studies), a systematic sonographic search for thyroid pathologies is essential in patients with the following recognized risk factors: (a) accidental irradiation, as at Chernobyl, where there has been an increase in the frequency of thyroid abnormalities (essentially thyroiditis and cystic lesions) and where the incidence of cancer is higher than in the normal population (HANCOCK et al. 1995; ITO et al. 1995; KUMPUSALO et al. 1996), and (b) a history of therapeutic irradiation of the head and neck in childhood (HEALY et al. 1996; CROM et al. 1997).

12.1.1.2 Etiology

The origin of nodular thryoid disease can be discussed in two manners. The first classification distinguishes between benign and malignant lesions:

- *Benign lesions:* multinodular goiter, Hashimoto's thyroiditis, simple or hemorrhagic colloid cyst, vesicular adenoma (orthoplastic, macrovesicular or colloid vesicular, microvesicular or fetal) solid microtrabecular, oxyphilic Hürthle cell adenomas
- *Malignant lesions:* papillary carcinoma (follicular variant, sclerosing, cystic adenocarcinoma), vesicular carcinoma (with minimal or massive invasion, oxyphilic), medullary carcinoma, undifferentiated carcinoma (anaplastic), non-Hodgkin lymphoma (NHL), metastasis, malignant hemangioendothelioma

The second approach is based on the solitary or multiple nature of nodules. As this data is provided by US, this is the classification used in this chapter:

- *Single thyroid nodule:* carcinoma, adenoma (including toxic adenoma), rarely cyst
- *Multinodular lesions:* multinodular goiter, Basedow's goiter, anaplastic carcinoma, lymphoma

12.1.1.3 Differential Diagnosis

US can differentiate a thyroid anomaly from a nonthyroidal pathology of the lateral neck such as lymphadenopathy or a cyst (FARWELL and BRAVERMAN 1996). As a result of US, the only remaining differential diagnosis for nodular thyroid disease is intrathyroid parathyroid adenoma, a rare localization accounting for only 1%–2% of cases. In patients with primary hyperparathyroidism, the thyroid lobe containing the nodule must be explored surgically, even in the absence of a sharp separation between the nodule and the adjacent thyroid parenchyma. This is especially true if the remainder of the cervical examination is normal. While there is no formal surgical indication, US-guided FNA may be helpful (SOLBIATI et al. 1995). Hyperparathyroidism is frequently associated with thyroid nodules (48% of cases according to FUNARI et al. 1992); this is not surprising in light of the elevated incidence of thyroid nodules.

Hypopharyngeal diverticulae (Zenker's diverticulae) are potentially one of the rare instances in which it may prove difficult to distinguish a thyroid nodule from a nonthyroid etiology. Dynamic analysis during deglutition usually allows differential diagnosis.

In practice, the difficulties encountered during sonographic evaluation of thyroiditis concern pseudonodular modifications in echotexture, particularly in chronic thyroiditis. The fibrous septa that image as hyperechoic bands traversing the thyroid gland may create a pseudonodular appearance. Colloid-filled follicles may image sonographically as microlesions several millimeters in size, but they are not pathologic (SOLBIATI et al. 1995; BRUNETON et al. 1996).

12.1.2 Sonographic Techniques for Thyroid Examination

12.1.2.1 Ultrasonography

For clinicians worldwide, US has become the first-line imaging modality for the thyroid (MASSOL et al. 1993). In addition to detection and accurate localization of thyroid nodules, US is highly effective in the guidance of FNA and in post-therapy follow-up (READING and GORMAN 1993; BRUNETON et al. 1996).

Currently available US units equipped with high-frequency transducers (7.5–13 MHz) provide images of remarkable clarity. However, this increase in transducer frequency does not always allow examination of the entire gland in patients with a large goiter. In contrast, high resolution permits detailed analysis of thyroid nodules and can visualize normal laterocervical nodes (BRUNETON et al. 1994a). The data provided by US has not changed significantly over the past decade (BRUNETON et al. 1996), but state-of-the art equipment allows identification of previously unrecognized anatomic structures, such as the laryngeal nerve (SOLBIATI et al. 1995).

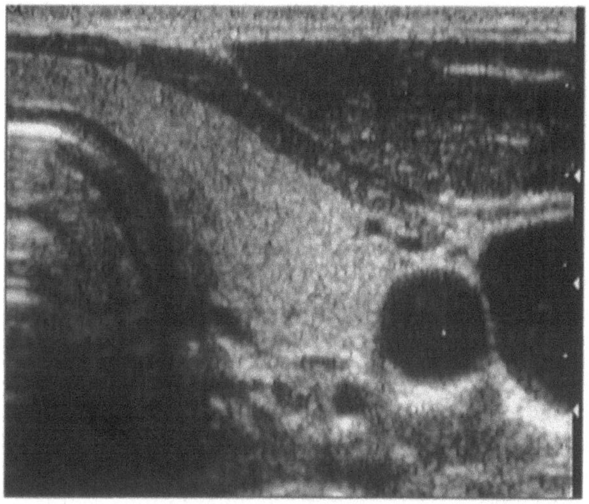

Fig. 12.1. Transverse scan: the left thyroid lobe appears homogeneous and hypoechoic relative to the sternocleidomastoid muscle

Transverse, longitudinal, and in certain cases coronal scans allow assessment of the thyroid gland, which has a fine echotexture that is more echoic than the adjacent muscles (Fig. 12.1). Before analyzing any nodules, the thyroid must be examined in its entirety. Thyroid volume and gland diameters vary considerably. In normal adults, the height ranges from 4 to 6 cm and the width from 1 to 2 cm. The anteroposterior diameter is a particularly interesting parameter because it is relatively constant from one individual to another. An anteroposterior diameter greater than 2 cm suggests an underlying pathology not visible by US. Anteroposterior diameters greater than 2.5 cm are frankly abnormal, regardless of the results of morphologic analysis of the gland. Thyroid volume can be determined from contiguous scans (mean, 10±4 ml) (YOKOYAMA et al. 1988; JARLOV et al. 1991).

A decrease in thyroid volume is common in the elderly, as are modifications in the echotexture, which becomes discretely inhomogeneous, combining variable proportions of anechoic colloid zones and small areas of fibrosis. These modifications do not signify a pathologic condition (GONCZI et al. 1994).

Thyroid US is completed by examination of the laterocervical neck in search of lymphadenopathy. Except for clinically evident lesions, this requires the use of a high-frequency transducer. The normal lymph node is oval and has an echogenic central hilum. An inflammatory node may present the entire spectrum of morphologic appearances, but remains oval. Metastatic nodes appear round, even when normal sized or smaller than normal, and lack an echogenic hilum (Bruneton et al. 1994b).

The presence of one or more thyroid nodules requires analysis of their echotexture (solid with an echotexture comparable to that of the healthy tissue, fluid zones, calcifications) and contours and determination of the extent of the normal parenchyma and the various thyroid diameters. Locoregional examination must include a search for lymphadenopathy and tracheal compression. Thyroid mobility should be assessed during deglutition. Very high frequency transducers allow evaluation of the capsule and the visceral sheath (Bruneton et al. 1994a; Solbiati et al. 1995).

The presence of multiple nodular lesions requires determination of the quantity of residual normal tissue. Particular attention must be paid to the upper portion of the thyroid lobes, because their status determines the possibility of subtotal thyroidectomy.

If diving goiter is suspected, US may be insufficient, even if the patient is examined with the neck hyperextended (which is not always easy in the elderly). Thus, even though the anterior mediastinum can be correctly examined by US (Wernecke and Diederich 1994), disease staging should be supplemented by another imaging modality for the mediastinum, i.e., computed tomography (CT) or magnetic resonance imaging (MRI).

12.1.2.2 Color Doppler and Power Doppler

CD and power Doppler (PD) provide comparable results for evaluation of thyroid disease (Fig. 12.2). PD does not provide any fundamentally new elements compared to CD, even though the depiction of intranodular vascularity is improved. Regardless of the method used, Doppler techniques are increasingly used as complements to conventional US, especially when nodular or functional anomalies are detected. CD consistently identifies the superior and inferior thyroid arteries; sporadic signals are detected within the thyroid gland (Kerr 1994; Clark et al. 1995). Doppler study of the inferior thyroid artery allows determination of the peak flow velocity (Schweiger et al. 1996). Venous structures are generally well identified, especially in the perithyroid region. As for other anatomic sites, CD of the thyroid is a source of intraobserver variations (around 30% for color pixel density and nearly 10% for mean color

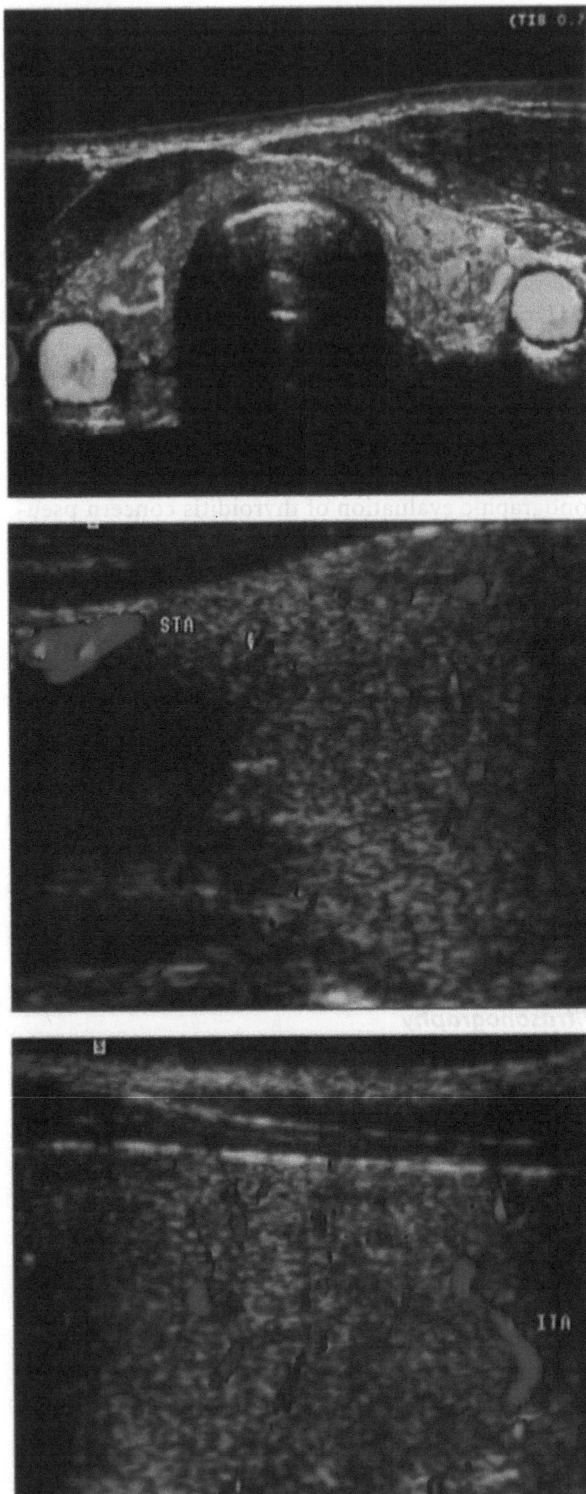

a
b
c

Fig. 12.2a–c. Thyroid vascularity. **a** Normal thyroid vascularity (power Doppler). **b** Superior thyroid artery (*STA*). **c** Inferior thyroid artery (*ITA*) value) (Delorme et al. 1995). Peak systolic velocity in the thyroid arteries remains below 40 cm/s. The high diastolic velocity is consistent with the thyroid's secretory nature (Clark et al. 1995).

12.1.2.3
Ultrasound-Guided Fine-Needle Aspiration

Despite its simplicity, US-guided FNA has been criticized because of the non-negligible frequency of uninformative results due to inadequate samples (Gharib et al. 1993; Hamburger 1994). In fact, the number of trained teams is increasing, and thyroid FNA will probably eventually play the essential role that certain teams already give it today. Thyroid FNA does, however, require close cooperation between the sonographer and the cytologist. The efficacy of US-guided FNA both in adults and in children makes it the initial diagnostic procedure for the management of nodular thyroid disease (Ito et al. 1995; Raab et al. 1995; Degnan et al. 1996).

Technique. A trajectory guidance device can be used to attach the needle to the transducer and guide it toward the target in the US beam. The trajectory of the needle shows up on the US unit screen. Such devices are available for use with linear-array, convex, or sector transducers. FNA can also be performed freehand without a guide. The operator him- or herself controls the path of the needle in the ultrasonic beam. Although a guidance device facilitates learning, most experienced operators use the freehand technique.

FNA is usually performed with a 21- to 26-gauge needle. To avoid altering the biopsy material, isotonic solution should be used as a coupling agent between the skin and the transducer rather than gel. Although this reduces image quality during the procedure, the thyroid gland and the nodule or nodules to be biopsied have already been localized and mapped during prior US examination (Tramalloni et al.1997). Few teams currently use an 18-G needle for core biopsy because of the need for local anesthesia. Taki et al. (1997), however, reported a sensitivity of 84%, a specificity of 95%, and an accuracy of 91% using an automated biopsy gun fitted with an 18-G needle. Incidents and hemorrhagic accidents have been reported with 18-G needles, whereas complications are very rare with aspiration biopsy (especially with US-guided FNA) (Fig. 12.3).

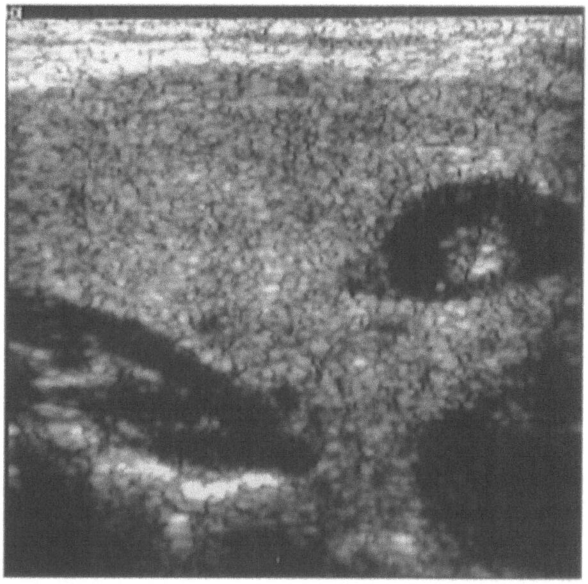

Fig. 12.3. Ultrasound (US)-guided fine-needle aspiration (FNA) of a partially cystic thyroid nodule with a solid internal structure: the tip of the needle appears more echoic than the intracystic mass

Palpation-Guided Aspiration and Ultrasound-Guided Fine-Needle Aspiration. US guidance permits aspiration biopsy of nonpalpable nodules. In the seven series of aspiration biopsies performed under palpation (18,183 cases) reviewed by Gharib and Goellner (1993), the results were as follows: mean sensitivity 83% (range, 65%–98%), mean specificity 92% (72%–100%), and overall accuracy of cytology over 90%.

The few studies comparing direct aspiration biopsy under palpation to US-guided sampling have often arrived at contradictory conclusions. Morosini et al. (1996) had more nonsignificant results with US guidance but diagnosed more cancers. Takashima et al. (1994) obtained better results with US guidance (3% initial failure rate versus 19% with palpation). Rosen et al. (1993) used US guidance when initial palpation-guided biopsy had failed as well as for nonpalpable nodules. Although the overall rate of nonsignificant results was 32%, these last authors obtained a cytologic response for 60% of the nodules. Finally, Yokozawa et al. (1996) used US guidance for repeat aspiration of nodules that had been considered benign by palpation-guided biopsy; 84.2% of the nodules were confirmed as benign, but 15.8% (n=107) were rediagnosed as malignant. The errors encountered with palpation-guided aspiration biopsy appear related to nodules that are difficult to palpate and necrotic or calcified neoplasms.

Evaluation of the true benefits of US guidance is often difficult because series are not comparable and a variety of methodologies have been used. Certain authors advocate US-guided FNA for all nonpalpable nodules, while others reserve it for cases where direct biopsy fails (Rosen et al. 1993).

Results. Compared to surgery, US-guided FNA has a sensitivity of 79.8%–96%, a specificity of 77.7%–100%, an accuracy of 81.8%–94%, a positive predictive value of 95%–100%, a negative predictive value of 75%–91.7%, and a nonsignificant rate of 3%–32% (Horvath et al. 1993; Rosen et al. 1993; Cochan-Priollet et al. 1994; Takashima et al. 1994; Yokozawa et al. 1995; Morosini et al. 1996; Lin et al. 1997b).

To better evaluate the efficacy of FNA and its utility for therapeutic decisions (surveillance versus surgery), several investigators have analyzed the outcome of nodules after biopsy. Hamburger (1987) repeated FNA for patients with lesions initially considered benign: 91% were confirmed as benign, but 6% were reclassified as suspicious and 3% were considered malignant. Kuma et al. (1994) followed up 134 patients for a mean of 10 years; 61 had undergone US-guided FNA. Among the initially benign cytologies, only one nodule became malignant.

In a personal study (Tramalloni et al. 1997), 311 patients were followed up for 2–7 years; 45% had undergone direct palpation-guided biopsy and 55% US-guided FNA. Palpation-guided biopsy gave nonsignificant results in 23% of cases; after repeat biopsy, this rate was reduced to 6%. None of the initially nonsignificant results were malignant at repeat FNA, but two suspicious results proved to be benign at surgery. In 3% of cases, the initially benign cytologies became suspicious, and four cancers were found at histologic examination.

Indications. Two significant benign biopsy samples must be obtained at an interval of several months before a nodule can be definitively considered benign. This is an important consideration for the management of thyroid nodules, especially because follicular carcinoma is difficult to diagnose histologically and FNA alone is not diagnostic. According to Okamoto et al. (1994), the sensitivity of FNA for follicular carcinoma is only 8% versus 88% for papillary carcinoma.

US-guided FNA has not proven superior to palpation-guided nodal sampling and is also more expensive. It should thus be reserved for nonpalpable nodules of sufficient size to allow accurate diagnosis (minimum, 8 mm).

US-guided FNA allows identification of those thyroid nodules that can merely be kept under surveillance and those warranting surgery. The resultant decrease in the number and percentage of surgical cases is associated with both a reduction in costs (Gimondo et al. 1994) and an increase in the number of carcinomas coming to surgery (Ng et al. 1990).

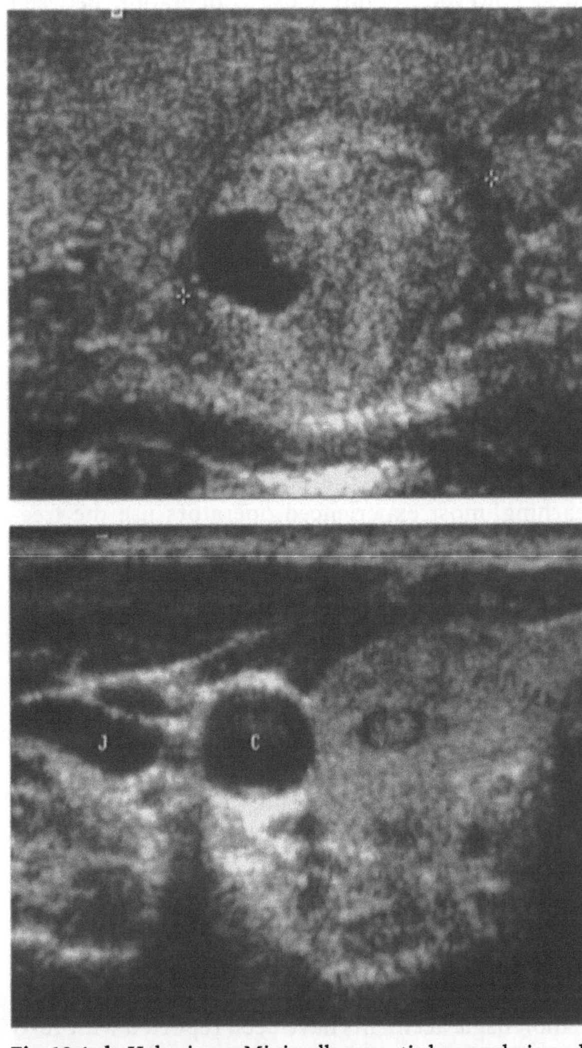

a

b

Fig. 12.4a,b. Halo sign. **a** Minimally necrotic hyperechoic nodule (18.8 mm between the two *crosses*) surrounded by a complete peripheral halo. An adenoma was found at surgery. **b** Micronodule due to follicular hyperplasia. *C*, common carotid artery; *J*, internal jugular vein

12.1.3 Results

12.1.3.1 *Ultrasound Patterns*

Gray Scale. Ultrasonography can demonstrate the location, size, number, echotexture, and margins of thyroid nodules. Very high frequency transducers improve analysis of nodule contours and can demonstrate parietal anomalies suggestive of a neoplastic process. A peripheral halo is almost unanim¡ously considered a sign of benignity, although only when complete (Fig. 12.4); a nodule with an incomplete halo may correspond to a neoplasm (Seya et al.1990).

Certain rare thyroid nodules have a completely fluid-like echotexture. Meticulous methodology is required to demonstrate an anechoic structure with posterior reinforcement and thin margins. Cysts may contain diffuse echoes; viscous fluid typically has a homogeneous echotexture. Actually, fluid-like nodules are usually not cysts at all; most correspond to solid lesions that have undergone necrosis or cystic degeneration (Fig. 12.5).

Solid nodules, which predominate, may be hypoechoic, hyperechoic, or isoechoic to the normal thyroid tissue. Hypoechoic nodules predominate (Fig. 12.6); isoechoic and hyperechoic nodules occur at similar frequencies (Viateau-Poncin 1992; Brkljacic et al. 1994; Solbiati et al. 1995). Hyperechogenicity is a good sign of benignity (Gooding 1993) because hyperechoic nodules are rarely malignant (only 2%–4% of cases according to Messina et al. 1996).

Certain apparently hyperechoic nodules are actually microcalcifications that have gone undetected by the examiner. These small echoic foci are too small to have an acoustic shadow. This may confuse the inexperienced sonographer, who may be misled by the reassuring sonographic pattern of the apparently hyperechoic nodule because microcalcifications are a characteristic feature of papillary carcinoma (Lee et al. 1993). Hyperechoic nodules often correspond to colloid-type follicles, whereas hypoechoic nodules frequently correspond to an adenoma composed of embryonal-type follicles (Chang et al. 1990). According to Ahuja et al. (1996), the comet-tail artifact is correlated in 85% of cases with the presence of colloid.

Complex nodules with an inhomogeneous echotexture (mixed pattern) account for approximately 25% of all thyroid nodules. A fluid component of variable size may be present. Complex nodules in which fluid accounts for at least two thirds of the volume are almost always necrotic, solid benign lesions (Viateau-Poncin 1992).

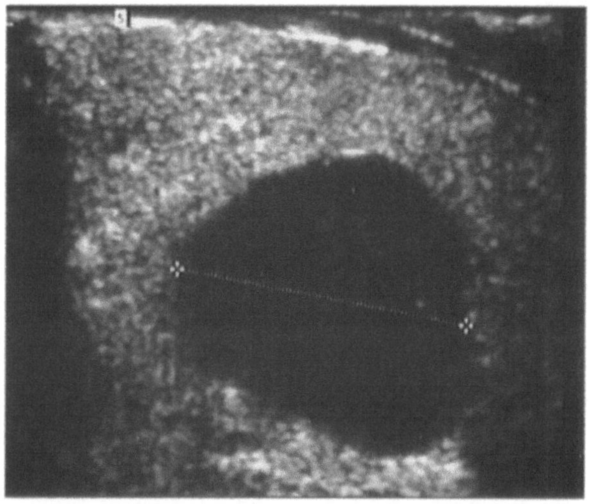

Fig. 12.5. Cystic lesion (17.2 mm between the two *crosses*) in the left thyroid lobe

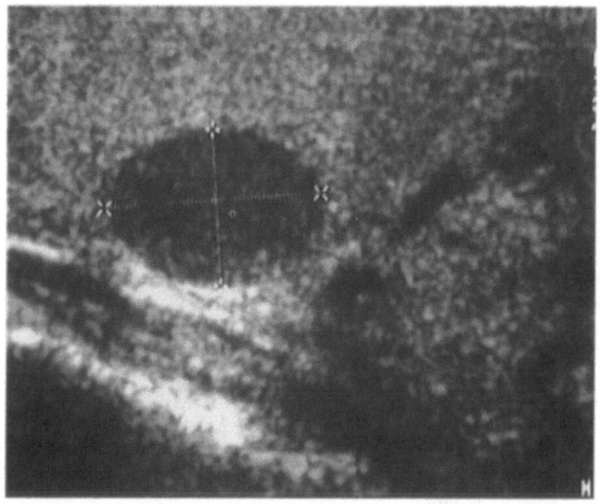

Fig. 12.6. Hypoechoic nodule 8.4+13.1 mm (*crosses*). At surgery, a small papillary cancer was found

Other architectural modifications may also be detected, in particular calcifications. Macrocalcifications are readily identified as highly echoic zones with an acoustic shadow. Microcalcifications often escape detection by US with a 7.5-MHz transducer. It was not until the introduction of higher-frequency transducers with a better sensitivity that microcalcifications were visualized as small, often punctate echoic foci, on rare occasions associated with an acoustic shadow (Fig. 12.7). As emphasized previ-

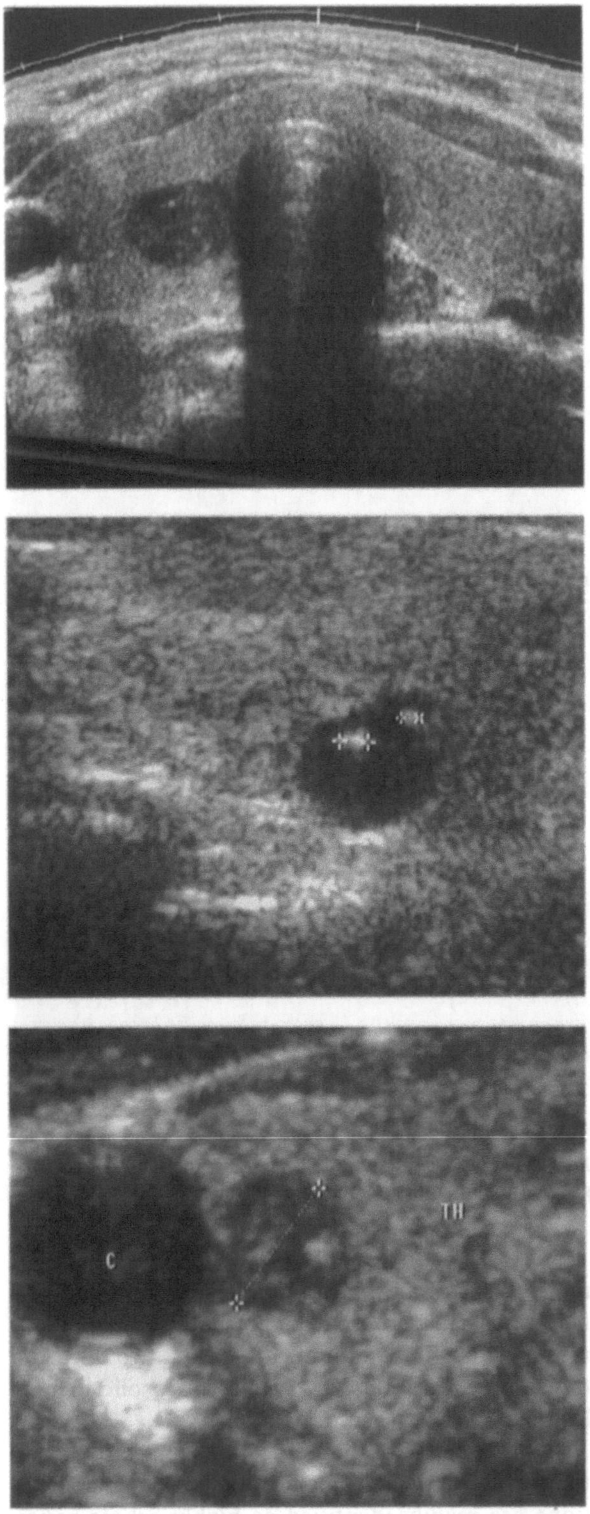

a b c

Fig. 12.7a–c. Intranodular microcalcifications: although these microcalcifications lack a posterior acoustic shadow, they must not be overlooked because they often correspond to a papillary cancer. **a** Transverse scan revealing a 15-mm hypoechoic nodule with fine echoes but no posterior shadowing: papillary cancer. **b** Small nodule with ill-defined anterior margins containing microcalcifications (1 and 1.5 mm, *crosses*): papillary cancer. **c** Small nodule (<5 mm, *crosses*) with numerous microcalcifications that prompted surgery: papillary cancer. *C*, right common carotid artery; *TH*, normal thyroid

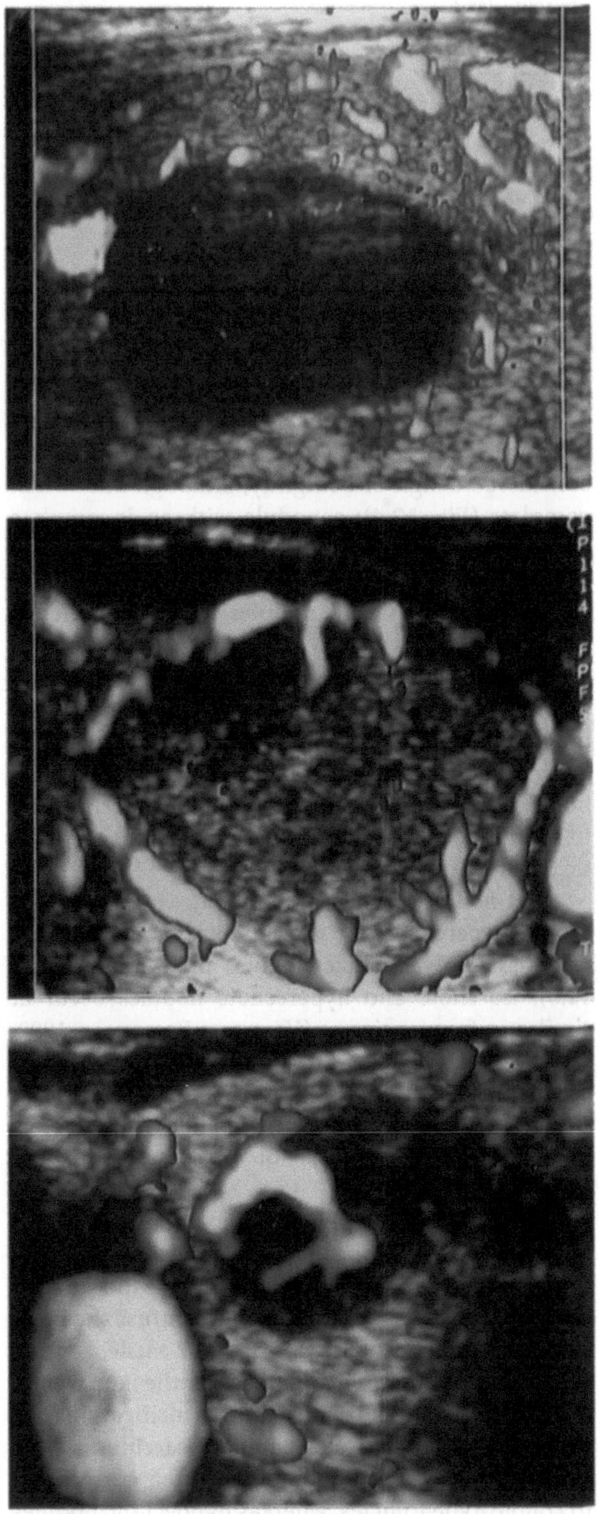

a b c

Fig. 12.8a–c. Power Doppler (PD) of thyroid nodules. **a** Cystic disease associated with avascularity. **b** Isoechoic lesion with a halo: PD demonstrated vascular structures within the hypoechoic perinodular halo. **c** Intranodular vascularity of a hypoechoic nodule: an adenoma was found at surgery ously, the detection of microcalcifications is important because they are highly suggestive of malignancy (specificity, 93%; positive predictive value, 70%). However, the overall sensitivity of US for the detection of microcalcifications is low (36% according to TAKASHIMA et al. 1995a).

Color Doppler and Power Doppler. According to SOLBIATI et al. (1995), CD and PD may assist in the differentiation between benign disease and malignancy by demonstrating three different patterns: (1) avascular lesion, (2) peripheral vascularity, and (3) peripheral and central vascularity (Fig. 12.8). While this latter pattern is associated with a high risk of malignancy (MESSINA et al. 1996), certain adenomas also show central hypervascularity. This pattern thus cannot be used to predict whether a nodule is benign or malignant. Avascular nodules are the only consistently benign lesions and generally correspond to follicular hyperplasia (ARGALIA et al. 1995). The other two patterns of vascularity do not allow differentiation between benign and malignant lesions (SHIMOMATO et al. 1993; ARGALIA et al. 1995; CLARK et al. 1995; HOLDEN 1995). CD demonstration of a complete halo containing vascular structures (usually venous rather than arterial) around an adenoma is highly suggestive of benignity (sensitivity, 96%; specificity; 93%; STERN et al. 1994). Awareness of the position of these vessels is helpful when biopsy is scheduled; small-caliber needles are required for hypervascular nodules, whereas poorly vascularized nodules can theoretically be biopsied with a large-caliber needle without any major risk of hemorrhage. This point is especially important for the minority of investigators who use 18-G needles.

Hot thyroid nodules are always hypervascular (CLARK et al. 1994; BECKER et al. 1997; Fig. 12.9).

There is no correlation between sonographic patterns, hypervascularity detected by CD or PD, and scintigraphic and laboratory data. Furthermore, 5-mm nodules are often poorly vascularized, and etiologic diagnosis remains difficult. Thus, although a peritumoral halo containing venous or arterial structures is highly suggestive of a benign process, biopsy or exeresis is indicated for all lesions with central hypervascularity (MESSINA et al. 1996).

CD and PD can facilitate treatment planning for nodular thyroid disease. Performed prior to FNA, these techniques also allow vascular workup that assists needle selection and helps prevent perforation of vascular structures. Spectral analysis of nodule vascularity does not appear to have any practical value (ARGALIA et al.1995; HOLDEN 1995).

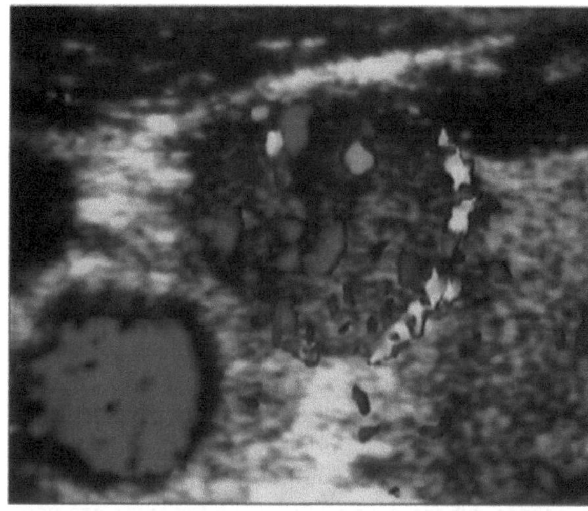

Fig. 12.9. Functional adenoma with hypervascularity on color Doppler (CD)

Reporting Results. As previously emphasized for CD and PD, interobserver differences must be taken into account when deciding to monitor thyroid nodules. In addition to the written report, an accurate map of the thyroid should be prepared, indicating all pertinent volumetric data and the position and maximum diameter of all nodules. This easily prepared document is an excellent means to convey information during follow-up (BRUNETON et al. 1987; MEYER 1991; JARLOV et al. 1993) and a valuable perioperative aid for the surgeon when lesions are not palpable (KRAIMPS and BARBIER 1993).

12.1.3.2 Solitary Thyroid Nodules

Sonographic Features Suggestive of Benignity or Malignancy. Ultrasonography can accurately localize thyroid nodules and determine whether or not they are solitary. Criteria exist in favor of benignity and malignancy, but each criterion taken separately has little predictive value. In contrast, a constellation of findings is helpful for patient management:

- A benign etiology is suggested by a hyperechoic or extensively cystic nodule (over two thirds of the nodule volume), presence of a complete halo, multiple lesions, absence of hypervascularity, and absence of laterocervical lymphadenopathy.
- Features in favor of a malignant process include a solitary hypoechoic nodule (LIN et al. 1997a), microcalcifications, ill-defined margins, an incom-

plete halo, cervical lymphadenopathy, central hypervascularity on CD or PD, a history of cervical irradiation, existence of a metastasis prompting a search for a primary cancer, young age, and male sex. According to KATAGIRI et al. (1994), presurgical diagnosis based on US patterns has a sensitivity of 82%, a specificity of 78%, and an accuracy of 80% for malignancy.

Thyroid Adenomas. These typically solitary and follicular benign lesions can cause difficulties for differentiation from adenocarcinoma by FNA. Thyroid adenomas are less frequent than hyperplastic lesions, accounting for under 10% of all nodular thyroid lesions. Half of all follicular lesions are isoechoic, whereas nonfollicular adenomas are usually hypoechoic. Regardless of the histologic type, other solid patterns can also be encountered. CD and PD demonstrate mixed vascularity (both peripheral and central), and there are thus no characteristic features suggesting the diagnosis.

Functional thyroid adenomas have no typical sonographic features, but exhibit marked central hypervascularity and an increased peak systolic velocity (SOLBIATI et al. 1995).

For nonsurgical adenomas that are merely kept under surveillance (possibly under suppressive therapy), US can usefully evaluate modifications in echotexture and especially size (VIATEAU-PONCIN 1992).

Cystic Lesions. True thyroid cysts are exceptional. Most cystic lesions in the thyroid are adenomas or hyperplastic lesions that have undergone hemorrhagic degeneration or necrosis.

Papillary Carcinoma of the Thyroid. As the most frequent thyroid malignancy (>70% of all series), papillary carcinoma usually affects young females. This carcinoma has three main features: (1) it has a propensity for lymphatic spread, (2) a slow growth rate, and (3) is often multifocal. It rarely metastasizes (to the lung) and is often curable; the prognosis is often excellent.

The most common US finding is a hypoechoic nodule (86.7% of cases according to LU et al. 1994). These nodules are always inhomogeneous once they reach 1 cm. Margins are poorly defined in 80% of patients; under half contain sonographically visible microcalcifications. Less frequent features include cystic degeneration (28.3%) and the halo sign (13.2%). Isoechoic and hyperechoic nodules (2%) are much rarer (LU et al. 1994). Laterocervical exploration, which must be performed systematically, may depict various forms of lymphadenopathy: round rather than oval nodes or disappearance of the central echoic hilum in small lesions. Nodal metastases are often hyperechoic to adjacent muscle (Fig. 12.10) and are usually homogeneous (81.2% according to AHUJA et al. 1995). Punctate peripheral calcifications are seen in over two thirds of patients. These calcifications, correlated with psammoma bodies, are characteristic of papillary carcinoma.

In addition to solitary hypoechoic lesions (GARRETTI et al. 1994), papillary cancer manifests on

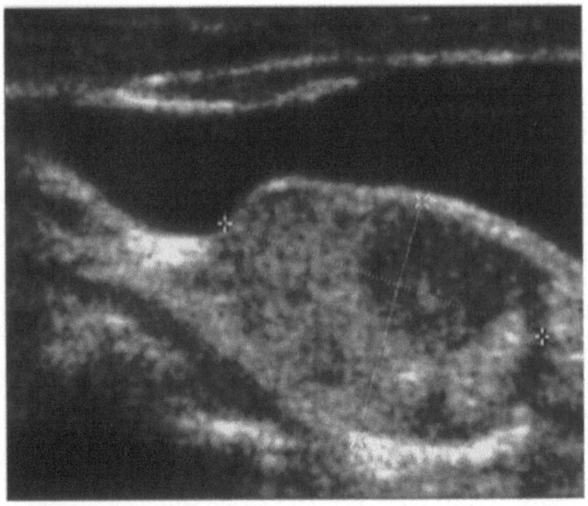

Fig. 12.10. Heterogeneous laterojugular node 19.9+13.4 mm (*crosses*) that at some points is hyperechoic compared with the adjacent muscles. At surgery, this proved to be a metastasis of a papillary cancer

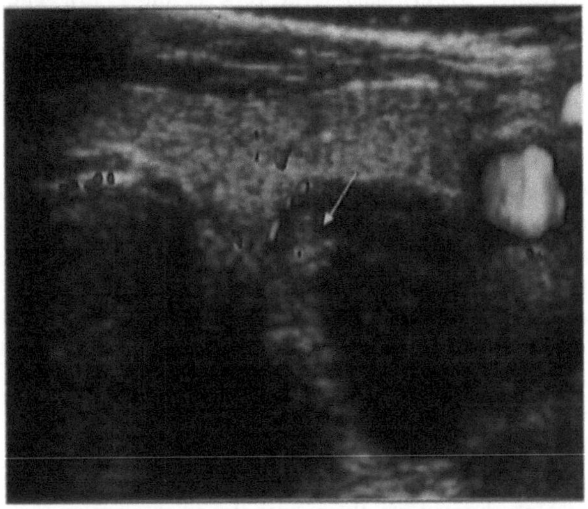

Fig. 12.11. Power Doppler (PD) of a small papillary cancer within a cystic lesion (*arrow*)

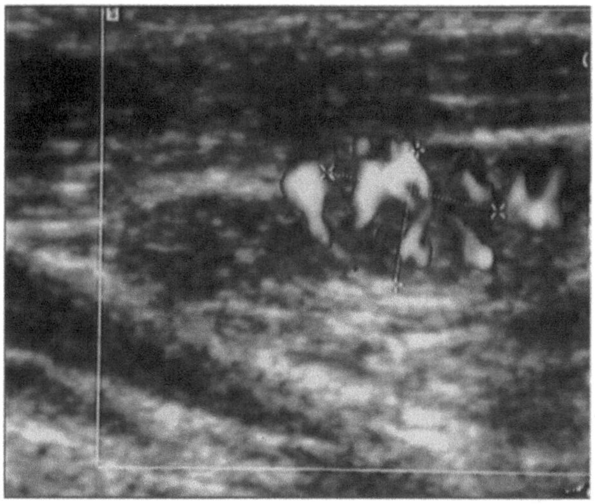

Fig. 12.12. Power Doppler (PD) of a small (5.3+7.5 mm, *crosses*) hypervascular laterocervical node. Fine-needle aspiration (FNA) cytology diagnosed a nodal metastasis of papillary cancer. Thyroid ultrasound was negative, but a small, 3-mm papillary cancer was found after resection of the homolateral thyroid lobe

rare occasions as a subcentimeter tissue mass within an apparently cystic lesion (Hiromura 1994; Fig. 12.11).

On other rare occasions, detection of one or more enlarged nodes prompts thyroid imaging. The differential diagnosis for necrotic or pseudocystic nodes is cystic lymphangioma. Ultrasonography may reveal a small homolateral and nonspecific intrathyroid lesion; in other cases, thyroid sonography is strictly normal (Fig. 12.12). US-guided FNA is indispensable in such cases and generally yields neoplastic tissue that confirms the need for surgery (Lee et al. 1993; Solbiati et al. 1995).

Regardless of the presentation of papillary cancer, CD demonstrates nonspecific central hypervascularity. Particular care should be paid to recognizing this feature, especially in predominantly cystic tumors (small hypervascular parietal zone).

Accurate evaluation of the contralateral lobe is essential because the thyroidectomy specimen often contains coexistent tumor, even though US is negative (Price et al. 1993). Contralateral cancers were recognized sonographically in only 12.8% of cases by Lu et al. (1994).

Follicular carcinoma represents less than 15% of all thyroid cancers. If the entire surgical specimen is not available for examination, a well-differentiated tumor may be confused with an adenoma because sparse tumoral emboli in peripheral veins may be the only signs of malignancy (Fig. 12.13). Follicular carcinomas often have a slow growth pattern and rarely spread to the lymph nodes.

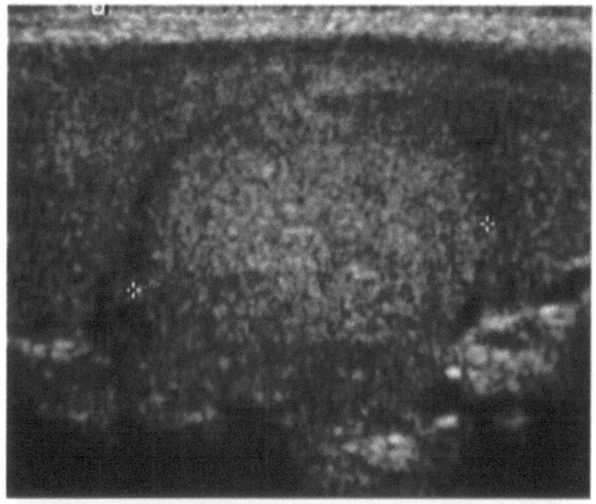

a

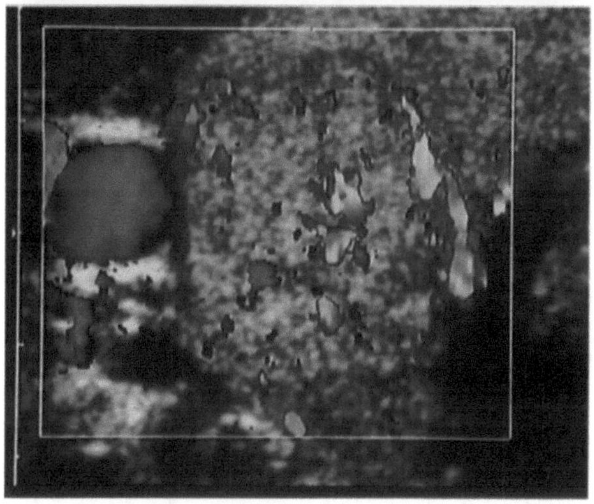

b

Fig. 12.13a,b. Follicular cancer. **a** Isoechoic lesion (21.8 mm between the two *crosses*) surrounded by a halo that is incomplete, particularly in its anterior portion. **b** Color Doppler (CD) demonstrated peripheral and internal vascularity

Two thirds of all follicular thyroid carcinomas are associated with goiter, and this creates problems for detection. If the tumor is hypervascular, CD and PD can theoretically suggest the etiologic diagnosis by demonstrating a suspicious zone within a multinodular goiter. This finding may indicate US-guided FNA.

This rare carcinoma may be isoechoic or, less often, hypoechoic. Neither calcification nor lymphadenopathy is present. Diagnosis of follicular thyroid cancer is thus particularly difficult; US-guided FNA rarely provides useful information (Okamoto et al. 1994), and these tumors often develop within benign multinodular lesions.

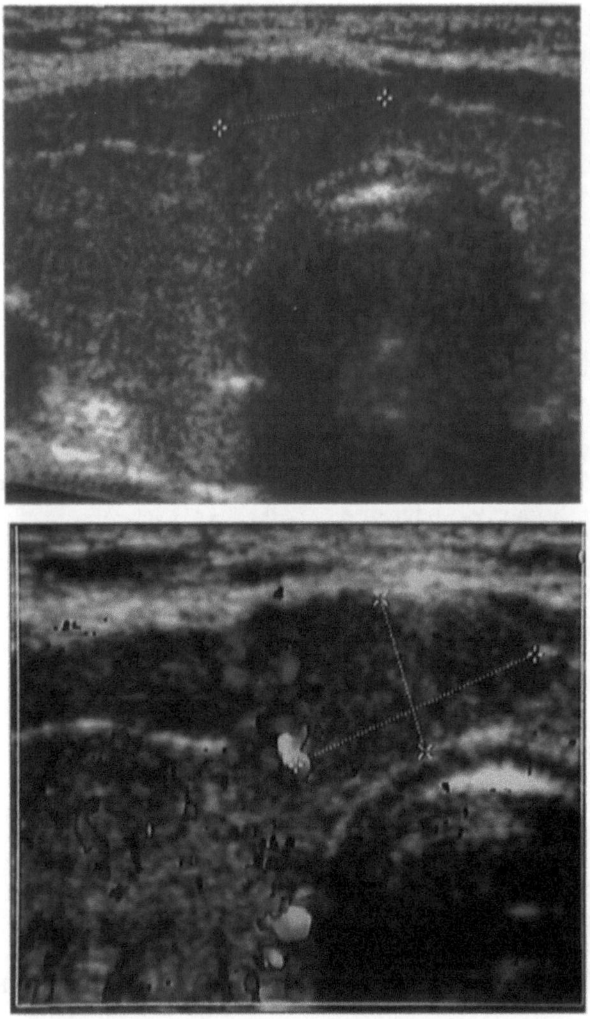

a

b

Fig. 12.14a,b. Medullary thyroid carcinoma detected during family screening. **a** Discretely hypoechoic nodule (10 mm between the two *crosses*) located on the right side of the thyroid isthmus. **b** Color Doppler (CD) demonstration of peripheral vascularity did not permit diagnosis. A medullary carcinoma was found at surgery

Medullary carcinoma, which accounts for less than 10% of all thyroid cancers, arises from the parafollicular cells that secrete calcitonin, which is thus the marker for medullary carcinoma.

Sonographically, medullary carcinomas tend to be hypoechoic (Fig. 12.14). Isoechoic tumors recognized by a halo are rare. Microcalcifications exist in 80%–90% of cases (GORMAN et al. 1987) and are correlated with the presence of amyloid substance. CD and PD demonstrate peripheral and central hypervascularity. Laterocervical lymphadenopathy is frequent. CT and MRI are helpful for demonstration of lymphatic spread to the mediastinum (CT can be performed with iodinated contrast material because medullary carcinoma is not treated by radioactive iodine).

Although most cases of medullary thyroid carcinoma are sporadic, 15% are autosomal dominant familial forms. Systematic familial screening by laboratory tests and US is thus indicated for the relatives of affected patients.

12.1.3.3
Multiple Thyroid Nodules

The foremost value of US is demonstration of whether cervical hypertrophy is due solely to thyroid enlargement or is associated with nodal lesions, as this completely modifies etiologic diagnosis.

Multinodular Goiter. Multinodularity is best evaluated by US, particularly because 70% of scintigraphically solitary lesions are multiple on sonograms, and because nearly one third of all thyroid cancers are discovered within multinodular goiters (SOLBIATI et al.1995).

Multinodular goiters are generally composed of hyperechoic zones that are highly suggestive of a benign process. This hyperechoic echotexture is due to their macrofollicular structure, which creates interfaces between the cells and the colloid substance (MULLER et al. 1985; SOLBIATI et al. 1995). Hypoechoic multinodular goiters with high cellularity are less frequent. There are no signs of invasion of adjacent structures, but areas of cystic or hemorrhagic degeneration may be present. Cystic degeneration may be complete or may create a fluid–fluid level due to the echotexture of the colloid

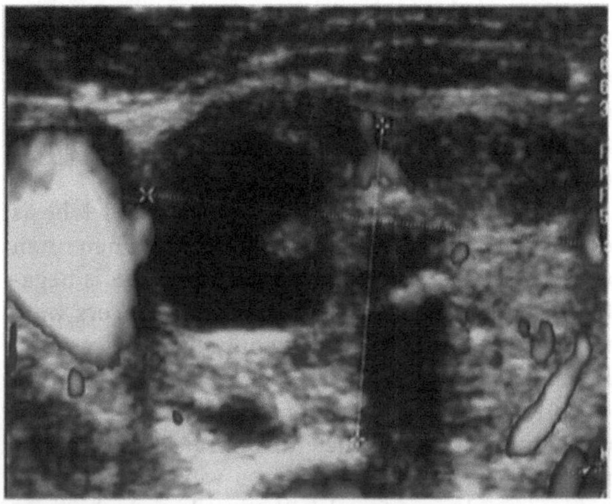

Fig. 12.15. Multinodular goiter with cystic zones and anarchic vascularity on power Doppler (PD) (13.3+21.3 mm nodule, *crosses*)

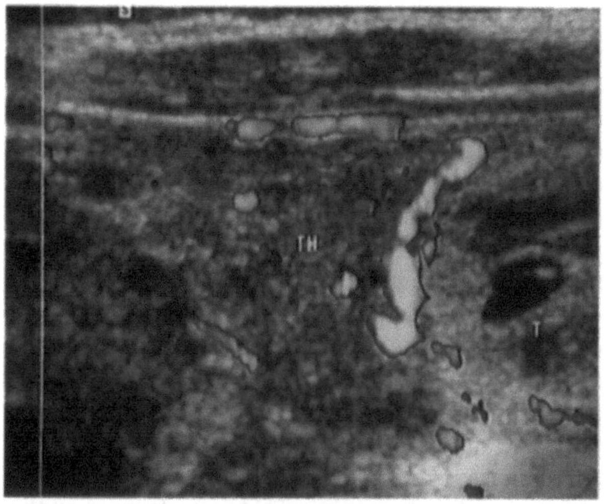

Fig. 12.16. Analysis of the superior portion of the right thyroid lobe (*TH*). The multinodular lesions (*T*) extend to within 2 cm of the upper part of the lobe. Color Doppler (CD) did not reveal any abnormal hypervascularity, but sonography demonstrated heterogeneity in this upper portion, prompting total thyroidectomy

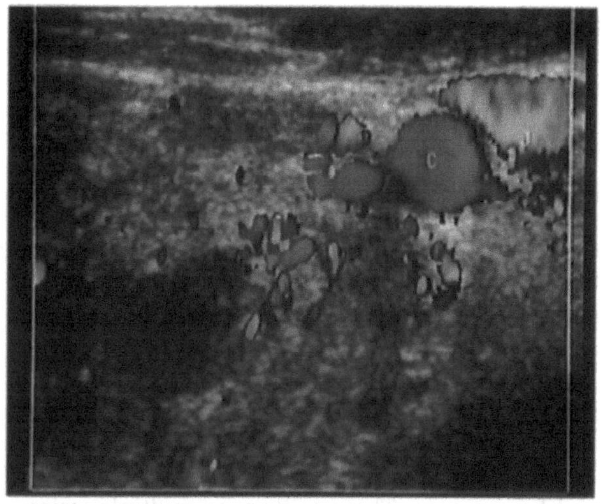

Fig. 12.17. Color Doppler (CD) of an anaplastic thyroid carcinoma with nonspecific anarchic vascularity. *C*, left common carotid artery; *J*, left internal jugular vein

substance. Coarse or "egg-shell" calcification may be observed.

CD often reveals anarchic vascularity (Fig. 12.15). Peak systolic velocities remain within normal limits except in patients with thyrotoxicosis (Kerr 1994; Solbiati et al. 1995).

Accurate mapping of lesions is essential prior to therapy. Multinodular goiter is usually bilateral and diffuse. The surgeon must keep this in mind before deciding to operate on a small and apparently unilateral lesion. Sonography should be performed to evaluate the status of the upper portion of the thyroid lobes (Fig. 12.16), as this determines the possibilities for subtotal or total thyroidectomy (Bruneton et al. 1987). If surgery seems advisable owing to the volume of the thyroid and clinical symptoms of compression, CT or MR imaging should be performed first.

Cancer Within a Multimodular Goiter. Although multinodular goiter involves less risk of malignancy than a solitary nodule, US alone usually cannot suggest the presence of cancer within a polyadenomatous goiter unless it is accompanied by laterocervical lymphadenopathy (Brkljacic et al. 1994). As mentioned previously, sonographic depiction and FNA of follicular cancers is difficult. Additional studies are required to determine whether focal zones of hypervascularity in a polyadenomatous goiter have any predictive value for malignancy.

Anaplastic carcinoma of the thyroid usually involves the entire gland and is seen predominantly in the elderly. Despite several reports of solitary anaplastic lesions, most patients have more or less diffuse invasion of the thyroid, and the course is rapidly unfavorable. Sonographically, anaplastic carcinoma manifests as a weakly echoic mass with a complex echotexture infiltrating the thyroid and spreading toward the adjacent muscle (and sometimes the vascular structures). Extension to the trachea is difficult to assess sonographically; it is best evaluated by other techniques, in particular CT. Laterocervical lymphadenopathy is present. CD and PD reveal variable degrees of vascularity, which often appears often poor compared to the extensive nature of the thyroid lesion (unless metastatic jugular thrombosis has resulted in an intrathyroid venous bypass network). US is basically used to confirm the findings of physical examination and to guide biopsy of nonnecrotic zones (Fig. 12.17).

Primary thyroid lymphoma accounts for approximately 4% of all thyroid cancers and is most prevalent in elderly women. Nearly all patients with thyroid lymphoma have coexistent Hashimoto's thyroiditis, but only a small percentage of individuals with Hashimoto's disease have lymphoma (Burke et al. 1977; Hamburger et al. 1983). The tumor generally invades the adjacent structures (esophagus, muscles, vessels). Weakly echoic enlarged nodes are common.

The sonographic patterns of primary thyroid lymphoma vary considerably. A weakly echogenic or fluid-like mass in a patient with Hashimoto's disease suggests the diagnosis and indicates aspiration biopsy. In the opinion of TAKASHIMA et al. (1995c), US is superior to CT and MRI for diagnosis of lymphoma during follow-up of patients with Hashimoto's thyroiditis, but is less effective for diagnosis of tumor spread to adjacent structures. Primary thyroid lymphoma may also image as multiple, very hypoechoic nodules, occasionally with posterior reinforcement, that may be associated with bilateral laterocervical lymphadenopathy (KOMATSU et al. 1994; TATSUNO et al. 1994).

Thyroid metastases are rare entities that occur late in the course of 2%–17% of all cancers (SHIMAOKA et al. 1962). The most frequently incriminated primaries are melanoma, breast cancer, and lung cancer. These solitary or multiple lesions are frequently large (up to 6 cm), do not undergo cystic degeneration, and are often associated with cervical lymphadenopathy and metastatic spread to the liver or lungs (AHUJA et al. 1994).

12.1.4 Strategy

Since the 1980s, a number of teams have addressed the problem of sonographic detection of one or more thyroid nodules (CARROL 1982; BRANDER et al. 1989). Clinically, these incidentalomas (TAN and GHARIB 1997) have been associated with widely variable risks of malignancy; rates of 0.45%–13% have been cited in the literature over the past 15 years (TAN and GHARIB 1997), whereas LIN et al. (1997) recently reported a rate of only 2.98%. Owing to the indolent course of papillary cancer and its favorable prognosis, the search for features that can aid treatment planning (follow-up versus surgery) appears justified.

In over 90% of patients, sonographic depiction of lesions is accurately correlated with their gross features. However, there are no pathognomonic signs of benignity or malignancy except, of course, in advanced cancers (cervical lymphadenopathy, anaplastic cancer, metastases). CD provides no conclusive elements for differentiation between benign and malignant tumors, even though central hypervascularity in a nodule suggests a neoplastic process. Scintigraphy has clearly seen its indications decrease, and there do not seem to be any broad diagnostic indications for CT or MRI. US is the first and often the only morphologic examination required for assessment of nodular thyroid disease, but all nodules larger than 8 mm should also undergo US-guided FNA.

Numerous management strategies have been proposed. Some are based on the palpable or nonpalpable nature of the thyroid nodule (PROYE 1993). The utility of complementary techniques can be evaluated by determining the cost, the frequency of cancers, the death rate, and postoperative iatrogenic complications (EECKHOUDT et al. 1993). GIUFFRIDA and GHARIB (1995) suggested mere US surveillance for nodules smaller than 1.5 cm; these authors reserved US-guided FNA for nodules larger than 1.5 cm. US-guided FNA can be performed in the office setting (RIFAT and RUFFIN 1994). For clinically asymptomatic and moderate nontoxic goiters, HURLEY and GHARIB (1996) proposed biological surveillance; if thyroid-stimulating hormone (TSH) assays reveal euthyroidism, FNA is performed on the largest nodule. Benign nodules are monitored by clinical examination and annual TSH assays. US is indicated for symptomatic patients (cervical swelling of rapid onset) and may demonstrate cystic change or hemorrhage in a nodule. Surgery remains indispensable for thyroid nodules larger than 3 or 4 cm, especially when signs of compression are present.

In addition to these approaches based on laboratory tests and aspiration cytology, a nonsurgical and nonhormonal therapeutic alternative has been developed for hot nodules, i.e., percutaneous ethanol ablation (PEA). Currently performed by only a few teams, PEA is indicated whenever diagnostic aspiration has formally identified a benign lesion. Along with its indications for hot nodules, PEA has recently confirmed its efficacy for predominantly cystic lesions, which are unlikely to be malignant (VERDE et al. 1994; ZINGRILLO et al. 1996b; KIM et al. 1997). PEA in one or more sessions successfully reduces nodule volume in over 80% of cases and is associated with a much lower recurrence rate than mere aspiration of cyst fluid (VERDE et al. 1994). Few trials have been conducted to date on cold nodules, which are much rarer (GOLETTI et al. 1993). In light of the major role that should be played by US-guided FNA in treatment planning, teams of sonographers and cytologists should be trained in order to improve the efficacy of the method and thus allow more widespread use.

12.2 Ultrasonography of Inflammatory and Functional Thyroid Disorders

J.N. BRUNETON, T. LIVRAGHI, and F. TRANQUART

In addition to its essential role for nodular thyroid disorders, ultrasonography has progressively demonstrated its value for the management of inflammatory and functional diseases of the thyroid. As for thyroid nodules, US is increasingly becoming the first-line imaging modality for these pathologies (TRANQUART et al. 1996).

12.2.1 Sonographic Features

Ultrasonographic evaluation of non-nodular thyroid disease may demonstrate modifications in gland volume and/or echotexture.

12.2.1.1 Normal or Enlarged Thyroid Gland

Isoechoic Parenchyma. The thyroid parenchyma is usually isoechoic in simple goiters; nodules or modifications in echotexture suggest progression to autoimmune or nodular thyroiditis (CLARK et al. 1992).

Hypoechoic Parenchyma. Regardless of the etiology, inflammatory processes are often associated with a hypoechoic parenchyma (VIATEAU-PONCIN 1992). Hypoechogenicity can be evaluated qualitatively by comparison with adjacent muscle, but quantitative evaluation is of no practical benefit for routine management (BENSON et al. 1983).

Focal hypogenicity may correspond to an infrequent form of subacute thyroiditis for which the differential diagnosis is nodular thyroid disease.

Global hypoechogenicity is encountered in three clinical situations that are usually associated with a functional goiter: subacute thyroiditis, chronic lymphocytic thyroiditis, and Basedow's goiter. Basedow's goiter never exhibits extensive hypoechogenicity, whereas this pattern is possible in subacute thyroiditis. If the clinical picture is not very suggestive (especially during early disease), US depiction of goiter associated with hypoechogenicity does not suggest the diagnosis. CD analysis of flow velocities in the inferior thyroid artery may allow diagnosis on the basis of vascular characteristics; Basedow's goiter is highly vascular as opposed to subacute thyroiditis and chronic lymphocytic thyroiditis, which are not, at least initially.

Inhomogeneous Parenchyma. An inhomogeneous echo pattern may be encountered in chronic lymphocytic thyroiditis, particularly during the early phase, before thyroid dysfunction becomes apparent. During this initial phase, the gland is enlarged and vascularity is at the upper limit of the normal range, probably due to inflammation.

12.2.1.2 Thyroid Gland of Reduced Volume

A thyroid of reduced volume is frequently observed in progressive hypothyroidism of the adult, whether idiopathic or the final stage of chronic lymphocytic thyroiditis. Echogenicity is extremely variable, but is usually normal or discretely diminished. Sonographic features often include a reduction in thyroid dimensions (especially the anteroposterior diameter), ill-defined contours, and poor differentiation from adjacent structures (difficulty in identifying the thyroid gland is suggestive of hypothyroidism).

12.2.2 Inflammatory Thyroid Disease

12.2.2.1 Subacute Granulomatous Thyroiditis (de Quervain's Thyroiditis)

Subacute granulomatous thyroiditis is a painful, self-limited inflammatory disease that develops after a viral infection of the upper respiratory tract and is often diagnosed clinically (FARWELL and BRAVERMAN 1996). Women in the second to fifth decades of life are affected most often. Clinical presentations vary between focal and diffuse disease.

US generally demonstrates extensive and diffuse hypoechogenicity (over 75% of the entire thyroid) with an increased mean thyroid volume. The hypoechoic zones are poorly delimited and do not appear nodular. Examination of the laterocervical neck may reveal inflammatory nodes (BIRCHALL et al. 1990; BENNEDBAEK and HEGEDUS 1997; HORVATH et al. 1997). There is usually no correlation between the extent of sonographic images and alterations in thyroid function. Vascularity may appear normal or decreased on CD, especially in

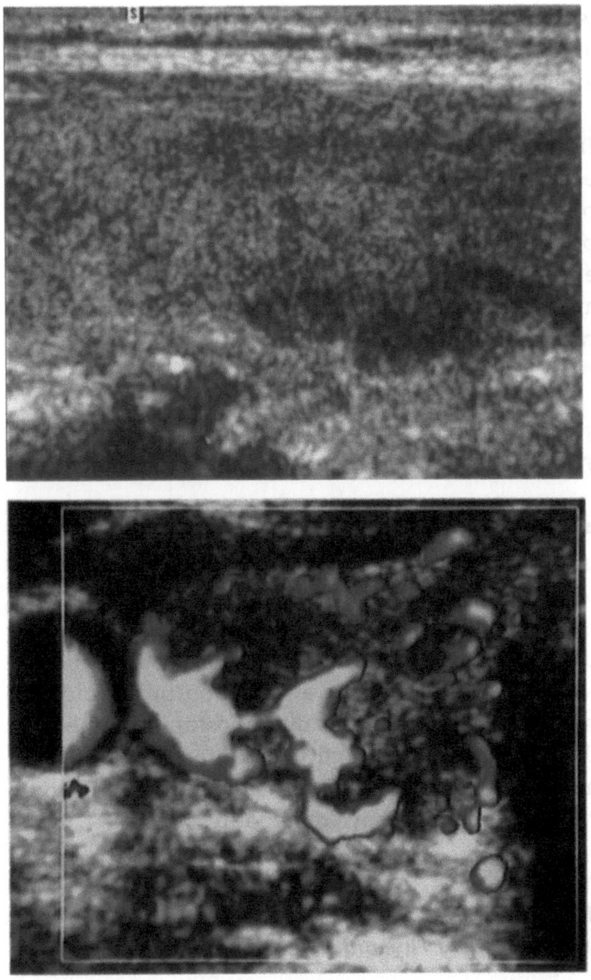

a

b

Fig. 12.18a,b. Subacute thyroiditis. **a** Sonogram of subacute thyroiditis with several hypoechoic zones. **b** Color Doppler (CD) of subacute thyroiditis with hypovascular foci in the hypoechoic zones

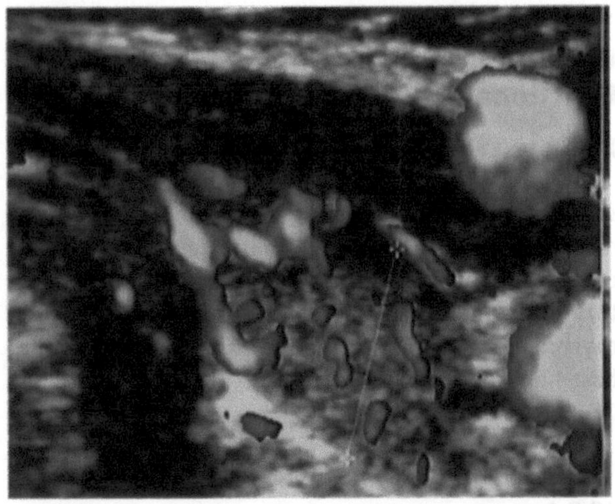

Fig. 12.19. Power Doppler (PD) of sequelae of subacute thyroiditis that had occurred 2 years earlier. Note the decreased size of the thyroid lobes (7.6 mm between the two *crosses*) due to secondary hypothyroidism

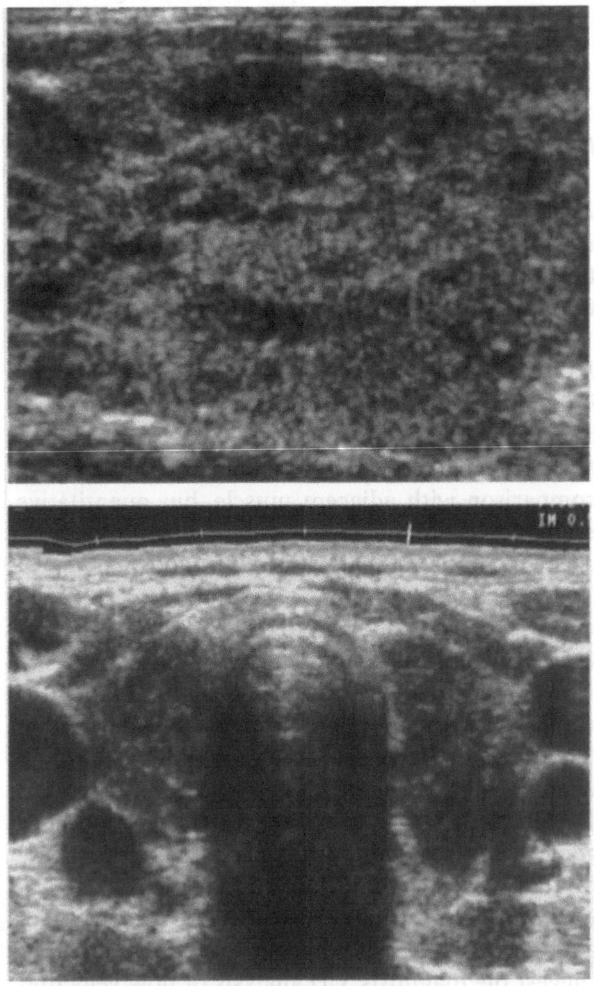

a

b

Fig. 12.20a,b. Sonogram of Hashimoto's disease. **a** Confluent micronodular lesions. **b** Late form: atrophic and heterogeneous pattern

hypoechoic zones (Solbiati et al. 1995; Fig. 12.18). The volume of the thyroid decreases during the course of the disease, but morphologic anomalies persist in 60% of cases. A rare form of de Quervain's thyroiditis presents as a painful but regressive solitary nodule; differential diagnosis from a true nodular pathology (which is more frequent) can be difficult, but US-guided FNA is diagnostic (Hardoff et al. 1995).

Subacute thyroiditis usually responds completely to treatment (Fig. 12.19). Possible recurrences image as an increase in the hypoechoic zones and thyroid volume.

12.2.2.2
Chronic Lymphocytic Thyroiditis (Hashimoto's Thyroiditis)

Chronic lymphocytic thyroiditis is an autoimmune syndrome with a predilection for middle-aged women that manifests in several manners: fibrous, atrophic, or asymptomatic thyroiditis, idiopathic myxedema, and an adolescent lymphocytic variety. Circulating antithyroglobulin or antimicrosomal antibodies are an almost consistent finding. One third of patients have an associated functional disorder such as hypo- or hyperthyroidism. The clinical presentation changes with the stage of the disease, varying from thyrotoxicosis in the early phase to atrophy.

Initial sonographic reports described almost consistent and durable hypoechogenicity that appeared homogeneous with early sonographic equipment (Hayashi et al. 1986; Viateau-Poncin 1992). State-of-the-art high-resolution transducers now depict micronodules as small as 1–6 mm in diameter (Set et al. 1996). These hypoechoic micronodules are surrounded by an echoic halo (Sostre and Reyes 1991) and are correlated with increased lobulation (Fig. 12.20). Such micronodules have a predictive value of 94.7% for the diagnosis of Hashimoto's disease (Yeh et al. 1996). According to Rubello et al. (1996), even though there is no strict correlation between hypothyroidism and hypoechogenicity, the prevalence of hypothyroidism increases with the extent of hypoechogenicity.

CD and PD are useful if an enlarged thyroid appears hypoechoic on sonograms and if problems exist in differentiating between Hashimoto's disease and Graves' disease. Vitti et al. (1995) defined four CD flow patterns ranging from normal to extensive hypervascularity. In Hashimoto's disease, the flow is normal in 49% of patients and slightly increased in 44%. This clearly distinguishes Hashimoto's disease from untreated Graves' disease, which always exhibits markedly increased vascularity. CD can thus easily distinguish between Hashimoto's disease and early Graves' disease in their initial stages.

Serial studies reveal a decrease in gland volume; the reduction is directly correlated with the extent of hypothyroidism. At this stage, CD and PD may demonstrate increased vascularity, especially in the fibrous septa (Solbiati et al. 1995; Romaldini et al. 1996). The possibility of progression to hypothyroidism is complicated by the risk of lymphoma (Podoloff 1996). Although routine screening is not feasible, any increase in the volume of the neck in a patient with Hashimoto's thyroiditis should prompt sonography and US-guided FNA (Fig. 12.21).

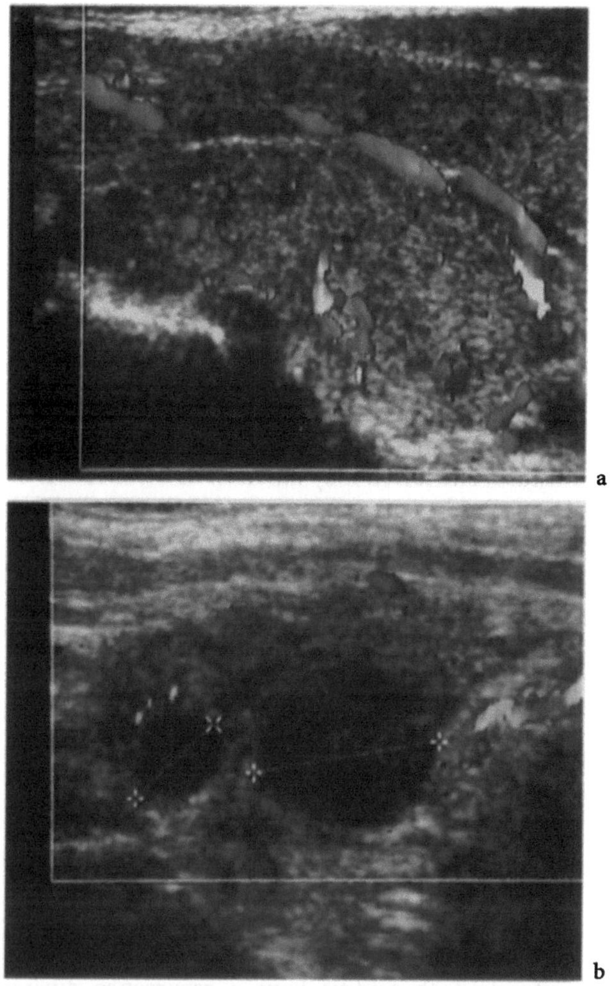

Fig. 12.21a,b. Ultrasound surveillance of Hasimoto's disease (color Doppler, CD). **a** The vascularity in the hyperechoic fibrous septa is readily depicted. **b** Appearance of avascular hypoechoic nodules corresponding to lymphoma

12.2.2.3
Invasive Fibrous Thyroiditis (Riedel's Thyroiditis)

Invasive fibrous thyroiditis is chronic inflammatory disease corresponding to an invasive fibrotic process that destroys all or part of the thyroid gland and invades the adjacent structures. Although its origin remains unclear, an association seems probable with other fibrosing conditions (retroperitoneal fibrosis, sclerosing cholangitis, mediastinal fibrosis). This rare disorder is responsible for less than 0.1% of all thyroidectomies (Mallote et al. 1991). Middle-aged women are affected predominantly. Pressure in the neck and pain may suggest carcinoma, especially anaplastic cancer. One third of all cases of Riedel's thyroiditis progress to hypothyroidism.

Sonography visualizes a hypoechoic mass in one of the lobes that often invades the adjacent muscle (FONTAN et al. 1993) or, occasionally, the vascular structures (JAMES et al. 1991).

12.2.2.4
Other Types of Thyroiditis

Suppurative thyroiditis is rare and should prompt a search for immunodepression or, in young subjects, a fistula. The lesion may manifest as a collection of viscous fluid (VIATEAU-PONCIN 1992) or a complex nodule, occasionally containing hyperechoic trabeculae, whereas the remainder of the thyroid is diffusely hypoechoic (GIMONDO et al. 1996). Owing to the difficulties in differential diagnosis from focal subacute thyroiditis (because of the associated pain), a hemorrhagic cyst, carcinoma, or lymphoma, aspiration biopsy is required for accurate diagnosis.

Silent or painless thyroiditis and postpartum thyroiditis are subacute forms of lymphocytic thyroiditis (LOEVNER 1996). The presence of antithyroid antibodies suggests an autoimmune origin. Early thyrotoxicosis usually progresses to transient hypothyroidism before its ultimate return to the euthyroid state. One out of 20 women who experience postpartum thyroiditis have a recurrence during subsequent pregnancies. Progression to a chronic form is possible.

Sonography reveals ill-defined patches of hypoechogenicity. The extent of these sonographic images allows assessment of the degree of thyroiditis (ADAMS et al. 1992; PARKES et al. 1996).

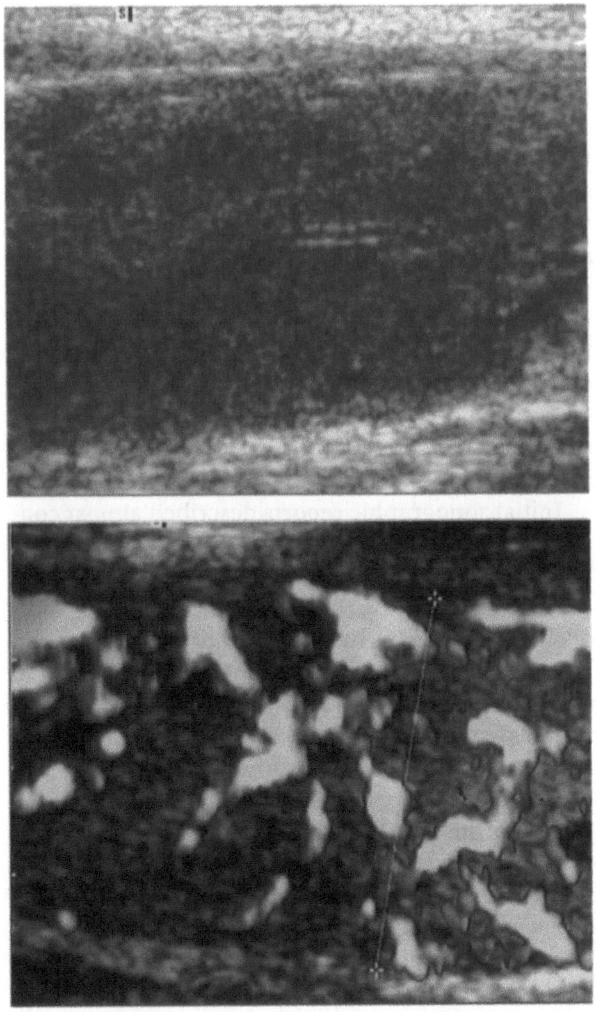

a

b

Fig. 12.22a,b. Graves' disease. **a** Moderate hypoechogenicity of the entire thyroid (sagittal scan of the right lobe): the small ductal structures correspond to hypertrophic vessels. **b** Power Doppler (PD) at the same level as Fig. 22a: the thyroid lobe is not enlarged (17.6 mm between the two *crosses*), but presents extensive hypervascularity

12.2.3
Functional Thyroid Disease

12.2.3.1
Basedow's Goiter

General Features. Basedow's goiter is the most frequent autoimmune disorder. In the United States, for example, it affects 0.4% of the general population (DE LELLIS 1989). Women in the fourth decade of life are affected most often, and a familial predisposition has been observed. Diffuse enlargement of the gland is associated with hypervascularity. Coexistence of other autoimmune disorders is possible. Treatment is based on synthetic antithyroid drugs, radioactive iodine treatment, and surgery.

Ultrasound Patterns. US depicts thyroid enlargement and hypoechogenicity in 86% of cases (VITTI et al. 1995). Increased flow is demonstrated in the inferior thyroid artery. SCHWEIGER et al. (1996) reported a correlation between the peak velocity and free triiodothyroxine (FT3) and free thyroxine (FT4). In the view of these authors, a velocity of less than 0.3 m/s corresponds to hypothyroidism, while a flow greater than 1.2 m/s is indicative of hyperthyroidism.

CD depicts gland hypervascularity as the "thyroid inferno" (Fig. 12.22) described by RALLS et al. (1988). This increased vascularity is due to arteriovenous shunts; the flow rate is generally greater than 70 ml/min (HODGSON et al. 1988).

CASTAGNONE et al. (1996) failed to observe any correlation between normalization of the vascularity and reduction in hormone secretion in response to treatment. However, patients in remission are at increased risk of relapse if the number of vessels per square centimeter is high and if the flow velocity increases in the inferior thyroid artery.

Follow-up of patients treated by methimazole must include a search for hypoechogenicity, which may exist early in the disease but is absent in overt Basedow's goiter. The absence of hypoechogenicity during treatment appears to be a favorable prognostic indicator of remission for hyperthyroidism, even though hypoechogenicity is not an indicator of recurrence (GEMMA et al. 1996; ZINGRILLO et al. 1996a).

Graves' Disease and Cancer. Coexistent Graves' disease and thyroid carcinoma is reported in 0.3%–16.6% of patients, with a higher incidence in toxic nodular goiter than in Graves' disease. The neoplasm is generally a small papillary carcinoma (follicular carcinomas are less common) that is identified only in the surgical specimen. The prognosis does not appear to be influenced by this association (NICOLOSI et al. 1994).

Thyrotoxicosis factitia (BOGAZZI et al. 1996), caused by use of exogenous thyroid hormones, can be diagnosed by elevated FT3 and FT4 levels, very low TSH and serum thyroglobulin, the absence of antithyroid antibodies, and the absence or very marked decrease in radionuclide uptake during scintigraphy. US reveals a gland of normal volume and echotexture. CD and PD may reveal several vascular foci without hypervascularity. The peak systolic velocity is at the lower limit of the normal range, a feature that differentiates this pathology from Graves' disease. When findings are equivocal, CD or PD can easily suggest the etiologic diagnosis.

12.2.3.2 Autonomous Thyroid Nodules and Percutaneous Ethanol Ablation

A thyroid nodule that appears hypervascular on CD or PD and is associated with reduced circulating TSH levels is an indication for scintigraphy, which usually reveals an autonomous thyroid nodule. Italian authors were the first to propose therapeutic intratumoral injection of ethanol for these lesions. The efficacy of PEA markedly reduces the incidence of post-therapy hypothyroidism compared to other methods, including surgery, especially radioactive iodine treatment (Figs. 12.23, 12.24).

LIPPI et al. (1996) reviewed a series of 429 patients, 56.4% of whom had a toxic adenoma treated by PEA. Patients underwent a mean of four sessions and received 1–8 ml per session with a cumulative dose of 2–50 ml. Surveillance was conducted by sonography (including CD), isotopic studies, and laboratory tests (TSH, FT3, FT4). After more than 1 year, these authors reported a success rate of 66.5% for toxic adenomas and 83.4% for pretoxic adenomas. All of the thyroid nodules had decreased in volume, but the efficacy of the technique decreased with nodule size. These authors consider PEA an excellent alternative to surgery for nodules less than 15 ml.

CD and PD are helpful for evaluation of response to therapy because toxic adenomas are always hypervascular (BRAUN and BLANK 1994; BECKER et al. 1997). Decreased echogenicity and modifications in nodule shape and volume have been observed after PEA (GONSORCIKOVA et al. 1996).

PEA preserves the function of the residual thyroid tissue and reduces the risk of post-therapy hypothyroidism (LIVRAGHI et al. 1994; OZDEMIR et al. 1994). The technique can also be proposed for larger hot nodules (even those over 30 ml). A mean of six sessions is required, and the total ethanol volume administered may exceed 50 ml. In 6–9 months, nodules may regress by 40%–80%. Autonomous nodules do not recur, but PEA is always painful (TARANTINO et al. 1997).

12.2.3.3 Hypothyroidism

Ultrasonography can assess the therapeutic response of reversible hypothyroidism of chemical, immunological, mixed, or postpartum origin (SATO et al. 1996). Response corresponds to a decrease of at least 50% in the initially elevated TSH concentration during iodine restriction over a 2- to 15-week period without replacement therapy. Sonographically, the preexistent hypoechogenicity disappears more rapidly in chemically induced hypothyroidism than in other etiologies. If imaging is required, US is sufficient for atrophic thyroiditis; sonograms demon-

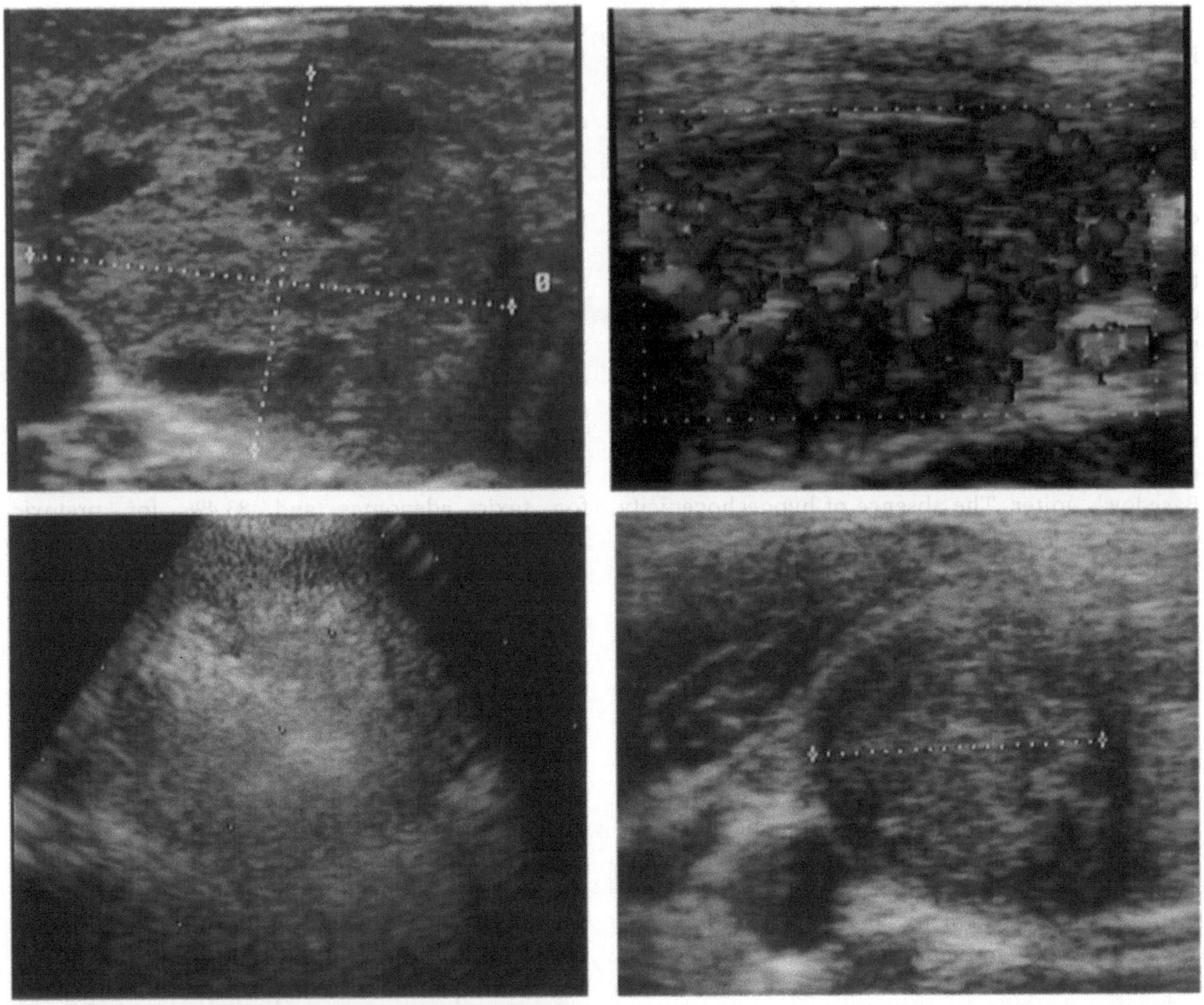

a b c d

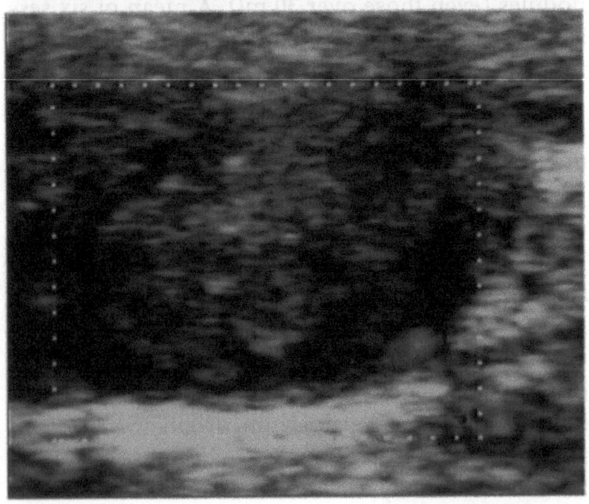

e

Fig. 12.23a–e. Percutaneous ethanol ablation (PEA) of a hot thyroid nodule. **a** Partially necrotic left thyroid nodule (28.8+20.9 mm, *crosses*). **b** The entire nodule appeared hypervascular on color Doppler (CD). **c** Sonographic control during ethanol injection: hyperechoic appearance of the alcohol within the nodule. **d** Control after 4 months: note the reduction in nodule size (21+13.6 mm, *crosses*). **e** CD revealed nearly complete disappearance of nodule vascularity

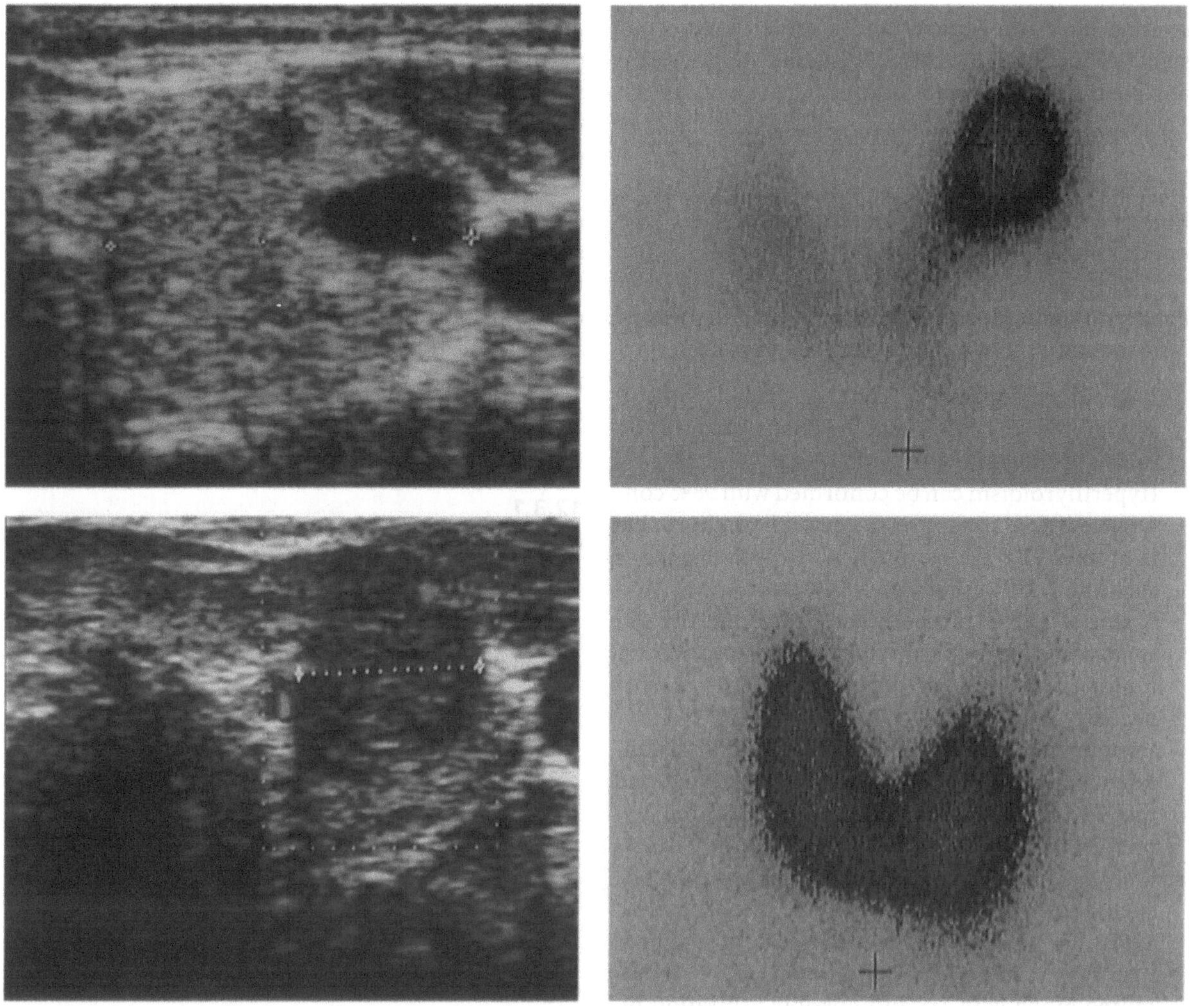

a b c d

Fig. 12.24a–d. Percutaneous ethanol ablation (PEA) of a hot nodule. **a** Solid nodule with minimal cystic degeneration (24 mm between the two *crosses*). **b** Scintiscan demonstrating the hot nodule and extinction of the normal gland. **c** Late post-therapy control (after 2 years) revealing marked reduction in nodule size (11 mm, *crosses*). **d** Follow-up scintiscan 15 months after PEA: diasappearance of the hot nodule and reappearance of normal thyroid tissue

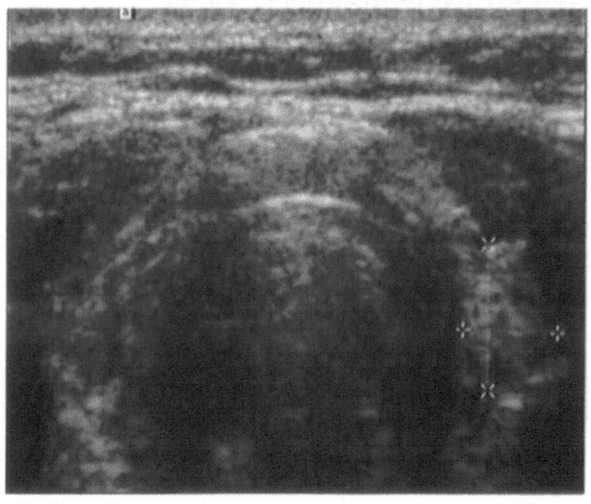

Fig.12.25. Severe hypothyroidism secondary to chronic thyroiditis (transverse diameter of the left lobe, 5.9 mm; thickness of the left lobe, 8.3 mm; *crosses*)

strating hypoechogenicity and a more or less constant reduction in thyroid volume (Fig. 12.25) obviate the need for scintigraphy (VITTI et al. 1994).

12.2.3.4
Role of Ultrasound in the Management of Functional Thyroid Disease

FELDKAMP and HORSTER (1995) defined the role of ultrasonography in various clinical settings:

- Thyroid dysfunction can be ruled out if sonograms are normal and the TSH concentration ranges from 0.4 to 4 mU/ml.
- Hyperthyroidism can be confirmed with 98% confidence if TSH is suppressed and triiodothyroxine (T3) and FT3 are elevated. If Graves' disease is suspected, US supplements laboratory tests (thyroxine, T4; TSH antibody receptors, and thyroid peroxidase antibodies). Scintigraphy and US are indicated if focal or diffuse autonomy is suspected.
- Hypothyroidism can be diagnosed with 98% confidence if the TSH concentration is elevated and the T4 concentration is low. In congenital hypothyroidism, US suffices in 50% of patients (TAKASHIMA et al. 1995d). If ectopia is suspected, scintigraphy is more effective (YOSHIMURA et al. 1995). For patients with symptoms of acquired hypothyroidism, TPO antibody assays are required along with US and possibly aspiration biopsy to rule out de Quervain's thyroiditis or Hashimoto's disease.

12.3
Non-ultrasonographic Imaging of Thyroid Disorders

F. TRANQUART, P.Y MARCY, and J.N. BRUNETON

In vivo isotopic exploration of the thyroid gland was one of the first scintigraphic examinations performed owing to the availability of iodine-131, a theoretically ideal radionuclide because it is the perfect tracer of natural iodine, a component of thyroid hormones. Scintigraphy was thus the gold standard for thyroid imaging for many years.

The introduction of new imaging modalities and refinement of laboratory techniques that now permit indirect and highly accurate analysis of thyroid disorders have markedly reduced the indications for diagnostic thyroid scintigraphy. Ultrasonography, in particular, offers much better spatial resolution. Assessment of thyroid function has, however, benefited from the development of new isotopic tracers. Improved knowledge about thyroid physiology has in turn prompted clinical trials using new techniques and new contrast agents. Recent research has been successful in cloning the thyroid iodine transporter, thereby helping to elucidate the mechanisms of iodine transport in healthy and diseased tissues. Similar clarification is under way concerning the mechanisms of regulation of thyroid hormone biosynthesis (CAVALIERI 1997).

12.3.1
Nuclear Medicine

12.3.1.1
Current Techniques

The scintillation cameras used for thyroid imaging are usually equiped with a pinhole collimator. While such units offer satisfactory resolution, the conical projection is a drawback that precludes imaging in actual dimensions. This can interfere with accurate localization of certain nodules.

Technetium (Tc 99m), used in the form of Tc 99m pertechnetate, is taken up by the thyroid but is not organified. This prevents true evaluation of thyroid function. Images are obtained 30 min after intravenous injection (usually 74 MBq), when contrast between the thyroid and background noise is maximum. The ready availability of this radionuclide explains its widespread use.

Owing to its similarity to natural iodine and its favorable dosimetric properties, iodine-123 is the nearly ideal tracer for assessment of thyroid function. This relatively expensive product has a short half-life (13 h), which precludes long-term storage. Scintigraphy is generally performed 3–24 h after intravenous injection (average dose, 3.7 MBq). Scanning during the early phase allows establishment of the curve of tracer uptake. Iodine-123 uptake at 3 h can also be determined.

Iodine-131, another analogue of natural iodine, is much less expensive but is currently reserved for certain indications because its involves non-negligible radiation exposure. Owing to its long half-life (8 days), iodine-131 is used to determine long-term uptake kinetics prior to treatment and for whole-body scanning of patients with thyroid cancer. Iodine-131 is also used for therapeutic metabolic irradiation of hyperthyroidism and thyroid cancer (TRANQUART et al. 1996).

12.3.1.2
Results

Elements Interfering with Iodine Uptake. The quality of scintigraphy and accurate interpretation of data are affected by several factors that interfere with iodine uptake by the thyroid:

- Prior overload with iodine must be taken into consideration. Scintigraphy should be performed before radiologic examinations requiring injection of iodinated contrast material. If this is not possible, an interval of at least 3 weeks is required after the radiologic examinations before scintigraphy is performed. Potential problems include isotope dilution, blockage of iodine organification due the Wolff-Chaikoff effect, which causes hypothyroidism with elevation of TSH levels, and iodine saturation with complete blockage of uptake (usually accompanied by hyperthyroidism).
- Numerous drugs (e.g., propylthiouracil, methimazole) interfere with thyroid metabolism of iodine and reduce the gland's uptake capacity (ALBERT et al. 1987).
- An elevated TSH level may produce a biphasic uptake curve.

Results with Iodine-123. A number of anomalies are associated with suppressed iodine-123 uptake, i.e., subacute thyroiditis, thyrotoxicosis factitia (COHEN et al. 1989), hyperthyroidism due to excess iodine (particularly after amiodarone administration) (ALBERT et al. 1987), certain forms of non-Basedow autoimmune thyroiditis, and postpartum thyroiditis.

Uptake is lowered, and usually accompanied by hypothyroidism, in chronic lymphocytic thyroiditis and hypothyroidism in the elderly.

Normal uptake in an enlarged thyroid is observed in simple goiter without associated thyroid dysfunction.

Increased uptake is often seen in diffuse hypertrophy of the entire gland. Homogeneous uptake is suggestive of Graves' disease, whereas inhomogeneous uptake suggests chronic lymphocytic thyroiditis.

Elevated uninodular uptake corresponds to a hot nodule that may be asymptomatic. Evaluation of uptake by the adjacent parenchyma can demonstrate no fixation. The presence of a hot nodule is usually a sign of benignity, but this does not exclude the possibility of a malignant nodule elsewhere in the thyroid (SHAMMA and ABRAHAMS 1992).

Absent or markedly decreased uninodular uptake corresponds to a cold nodule. This feature may be difficult to determine for posterior or isthmic nodules. The term "cold nodule" actually refers to a variety of entities ranging from a colloid nodule to cancer (TENNVALL et al. 1981).

In multinodular disease, uptake may remain within normal limits or be decreased, even if true hot nodules are present. The entire spectrum of appearances is possible, from the presence of cold or hot nodules to a combination of the two.

12.3.1.3
Current Indications for Scintigraphy

Until recently, scintigraphy was sometimes still considered the next logical step after US. Owing to the efficacy of sonography and the accuracy of laboratory tests, its indications have declined considerably, especially because it usually proves unnecessary (Fig. 12.26).

The "maximalist" approach for subcentimeter lesions that resulted in unnecessary scintigraphy (unnecessary because it is consistently negative) is increasingly being replaced by a "minimalist" approach consisting in US-guided FNA followed by adaptation of the indications for scintigraphy to the circulating TSH level. If the TSH concentration is low, scintigraphy is performed to search for a hot nodule (TOURNIAIRE et al. 1997); this allows differentiation of a toxic adenoma from a cold nodule in Graves' disease (DUQUENNE et al. 1997). Scintigraphy may be unnecessary if the nodule is smaller than 1 cm, if it is not extinctive, or if sonograms demonstrate cystic changes in at least half the volume of the nodule.

Scintigraphy does not provide any fundamental data for assessment of inflammatory thyroid disorders, which are diagnosed by laboratory tests. The required morphologic information is provided by sonography. The results of recent scintigraphy studies concerning acute and chronic inflammatory thyroid disease are too variable for diagnostic guidelines to be established (PRICE 1993; LOEVNER 1996).

US, associated with CD and PD, even appears capable of replacing scintigraphy for differential diagnosis of thyroid gland dysfunction (Graves' disease versus an inflammatory pathology), especially because it is faster and more economical.

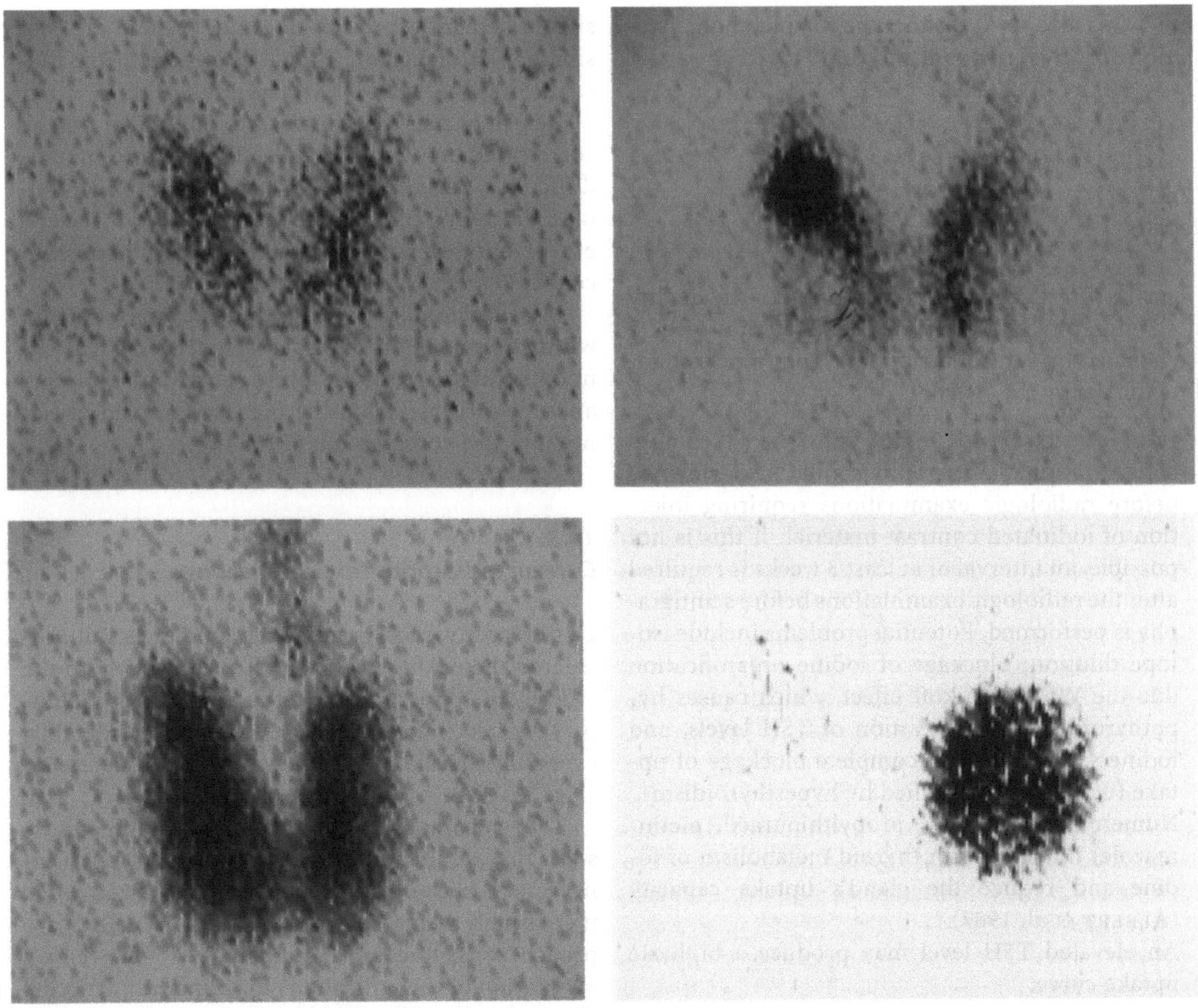

a b c d

Fig. 12.26a–d. Scintigraphic images observed in thyroid disease. **a** Weak thyroid uptake of iodine-123 due to hypothyroidism (chronic lymphocytic thyroiditis). **b** Heterogeneous thyroid uptake due to a hot nodule in the upper part of the right lobe and bilateral cold micronodules. **c** Increased uptake in Graves' disease. **d** Toxic adenoma of the left thyroid lobe

12.3.1.4
Recent Applications of Scintigraphy

Thallium-201 scintigraphy has proven disappointing for demonstration of nodule malignancy. Derebek et al. (1996) concluded that early and delayed thallium-201 imaging have no utility for definition of the benign or malignant nature of a cold nodule. According to Kume et al. (1996), delayed thallium-201 scans reflect proliferative tumor activity, but delayed thallium uptake is also seen in thyroiditis and parathyroid pathologies, and few teams currently use this technique routinely.

Tc 99m-methoxyisobutylisonitrile (MIBI) using a dual-phase acquisition protocol (at 30 min and 2 h) has also been used in attempts to determine the etiology of cold nodules (Kresnik et al. 1997). Prolonged retention of MIBI is generally not considered specific for cancer because it is even more frequent in adenomas, although this is debated by some authors (Alonso et al. 1996).

Due to its high resolution (up to 6–7 mm), single photon emission CT (SPECT) can accurately depict cold nodules that are usually surrounded by more intense peripheral activity (Wanet et al. 1996). Thyroid volumetry appears more accurate than planar imaging (Zaidi 1996).

Future applications may develop thanks to new contrast agents such as octreotide or fluorodeoxyglucose. At present, however, these agents are essentially reserved for the detection of metastases of thyroid cancer and are not used for pretherapy disease staging (Reinhardt and Moser 1996).

12.3.2
Computed Tomography

12.3.2.1
Indications and Limitations of Computed Tomography

Injection of an iodinated contrast material compromises the efficacy of radioiodine therapy for differentiated thyroid carcinoma by saturating the thyroid gland and any metastases with iodine. Iodinated injections should therefore be avoided during thyroid investigations unless the diagnosis has already been established (anaplastic carcinoma, medullary carcinoma).

CT has the advantage of permitting cervicomediastinal asessment (along with subdiaphragmatic evaluation in the case of medullary carcinoma) and, due to the use of thin slices, three-dimensional image reconstruction. However, the spatial resolution of CT is lower than that of high-resolution US. In addition, there are no CT features allowing differentiation between benign and malignant nodules except for indirect signs such as lymphadenopathy and muscle or vascular invasion.

CT thus cannot be relied on for characterization of thyroid nodules (Hopkins and Reading 1995). However, unenhanced CT with contiguous slices 5 mm thick allows determination of thyroid volume (mean error compared to surgical specimens, ±12%), based on the assumption that 1 cm^3 thyroid tissue weighs 1 g (Hermans et al. 1997). This information is beneficial when adjusting radioiodine therapy to the volume of the gland.

12.3.2.2
Features of Thyroid Disease on Computed Tomography

CT characterization of thyroid nodules is not routine practice, even though certain authors emphasize the technique's value for helping to suggest benignity or malignancy (Sashi et al. 1997). Cervical lymphadenopathy, with or without venous thrombosis (visible by US), and tracheal, esophageal, or bone invasion are the only signs of a malignant process. CT thus has no indications for the workup of differentiated, curable carcinomas, which account for the majority of thyroid cancers.

Anaplastic carcinomas, which represent approximately 10% of all thyroid cancers (Bittman et al. 1992), are diagnosed clinically in cases of diffuse involvement that manifests as rapid swelling of the neck, sometimes accompanied by lung or bone metastases. US can confirm the highly suspicious nature of these lesions (tumor mass and cervical lymphadenopathy, invasion of adjacent structures) and be used to guide FNA. Subsequent CT is indicated for rapid assessment of cervicomediastinal spread in patients with symptoms of respiratory compression, because it can demonstrate locoregional extranodal invasion better than US (Hopkins and Reading 1995).

NHL of the thyroid is rare, accounting for only 2.5% of all extranodal NHL, and is generally associated with laterocervical nodal disease. Biopsy is usually performed before any therapeutic procedure is carried out. If thyroid NHL is diagnosed, thoracic and abdominopelvic CT are indicated. Contrast-enhanced cervical CT may demonstrate isodense or hypodense zones corresponding to the hypoechoic areas seen on sonograms (Takashima et al. 1995c).

CT is of no practical value for workup of thyroiditis unless sonograms or clinical findings suggest malignancy (Kamijo 1994), as in Riedel's thyroiditis that has invaded adjacent structures (Fontan et al. 1993).

Except for the evaluation of exophthalmos, CT has no diagnostic value for Basedow's goiter.

If US demonstrates mediastinal involvement in a patient with multinodular goiter, CT may be helpful if surgery is envisaged because it can accurately demonstrate relations with the trachea, anterior or posterior mediastinal spread, and the generally symmetrical displacement of the vessels, without infiltration (Fig. 12.27).

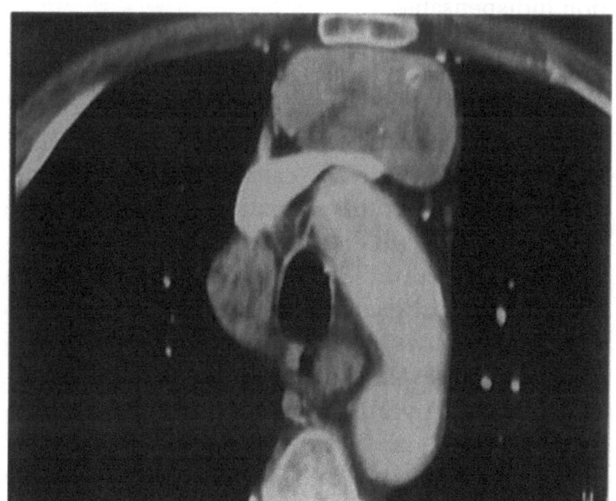

Fig. 12.27. CT scan of a goiter with mediastinal spread and posterior and anterior extension: no signs of invasion

12.3.3 Magnetic Resonance Imaging

MRI has an advantage over CT because it does not require injection of iodinated agents and allows multiplanar imaging as well as cervicomediastinal workup. However, its more limited availability, higher cost, and the duration of acquisition times together with a number of contraindications and artifacts restrict the indications for pretherapy MRI of thyroid disorders.

On T_1-weighted sequences, the thyroid appears homogeneous and discretely hyperintense to muscle. On T_2-weighted sequences, the gland appears hyperintense to muscle; gadolinium injection results in diffuse homogeneous enhancement (LOEVNER 1996).

12.3.3.1 Nodular Thyroid Disease

The frequency of thyroid nodules, the problems involved in management, and the risk of cancer have prompted numerous investigations on the utility of MRI for nodular thyroid disease. To date, MRI has not proven conclusive for differential diagnosis of benign and malignant lesions. RENARD et al. (1991) described features associated with benign thyroid nodules, and absence of these features is suggestive of a malignant process. However, the frequency of false-positive results (linked to the cystic or hemorrhagic nature of a nodule) and false-negative results (encapsulated cancer, lymphoma associated with thyroiditis) continues to render histologic examination indispensable.

In addition, MRI cannot detect the microcalcifications that are typical of papillary carcinoma. KUSUNOKI et al. (1994) studied "uncomplicated" nodules without any secondary modifications such as hemorrhage, necrosis, calcification, or fibrosis. While the grade of differentiation and proliferative cellular activity could be recognized on T_1- and T_2-weighted images, these features did not establish the benignity or malignancy of a nodule.

Adenomas may appear hyperintense on T_1-weighted images and enhance after gadolinium administration. Thyroid carcinoma also enhances with gadolinium, but may have irregular margins (STERN et al. 1994). NAKAHARA et al. (1997) failed to observe any difference between benign and malignant nodules on T_1- and T_2-weighted images or gadolinium-enhanced scans (Fig. 12.28).

MRI has an accuracy of 80% for detection of lymphadenopathy (TAKASHIMA et al. 1997). For SOM et al. (1994), nodal metastases have an intermediate-intensity signal on T_1-weighted images and high-intensity signal on T_2-weighted images. According to these authors, areas of high attenuation on T_1-weighted images reflect an elevated thyroglobulin concentration.

If medullary carcinoma has been diagnosed preoperatively, MRI may be useful for pretherapy staging. These lesions are isointense or hyperintense on T_1-weighted images and hyperintense on T_2-weighted sequences. Malignant nodes are hypointense to fat on T_1-weighted sequences and hyperintense on T_2-weighted sequences. Medullary carcinoma enhances discretely after gadolinium injection (Fig. 12.29). Increased amyloid deposits and tissue cellularity appear to increase the T_2 signal (WANG et al. 1997).

Literature data concerning primary thyroid lymphoma are rather variable. The lesions are often isointense on T_1-weighted sequences, and half enhance after gadolinium injection. On T_2-weighted images, thyroid lymphomas are hyperintense in 50% of cases, but they may also have a complex or isointense signal (TAKASHIMA et al. 1995c; NAKAHARA et al. 1997). MRI has not proven more useful than CT in thyroid lymphoma.

12.3.3.2 Other Applications

MRI appears more accurate than scintigraphy for analysis of tumor volume in patients with a large goiter (HUYSMANS et al. 1994; Fig. 12.30).

It can also optimize assessment of ophthalmologic involvement in Graves' disease. LAITT et al. (1994) used short tau inversion recovery (STIR) sequences in addition to visual assessment of muscle size. The increased signal intensity is due to edema secondary to inflammation. STIR sequences with retro-orbital fat suppression permit excellent analysis of modifications in the muscles. In the opinion of these authors, this technique can predict which patients will respond to anti-inflammatory therapy. ONISHI et al. (1994) investigated measurement of the T_2 relaxation time; in their study, the probability of response to treatment increased with augmentation of the mean T_2 relaxation time of the extraocular muscles.

Examination of thyroiditis by MRI does not provide any truly valuable information, in particular for

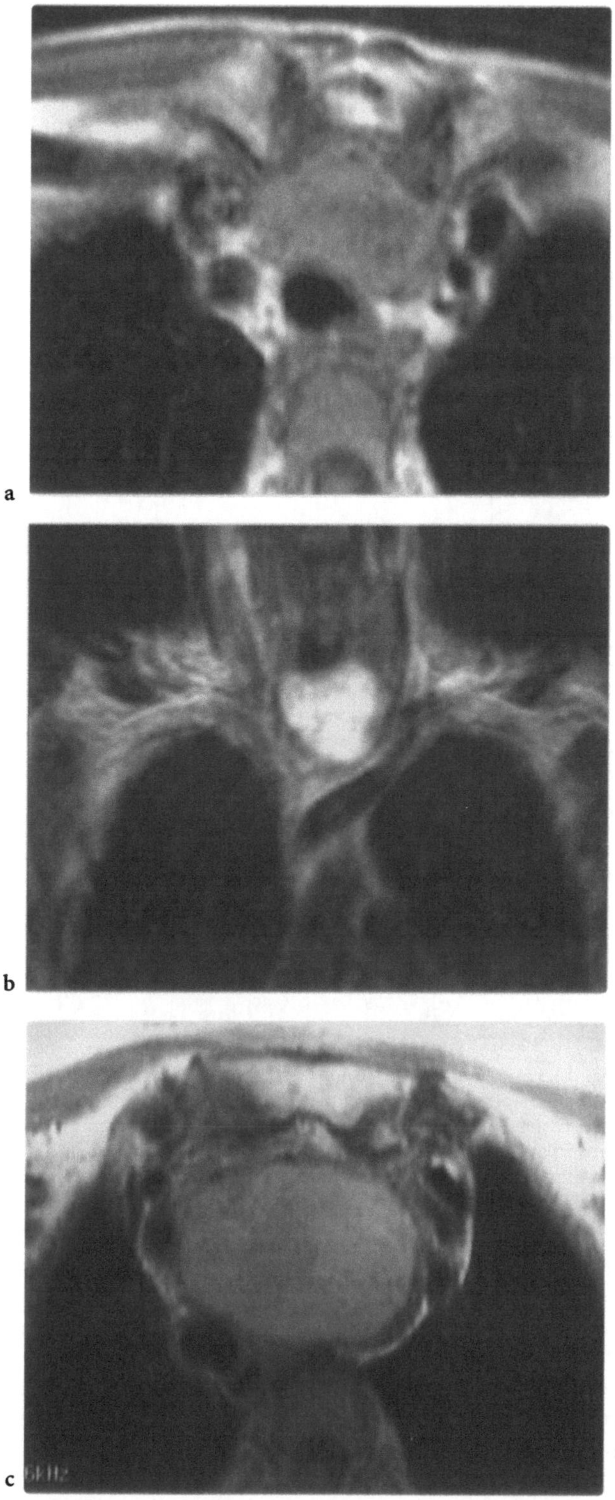

Fig. 12.28a–c. MRI of anaplastic thyroid carcinomas. **a** T_1-weighted turbo spin-echo (TSE) sequence of an undifferentiated cancer in the lower pole of a goiter; demonstration of the close relations between the tumor and the anterior aspect of the trachea. **b** Coronal T_2-weighted TSE image demonstrating the hyperintense tumor mass located above the left innominate venous trunk (same patient as in Fig. 12.28a). **c** T_2-weighted image of anaplastic thyroid carcinoma displacing but not invading the adjacent structures. This lesion proved unresectable at surgery

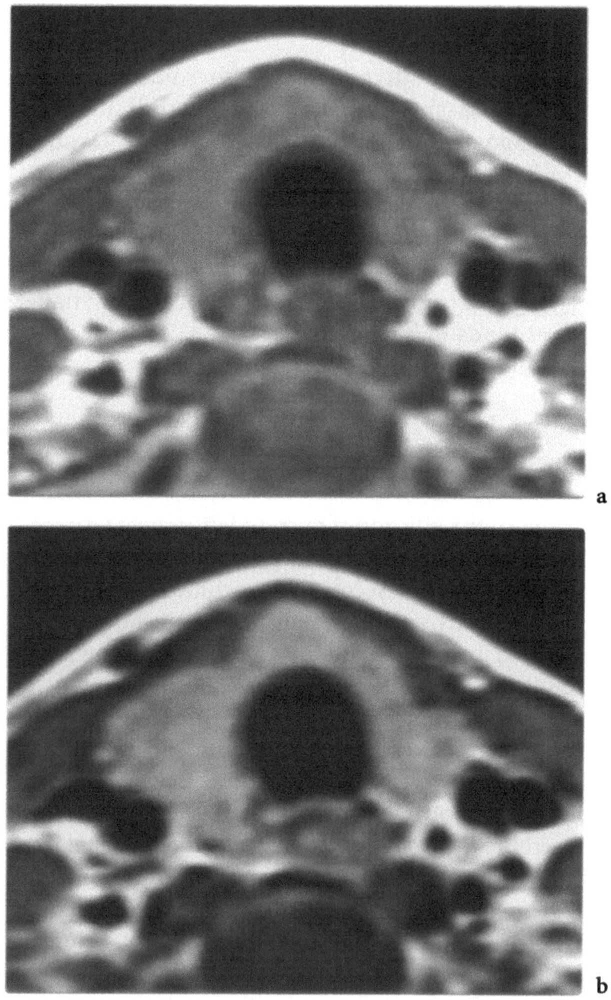

Fig. 12.29a,b. MRI of a medullary carcinoma (same patient as in Fig. 12.14). **a** The T_1-weighted sequence did not allow clear differentiation of the isthmic tumor from the normal thyroid tissue. **b** Gadolinium injection revealed discrete hypervascularity of the tumor lying anterior to the trachea

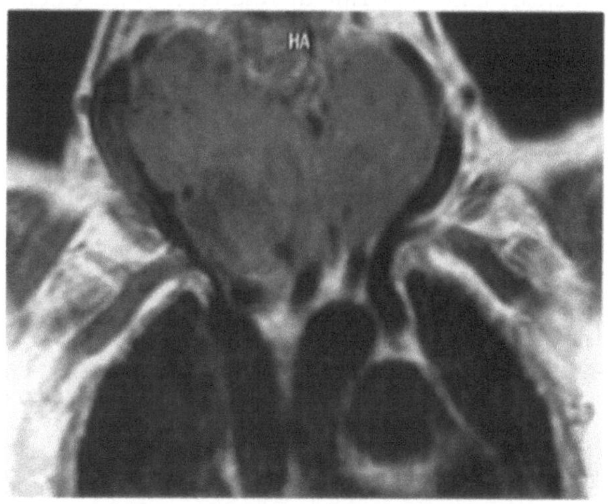

Fig. 12.30. Coronal MRI scan of a goiter that merely displaces the vascular structures. *HA*, head anterior (i.e., not strictly coronal but slightly oblique)

subacute thyroiditis and Riedel's thyroiditis, because MRI has the same limitations as other techniques for morphologic analysis (Fontan et al. 1993; Otsuka et al. 1994). Takashima et al. (1995b), however, reported that signal intensity ratios were valuable for Hashimoto s thyroiditis. For these authors, a ratio of 1.54 or higher suggests hypothyroidism, while a T_2-weighted signal intensity ratio of 5.8 or higher corresponds to lymphoma.

12.3.4 Conclusion

Owing to the efficacy of current laboratory tests and the morphologic data provided by US, other imaging modalities remain second-line techniques. Scintigraphy, previously the sole morphologic examination, has seen its indications decrease, even though the examination is still often carried out merely out of habit. Following TSH assays and US, scintigraphy can be used to search for a hot nodule. Scintigraphy can also be used to determine the efficacy of percutaneous ethanol injection, which is increasingly proposed as an alternative to surgery. Outside of clinical trials and research on new contrast agents, scintigraphy often serves merely to confirm the diagnostic hypotheses formulated by US techniques (including CD, PD, and US-guided FNA). The indications for CT and MRI are similar, and either technique may be used, depending on unit availability. Contrast-enhanced CT or MRI is indicated for preoperative staging of recognized medullary carcinoma (analysis of mediastinal nodes and abdominal examination in search of multiple endocrine neoplasia: adrenals, pancreas) and anaplastic thyroid carcinoma. Unenhanced CT or MRI may be useful for goiters with mediastinal involvement if surgery is being planned.

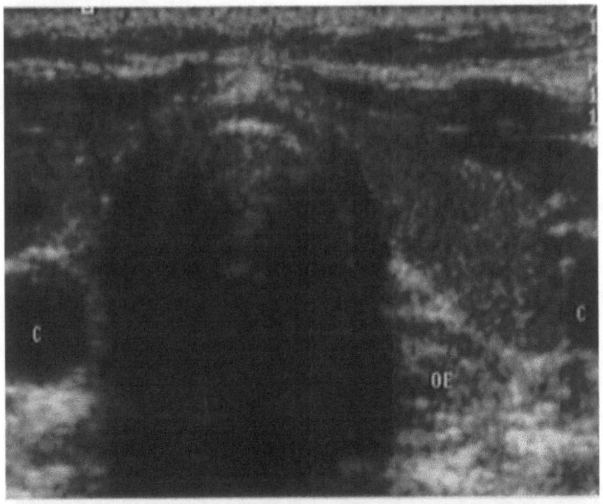

a

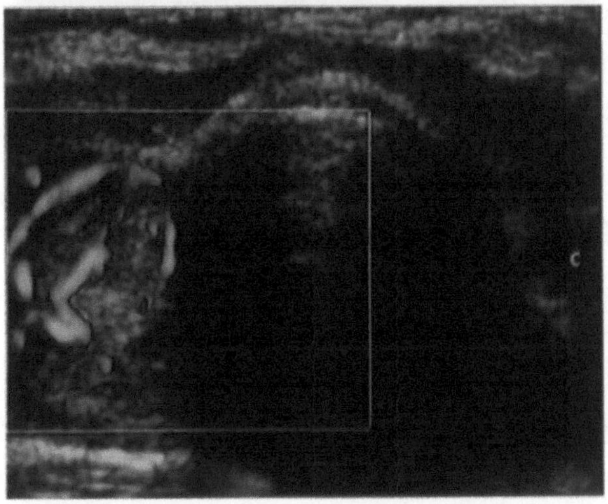

b

Fig. 12.31a,b. Follow-up sonogram after lobo-isthmectomy. **a** Normal appearance after right lobo-isthmectomy: the right carotid artery lies against the aerodigestive tract. *C*, common carotid artery; *OE*, esophagus. **b** Color Doppler (CD) of a nodule that developed in the remaining right lobe: power Doppler (PD) revealed peripheral and central hypervascularity. An adenoma was diagnosed by fine-needle aspiration (FNA)

12.4 Post-therapy Follow-Up of Thyroid Tumors

P.Y. Marcy, J.N. Bruneton, and J. Darcourt

12.4.1 Benign Thyroid Pathologies

12.4.1.1 Nonsurgical Thyroid Disease

Nonsurgical thyroid pathologies include lesions that are merely followed up after FNA and thyroid disease managed by hormone therapy. Using the thyroid map established during initial workup for comparative purposes, US can reveal progression or regression in nodule size.

12.4.1.2 Postsurgical Follow-Up

After loboisthmectomy or nodule enucleation, US can demonstrate the appearance of any new nodules. This is particularly helpful after surgery for colloid goiter or multinodular goiter. Optimum diagnostic accuracy is obviously required to avoid repeat surgery that would result in subtotal or total thyroidectomy for benign disease (Fig. 12.31). US has no indications in the follow-up of total thyroidectomy performed for a nonmalignant lesion.

12.4.2 Curable Differentiated Thyroid Cancers

12.4.2.1 Natural History of Differentiated Thyroid Cancer

Papillary carcinomas have a propensity for lymphatic spread. Their main risk is local recurrence in the form of neoplastic grafts in the thyroidectomy bed. Recurrence is most common in elderly patients with an aggressive tumor. Nodal recurrence (less than 10% of cases) occurs secondarily if a micrometastasis is left in situ; nodes at the limits of high cervical, spinal, and superior mediastinal curettage are involved most often (CANNONI and DEMARD 1995). Visceral metastases are rare; miliary and micronodular pulmonary metastases predominate. These lesions take up iodine and have a favorable prognosis (SCHLUMBERGER et al. 1988; WITTERICK et al. 1993).

Local recurrence of follicular cancer is exceptional and is usually due to incomplete resection of extracapsular lesions. The prognosis is primarily determined by the existence of visceral metastases, which are present in 20% of patients (ZOHAR and STRAUSS 1994). These lung and bone metastases do not always exhibit intense uptake and hypervascularity. The mortality rate at 5 years is 60% despite radioiodine therapy or external irradiation.

12.4.2.2 Follow-Up of Differentiated Thyroid Cancers

In the postsurgical setting, the extent of thyroid ablation can usefully be evaluated by quantification of neck uptake. Follow-up is based on iodinated whole-body scintigraphy studies combined with thyroglobulin assays. The association of these two methods has an estimated diagnostic accuracy of 96.7% (RONGA et al. 1990). Whole-body scintiscans can localize histologically well-differentiated metastases in a two-dimensional plane after suppressive therapy. Doses (usually 5–10 mCi) can reach 100–150 mCi (SCHLUMBERGER et al. 1988); this has the advantage of being both diagnostic and therapeutic (Fig. 12.32).

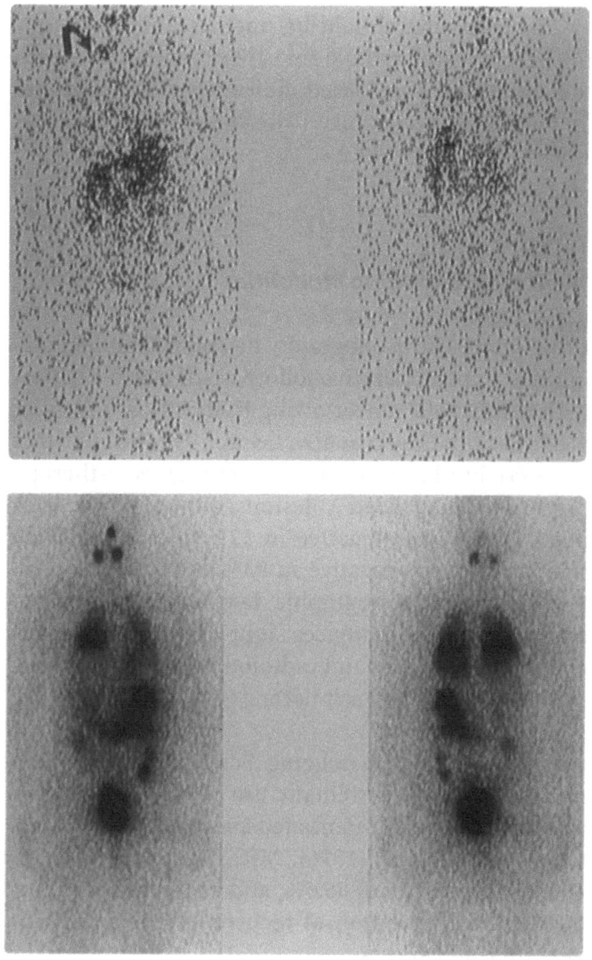

a

b

Fig. 12.32a,b Whole-body scintiscan (iodine-131) after total thyroidectomy for papillary carcinoma. **a** Discrete right cervical thyroid remnant. **b** Pulmonary and bone metastases

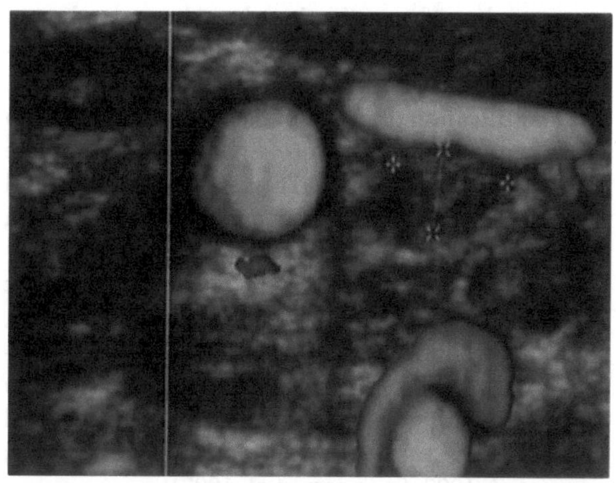

Fig. 12.33. Power Doppler (PD) of the laterocervical region in a patient treated for papillary carcinoma. Appearance of a 3.2+4.9 mm node (*crosses*) that was not visible on the follow-up scintiscan. Ultrasound (US)-guided fine-needle aspiration (FNA) led to diagnosis of a nodal metastasis

Thyroglobulin should be undetectable after thyroidectomy and radioiodine treatment. Any elevation should be considered indicative of locoregional or metastatic recurrence (Sweeney and Johnston 1995; Cavalieri 1996).

12.4.2.3
Nonisotopic Imaging Modalities

Ultrasound. Ultrasonography has played an increasing role in postoperative follow-up of curable differentiated thyroid cancer owing to its efficacy for cervical examination (Solbiati et al. 1992; Bolland et al. 1993). For Franceschi et al. (1996), post-therapy cervical US visualized 23 lesions, although thyroglobulin levels were negative in 52% and whole-body scintiscans were negative in 83%. Antonelli et al. (1995) reported sonographic detection of 16 cervical anomalies (12 recurrences, four cases of lymphadenitis) after surgery and radioiodine therapy despite normal whole-body scintiscans (Fig. 12.33).

Magnetic Resonance Imaging. Few studies have been published on the systematic use of MRI for surveillance of curable differentiated cancers. According to Cyna-Gorse et al. (1996), MRI has a sensitivity of 100%, a specificity of 66.6%, and an overall accuracy of 82.6% for detection of recurrences of differentiated thyroid cancers.

Perspectives. Although US appears to be the sole nonscintigraphic technique of any practical complementary value owing to its sensitivity and availability, a number of investigations have been conducted with new isotopic techniques in an attempt to improve the efficacy of whole-body scintigraphy.

Quantification of neck uptake appears superior to visual assessment. Ablation is considered complete when uptake is under 1%. This is all the more useful because visual evaluation overestimates uptake in 22% of cases (Chopra et al. 1996).

Although not yet widely available, diagnostic scanning using new radioisotopes such as octreotide, fluorodeoxyglucose ([^{18}F]FDG-PET), and Tc 99m-tetrofosmin reportedly reveals metastases even when iodinated scintigraphy is normal (Reinhardt and Moser 1996; Conti et al. 1997; Fridrich et al. 1997; Lind et al. 1997; Seabold et al. 1997).

According to Kobayashi et al. (1997), MIBI markedly improves the sensitivity of conventional scintigraphic techniques for the detection of recurrence, especially when coupled with SPECT.

In addition to searching for means to improve results, Reynolds and Robbins (1997) investigated ways to reduce the discomfort caused by the symptoms of hypothyroidism. They proposed that patients be pretreated by recombinant human TSH (rhTSH) prior to imaging with iodine-131. A number of questions remain, however, concerning the iodine-131 dose for follow-up scintiscans (conventional doses versus a more modern approach using iodine-123) and the percentage of iodine-31 uptake required for effective therapy (no clear correlation was found between iodine-31 uptake and the therapeutic outcome, even though the correlation is better with the percent uptake per gram) (Reynolds and Robbins 1997).

Scott et al. (1995) demonstrated the interest of sensitive isotopic imaging combined with morphologic analysis by CT or MRI.

Overall, follow-up of curable differentiated cancers has changed very little. The main source of progress concerns complementary cervical US. The role of new contrast agents has not yet been conclusively established, but [^{18}F]FDG-PET and MIBI have recently proven superior to the conventional technique for patients with increased thyroglobulin levels not explained by scintigraphy.

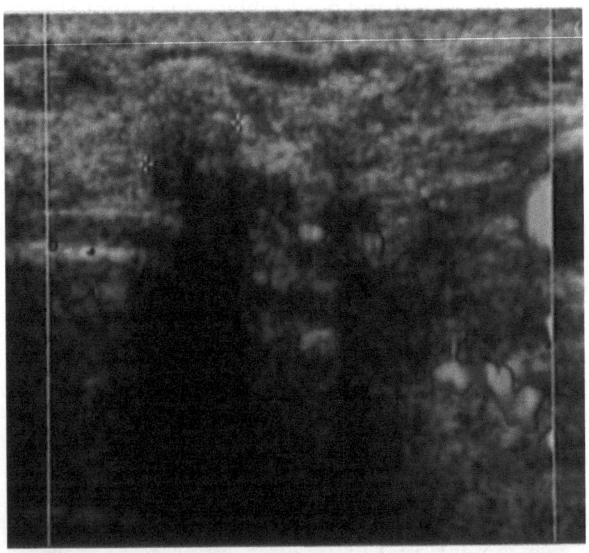

Fig. 12.34. Follow-up of medullary carcinoma. Biochemical abnormalities prompted cervicothoracic and abdominal imaging. Ultrasound detected an attenuating lesion (6.3 mm between the two *crosses*) corresponding to a tumor recurrence

12.4.3
Medullary Thyroid Carcinoma

12.4.3.1
Course of Disease

Whether sporadic, familial, an isolated form, or associated with a multiple endocrine neoplasia (MEN) syndrome (IIa or IIb), medullary carcinoma does not take up iodine and can only be treated by surgery (primary cancer, metastases). Medullary carcinoma metastasizes to the lymph nodes and the liver; metastases are often calcified by amyloid deposits and calcium. Optimum follow-up is based on assays of calcitonin, an excellent marker of locoregional and distant tumor progression. Any elevation in calcitonin should prompt imaging studies (Bourguignat et al. 1997; Fig. 12.34).

12.4.3.2
Post-therapy Imaging Follow-Up

While scintigraphic methods using various isotopes may detect subradiologic and subclinical metastases, they remain of low value compared to selective venous sampling (Lupoli et al. 1991; Dorr et al. 1993; Abdelmoumene et al. 1994). Tc 99m (V)-dimercaptosuccinic acid (DSMA) is reportedly superior to MIBI and thallium-201 for diagnosis of secondary disease sites (Ugur et al. 1996).

Cervicomediastinal examination in search of nodal lesions can be performed by MRI, which can differentiate tumor recurrence from fibrosis (Aufferman et al. 1988; Van Den Brekel et al. 1990; Som 1992).

Hepatic metastases are identified by US and characterized by CT or MRI. Sonographically, hepatic metastases of medullary thyroid cancer image as one or more homogeneous hyperechoic nodules that may suggest an angioma (frequency, 91.3%; Leclere et al. 1993). T_2-weighted sequences can distinguish the increasing hypersignal of hemangioma from the stable and less intense signal of a metastasis.

Follow-up of medullary thyroid carcinoma is essentially performed by tumor markers, i.e., calcitonin and carcinoembryonic antigen (CEA) assays. Depending on results, imaging studies may be indicated. US usually suffices for cervical and hepatic examination, but CT or MRI are required for thoracoabdominal workup.

12.4.4
Undifferentiated Thyroid Carcinomas

Undifferentiated thyroid carcinomas have a very poor prognosis, and examinations should be kept to a minimum. Cervicomediastinal CT appears to be the best approach. Other examinations in search of secondary localizations are dictated by clinical symptoms.

12.5
Conclusion

Overall, modern imaging modalities have not essentially changed management of tumoral thyroid pathologies:

- For benign thyroid disease, US initially led to an increase in the number of surgical procedures, but has not solved the problem of multinodular thyroid disease. The fact that excessive recourse to surgery often revealed only benign disease underscores the importance of US-guided FNA.
- Post-therapy follow-up of medullary carcinoma is based on laboratory tests; imaging is reserved for second-line use.
- The rapidly progressive course of anaplastic cancers requires use of the fastest and least invasive techniques whenever follow-up by imaging is warranted.
- The effectiveness but also the limitations of whole-body scintigraphy for differentiated cancers have prompted searches for new contrast agents. The encouraging results obtained with a combination of PET scans and [^{18}F]FDG have raised hopes for early detection of metastases and recurrence. Although this approach allows recognition of lesions before other imaging modalities (Seabold 1997), its sensitivity is associated with nonspecific contrast uptake in the thyroid that is also seen in individuals without thyroid cancer (Conti et al. 1997). MIBI has proven effective, is not overly expensive, and does not require interruption of hormone therapy (Fridrich et al. 1997). Further research on these new diagnostic techniques may rapidly modify post-therapy follow-up of differentiated thyroid cancer.

References

Abdelmoumene N, Schlumberger M, Gardet P et al (1994) Selective venous sampling catheterisation for localization of persisting medullary thyroid carcinoma. Br J Cancer 69:1141–1144

Adams H, Jones MC, Othman S et al (1992) The sonographic appearances in postpartum thyroiditis. Clin Radiol 45:311–315

Aghini-Lombardi F, Antonangeli L, Pinchera A et al (1997) Effect of iodized salt on thyroid volume of children living in an area previously characterized by moderate iodine deficiency. J Clin Endocrinol Metab 82:1136–1139

Ahuja A, Chick W, King W, Metreweli C (1996) Clinical significance of the comet-tail artifact in thyroid ultrasound. J Clin Ultrasound 24:129–133

Ahuja AT, King W, Metreweli C (1994) Role of ultrasonography in thyroid metastases. Clin Radiol 49:627–629

Ahuja AT, Chow L, Chick W et al (1995) Metastatic cervical nodes in papillary carcinoma of the thyroid: ultrasound and histological correlation. Clin Radiol 50:229–231

Albert SG, Alves LE, Rose EP (1987) Thyroid dysfunction during chronic amiodarone therapy. J Am Coll Cardiol 9:175–183

Alonso O, Lago G, Mut F et al (1996) Thyroid imaging with Tc-99m MIBI in patients with solitary cold nodules on pertechnetate imaging. Clin Nucl Med 21:363–367

Antonelli A, Miccoli P, Ferdeghini M et al (1995) Role of neck ultrasonography in the follow-up of patients operated on for thyroid cancer. Thyroid 5:25–28

Argalia G, D'Ambrosio F, Lucarelli F et al (1995) L'eco Doppler nella caratterizzazione della patologia nodulare tiroidea. Radiol Med 89:651–657

Auffermann W, Clark OH, Thurnher S, Galante M, Higgings CB (1988) Recurrent thyroid carcinoma: characteristics on MRI. Radiology 168:753–757

Becker D, Bair HJ, Becker W et al (1997) Thyroid autonomy with color-coded image-directed Doppler sonography: internal hypervascularization for the recognition of autonomous adenomas. J Clin Ultrasound 25:63–69

Bennedbaek FN, Hegedus L (1997) The value of ultrasonography in the diagnosis and follow-up of subacute thryoiditis. Thyroid 7:45-50

Benson DM, Rifkin MD, Rose JL et al (1983) Characterization of benign and malignant tissues of the thyroid gland. An ultrasonic approach using RF waveform analysis and pattern recognition. Invest Radiol 18:459–462

Birchall IWJ, Chow CC, Metreweli C (1990) Ultrasound appearance of de Quervain's thyroiditis. Clin Radiol 41:57–59

Bittman O, Bruneton JN, Fenart D et al (1992) Imagerie des cancers anaplasiques de la thyroïde. J Radiol 73:35–38

Bogazzi F, Bartalena L, Vitti P, Rago T, Brogioni S, Martino E (1996) Color flow Doppler sonography in thyrotoxicosis factitia. J Endocrinol Invest 19:603–606

Bolland GW, Lee MJ, Mueller PR, Mayo-Smith W, Dawson SL, Simenone JF (1993) Efficacy of sonographically-guided biopsy of thyroid masses and cervical lymph nodes. AJR 161:1053–1056

Bourguignat E, Marcy PY, Bobin S, Bruneton JN (1997) Cancers de la thyroïde. In : Lavayssière R, Vannetzel JM, Cabée AE (eds) TDM et IRM en carcinologie de l'adulte. Vigot, Paris, pp 140–156

Brander A, Viikinkoski P, Nickels J, Kivisaari L (1989) Thyroid gland: US screening in middle-aged women with no previous thyroid disease. Radiology 173:507–510

Brander A, Viikinkoski P, Tuuhea J, Voutilainen L, Kivisaari L (1992) Clinical versus ultrasound examination of the thyroid gland in common clinical practice. J Clin Ultrasound 20:37–42

Braun B, Blank W (1994) Color Doppler sonography-guided percutaneous alcohol instillation in the therapy of functionally autonomous thyroid nodules. Dtsch Med Wochenschr 119:1607–1612

Brkljacic B, Cuk V, Tomic-Brzac H, Bence-Zigman Z, Delic-Brkljacic D, Drinkovic I (1994) Ultrasonic evaluation of benign and malignant nodules in echographically multinodular thyroids. J Clin Ultrasound 22:71–76

Bruneton JN, Santini N, Santini J (1987) Medical ultrasound equipment, examination techniques, and ultrasonography of the normal neck. In: Bruneton JN (ed) Ultrasonography of the neck. Springer, Berlin Heidelberg New York, pp 1–21

Bruneton JN, Balu-Maestro C, Marcy PY, Melia P, Mourou MY (1994a) Very high frequency (13 Mhz) ultrasonographic examination of the normal neck: detection of normal lymph nodes and thyroid nodules. J Ultrasound Med 13:87–90

Bruneton JN, Maestro C, Marcy PY, Padovani B (1994b) Echographie des ganglions superficiels. J Radiol 75:373–381

Bruneton JN, Marcy PY, Maestro C, Raffaelli C (1996) Echographie des nodules thyroïdiens. In: Bruneton JN, Padovani B (eds) Imagerie en endocrinologie. Masson, Paris, pp 48–54

Burke JS, Burke JJ, Fuller LM (1977) Malignant lymphoma of the thyroid: a clinical pathologic study of 35 patients including ultrastructural observations. Cancer 39:1587–1602

Cannoni M, Demard F (1995) Les nodules thyroïdiens du diagnostic à la chirurgie. Arnette, Paris

Carrol BA (1982) Asymptomatic thyroid nodules: incidental sonographic detection. AJR 133:499–501

Castagnone D, Rivolta R, Rescalli S, Baldini MI, Tozzi R, Cantalamessa L (1996) Color Doppler sonography in Graves' disease: value in assessing activity of disease and predicting outcome. AJR 166:203–207

Cavalieri RR (1996) Nuclear imaging in the management of thyroid carcinoma. Thyroid 6:485–492

Cavalieri RR (1997) Iodine metabolism and thyroid physiology: current concepts. Thyroid 7:177–181

Chang TC, Hong CT, Chang SL, Hsieh HC, Liaw KY, How SW (1990) Correlation between sonography and pathology in thyroid diseases. J Formos Med Assoc 89:777–783

Chopra S, Wastie ML, Chan S et al (1996) Assessment of completeness of thyroid ablation by estimation of neck uptake of 131I on whole-body scans: comparison of quantification and visual assessment of thyroid bed uptake. Nucl Med Commun 17:687–691

Clark KJ, Cronan JJ, Scola FH (1995) Color Doppler sonography: anatomic and physiologic assessments of the thyroid. J Clin Ultrasound 23:215–223

Cochan-Priollet B, Guillausseau PJ, Chagnon S et al (1994) The diagnostic value of fine-needle aspiration biopsy under ultrasonography in nonfunctional thyroid nodules: a prospective study comparing cytologic and histologic findings. Am J Med 97:152–157

Cohen JH, Ingbar SH, Braverman LE (1989) Thyrotoxicosis due to ingestion of excess thyroid hormone. Endocr Rev 10:113–124

Conti PS, Durski JM, Singer PA (1997) Incidence of thryoid gland uptake of F-18 FDG in cancer patients. Radiology 205 (P):220

Crom DB, Kaste SC, Tubergen DG, Greenwald CA, Sharp GB, Hudson MM (1997) Ultrasonography for thyroid screening

after head and neck irradiation in childhood cancer survivors. Med Pediatr Oncol 28:15–21
Cyna-Gorse F, Toubert ME, Zagdanski AM et al (1996) Récidives cervico-médiastinales des cancers thyroïdiens différenciés: valeur de l'IRM. J Radiol 77:1195–1200
Danese D, Schiacchitano S (1993) Il nodulo tiroideo. Considerazioni diagnostiche. Minerva Endocrinol 18:129–13337
De Lellis RA (1989) The endocrine system. In: Cotram R, Kumar V, Robbins SL (eds) Robbins pathologic basis of disease, 4th edn. Saunders, Philadelphia, pp 1214–1242
Degnan BM, McClellan DR, Francis GL (1996) An analysis of fine-needle aspiration biopsy of the thyroid in children and adolescents. J Pediatr Surg 31:903–907
Delorme S, Weisser G, Zuna I, Fein M, Lorenz A, Van Kaick G (1995) Quantitative characterization of color Doppler images: reproducibility, accuracy, and limitations. J Clin Ultrasound 23:537–550
Derebek E, Biberoglu S, Kut O et al (1996) Early and delayed thallium-201 scintigraphy in thyroid nodules: the relationship between early thallium-201 uptake and perfusion. Eur J Nucl Med 23:504–520
Dorr V, Wurstlin S, Franck-Raue K et al (1993) Somastatin receptor scintigraphy (SRS) and MRI in recurrent medullary thyroid carcinoma: a comparative study. Horm Metab Res 27:48–55
Duquenne M, Rohmer V, Guyetant S et al (1997) Nodule thyroïdien isolé. Intérêt de la cytoponction et de la scintigraphie. Presse Méd 26:507–511
Eeckhoudt L, Hermans J, Merlo P et al (1993) Analyse économique des approches diagnostiques et thérapeutiques du nodule froid de la thyroïde. Ann Endocrinol 54:293–296
Erom DB, Kaste SC, Tubergen DG, Greenwald CA, Sharp GB, Hudson MM (1997) Ultrasonography for thyroid screening after head and neck irradiation in childhood cancer survivors. Med Pediatr Oncol 28:15–21
Ezzat S, Sarti DA, Cain DR, Braunstein GD (1994) Thyroid incidentalomas. Prevalence by palpation and ultrasonography. Arch Intern Med 154:1838–1840
Farwell AP, Braverman LE (1996) Inflammatory thyroid disorders. Otolaryngol Clin North Am 29:541–557
Feldkamp J, Horstser FA (1995) Rationelle Diagnostik von Schilddrusen Funktionsstörungen. Z Arztl Fortbild 89:21–25
Fontan FJP, Carballido FC, Felipe FP, Oses JM, Martin CV (1993) Riedel thyroiditis: US, CT, and MR evaluation. J Comput Assist Tomogr 17:324–325
Franceschi M, Kujic Z, Franceschi D, Lukinac L, Roncevic S (1996) Thyroglobulin determination, neck ultrasonography and iodine-131 whole-body scintigraphy in differentiated thyroid carcinoma. J Nucl Med 37:446–451
Freitas JE, Freitas AE (1994) Thyroid and parathyroid imaging. Semin Nucl Med 24:234–245
Fridrich L, Messa C, Landoni C et al (1997) Whole-body scintigraphy with 99 Tcm-MIBI, 18 F-FDG and 131I in patients with metastatic thyroid carcinoma. Nucl Med Commun 18:3–9
Funari M, Campos Z, Gooding GA, Higgins CG (1992) MRI and ultrasound detection of asymptomatic thyroid nodules in hyperparathyroidism. J Comput Assist Tomogr 16:615–619
Gandon J, Ledoux-Robert J (1995) Les cancers du corps thyroïde. Actualités en cancérologie cervicofaciale. Masson, Paris
Garretti L, Cassinis MC, Cesarini F, Drogo M, Papotti M, Ragona R (1994) Attendibilita della diagnosi ecotomografica nella valutazione delle lesioni della tiroide. Confronto con la citologia e l'istologia. Radiol Med 88:598–605
Gemma R, Nakamura H, Mori T, Andoh S, Suzuki Y, Yoshimi T (1996) The change in 123 I-uptake between 3- and 24-hours is useful in predicting early response to methimazole in patients with Graves' disease. Endocr J 43:61–66
Gharib H (1994) Fine-needle aspiration biopsy of thyroid nodules: advantages, limitations and effect. Mayo Clin Proc 69:44–49
Gharib H, Goellner JR (1993) Fine-needle aspiration biopsy of the thyroid: an appraisal. Ann Intern Med 118:282–289
Gharib H, Goellner JR, Johnston DA (1993) Fine-needle aspiration cytology of the thyroid: a 12-year experience with 11,000 biopsies. Clin Lab Med 13:669–709
Gimondo P, Messina G, Caratozzolo M, Tomei A (1994) Analisi del ruelo della citologia agoaspirativa ecoguidata quale criterio di selezione nella terapia chirurgica delle malattie tiroidee. Studio retrospettivo multicentrico su 5109 pazienti. Radiol Med 87:648–652
Gimondo P, Messina G, Gimondo S (1996) Raro caso di tiroidite acuta suppurativa. Minerva Med 87:475–478
Giuffrida D, Gharib H (1995) Controversies in the management of cold, hot, and occult thyroid nodules. Am J Med 99:642–650
Goletti O, Lenziardi M, Lippolis PV et al (1993) Alcolizzazione percutanea ecoguidata dei noduli tirodei freddi non neoplastici. Radiol Med 85:827–830
Gonczi J, Szabolcs I, Kovacs Z, Kakosy T, Goth M, Szilagyi G (1994) Ultrasonography of the thyroid gland in hospitalized, clinically ill geriatric patients: thyroid volume, its relationship to age and disease, and the prevalence of diffuse and nodular goiter. J Clin Ultrasound 22:257–261
Gonsorcikova V, Trebjbal D, Tajtakova M et al (1996) Treatment of autonomous thyroid gland nodules using percutaneaous injections of ethanol under ultrasonography control. Initial experience. Vnitr Lek 42:166–170
Gooding GA (1993) Sonography of the thyroid and parathyroid. Radiol Clin North Am 31:967–989
Gorman B, Charboneau JW, James EM et al (1987) Medullary thyroid carcinoma: role of high-resolution US. Radiology 162:147–150
Hamburger JI (1987) Consistency of sequential needle biopsy findings for thyroid nodules. Arch Intern Med 147:97–99
Hamburger JI (1994) Diagnosis of thyroid nodules by fine-needle biopsy: use and abuse. J Clin Endocrinol Metab 79:335–339
Hamburger JI, Miller JM, Kini SR (1983) Lymphoma of the thyroid. Ann Intern Med 99:685–693
Hancock SL, McDougall IR, Constine LS (1995) Thyroid abnormalities after therapeutic external radiation. Int J Radiat Oncol Biol Phys 31:1165–1170
Hardoff R, Baron E, Sheinfeld M, Luboshitsky R (1995) Localized manifestations of subacute thyroiditis presenting as solitary transient cold thyroid nodules. A report of 11 cases. Clin Nucl Med 20:981–984
Hayashi N, Tamaki N, Konishi J et al (1986) Sonography of Hashimoto's thyroiditis. J Clin Ultrasound 14:123–126
Healy JC, Shafford EA, Reznek RH et al (1996) Sonographic abnormalities of the thyroid gland following radiotherapy in survivors of childhood Hodgkin's disease. Br J Radiol 69:671–623
Hermans R, Bouillon R, Laga K et al (1997) Estimation of thyroid gland volume by spiral computed tomography. Eur Radiol 7:214–216
Hiromura T (1994) Ultrasonography of cystic thyroid nodules: sonographic-pathologic correlation. Nippon Igaku Hoshasen Gakkai Zasshi 54:500–509
Hodgson KJ, Lazarus JH, Wheeler MH et al (1988) Duplex scan-derived thyroid blood flow in euthyroid and hyperthyroid patients. World J Surg 12:470–475

Holden A (1995) The role of colour and duplex Doppler ultrasound in the assessment of thyroid nodules. Australas Radiol 39:343–349
Hopkins CR, Reading CC (1995) Thyroid and parathyroid imaging. Semin Ultrasound CT MR 16:279–295
Horlocker TT, Hay JE, James EM, Reading CC, Charboneau JW (1986) Prevalence of incidental nodular thyroid diseases detected during high resolution parathyroid ultrasonography. In: Medeiros-Neto A, Gaitan E (eds) Frontiers of thyroidology, vol 2. Plenum, New York, pp 1309–1312
Horvath E, Majilis S, Yanez P et al (1997) Thyroidite de de quervain: diagnostic en échographie. J Radiol 78:897
Horvath F, Capuano LG, Lippolis G et al (1993) In tema di diagnosi di natura preoperatoria del nodulo tiroideo. Minerva Chir 48:1279–1281
Hurley DL, Gharib H (1996) Evaluation and management of multinodular goiter. Otolaryngol Clin North Am 29:527–540
Huysmans DA, De Haas MM, Van Den Broerk WJ et al (1994) Magnetic resonance imaging for volume estimation of large multinodular goitres: a comparison with scintigraphy. Br J Radiol 67:519–523
Ito M, Yamashita S, Ashizawa S et al (1995) Childhood thyroid diseases around Chernobyl evaluated by ultrasound examination and fine-needle aspiration cytology. Thyroid 5:365–368
James EM, Charboneau JW, Hay ID (1991) The thyroid. In: Rumack CM (ed) Diagnostic ultrasound, vol 1. Mosby, St Louis, pp 507–523
Jarlov AE, Hegedus L, Gjorup T, Hansen JEM (1991) Accuracy of the clinical assessment of thyroid size. Dan Med Bull 38:87–89
Jarlov AE, Nygard B, Hegedus L, Kastrup S, Hansen JM (1993) Observer variation in ultrasound assessment of the thyroid gland. Br J Radiol 66:625–627
Kamijo K (1994) Clinical studies on thyroid CT number in chronic thryoiditis. Endocr J 41:19–23
Katagiri M, Harada T, Kiyono T (1994) Diagnosis of thyroid carcinoma by ultrasonic examination: comparison with diagnosis by fine-needle aspiration cytology. Thyroidology 6:21–26
Kerr L (1994) High resolution thyroid ultrasound: the value of color Doppler. Ultrasound Q 12:21–43
Kim JK, Lee HK, Ahn IM, Lee MJ, Choi CG, Suh DC (1997) Treatment of benign cold thyroid nodules: efficacy and safety of sonographically guided percutaneous ethanol injection. Radiology 205 (P):531
Kobayashi M, Mogami T, Uchiyama M et al (1997) Usefulness of 99 mTc-MIBI SPECT in the metastatic lesions of thyroid cancer. Nippon Igaku Hoshasen Gakkai Zasshi 57:127–132
Komatsu M, Kobayashi S, Ito N, Sugenoya A, Ida F (1994) Ultrasonography in the diagnosis of malignant lymphoma of the thyroid. Nippon Geka Gakkai Zasshi 95:187–191
Kraimps JL, Barbier J (1993) Apport de l'échographie peropératoire. Ann Endocrinol 54:235–236
Kresnik E, Gallowitsch HJ, Mikosch P, Gomez I, Lind P (1997) Technetium-99m-MIBI scintigraphy of thyroid nodules in an endemic goiter area. J Nucl Med 38:62–65
Kuma K, Matzsuzuka F, Yokozawa T, Miyauchi A, Sugawara M (1994) Fate of untreated benign thyroid nodules: results of long term follow-up. World J Surg 18:495–498
Kumar A, Aggarwal S, Pham DH (1994) Pharyngoesophageal (Zenker's) diverticulum mimicking thyroid nodule on ultrasonography: report of two cases. J Ultrasound Med 13:313–322
Kume N, Suga K, Nishigauchi K, Kawamura M, Matsunaga N (1996) Relationship between thallium-201 uptake and tumour proliferative ability in thyroid nodules. Eur J Nucl Med 23:376–382
Kumpusalo L, Kumpusalo E, Soimakallio S et al (1996) Thyroid ultrasound findings 7 years after the Chernobyl accident. A comparative epidemiological study in the Bryansk region of Russia. Acta Radiol 37:904–909
Kusunoki T, Murata K, Nishida S, Tomura T, Inoue M (1994) Histopathological findings of human thyroid tumors and signal intensities of MRI. Nippon Jibiinkoka Gakkai Kaiho 97:1406–1411
Laitt RD, Hoh B, Wakeley C et al (1994) The value of the short tau inversion recovery sequence in magnetic resonance imaging of thyroid eye disease. Br J Radiol 67:244–247
Leclere J, Sidibe S, Lassau N et al (1996) Aspects échographiques des métastases hépatiques des cancers médullaires de la thyroïde. J Radiol 77:99–103
Lee MJ, Ross DS, Mueller PR, Daniels G, Dawson SL, Simeone JF (1993) Fine needle aspiration biopsy of cervical lymph nodes in patients with thyroid cancer: a prospective comparison of cytopathologic and tissue marker analysis. Radiology 187:851–854
Lin JD, Hsueh C, Chao TC, Weng HF, Huang BY (1997a) Thyroid follicular neoplasms diagnosed by high-resolution ultrasonography with fine-needle aspiration cytology. Acta Cytol 41:687–691
Lin JD, Huang BY, Weng HF, Jeng LB, Hsuem C (1997b) Thyroid ultrasonography with fine-needle aspiration cytology for the diagnosis of thyroid cancer. J Clin Ultrasound 25:111–118
Lind P, Gallowitsch HJ, Langsteger W, Kresnik E, Mikosch P, Gomez I (1997) Technetium-99m-tetrofosmin whole-body scintigraphy in the follow-up of differentiated thyroid carcinoma. J Nucl Med 38:348–352
Lippi F, Ferrari C, Manetti L et al (1996) Treatment of solitary autonomous thyroid nodules by percutaneous ethanol injection: results of an Italian multicenter study. The Multicenter Study Group. J Clin Endocrinol Metab 81:3261–3264
Livraghi T, Paracchi A, Ferrari C, Reschini E, Macchi RM, Bonifacino A (1994) Treatment of autonomous thyroid nodules with percutaneous ethanol injection: 4-year experience. Radiology 190:529–533
Loevner LA (1996) Imaging of the thyroid gland. Semin Ultrasound CT MRI 17:539–562
Lu C, Chang TC, Hsiao YL, Kuo MS (1994) Ultrasonographic findings of papillary thyroid carcinoma and their relation to pathologic changes. J Formos Med Assoc 93:933–938
Lupoli G, Lombardi G, Panza N et al (1991) MIBG scintigraphy and selective venous catheterization after thyroidectomy for MTC. Med Oncol Tumor Pharmacother 13:8101–8107
Malotte MS, Chonkich GD, Zuppan CW (1991) Riedel's thyroiditis. Arch Otolaryngol Head Neck Surg 117:214–217
Massol J, Pazart L, Aho S, Strauch G, Leclere J, Durieux P (1993) Prise en charge de nodule thyroïdien. Résultats préliminaires d'une enquête de pratiques auprès de 685 médecins généralistes et spécialistes. Ann Endocrinol 54:220–225
Messina G, Viceconti N, Trinti B (1956) Ecotomografia e color-Doppler nella diagnosi di carcinoma teroideo. Ann Ital Med Int 11:263–267
Meyer D (1991) Bewertung der Schilddrusenszintigraphie sowie der Schilddrusensonographie aus chirurgischer Sicht. Zentralbl Chir 116:935–942
Miki H, Oshimo K, Inoue H et al (1993) Incidence of ultrasonographically-detected nodules in healthy adults. Tokushima J Exp Med 40:43–46
Morosini P, Mancini V, Filipponi S et al (1996) Cytological diagnosis of thyroid nodules. Comparison of results ob-

tained with guided echography with those from a blind biopsy. Minerva Endocrinol 21:18–25
Muller NW, Schroder S, Schneider C, Seifert G (1985) Sonographic tissue characterization in thyroid gland diagnosis. Klin Wochenschr 63:706–710
Nakada K, Kasai K, Watanabe Y et al (1996) Treatment of radioiodine-negative bone metastasis from papillary thyroid carcinoma with percutaneous ethanol injection therapy. Ann Nucl Med 10:441–444
Nakahara H, Noguchi S, Murakami N et al (1997) Gadolinium-enhanced MR imaging of thyroid and parathyroid masses. Radiology 202:765–772
Ng EH, Tan Sk, Nambiar R (1990) Impact of fine-needle aspiration cytology on the management of solitary thyroid nodules. Aust N Z J Surg 60:463–466
Nicolosi A, Addis E, Calo PG, Tarquini A (1994) Ipertiroidismo e cancro della tiroide. Minerva Chir 49:491–495
Okamoto T, Yamashita T, Harasawa A et al (1994) Test performances of three diagnostic procedures in evaluating thyroid nodules: physical examination, ultrasonography and fine-needle aspiration cytology. Endocr J 41:243–247
Onishi T, Noguchi S, Murakami N et al (1984) Extraocular muscles in Graves' ophtalmopathy: usefulness of T2 relaxation time measurements. Radiology 190:857–862
Otsuka N, Nagai K, Morita K et al (1994) MRI of subacute thyroiditis. Radiat Med 12:273–276
Ozdemir H, Iigit ET, Yucel C et al (1994) Treatment of autonomous thyroid nodules: safety and efficacy of sonographically guided percutaneous injection of ethanol. AJR 163:929–932
Parkes AB, Adams H, Othman S, Hall R, John R, Lazarus JH (1996) The role of complement in the pathogenesis of postpartum thyroiditis: ultrasound echogenicity and the degree of complement-induced thyroid damage. Thyroid 6:177–182
Podoloff DA (1996) Is there a place for routine surveillance using sonography, CT, or MR imaging for early detection (notably lymphoma) of patients affected by Hashimoto's thyroiditis. AJR 167:1337–1338
Price DC (1993) Radioisotopic evaluation of the thyroid and parathyroids. Radiol Clin North Am 31:991–1015
Price R, Horvath K, Moore FD Jr (1993) Surgery for solitary thyroid nodules: assessment of methods to select patients at low risk for unsuspected malignancy in the unaffected lobe and the possible utility of preoperative thyroid ultrasound. Thyroid 3:87–92
Proye C (1993) Prise en charge du nodule thyroïdien isolé. Conclusion. Ann Endocrinol (Paris) 54:297–300
Raab SS, Silverman JF, Elsheikh TM et al (1995) Pediatric thyroid nodules: disease demographics and clinical management as determined by fine-needle aspiration biopsy. Pediatrics 95:46–49
Ralls PW, Mayekawa DS, Lee KP et al (1988) Color-flow Doppler sonography in Graves' disease: «thyroid inferno». AJR 150:781–784
Reading CC, Gorman CA (1993) Thyroid imaging techniques (review). Clin Lab Med 13:711–724
Reinhardt MJ, Moser E (1996) An update on diagnostic methods in the investigation of diseases of the thyroid (Review). Eur J Nucl Med 23:587–594
Renard E, Jaffiol C, Rouanet JP, Lamarque JL (1991) Nodules thyroidiens et goitres non fonctionnels. Apport diagnostique de l'imagerie par résonance magnétique. Presse Méd 20:214–298
Reynolds JC (1997) Percent 131 I uptake and post-therapy 131I scans: their role in the management of thyroid cancer. Thyroid 7:281–284
Reynolds JC, Robbins J (1997) The changing role of radioiodine in the management of differentiated thyroid cancer. Semin Nucl Med 27:152–164
Rifat SF, Ruffin MT IV (1994) Management of thyroid nodules. Am Fam Physician 50:785–790
Romaldini JH, Biancalana MM, Figueiredo DI, Farah CS, Mathias PC (1996) Effect of L-thyroxine administration on antithyroid antibody levels, lipid profile, and thyroid volume in patients with Hashimoto's thyroiditis. Thyroid 6:183–188
Ronga G, Fiorentino A, Paserio E et al (1990) Can iode 131 whole-body scan be replaced by thyroglobulin measurement in the postsurgical follow-up of differentiated thyroid carcinoma? J Nucl Med 31:1766–1771
Rosen IB, Azadian A, Walfish PG, Salem S, Lansdown E, Bedard YC (1993) Ultrasound-guided fine-needle aspiration biopsy in the management of the thyroid disease. Am J Surg 1766:346–349
Ross DS (1991) Evaluation of the thyroid nodule. J Nucl Med 32:2181–2192
Rubello D, Gasparoni P, Roth G et al (1996) Functional meaning of scintigraphic and echographic patterns, and of circulating anti-peroxidase antibodies in asymptomatic chronic thyroiditis. Q J Nucl Med 40:359–364
Sadoul JL (1995) Génèse des nodules thyroïdiens. Mécanismes physiologiques et pathologiques, implications cliniques. Ann Endocrinol 56:5–22
Sashi R, Tomura N, Hashimoto M, Kobayashi M, Watarai J (1997) Growth patterns of benign and malignant thyroid tumors estimated by CT. Radiat Med 15:7–11
Sato K, Okamura K, Hirata T et al (1996) Immunological and chemical types of reversible hypothyroidism; clinical characteristics and long-term prognosis. Clin Endocrinol 45:519–528
Schlumberger M, Archangioli O, Peirarski JD, Tubiana M, Parmentier C (1988) Detection and treatment of lung metastases of differentiated thyroid carcinoma in patients with normal chest X-rays. J Nucl Med 29:1790–1794
Schweiger U, Hosten N, Cordes M et al (1996) Die Duplexsonographie in der Schilddrusenfunktionsdiagnostik. Rofo Fortschr Geb Rontgenstr Neuen Bildgeb Verfahr 164:114–118
Scott AM, Macapinlac H, Zhang J et al (1995) Image registration of SPECT and CT images using an external fiduciary band and three-dimensional surface fitting in metastatic thyroid cancer. J Nucl Med 36:100–103
Seabold JE, Lawson MA, Guril NJ et al (1997) F-18 FDG PET scans in thyroid cancer patients with negative total body diagnostic I-131 scans. Radiology 205(P):399
Set PA, Oleszczuk-Raschke K, Von Lengerke JH, Bramswig J (1996) Sonographic features of Hashimoto thyroiditis in childhood. Clin Radiol 51:167–169
Seya A, Oeda T, Terano T et al (1990) Comparative studies in fine-needle aspiration cytology with ultrasound scanning in the assessment of thyroid nodule. Jpn J Med 29:478–480
Shamma FN, Abrahams JJ (1992) Imaging in endocrine disorders. J Reprod Med 37:39–45
Shimaoka K, Sokal IE, Pickren JW (1962) Metastatic neoplasms in the thyroid gland: pathological and clinical findings. Cancer 15:557–565
Shimomato K, Endo T, Ishigaki T, Sakuma S, Makino N (1993) Thyroid nodules: evaluation with color Doppler ultrasonography. J Ultrasound Med 12:673–678
Singer PA, Cooper DS, Daniels GH et al (1996) Treatment guidelines for patients with thyroid nodules and well-differentiated thyroid cancer. American Thyroid Association. Arch Intern Med 156:2165–2172

Solbiati L, Cioffi V, Ballarati E (1992) Ultrasonography of the neck. Radiol Clin North Am 30:951–954
Solbiati L, Livraghi T, Ballarati E, Ierace T, Crespi L (1995) Thyroid gland. In: Solbiati L, Rizzatto G (eds) Ultrasound of superficial structures. High frequencies, Doppler and interventional procedures. Churchill Livingstone, Edinburgh, pp 49–85
Som P (1992) Detection of metastasis in cervical lymph nodes: CT and MR criteria and differential diagnosis. AJR 158:961–969
Som PM, Brandwein M, Lidov M, Lawson W, Biller HF (1994) The varied presentations of papillary thyroid carcinoma cervical nodal disease: CT and MR findings. AJNR 15:1123–1128
Sostre J, Reyes MM (1991) Sonographic diagnosis and grading of Hashimoto' thyroiditis. J Endocrinol Invest 14:115–121
Stern WD, Laniado M, Vogl W et al (1994) Farbkodierte Duplexsonographie und konstrastverstarkte Magnetresonanztomographie szintigraphisch kalter Schilddrusenknoten. Rofo Fortschr Geb Rontgenstr Neuen Bildgeb Verfahr 160:3–10
Sweeney DC, Johnston GS (1995) Radioiodine therapy for thyroid cancer. Endocrinol Metab Clin North Am 24:803–809
Takashima S, Fukuda H, Kobayashi T (1994) Thyroid nodules: clinical effects of ultrasound-guided fine-needle aspiration biopsy. J Clin Ultrasound 22:535–542
Takashima S, Fukuda H, Nomura N, Kishimoto H, Kim T, Kobayashi T (1995a) Thyroid nodules: re-evaluation with ultrasound. J Clin Ultrasound 23:179–184
Takashima S, Fukuda H, Tomiyama N, Fujita N, Iwatani Y, Nakamura H (1995b) Hashimoto thyroiditis: correlation of MR imaging signal intensity with histopathologic findings and thyroid function test results. Radiology 197:213–219
Takashima S, Nomura N, Noguchi Y, Matsuzuka F, Inoue T (1995c) Primary thyroid lymphomas: evaluation with US, CT, and MRI. J Comput Assist Tomogr 19:282–288
Takashima S, Nomura N, Tanaka H, Itoh Y, Miki K, Harada T (1995d) Congenital hypothyroidism: assessment with ultrasound. AJNR 16:1117–1123
Takashima S, Sone S, Takayama F, Maruyama Y, Hasegawa M, Wang Q (1997) Differentiated thyroid carcinomas: prediction of tumor invasion into surrounding structures with MR imaging. Radiology 205 (P):604
Taki S, Kakuda K, Kakuma K et al (1997) Thyroid nodules: evaluation with US-guided core biopsy with an automated biopsy gun. Radiology 202:874–877
Tan GH, Gharib H (1997) Thyroid incidentalomas: management approaches to nonpalpable nodules discovered incidentally on thyroid imaging. Ann Intern Med 126:226–231
Tan GH, Gharib H, Reading CC (1995) Solitary thyroid nodule. Comparison between palpation and ultrasonograhy. Arch Intern Med 155:2418–2423
Tarantino L, Giorgio A, Perotta A, Aloisio V, Forestieri MC (1997) Percutaneous ethanol injection (PEI) of large autonomous hyperfunctioning thyroid adenoma. Radiology 205 (P):531
Tatsuno S, Miyamoto Y, Ishihara K, Irie T, Kobori K, Tada S (1994) Ultrasonography in primary malignant lymphoma of the thyroid. Nippon Igaku Hoshasen Gakkai Zasshi 54:853–859
Tennvall J, Palmer J, Cederquist E et al (1981) Scintigraphic evaluation and dynamic studies with thallium-201 in thyroid lesions with suspected cancer. Eur J Nucl Med 6:295–300
Tourniaire J, Nicolas MH, Paulin C et al (1997) Nodules thyroïdiens: dosage d'hormone thyréotrope sérique et cytoponction versus scintigraphie comme examens de première intention. Etude prospective de 150 dissections. Presse Med 26:752–755
Tramalloni J, Swagier-Uzan C, Moreau JF (1997) Etude de l'efficacité de la cytoponction échoguidée des nodules thyroïdiens en fonction de leur taille. J Radiol 78:897
Tranquart F, Girard JJ, Baulieu JL, Pourcelot L (1996) Echographie de la pathologie inflammatoire et fonctionnelle de la thyroïde. In: Bruneton JN, Padovani B (eds) Imagerie en endocrinologie. Masson, Paris, pp 60–63
Ugur O, Kostakglu L, Guler N et al (1996) Comparison of 99m Tc (V)-DMSA, 201 TI and 99m Tc-MIBI imaging in the follow-up of patients with medullary carcinoma of the thyroid. Eur J Nucl Med 23:1367–1371
Van den Breckel MWM, Stel HV, Castelijns J et al (1990) Cervical lymph node metastasis: assessment of radiologic criteria. Radiology 177:373–384
Verde G, Papini E, Pacella CM et al (1994) Ultrasound guided percutaneous ethanol injection in the treatment of cystic thyroid nodules. Clin Endocrinol 41:719–724
Viateau-Poncin J (1992) Echographie de la thyroïde, 2nd edn. Vigot, Paris
Vidone RA, Silverberg SG (1966) Carcinoma of the thyroid in surgical and post-mortem material. Ann Surg 164:291–299
Vitti P, Lampis M, Piga M et al (1994) Diagnostic usefulness of thyroid ultrasonography in atrophic thyroiditis. J Clin Ultrasound 22:375–379
Vitti P, Rago T, Mazzeo S et al (1995) Thyroid blood flow evaluation by color-flow Doppler sonography distinguishes Graves' disease from Hashimoto's thyroiditis. J Endocrinol Invest 18:857–861
Wanet PM, Sand A, Abramovici J (1996) Physical and clinical evaluation of high-resolution thyroid pinhole tomography. J Nucl Med 37:2017–2020
Wang Q, Takashima S, Sone S, Takayama F, Maruyama Y, Hasegawa M (1997) MR imaging of medullary thyroid carcinoma: correlation with pathologic findings. Radiology 205 (P):604
Wernecke K, Diederich P (1994) Sonographic features of mediastinal tumors. AJR 163:1357–1364
Witterick IJ, Abel SM, Noyek AM et al (1993) Non palpable occult and metastatic papillary thyroid carcinoma. Laryngoscope 103:149–155
Yeh HC, Futterweit W, Gilbert P (1996) Micronodulation: ultrasonographic sign of Hashimoto thyroiditis. J Ultrasound Med 12:813–819
Yokoyama N, Nagayama Y, Kakezono F et al (1988) Determination of the volume of the thyroid gland by a high resolution ultrasonic scanner. J Nucl Med 27:1475–1479
Yokozawa T, Fukata S, Kuma R et al (1996) Thyroid cancer detected by ultrasound-guided fine-needle aspiration biopsy. World J Surg 20:848–853
Yoshimura R, Kodama S, Nakamura H (1995) Classification of congenital hyperthyroidism based on scintigraphy, ultrasonography and the serum thyroglobulin level. Kobe J Med Sci 41:71–82
Zaidi H (1996) Comparative methods for quantifying thyroid volume using planar imaging and SPECT. J Nucl Med 37:1421–1426
Zingrillo M, D'Aloiso L, Ghiggi MR et al (1996a) Thyroid hypoechogenicity after methimazole withdrawal in Graves' disease: a useful index for predicting recurrence? Clin Endocrinol 45:201–206
Zingrillo M, Torlontano M, Ghiggi MR et al (1996b) Percutaneous ethanol injection of large thyroid cystic nodules. Thyroid 6:403–408
Zohar Y, Strauss M (1994) Occult distant metastases of well differentiated thyroid carcinoma. Head Neck 16:438–442

13 Parathyroid Glands

F. Bussière, J. Darcourt, J. Drouillard, V. Gense, M. Gray, and R. Lecesne

Contents

13.1 Non-isotopic Imaging

R. Lecesne, V. Gense, and J. Drouillard

Evaluation of parathyroid morphology is performed essentially for patients in whom the clinical and biochemical presentation of hyperparathyroidism is dominated by hypercalcemia. These clinical and biological anomalies are usually due to a parathyroid adenoma or, less often, to hyperplasia. As a result of their capability to localize abnormal parathyroid glands in the neck and/or mediastinum, imaging studies permit accurate preoperative mapping (Loevner 1996).

A review of the embryology and anatomy of the parathyroid glands is followed by a brief description of their function and the various noninvasive techniques available for examination, i.e., ultrasound, computed tomography (CT), magnetic resonance imaging (MRI), and invasive and interventional procedures. A discussion of the chronology of imaging techniques as a function of the clinical image concludes this chapter.

13.1.1 Embryology

The parathyroid glands arise from the third and fourth branchial pouches. The superior parathyroids arise from the fourth branchial pouch along with the lateral thyroids. Attached to the thyroid, their positions are relatively constant, with only 2% lying in an ectopic position. The inferior parathyroids arise from the third branchial pouch and form a bilobar complex with the thymic lobe. During embryonic descent, the inferior parathyroid glands may migrate into the anterior mediastinum as far down as the pericardium.

13.1.2 Anatomy

Most individuals (84%) have four parathyroid glands (range, two to 12). The average normal parathyroid gland weighs 20–40 g and averages 3–6 mm in length, 2–4 mm in width, and 1–3 mm in thickness. The glands are often located symmetrically relative to the midline (Akerström et al. 1984).

The superior parathyroids are usually located on the posterior aspect of the midportion of the thyroid

F. Bussière, J. Darcourt, Service de Médecine Nucléaire, Centre Antoine-Lacassagne, 33 avenue de Valombrose, 06189 Nice, France
J. Drouillard, V. Gense, R. Lecesne, Service de Radiodiagnostic, Hôpital Du Haut Lévèque, avenue de Magellan, 33604 Pessac, France
M. Gray, Institut Arnault Tzanck, avenue du Docteur Monot, 06700 Saint Laurent du Var, France

lobe (75%). They may lie more or less posterior to the thyroid or in a latero- or retroesophageal, intertracheoesophageal, or retropharyngeal position. Less often, they are found in an ectopic position in the posterior mediastinum at the level of the tracheoesophageal groove.

The inferior parathyroids generally lie at the posteroinferior poles of the thyroid lobes (50%). In 15% of cases, they are located within 1 cm of the lower aspect of the thyroid lobes. In 35% of cases, they lie in a high cervicomediastinal position in the anterior mediastinum, connected to the remnants of the thymus. The lower parathyroids can basically be found anywhere between the angle of the jaw and the pericardium. The parathyroid glands may be related to the various anatomic structures of the infrahyoid sector of the neck, namely the recurrent laryngeal nerves and the jugulocarotid bundle containing the vagus nerve (WANG 1976; DOPPMAN et al. 1994).

The parathyroids occasionally lie inside the thyroid capsule (3.5%), in which case they are difficult to distinguish from thyroid nodules (THOMPSON 1988; PROYE et al. 1994).

The arterial supply of the superior and inferior parathyroid glands is ensured by branches of the inferior thyroid artery (BISMUTH et al. 1975). Ectopic glands in the mediastinum are fed by the inferior thyroid artery or a mediastinal artery such as the internal mammary artery or the thymic artery.

Venous return from the parathyroids is usually ensured by thyroid veins that drain into the brachiocephalic venous trunks or the internal jugular vein, but there are numerous anatomic variations. Ectopic parathyroid glands may drain into the inferior thyroid veins or the azygos vein.

Innervation of the parathyroid glands is via the cervical ganglia of the autonomic nervous system.

13.1.3
Clinical and Biological Features

The parathyroid glands secrete parathyroid hormone (PTH), which regulates the calcium ion concentration in extracellular fluids (BARDIN 1994). When the calcium concentration drops, the rate of PTH secretion increases. This has three consequences: (1) increased mobilization of bone calcium, (2) reduction in urinary excretion, and (3) acceleration of intestinal absorption of calcium.

When the calcium concentration is high, PTH secretion is normally suppressed. Hypercalcemia with a normal or elevated PTH level corresponds to hyperparathyroidism. The clinical manifestations of hyperparathyroidism include bone pain, recurrent nephrolithiasis, and, less often, psychoneurologic disorders. Hyperparathyroidism may be primary or secondary.

13.1.2.1
Primary Hyperparathyroidism

Parathyroid adenomas are the most frequent cause of primary hyperparathyroidism (80%–85% of patients). These lesions are usually solitary and can range in size from 1 to several centimeters. Parathyroid hyperplasia involving all four glands is less common (10%–20% of patients). Asymmetrical enlargement of two or three parathyroid glands may create confusion with multiple parathyroid adenomas (2%–3% of patients). One third of all patients with primary hyperplasia have familial hyperparathyroidism or multiple endocrine neoplasia (MEN) (LIVOLSI and HAMILTON 1994). Parathyroid carcinoma (1% of patients) usually presents as an adherent cervical mass associated with vascular invasion (LOEVNER 1996).

13.1.2.2
Secondary Hyperparathyroidism

In patients with chronic renal failure, hyperplasia of the parathyroid glands causes secondary hyperparathyroidism. Chronic oversecretion of PTH secondary to hypocalcemia causes various degrees of hypertrophy of all four glands. The presence of supernumerary glands, often in unusual locations, is more common in this population and is thought to be related to overstimulation of embryonal rests disseminated throughout the cervical and mediastinal fat (LOSSEF et al. 1993). In these patients, phosphate retention in the kidneys and decreased calcium absorption from the intestine results in hypocalcemia. Excessive PTH secretion causes the radiologically and histologically demonstrable lesions of osteitis fibrosa cystica. Secondary hyperparathyroidism is one of the most frequent complications of chronic renal failure (BEN HAMIDA et al. 1994).

Tertiary hyperparathyroidism corresponds to autonomous growth of a hypertrophic parathyroid gland (LOSSEF et al. 1993).

13.1.2.3 Therapy

Treatment of primary hyperparathyroidism consists in surgical ablation. If an adenoma is discovered during neck exploration, the surgeon resects the lesion; if hyperplasia is found, total or subtotal parathyroidectomy is indicated. If neck exploration is unproductive, the procedure must be supplemented by mediastinotomy to search for an ectopic parathyroid gland in the thorax (Sarfati et al. 1994). Therapeutic interventional radiology has proven successful for patients with parathyroid adenomas who are poor candidates for surgery. Interventional procedures include ultrasound-guided percutaneous ethanol injection and angiographic ablation of ectopic adenomas (Solbiati et al. 1985; Miller et al. 1987a). Response to treatment is confirmed by normalization of serum calcium and PTH concentrations. Persistent or recurrent hyperparathyroidism after surgery suggests the existence of an unidentified or ectopic gland that must be localized by imaging.

13.2 Noninvasive Imaging

No available imaging modality can identify the normal parathyroid glands. The non-negligible frequency of ectopic glands and the possibility of multigland disease (hyperplasia) explain the low sensitivity and lack of specificity of the various techniques used alone.

13.2.1 Parathyroid Sonography

Noninvasive, economical, and rapid ultrasound is the imaging modality of choice for initial examination. Despite its insufficiencies for the detection of ectopic parathyroid glands, ultrasound can accurately assess the cervical region if performed by an experienced sonographer.

Parathyroid ultrasound must be performed with a high-resolution (7.5- to 10-MHz) linear-array transducer. Examination includes thorough analysis of the entire cervical region, from the hyoid bone down to the sternal notch. Cervical rotation and scanning during swallowing facilitate detection of laterotracheal and lateroesophageal glands. Use of 5-MHz transducers may allow detection of infrathyroid and cervicomediastinal glands (Gooding 1994).

Although it does not provide any information for histologic characterization, ultrasound demonstrates diffuse gland enlargement. In over 80% of patients, a hypoechoic solid mass is seen anterior to the long muscle of the neck. The oval-shaped parathyroids are usually located posterior to the thyroid lobes, from which they are separated by a hyperechoic interface (Figs. 13.1, 13.2). The glands may project just below the inferior pole of the thyroid lobes, in which case they tend to be nodular. Except for malignant etiologies with locoregional extension, the parathyroid glands are mobile during deglutition (Stark et al. 1983; Hopkins and Reading 1995).

In less than 20% of patients, the parathyroid gland is isoechoic relative to the thyroid parenchyma, exhibits cystic changes, or appears inhomogeneous due to necrotic or hemorrhagic degeneration. Calcifications are common in secondary hyperparathyroidism, and the parathyroid may be bilobar or multilobar (Fuggazola et al. 1995).

Color Doppler (CD) allows analysis of parathyroid vascularity. Although it does not improve the sensitivity of ultrasound for the detection of adenomas, CD can help differentiate an adenoma from an enlarged node by demonstrating a vascular arc

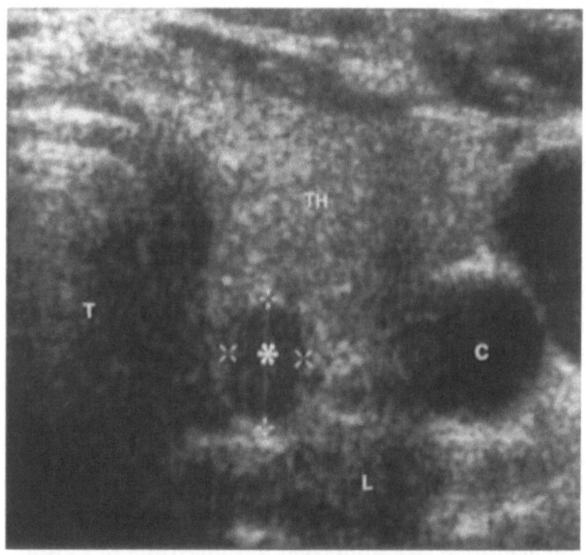

Fig. 13.1. Parathyroid adenoma. Typical sonographic pattern. Transaxial scan through the left thyroid lobe (*TH*). The left superior parathyroid adenoma (*asterisk*) is homogeneous and hypoechoic relative to the thyroid. It lies medial to the common carotid artery (*C*), anterior to the long muscle of the neck (*L*), and abuts the trachea (*T*)

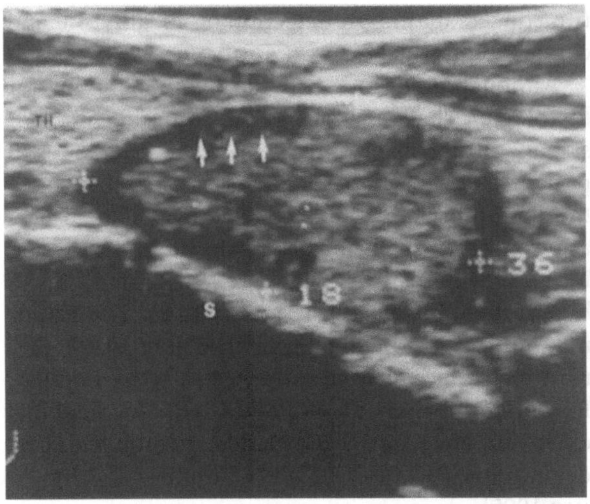

Fig. 13.2. Left inferior parathyroid adenoma. Atypical sonographic pattern. Paramedian sagittal scan through the left thyroid lobe (*TH*). This large (36+18 mm) left inferior parathyroid adenoma abutting the cervical spine (*S*) is hypoechoic relative to the left thyroid lobe and inhomogeneous. Note the hyperechoic center and the hypoechoic periphery (*arrows*).

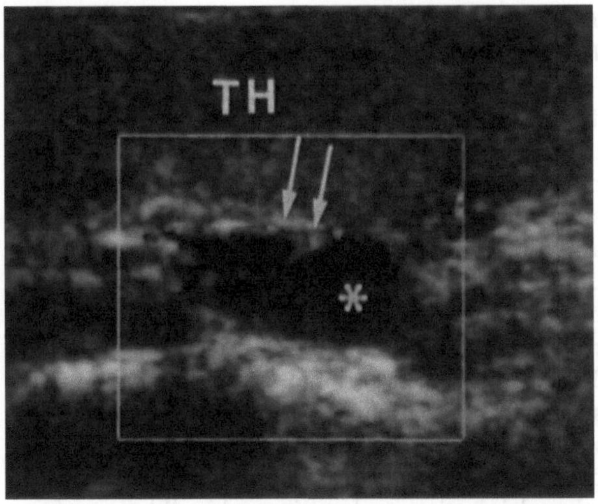

Fig. 13.3. Parathyroid adenoma. Color Doppler (CD). Parasagittal scan through the right thyroid lobe. The parathyroid adenoma (*asterisk*) is separated from the thyroid (*TH*) by a hyperechoic interface. Note the characteristic perinodular arc-like CD signal (*arrows*)

arising from the inferior thyroid artery that partially surrounds the gland (Fig. 13.3). The low-resistance flow in the inferior thyroid artery has both systolic and diastolic components (Wolf et al. 1994).

Ultrasound has a specificity of approximately 90% for the detection of abnormal parathyroid glands. Sensitivity ranges from 38% to 92% (Freitas and Freitas 1994; Bruneton et al. 1996). When performed by an experienced examiner using a high-resolution transducer, ultrasound has a sensitivity of 70%–80% for preoperative localization in patients with primary hyperparathyroidism (Hopkins and Reading 1995; Giron et al. 1996; Okada et al. 1997).

Despite a sensitivity of up to 90% for adenomas, sonography is less effective for detection of hyperplasia (50%–70%). This is probably due to the small size of hyperplastic glands and the difficulties in identifying multigland involvement (Doppmann and Miller 1991).

The main limitations of ultrasound are topographic. Laterocarotid parathyroids involve problems for differential diagnosis from enlarged lymph nodes. Furthermore, ultrasound cannot depict retrotracheal or retroesophageal parathyroids or ectopic glands in the mediastinum.

The lower sensitivity of ultrasound for re-exploration of persistent or recurrent hyperparathyroidism is attributable to artifacts caused by locoregional modifications following surgery and the higher frequency of ectopic glands. The estimated sensitivity of ultrasound in this clinical setting ranges from 47% (Stark et al. 1983) to 63% (Hopkins and Reading 1995). Endoesophageal ultrasound (Henry et al. 1990) reportedly allows detection of ectopic glands (Fig. 13.4), but the efficacy of this more invasive procedure remains to be evaluated.

A coexistent thyroid pathology may be responsible for false-positive or false-negative results. For example, the associated thyroid goiter found in 28%–46% of patients can interfere with examination of the cervical region. Similarly, the presence of a posterior intrathyroid nodule creates problems for differential diagnosis from a parathyroid mass. On rare occasions, the possibility of an intrathyroid ectopic gland must be entertained. All thyroid anomalies must be indicated in the examination report, because the surgeon may decide to perform a lobectomy if neck exploration remains negative (Bainbridge and Barnes 1982).

13.2.2 Computed Tomography

Like MRI, CT is reserved for second-line use, but the quality of CT scans appears more consistent, especially for patients with a short neck. In contrast to

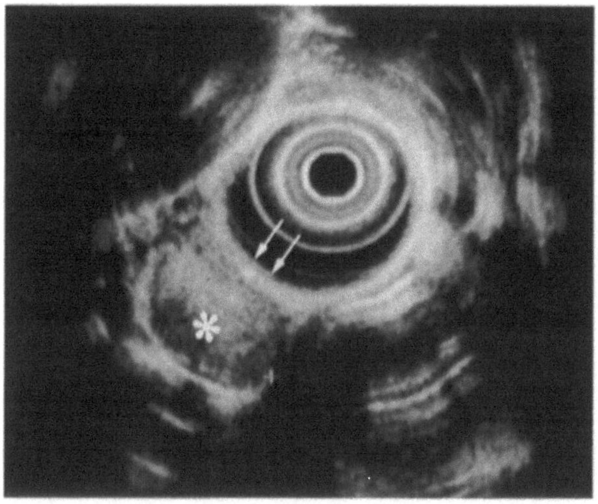

Fig. 13.4. Lateroesophageal left inferior parathyroid adenoma. Endosonography. The transducer placed in the esophagus readily demonstrates this large (2 cm) adenoma (*asterisk*) in contact with the esophageal wall (*arrows*)

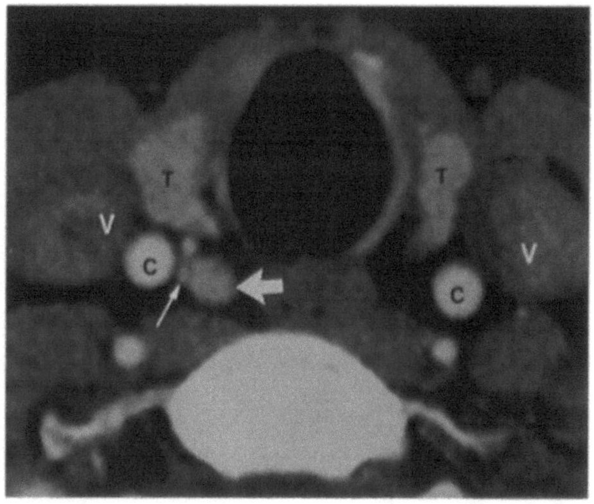

Fig. 13.5. Parathyroid adenoma. Contrast-enhanced helical CT in the arterial phase. The internal jugular veins are not yet enhanced (*V*), whereas the common carotid arteries (*C*) are enhanced. Enhancement of the parathyroid adenoma (*large arrow*) is identical to that of the right upper parathyroids and the thyroid gland (*T*). The inferior thyroid artery appears distinctly on the arterial phase (*small arrow*)

ultrasonography, CT can localize ectopic parathyroid glands in the mediastinum (Drouillard et al. 1983).

Whether performed with dynamic scanning or helical acquisition, CT scans must be obtained from the base of the skull down to the thorax. Overlapping or contiguous thin sections (3–5 mm) are required. The following CT protocol can be recommended to search for adenoma or parathyroid hyperplasia:

1. Unenhanced cervical CT scans. In thin patients, this permits visualization of adenomas susceptible to becoming isodense to the thyroid after contrast administration, because 25% of all adenomas enhance (Stark et al. 1983).
2. Cervical and mediastinal scans after administration of an iodinated contrast agent (240 mg/ml). With helical CT, both cervical and mediastinal scans are required. A total of 60 ml contrast material is injected at a rate of 3 ml/s for each acquisition. The ideal interval appears to be 15–20 s. Data acquisition must be obtained with the breath-hold technique, and the patient must be instructed not to swallow during cervical acquisition.

Scanning in the arterial phase (8–10 s after contrast administration) does not improve the detection of adenomas, but facilitates identification of their arterial pedicle.

Scanning is optimal when there is maximum jugulocarotid vascular enhancement. On unenhanced CT scans, adenomas appear round or oval, homogeneous, and isodense to the adjacent muscles (Drouillard et al. 1983).

After contrast injection, adenomas enhance in a variable manner (Figs. 13.5, 13.6). They are usually hypodense to the vessels and the thyroid (Cates et al. 1988), but may also be isodense to the thyroid (Higgins and Auffermann 1988). In the latter case, differentiation from the thyroid is difficult if there is no rim of fat between the two structures. Cervical nodes, vascular tortuosity, and the esophagus are the most frequent causes of false-positive results for adenoma. Analysis of supra- and subjacent scans usually corrects the diagnosis in the latter two cases, but differentiation from enlarged lymph nodes is more difficult (Drouillard et al. 1990).

It is impossible to differentiate an intrathyroid adenoma from a thyroid nodule; they have identical CT appearances, and hyperparathyoidism is often associated with thyroid disease (20% of patients; Bainbridge and Barnes 1982). Intrathyroid adenomas may be calcified and contain cystic, hemorrhagic, or necrotic components (Cates et al. 1988). In primary hyperparathyroidism, approximately 75% of all adenomas and cases of cervical hyperplasia are diagnosed by CT (Okada et al. 1997). Ultrasound is equally effective for cervical examination, but CT appears superior for detection of adenomatous disease of the superior parathyroid glands

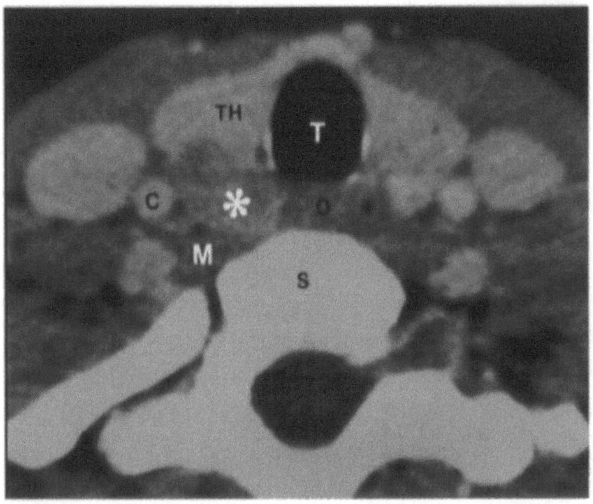

Fig. 13.6. Parathyroid adenoma. Dynamic CT acquisition in the arteriovenous phase after contrast administration. The right superior parathyroid adenoma (*asterisk*) is hypodense relative to the right thyroid lobe (*TH*), with which it is closely related. This adenoma is also related to the trachea (*T*), the esophagus (*O*), the cervical spine (*S*), the long muscle of the neck (*M*), and the right common carotid artery (*C*)

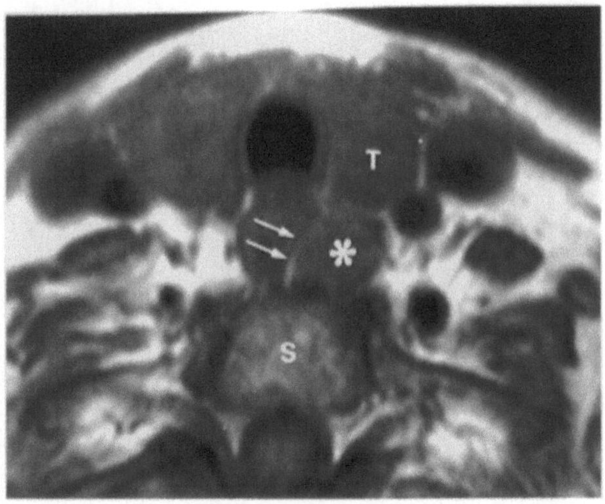

Fig. 13.7. Transaxial T_1-weighted MR sequence. This parathyroid adenoma (*asterisk*) displaces the esophageal wall (*arrows*) medially. It is also connected to the cervical spine posteriorly (*S*) and the left thyroid lobe anteriorly (*T*)

and ectopic parathyroid adenomas, which predominate in the mediastinum (Miller et al. 1987c).

CT can be used to guide diagnostic and therapeutic percutaneous interventional procedures (Doppmann et al. 1983; O'Doherty et al. 1992; Moinuddin and Whynott 1996). For example, CT can be used to verify angiographic ablation of mediastinal adenomas (Miller et al. 1987a) due to selective opacification using high-osmolarity contrast agents. Persistent opacification of an adenoma on a CT scan obtained 24 h after surgery is predictive of a successful procedure in 90% of patients.

13.2.3 Magnetic Resonance Imaging

Like CT, MRI is reserved for second-line imaging of parathyroid abnormalities after ultrasound. The protocol includes cervical examination with a surface transducer and mediastinal examination with a phased-array coil. Contiguous, thin (4–5 mm) slices are required in both transaxial and coronal planes, with an imaging volume extending from the hyoid bone to the lung apex.

T_1-weighted spin echo (SE) sequences and short tau inversion recovery (STIR) sequences are the most useful. These sequences actually complement each other. T_1-weighted sequences offer excellent spatial resolution, particularly for the mediastinum, as they benefit from the natural contrast between the hyperintense fat and the hypointense circulating vascular structures, while STIR sequences increase the contrast between the abnormal parathyroid gland and its surroundings, although spatial resolution is lower.

T_2-weighted sequences and gadolinium-enhanced T_1-weighted images are less effective, because the contrast between the parathyroid gland and adjacent structures is not optimal.

In the absence of adequate STIR sequences, T_2-weighted sequences with fat saturation are advisable (Goddard 1994; Bruneton et al. 1996).

Regardless of the sequence used, MRI can only reveal gland enlargement; it cannot differentiate between adenomas, hyperplasia, and parathyroid carcinoma. Vascular invasion is suggestive of parathyroid carcinoma.

The variable MRI features of parathyroid adenoma and hyperplasia are not correlated with histology (Higgins 1993). The most common pattern (occurring in approximately 70% of patients) is a mass of intermediate signal intensity that is isointense to muscle and the thyroid on T_1-weighted images (Figs. 13.7, 13.8) and isointense or hyperintense to fat on T_2-weighted sequences (Fig. 13.8).

On STIR sequences, an abnormal parathyroid gland is easily detectable as an extremely hyperintense structure within the suppressed fat (Fig. 13.8). This contrast phenomenon is also ob-

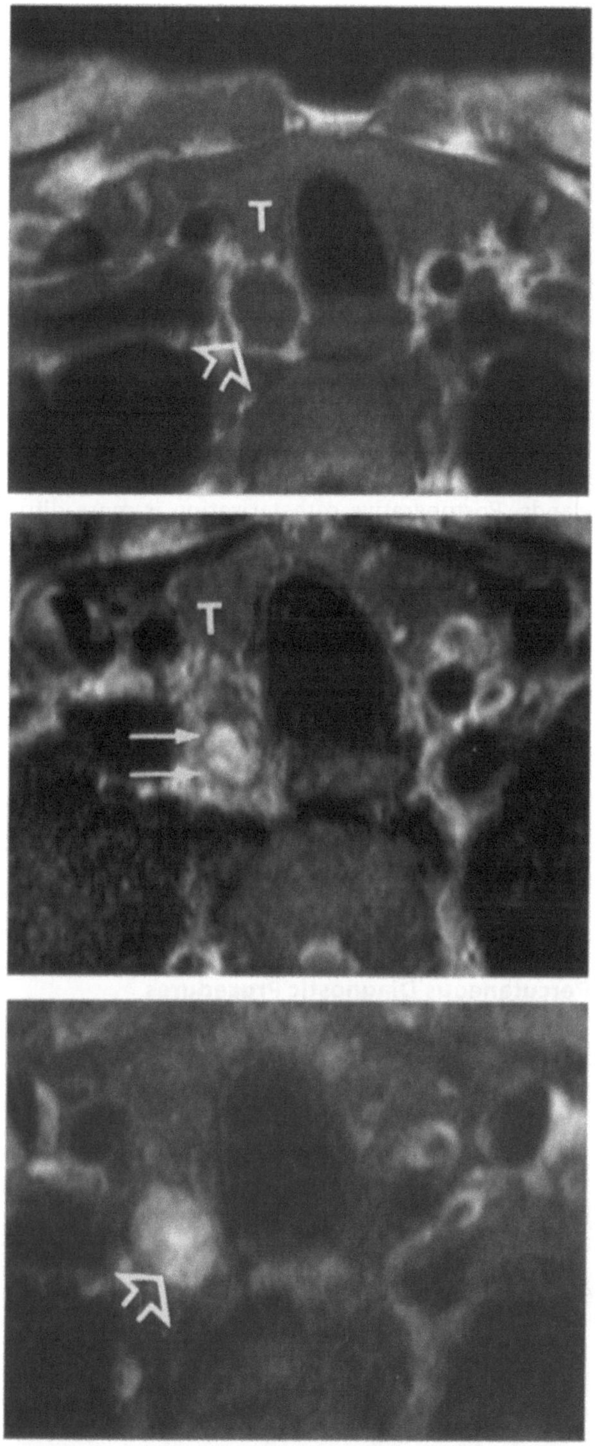

a
b
c

Fig. 13.8a–c. Paratracheal right inferior parathyroid adenoma. a T_1-weighted MR image. This homogenenous, solid 2-cm adenoma (*arrow*) is isointense to the thyroid gland (*T*). b Transaxial T_2-weighted MR image. The parathyroid adenoma is hyperintense to the thyroid (*T*), but isointense to the retrothyroid and paratracheal fat. The capsule of the adenoma (*arrows*) allows differentiation from cervical fat. c Short tau inversion recovery (STIR) sequence. Fat saturation creates excellent contrast between the hyperintense adenoma (*arrow*) and the hypointense peripheral fat

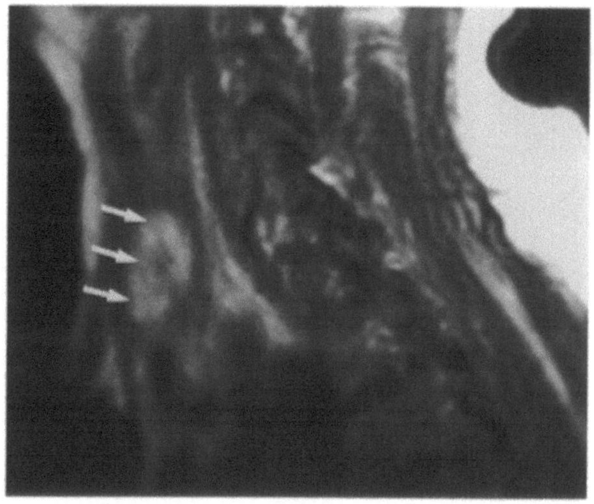

Fig. 13.9. Left inferior parathyroid adenoma. Gadolinium-enhanced T_1-weighted MR image. This left paramedian sagittal scan reveals inhomogeneous enhancement of the parathyroid adenoma (*arrows*)

tained with T_2-weighted sequences with fat saturation, although contrast is not as good because fat saturation is not homogeneous.

Several diagnostic pitfalls must be avoided. For example, the esophagus or vessels containing slow flow may also appear hyperintense on these sequences (LEGMANN et al. 1995). Intravenous gadolinium injection usually enhances the signal of the mass (Fig. 13.9) but does not improve detection, especially because of the frequency of numerous artifacts (NAKAHARA et al. 1997). Aproximately 30% of lesions appear hyperintense or isointense on T_1-weighted sequences and isointense on T_2-weighted sequences. This is particularly true for lesions with high cellularity and those that have undergone hemorrhagic degeneration (BRUNETON et al. 1996). A combination of transaxial and coronal images improves definition of the anatomic relations of these lesions (Fig. 13.10).

MRI is a sensitive technique that has similar efficacy for preoperative workup of primary and recurrent hyperparathyroidism. In the literature, the sensitivity of MRI varies from 65% to 80% preoperatively and is estimated at 75% postoperatively (HIGGINS 1993; BRUNETON et al. 1996; MCDERMOTT et al. 1996). Sensitivity is higher (84%–88%) with STIR sequences and T_2-weighted sequences with fat saturation (MCDERMOTT et al. 1996).

False-positive results may be related to nodular thyroid disease or lymphadenopathy (HIGGINS and

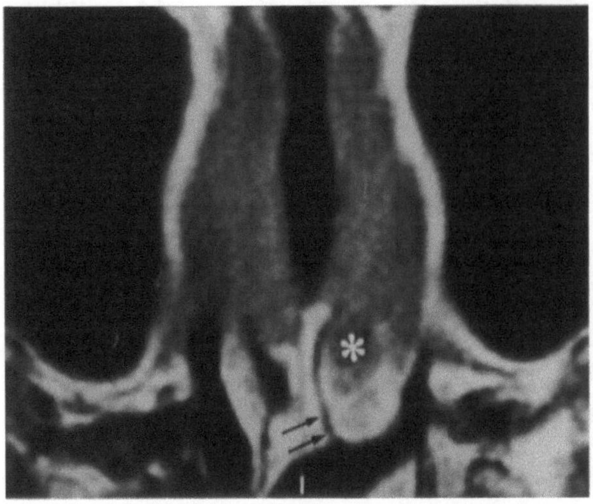

Fig. 13.10. Left inferior parathyroid adenoma. Coronal T_1-weighted MR scan. The parathyroid adenoma (*asterisk*) is in contact with an inferior thyroid vein (*arrows*) that drains directly into the left brachiocephalic trunk (*I*)

Auffermann 1988; Bruneton et al. 1996; Loevner 1996). MRI has equivalent value for depiction of cervical and mediastinal lesions (Stevens et al. 1993). False-negative results are attributable to the small size of certain lesions, the existence of multiple lesions, and an atypical signal (isointense on T_2-weighted sequences). Because they tend to be larger, adenomas are easier to detect than hyperplasia. However, volume may not be the sole factor because atypical signals are more frequent in hyperplasia than in adenoma (McDermott et al. 1996).

13.3 Invasive Imaging

13.3.1 Arteriography

Arteriography requires selective catheterization of the feeding arteries of the parathyroid glands; the superior and inferior thyroid arteries (Fig. 13.11) are the predominant vessels at the cervical level. Search for an ectopic thoracic adenoma requires selective catheterization of the internal thoracic arteries. The normal parathyroid glands are not visible, whereas an adenoma or hyperplasia creates an arteriographic blush. The sensitivity of arteriography is 60% (Brennan et al. 1982).

13.3.2 Venous Sampling

Percutaneous puncture of the femoral vein allows selective catheterization of the thyroid veins (superior, middle, and inferior) and the thymic, vertebral, and internal thoracic veins. The technique may be performed alone or as a complement to arteriography. Venous sampling allows demonstration of a PTH gradient in blood samples taken in one or more of the veins draining an adenoma or hyperplasia compared to the other veins catheterized. The gradient is considered significant if the PTH peak is twice the baseline value. A chart is prepared indicating the localization of the abnormal parathyroid gland or glands. Postoperative catheterization is more difficult owing to the presence of ligations and anastomoses. Venous sampling has a reported sensitivity of approximately 80% (Miller et al. 1987b).

13.4 Interventional Procedures

Interventional procedures are reserved for persistent or recurrent hyperparathyroidism after surgery and certain forms of secondary hyperparathyroidism.

13.4.1 Percutaneous Diagnostic Procedures

Fine-needle aspiration (FNA) or percutaneous biopsy under ultrasound or CT guidance with immunoradiometric assay of PTH can confirm the parathyroid nature of a cervical mass. These well-tolerated procedures, which can be performed on an outpatient basis, have a sensitivity of 96% and a specificity of 100% (Doppman et al. 1983; Karstrup et al. 1993; Sacks et al. 1994). Systematic use of these procedures has been proposed during workup of suspicious cervical masses prior to repeat surgery (Gooding 1993).

13.4.2 Percutaneous Treatment Procedures

A therapeutic alternative for poor surgical candidates and for secondary hyperparathyroidism in patients with chronic renal failure is percutaneous ethanol ablation (PEA), which is performed under ultrasound guidance. A small (22G or 25G) needle is

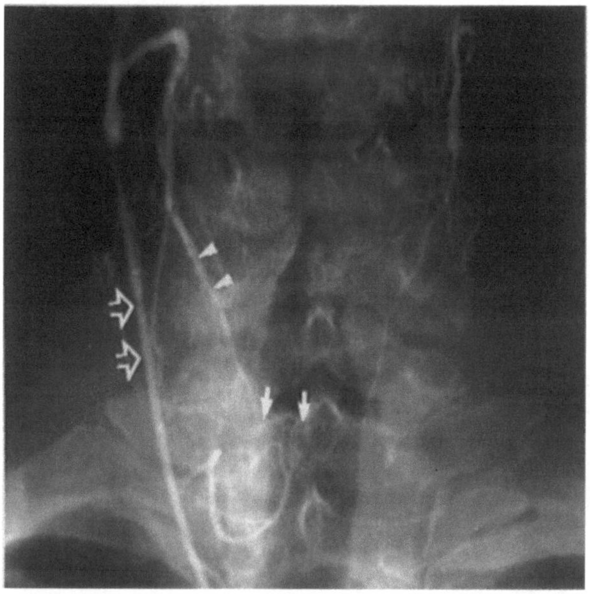

Fig. 13.11. Right inferior parathyroid adenoma. Cervical arteriography. Selective catheterization of the right thyrocervical trunk (*open arrows*) opacified the inferior thyroid arteries (*arrowheads*). The vascular plexus (*small arrows*) is related to a right inferior parathyroid adenoma

used to inject 96% ethanol into multiple areas of the mass. The amount of alcohol injected is equal to approximately one half the volume of the mass, but no more than 1 ml is injected during any one session. Treatment efficacy is judged by normalization of serum calcium and PTH concentrations.

The main potential complication of PEA is vocal cord paralysis, which is usually transient. A fibrotic reaction has been reported in the perilesional soft tissues of patients who have subsequently undergone repeat surgery. This iatrogenic fibrosis apparently does not complicate the surgical procedure. Normalization of biochemical parameters has been reported in more than 50% of patients (Solbiati et al. 1985; Verges et al. 1993).

13.4.3 Angiographic Embolization

Following superselective catheterization of the artery supplying the adenoma, embolization is achieved with a hyperosmolar contrast agent. CT verification 24 h after the procedure demonstrates persistence of the contrast material in the adenoma. Miller et al. (1987a) reported a success rate of 71% at 5 years using this technique to treat mediastinal adenomas.

13.5 Diagnostic Strategy and Role of Imaging

Diagnosis of hyperparathyroidism is based on clinical and biochemical findings. Regardless of the modality used, imaging is effective solely for lesion localization. A positive imaging study does not necessarily mandate surgery, and a negative imaging study does not exclude the possibility of hyperparathyroidism.

Parathyroid embryology explains the multiplicity of ectopic sites anywhere from the angle of the jaw down to the pericardium as well as the possibility of supernumerary glands. The parathyroid glands are small, and several may be diseased, which explains surgical difficulties. It also explains the lack of sensitivity and specificity of the imaging techniques, which have to examine the entire cervical and mediastinal region with high spatial resolution. No consensus has yet been reached concerning diagnostic procedures. However, certain strategies can be suggested as a function of the clinical picture and examiner preference.

13.5.1 Primary Hyperparathyroidism

13.5.1.1 Initial Preoperative Workup

The role of imaging for preoperative workup of primary hyperparathyroidism has been extensively debated in recent years. This is due primarily to the excellent results of parathyroid surgery (reported efficacy, 95%), especially when bilateral neck exploration is performed by an experienced surgeon (Sarfati et al. 1994). Most surgical failures are due to ectopic glands and multigland disease (Bruining and Ong 1987; Higgins and Auffermann 1988).

Despite general agreement that systematic preoperative imaging does not eliminate the need for bilateral exploration of the cervical node-bearing regions, the 5%–10% of nonproductive explorations may lead the surgeon to perform thyroid lobectomy (if imaging has demonstrated a thyroid nodule) (Proye et al. 1994) or complementary mediastinotomy.

Preoperative imaging studies are especially beneficial for patients with “malignant” hypercalcemia who respond poorly to medical treatment and for whom unsuccessful surgical failure would be especially prejudicial (Moinuddin and Whynott 1996).

Patients who are poor candidates for surgery may benefit from PEA or angiographic embolization. Elderly or fragile patients may benefit from an interventional procedure on an abnormal gland under local anesthesia (CHAPUIS et al. 1994). In these latter two settings, accurate lesion localization is essential, and care must be taken to confirm its unilateral nature (SARFATI et al. 1994). Cervical ultrasound is the initial imaging modality of choice in such cases; this inexpensive modality has a specificity of approximately 90% and a mean sensitivity of 70% for detection of pathological cervical parathyroids.

While some authors feel that workup may be stopped at this point in the absence of clinical and anamnestic data suggesting hyperplasia (familial antecedents, MEN), others combine ultrasound with Tc 99m- methoxyisobutylisonitrile (MIBI) scintigraphy (SADOUL 1996). However, owing to the poor spatial resolution of this approach, workup should be completed by CT or MRI if mediastinal uptake suggests a parathyroid lesion.

13.5.1.2 Persistent or Recurrent Hyperparathyroidism After Surgery

If hypercalcemia persists or recurs after surgery for hyperparathyroidism, the adenoma responsible for the biochemical and clinical anomalies must be localized. The adenoma may have been overlooked during the first operation (30%–75% of patients) or may occupy an ectopic position (anterior mediastinum, within the thyroid, or in the deep cervical region) (MILLER 1991; RODRIGUEZ et al. 1994). Imaging is recommended in these clinical settings (Fig. 13.12), where it improves the success rate of reoperation by approximately 20%–30% (GRANT et al. 1986; PRICE 1993). Noninvasive techniques such as scintigraphy and MRI usually succeed in localizing the adenoma (O'DOHERTY et al. 1992). If these noninvasive methods are negative or equivocal, angiographic techniques can be performed. A combination of arteriography and venous sampling is recommended to optimize mapping of lesions.

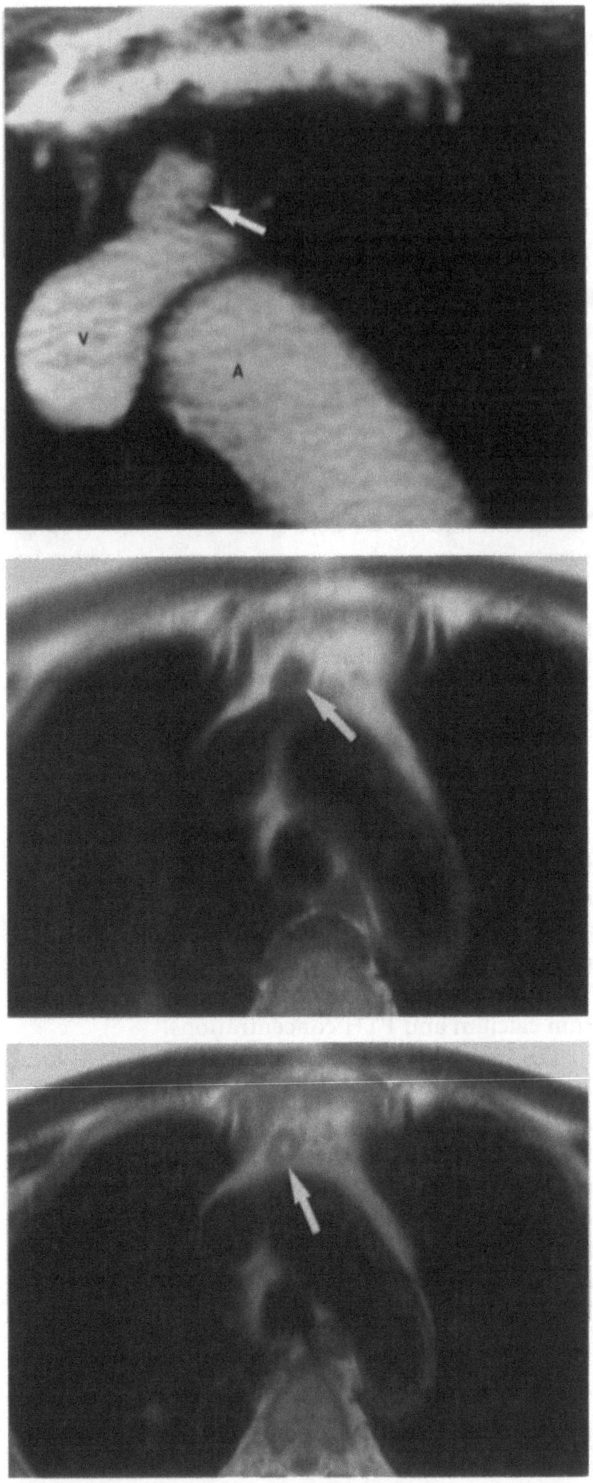

a b c

Fig. 13.12a–c. Persistent hyperparathyroidism with ectopic parathyroid adenoma in the thymic bed. **a** Contrast-enhanced axial CT scan through the aortic arch. This hypervascular adenoma (*arrow*) appears isodense to the superior vena cava (*V*) and the thoracic aorta (*A*) on the arteriovenous phase. **b** T_1-weighted MR image. On this scan passing through the same level, the adenoma (*arrow*) has a homogeneous intermediate signal intensity. **c** T_2-weighted MR image. The adenoma (*arrow*) appears inhomogeneous, with a hyperintense center

13.5.2 Secondary (or Tertiary) Hyperparathyroidism

Secondary (or tertiary) hyperparathyroidism is the most frequent disorder of calcium and phosphorus metabolism in chronic renal failure (Fig. 13.13). Even if only one or two parathyroid glands appear enlarged, all four glands are hyperplastic histologically, as in primary hyperparathyroidism (LIVOLSI and HAMILTON 1994). Parathyroid enlargement is manifest is patients refractory to medical treatment and is detectable by imaging (BEN HAMIDA et al. 1994).

Ultrasound is of no interest for the detection of gland anomalies because the clinical presentation and elevation of PTH are sufficiently suggestive of the diagnosis (BAQUE et al. 1994).

Clinicians may request imaging studies if subtotal or total parathyroidectomy is envisaged for patients who fail to respond to medical treatment.

Preoperative radiologic workup must include cervical and mediastinal exploration. An association of ultrasound, Tc 99m-sestamibi scintigraphy, and MRI appears useful because the combined sensitivity of these three noninvasive techniques is estimated at 92% (NUMEROW et al. 1995). MRI appears preferable to CT because it does not require injection of an iodinated contrast agent in these patients with chronic renal failure.

For patients with recurrent secondary hyperparathyroidism, imaging is used to detect a recurrence on the gland fragment left in place following subtotal parathyroidectomy (it can usually be localized by a metal clip). A supernumerary gland should be searched for. Hyperplasia of a graft implanted in the forearm after total parathyroidectomy is also possible. This complication is suggested sonographically if a hypoechoic nodule larger than 3 mm is depicted at the site of the autograft (WINKELBAUER et al. 1993).

A similar diagnostic strategy associating ultrasound, MIBI scintigraphy, and MRI can be proposed for patients with secondary hyperparathyroidism. Complementary diagnostic ultrasound-guided FNA is required for indeterminate cervical masses. If imaging is inconclusive or if the workup remains negative, invasive techniques are required, in particular venous sampling.

For patients with refractory or recurrent hyperparathyroidism, PEA of accessible lesions depicted by ultrasound has been proposed as an alternative to surgery. This technique reportedly reduces PTH and alkaline phosphatase levels, improves the manifestations of osteodystrophic lesions, and reduces gland size by 20%–50% 6 months after the intervention (SOLBIATI et al. 1985; KITAOKA et al. 1994).

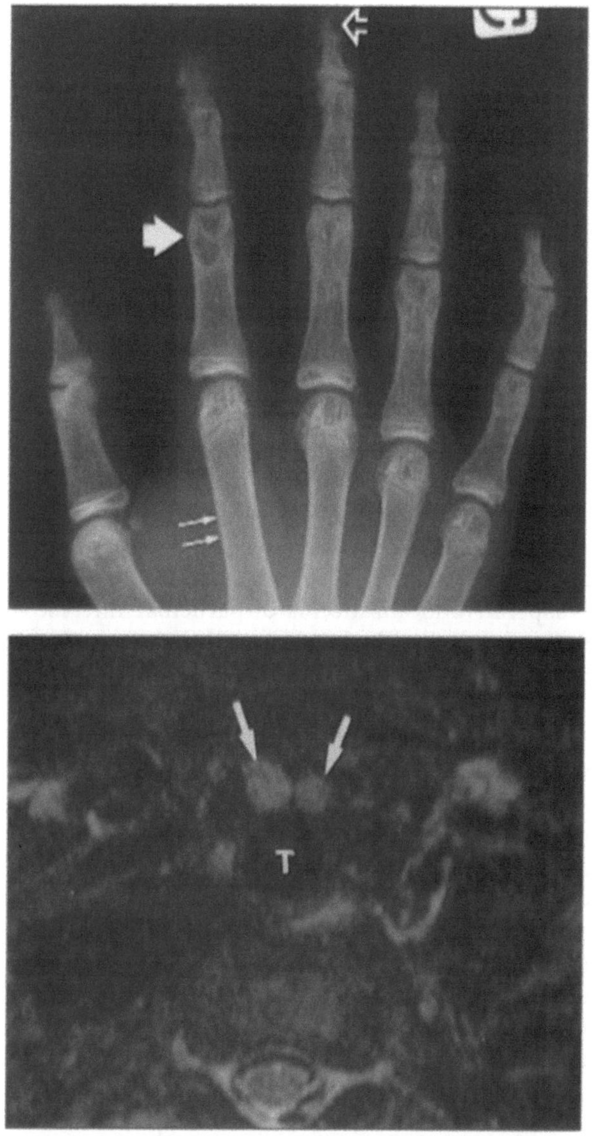

a

b

Fig. 13.13 a,b. Secondary hyperparathyroidism in an 18-year-old patient with chronic renal failure. **a** Plain film: anteroposterior view of the right hand. Delayed growth; diffuse bone demineralization with thinning of the cortical bone associated with a reticular aspect of the bone trabeculae (*small arrows*); typical subperiosteal resorption manifesting as erosion of the cortical bone of the phalangeal tufts, namely on the third finger (*open arrow*); geode-like appearance of the epiphysis of the first phalange of the index finger bulging against the cortical bone, related to a brown tumor lacuna (*solid arrow*). **b** Transaxial short tau inversion recovery (STIR) sequence. Hyperintensity and hypertrophy of both inferior parathyroid glands (*arrows*) located anterior to the trachea (*T*)

13.6 Scintigraphy

J. Darcourt, M. Gray, and F. Bussière

Radionuclide studies of the parathyroid glands are indicated solely for preoperative localization of hyperfunctioning parathyroid tissue responsible for hyperparathyroidism. The need for imaging tests for localization actually remains controversial, because 90%–95% of parathyroid abnormalities are found by experienced surgeons during total thyroid bed exploration. Certain authors have thus concluded that imaging for localization is unnecessary (Consensus Development Conference Panel 1991). Other investigators advocate imaging studies because of the frequency of ectopic parathyroid glands and/or savings in operative time and decreased morbidity (Davis et al. 1990; Wei and Burke 1995). Preoperative localization is of particular interest if repeat surgery is scheduled because such procedures have a higher risk of failure (Miller 1991).

In any case, whenever diagnostic localization appears necessary, the most effective method must obviously be selected. Unbiased comparison of available techniques is difficult. However, no currently available imaging modality has any definite advantage over radionuclide studies, which are generally performed during initial workup, often in combination with ultrasonography of the neck (Hopkins and Reading 1995). Imaging techniques are constantly being improved, however, and exploration strategies are subject to rapid change. Radionuclide techniques themselves have undergone notable improvements since the initial technetium–thallium subtraction scanning technique described by Ferlin et al. (1983) as a result of the development of new tracers and data analysis methods.

Radionuclide studies can be subdivided into dual-isotope methods, in which the uptake of two different radionuclides is compared by subtraction, and dual-phase approaches, which involve early and delayed imaging using a single imaging agent. The following review of standard radionuclide techniques and results is completed by a brief description of novel approaches.

13.6.1 Subtraction Techniques

13.6.1.1 Principle

No specific radiotracer exists for the parathyroid glands. "Mixed" tracers are taken up by both the thyroid and parathyroid cells (T+P), whereas "selective" imaging agents are taken up only by thyroid cells (T). Scintiscanning is first performed with both agents (T+P and T). Subtraction of the resultant images ([T+P]–T) provides an image of the parathyroid tissue. Owing to their small size (20–40 mg), normal parathyroid glands cannot be detected by this procedure. Any tracer uptake on the subtraction image thus corresponds to abnormal parathyroid tissue. Subtraction is best performed by computer-based systems or visual comparison of the T+P and T images.

13.6.1.2 Tracers

The two standard thyroid-specific imaging agents are iodine-123 and technetium - 99m pertechnetate. Both radionuclides are concentrated in the thyroid cells by the iodine pump. Mixed tracers taken up by both thyroid and parathyroid cells were originally developed for myocardial imaging; thallium-201 and 99m Tc-labeled MIBI. Cellular uptake of these two tracers is nonspecific; it depends on the sodium/

Table 13.1. Radiotracer doses

Tracer	Dose		Interval between injection and scan	Effective dose equivalents[a]
	(MBq)	(mCi)		(mSv)
Thallium-201	37–111	1–3	5 min	9.2–27.7
Tc 99m MIBI	200–740	5–20	5 min (+3 h)[b]	2–7.4
Tc 99m pertechnetate	37–300	1–8	20 min	0.5–1.4
Iodine-123	11–20	0.3–0.5	4 h	1.6–3

[a]After Perkins (1996). [or]

potassium pump for thallium-201 and on transmembrane potentials (namely at the mitochondrial level) for 99m Tc-MIBI. Standard doses are listed in Table 13.1.

13.6.1.3
Protocols

Two scintiscans are obtained in the anterior projection. The gamma camera is equipped with a parallel or, even better, a pinhole collimator (KIPPER et al. 1997). To avoid the need to readjust the cervical images, scans must be obtained successively, taking care to avoid patient motion between the two films. Studies of the neck are systematically completed by mediastinal views to search for ectopic parathyroid tissue. The cervical images are then subtracted pixel by pixel. Subtraction is performed after verification of data alignment (and readjustment where necessary) and scaling of the two examinations. Particular care is required during these steps to avoid artifacts (LIEHN et al. 1988).

The various scanning protocols developed all involve different compromises between practical difficulties (prolonged patient immobilization) and image "purity". The examination time is shorter if the pertechnetate is injected first or if the two energy peaks are acquired simultaneously, but this is to the detriment of a pure thallium image. During conventional scanning using single photon emission tracers, the diffused radiation is eliminated by spectrometry. If several radionuclides are used, however, diffusion of the highest-energy tracer (99m Tc) "contaminates" the image of the lower-energy agent (thallium-201). This explains why the early technetium–thallium scanning procedure, later improved by subtraction of diffusion, has been supplanted by a technetium–thallium protocol that allows visualization of parathyroid tumors on the thallium-201 scan without interference by the 99m Tc, which is injected afterwards. The major drawback of this new protocol is the need for prolonged patient immobilization (at least 45 min) (Fig. 13.14).

99m Tc-MIBI scintigraphy involves similar problems because the energy of thyroid tracers is greater than or equal to that of pure thyroid traceis. If iodine-123 is selected for thyroid imaging, the 4-h interval required between injection and stable thyroid uptake generally leads to injection of this tracer first. If 99m Tc is preferred, 99m Tc-MIBI can be injected first, but mastery of image readjustment is necessary to take advantage of the kinetics of MIBI (SCHVARTZ et al. 1996).

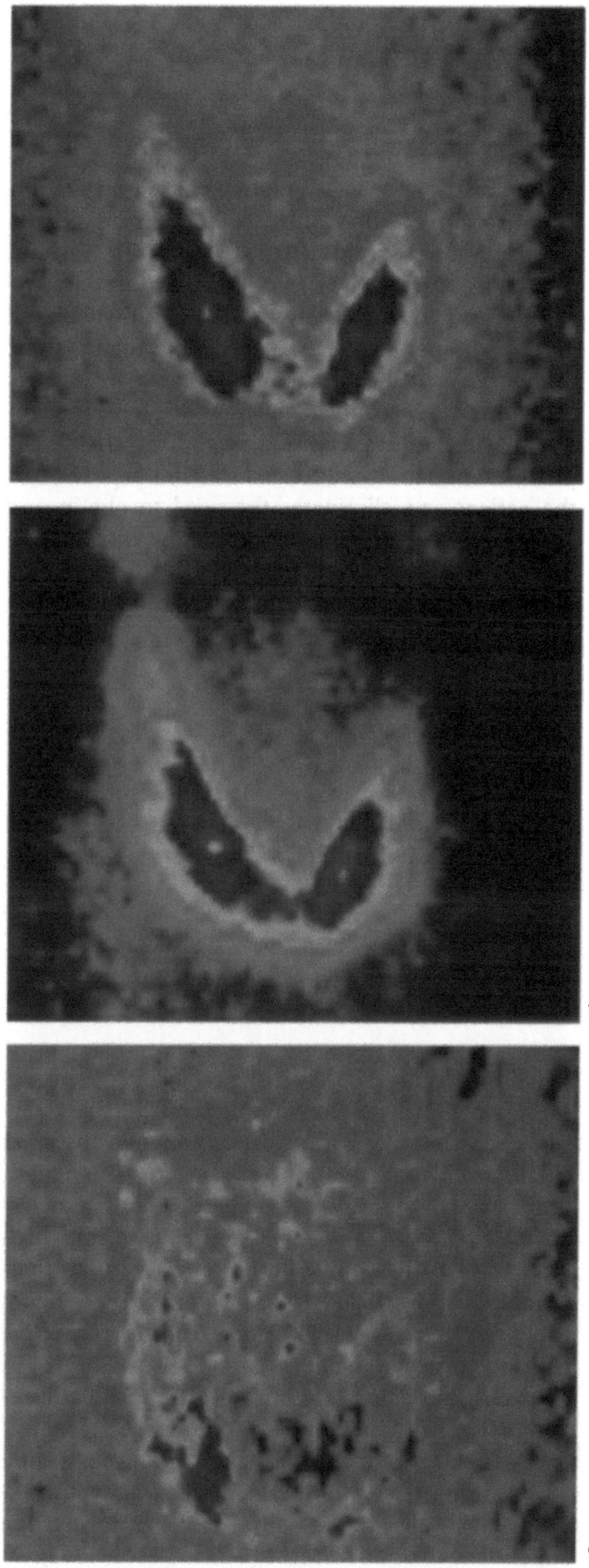

a

b

c

Fig. 13.14 a–c. Thallium-201/99m Tc subtraction examination. Subtraction reveals a focus of thallium-201 uptake in the right lower pole. Surgery confirmed the existence of a parathyroid adenoma at this point. **a** Thallium-201 image. **b** 99m Tc image. **c** Subtraction image

13.6.2 Dual-Phase Techniques

First proposed in 1992 by TAILLEFER et al. (1992), following the initial description by O'DOHERTY et al. (1992), dual-phase scintigraphy is based on the differential rates of 99m Tc-MIBI washout from the parathyroid and thyroid tissues. As tracer washout occurs faster from thyroid cells than from parathyroid tumors, contrast between the parathyroid and thyroid tissue increases significantly with time. Comparison of delayed scans taken 2 to 3 h after injection with early images obviates the need for subtraction techniques. Use of a single tracer for dual-phase examination reduces irradiation exposure for the patient and eliminates the need to obtain and then subtract a pure thyroid image. The examination is considered positive if a focus of MIBI uptake on early scans persists or enhances on delayed scans.

13.6.3 Technique Selection

Following selection of the mixed tracer (thallium-201 or 99m Tc-MIBI), the protocol must be selected (subtraction or dual-phase imaging with 99m Tc-MIBI).

13.6.3.1 Tracer Selection

Thallium-201 is gradually being replaced by 99m Tc-MIBI, which has more favorable physical characteristics allowing use of considerably higher doses yet entailing lower irradiation exposure for the patient (Table 13.1). These two advantages are particularly valuable for localization of ectopic lesions, for which 99m Tc-MIBI has proven more effective than thallium-201 (MOINUDDIN and WHYNOTT 1996). O'DOHERTY et al. (1992) analyzed the respective clinical efficacy of thallium-201 and 99m Tc-MIBI in a series of 55 patients. 99m Tc-MIBI and thallium-201 had sensitivities of 97.5% and 92.5%, respectively, for localization of 40 adenomas and 53.3% and 48.3%, respectively, for localization of 60 hyperplastic glands. Subsequent studies have confirmed the superiority of 99m Tc-MIBI (GEATTI et al. 1994).

13.6.3.2 Protocol Selection

The dual-phase protocol proposed in 1992 by TAILLEFER et al. (1992) has gained widespread acceptance owing to its relative simplicity and efficacy (LEE et al. 1995; KEZACHIAN et al. 1997). Several recent publications, however, have emphasized the potential insufficiency of the technique, and their authors advocate complementary subtraction methods (HUGLO et al. 1996; SCHVARTZ et al. 1996; CHEN et al. 1997). Proponents of complementary examinations point out that 99m Tc-MIBI washout from parathyroid cells is not only variable but sometimes also very rapid (CALENDINI-VIALLET et al. 1997). In such cases, the very principle of dual-phase imaging is negated, and a thyroid image is required to identify the lesion on the early scan.

13.6.4 Results

Regardless of the radiotracer or tracers and protocol used, three situations can be distinguished.

1. Scintigraphic detection of ectopic adenomas is fairly simple because it does not depend on subtraction techniques. The sensitivity and specificity of scintiscanning for adenomas are thus quite high, ranging from 90% to 100% for 99m Tc-MIBI (Table 13.2).
2. Hyperplastic parathyroid glands, in contrast, are difficult to localize on radionuclide scans. The infrequency of such lesions complicates evaluation of diagnostic efficacy, but the sensitivity of scintigraphy is generally considered to be of the order of only 60%, even with 99m Tc-MIBI. The specificity is high, though, and comparable to that for adenomas.
3. Retrothyroid adenomas, the most common cause of hyperparathyroidism, are consistently detected with a high specificity, regardless of the method or the series. Literature reviews concerning both thallium-201 and 99m Tc-MIBI techniques all report a specificity of around 95% (HAUTY et al. 1987; GORIS et al. 1991; SCHVARTZ et al. 1996). False-positive results are infrequent and are essentially due to tracer uptake by thyroid nodules. In contrast, the sensitivity of radionuclide scans for retrothyroid adenomas varies considerably. GORIS et al. (1991) reported sensitivities of 26%–94% for thallium-201 scanning, while HAUTY et al.

Table 13.2. Meta-analysis: sensitivity of Tc 99m methoxyisobutylisonitrile (MIBI) in hyperparathyroidism

Reference	Adenoma			Hyperplasia			Ectopic adenoma		
	TP	FN	Lesions (*n*)	TP	FN	Lesions (*n*)	TP	FN	Lesions (*n*)
O'Doherty et al. 1992	39	1	40	53	7	60	–	–	–
Taillefer et al. 1992	19	2	21	–	–	–	–	–	–
Geatti et al. 1994	40	2	42	–	–	–	–	–	–
Lee et al. 1995	28	2	30	18	12	30	–	–	–
Huglo et al. 1996	38	9	47	12	28	40	8	1	9
Moinuddin and Whynott 1996	–	–	–	–	–	–	4	0	4
Chen et al. 1997	41	3	44	19	19	38	6	1	7
Hindie et al. 1997	53	3	56	12	3	15	3	0	3
Ishibashi et al. 1997	–	–	–	–	–	–	3	0	3
Kezachian et al. 1997	21	3	24	2	3	5	1	0	1
Total	279	25	304	116	72	188	25	2	27
Sensitivity		91.8%			61.7%			92.6%	

TP, true positives; FN, false negatives.

(1987) cited a mean sensitivity of 82%. The sensitivities in studies using 99m Tc-MIBI vary to a lesser degree (from 81% to 97%). The meta-analysis of 318 adenomas reported in the literature allowed calculation of an overall sensitivity of 91.8% (Table 13.2). This variability in sensitivity is attributable more to the variation in tracer uptake by parathyroid lesions than to differences between the protocols themselves (Fig. 13.15).

For a given tracer concentration, uptake depends on the lesion's weight. Experimental studies indicate a lower limit of detectability of 400 mg (Brownless and Gimiette 1989). In practice, the smallest scintigraphically detected lesions reported in the literature weighed considerably less. Huglo et al. (1996) set the lower threshold at 225 mg with 99m Tc MIBI.

Even taking account of lesion size, the variable efficacy of radionuclide studies highlights the importance of the radiotracer concentration, which is linked to intracellular tracer accumulation. The parathyroid glands are normally composed of chief cells and oxyphil cells (the latter representing only 4%–

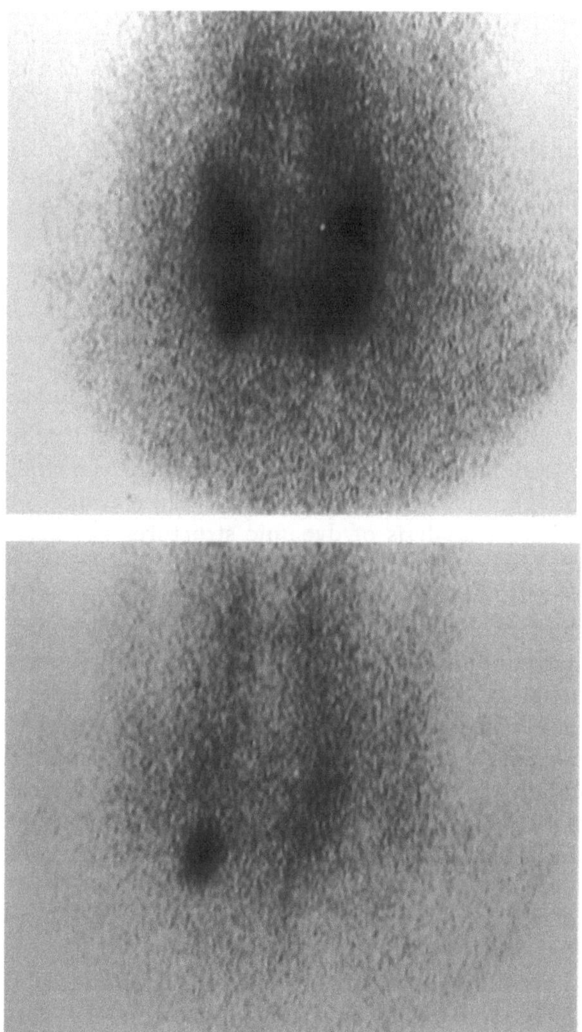

a

b

Fig. 13.15. Tc 99m-methoxyisobutylisonitrile (MIBI) examination. Note the focus of high MIBI uptake in the right lower pole that increased 2 h after injection. Surgery confirmed the presence of a right inferior parathyroid adenoma. **a** Thyroid image obtained 10 min after injection. **b** Thyroid image obtained 2 h after injection

5%). Adenomas and hyperplasia generally affect PTH-secreting chief cells. Oxyphil cells are rarely involved, except in oncocytic adenomas, where they are present exclusively. As oxyphil cells contain large numbers of mitochondria, it has been postulated that they may have a higher potential for uptake and accumulation of thallium-201 (Sandrock et al. 1993) and especially 99m Tc-MIBI, which has a predilection for mitochondria (Benard et al. 1995). Huglo et al. (1996), however, failed to confirm this hypothetical mechanism in their study of the relations between MIBI accumulation and the oxyphil cell concentration. The intracellular calcium ion concentration might also explain reduced 99m Tc-MIBI uptake (Calendini-Viallet et al. 1997). Parathyroid carcinomas take up 99m Tc-MIBI in a similar manner to adenomas, which prevents differential diagnosis. Finally, although radionuclide studies can be used for disease staging, tracer uptake by brown tumors and bone metastases has also been reported (Lu et al. 1995).

In conclusion, regardless of the technique used, 99m Tc-MIBI scintigraphy is highly effective for localization of retrothyroid and ectopic adenomas. By contrast, its sensitivity is relatively low for the detection of hyperplasia.

13.6.5 Recent Developments

A number of complementary methods are under investigation in an attempt to improve the sensitivity of radionuclide scanning for parathyroid tumor detection. These approaches are still experimental, though, and no consensus has yet been reached.

Factor analysis of dynamic structures has been advocated as a means to potentiate dual-phase 99m Tc-MIBI. This image analysis method reportedly shortens the surgical time and is more sensitive than conventional scintigraphy without any loss in specificity (Billotey et al. 1994). 99m Tc-tetrofosmin, a more recent technetium-labeled radionuclide developed for cardiac imaging, has also been tested for parathyroid imaging. This radiopharmaceutical gives equivalent results on early images, but without the differential washout phenomenon available with 99m Tc-MIBI (Fjeld et al. 1997). 99m Tc-tetrofosmin can thus only be used for single-phase studies.

Single photon emission computed tomography (SPECT) following injection of 99m Tc-MIBI has been described by several authors. SPECT-MIBI appears useful particularly in the early phase (Chen et al. 1997), offering improved anatomic localization of lesions and accuracy, especially for recurrent lesions and ectopic parathyroid glands (Billotey et al. 1996). When associated with intraoperative measurement of circulating PTH, SPECT-MIBI shortens surgery time. A recent study reported that simultaneous iodine-123/99m Tc sestamibi SPECT subtraction was superior to dual-phase 99m Tc-sestamibi SPECT with 99m Tc-MIBI alone for preoperative localization of hyperfunctioning parathyroid tissue in primary hyperparathyroidism (Neumann et al. 1997).

Trials have also been conducted with positron-emitting isotopes fluorodeoxyglucose-19 (^{19}FDG) (Neumann et al. 1994) and L-^{11}C-methionine (Sundin et al. 1996). Although initial results are encouraging, the diagnostic gain does not appear to justify the complicated nature of the examination procedure.

Finally, certain authors have proposed use of scintigraphic methods for assessment of parathyroid tissue transplanted into the forearm (Kilgore et al. 1996).

13.7 Conclusion

Numerous imaging techniques have been used for localization of hyperfunctioning parathyroid tissue responsible for hyperparathyroidism. Unbiased systematic comparison of available methods is difficult, but no imaging modality seems to have any definite advantage over radionuclide studies (O'Doherty et al. 1997).

Regardless of the radionuclide technique adopted, systematic exploration of the mediastinum is required for detection of ectopic adenomas. Scintigraphy appears more effective than CT or MRI for this purpose (Ishibashi et al. 1997). For cervical exploration, 99m Tc-MIBI has in most cases superseded thallium-201, because its differential washout characteristics increase the contrast of parathyroid lesions on delayed images. Nevertheless, a pure thyroid image is still recommended to assist in analysis of early scans, either by subtraction techniques or visual comparison.

Radionuclide studies are effective for diagnostic localization of adenomas (sensitivity and specificity, >90%), but are insufficient for hyperplasia. For patients with secondary hyperparathyroidism, scintigraphy serves solely to rule out the existence of an ectopic gland. Specificity is the most consistent quality of scintigraphy. Sensitivity should therefore be favored during interpretation (GORIS et al. 1991; SCHVARTZ et al. 1996). Recurrence following surgery requires particular efforts to localize the lesion. SPECT is especially indicated in such cases (O'DOHERTY et al. 1997), as are complementary imaging techniques such as CT and MRI. Aside from such situations, scintigraphy associated with cervical ultrasound is generally sufficient whenever preoperative localization seems justified by the expected reduction in morbidity and shorter operating time.

References

Akerström G, Malmaeus J, Bergstrom R (1984) Surgical anatomy of human parathyroid glands. Surgery 95:14–21

Bainbridge ET, Barnes AD (1982) Primary hyperparathyroidism due to overactive intrathyroid parathyroid glands: a potential of failed exploration. Br J Surg 69:200–202

Baque MC, Bruneton JN, Padovani B et al (1994) Parathyroid echography in dialysed patients with chronic renal failure. J Radiol 75:559–560

Bardin T (1994) Hyperparathyroïdie primitive: aspects cliniques épidémiologiques et histologiques. Ann Endocrinol 55:143–146

Ben Hamida F, Ghazali A, Boudzernidj M et al (1994) Hyperparathyroïdie secondaire à l'insuffisance rénale. Physiopathologie, aspects clinicoradiologiques et traitement. Ann Endocrinol 55:147–158

Bénard F, Lefebvre B, Beuvon F, Langlois MF, Bisson G (1995) Rapid washout of technetium-99m-MIBI from a large parathyroid adenoma. J Nucl Med 36:241–243

Billotey C, Aurengo A, Najean Y et al (1994) Identifying abnormal parathyroid glands in the thyroid uptake area using technetium-99m-sestamibi and factor analysis of dynamic structures. J Nucl Med 35:1631–1636

Billotey C, Sarfati E, Aurengo A et al (1996) Advantages of SPECT in technetium-99m-sestamibi parathyroid scintigraphy. J Nucl Med 37:1773–1778

Bismuth V, Fendler JP, Grellet J et al (1975) Le diagnostic artériographique des adénomes parathyroïdiens. A propos de 45 cas. J Radiol Electrol Med Nucl 56:235–244

Brennan MF, Doppman JL, Kurdy AG, Marx SJ, Spiegel AM, Auerbach GD (1982) Assessment of techniques for preoperative parathyroid gland localization in patients undergoing reoperation for hyperparathyroidism. Surgery 91:6–11

Brownless SM, Gimiette TDM (1989) Comparison of techniques for thallium-201-technetium-99m parathyroid imaging. Br J Radiol 62:532–535

Bruining HA, Ong GL (1987) Cause des échecs en chirurgie parathyroïdienne. Expérience de 862 interventions en 30 ans. Chirurgie 113:549–555

Bruneton JN, Laurent F, Chevallier P, Drouillard J (1996) Imagerie non isotopique des parathyroïdes. In: Bruneton JN, Padovani B (eds) Imagerie en endocrinologie. Masson, Paris, pp 84–94

Calendini-Viallet C, Bussy E, Lescout JM, Rinaldi JP (1997) Adénomes parathyroïdiens à «cinétique rapide»: à propos de deux observations. Med Nucl 21:439–443

Cates JD, Thorsen MK, Lawson TL et al (1988) CT evaluation of parathyroid adenomas: diagnostic criteria and pitfalls. J Comput Assist Tomogr 12:626–629

Chapuis Y, Richard B, Fulla Y et al (1994) Chirurgie de l'hyperparathyroïdie primaire par abord unilatéral sous anesthésie locale et dosage per-opératoire de la PTH 1-84. Ann Endocrinol 55:171–174

Chen CC, Holder LE, Scovill WA, Tchan AM, Gann DS (1997) Comparison of parathyroid imaging with technetium-99m-pertechnetate/sestamibi and technetium-99m-sestamibi SPECT. J Nucl Med 38:834–839

Consensus Development Conference Panel (1991) Diagnosis and management of asymptomatic primary hyperparathyroidism: consensus development conference statement. Ann Intern Med 114:593–597

Davis RK, Hoffmann J, Dart D et al (1990) Unilateral parathyroidectomy. Otolaryngol Head Neck Surg 102:635–638

Doherty GM, Doppman JL, Miller DL et al (1992) Results of a multidisciplinary strategy for management of mediastinal parathyroid adenomas as a cause of persistent primary hyperparathyroidism. Ann Surg 215:101–106

Doppman JL, Miller DL (1991) Localization of parathyroid tumors in patients with asymptomatic hyperparathyroidism and no previous surgery. J Bone Miner Res 6 [Suppl 2]:S153–S159

Doppman JL, Krudy AG, Marx SJ et al (1983) Aspiration of enlarged parathyroid glands for parathyroid hormone assay. Radiology 148:31–35

Doppman JL, Shawker TH, Fraker DL et al (1994) Parathyroid adenoma within the vagus nerve. AJR 163:943–945

Drouillard J, Philippe JC, Eresue J et al (1983) Place de la scanographie dans le diagnostic des adénomes parathyroïdiens. A propos de 27 cas. J Radiol 64:381–390

Drouillard J, Laurent F, Bruneton JN, De Verbizier G (1990) Les parathyroïdes. In: Vasile N (ed) Tomodensitométrie corps entier. Vigot, Paris, pp 25–34

Ferlin G, Borsato N, Camerani M, Conte N, Zotti D (1983) New perspectives in localizing enlarged parathyroids by technetium-thallium subtraction scan. J Nucl Med 24:438–441

Fjeld JG, Erichson K, Pfeffer PF et al (1997) Technetium-99m-tetrofosmin for parathyroid imaging: comparison with sestamibi. J Nucl Med 38:834–839

Freitas JE, Freitas AE (1994) Thyroid and parathyroid imaging. Semin Nucl Med 24:234–245

Fuggazola C, Bergamo-Andreis I, Solbiati L (1995) Parathyroid glands. In: Solbiati L, Rizzato G (eds) Ultrasound of superficial structures: high frequencies, Doppler and interventional procedures. Churchill Livingstone, Edinburgh, pp 87–113

Geatti O, Shapiro B, Orsolon PG et al (1994) Localization of parathyroid enlargement: experience with technetium-99m methoxyisobutylisonitrile and thallium-201 scintigraphy, ultrasonography and computed tomography. Eur J Nucl Med 21:17–22

Giron J, Ouhayoun E, Dahan M et al (1996) Imaging of hyperparathyroidism US, CT, MRI and MiBi scintigraphy. Eur J Radiol 21:167–173

Goddard PR (1994) Localization of abnormal parathyroid glands: value of fat suppression. Radiology 190:903

Gooding GA (1994) Sonography of the thyroid and parathyroid. Radiol Clin North Am 31:967–989

Goris ML, Basso LV, Keeling C (1991) Parathyroid imaging. J Nucl Med 32:887–889

Grant CS, Van Heerden JA, Charboneau JW et al (1986) Clinical management of persistent and/or recurrent primary hyperparathyroidism. World J Surg 10:555–565

Hauty M, Swartz K, Mac Lung M et al (1987) Technetium-thallium scintiscanning for localization of parathyroid adenomas and hyperplasia, a reappraisal. Am J Surg 153:479–486

Henry JF, Audiffret J, Denizot A et al (1990) Endosonography in the localization of parathyroid tumors: a preliminary study. Surgery 108:1021–1025

Higgins CB (1993) Role of magnetic resonance imaging in hyperparathyroidism. Radiol Clin North Am 31:1017–1028

Higgins CB, Auffermann W (1988) MR imaging of thyroid and parathyroid glands: a review of current status. AJR 151:1095–1106

Hindié E, Mellière D, Perlemuter L, Jeanguillaume C, Galle P (1997) Primary hyperparathyroidism: higher success rate of first surgery after preoperative Tc-99m sestamibi-I-123 subtraction scanning. Radiology 204:221–228

Hopkins CR, Reading CC (1995) Thyroid and parathyroid imaging. Semin Ultrasound CT MR 16:279–295

Huglo D, Nocaudie M, Lecompte-Houcke M et al (1996) Localisation préopératoire des lésions parathyroïdiennes par la scintigraphie 99m Tc MIBI/iode 123. Presse Méd 25:2017–2021

Ishibashi M, Nishida H, Hiromatsu Y, Kojima K, Uchida M, Hayabucchi N (1997) Localization of ectopic parathyroid glands using technetium-99m sestamibi imaging: comparison with magnetic resonance and computed tomography imaging. Eur J Nucl Med 24:197–201

Karstrup S, Hegedüs L, Holm (1993) Ultrasonically guided chemical parathyroidectomy in patients with primary hyperparathyroidism: a follow-up study. Clin Endocrinol 38:523–530

Kézachian B, Gray M, Bussière F, Freychet P, Sadoul JL (1997) Localisation préopératoire dans l'hyperparathyroïdie primitive: valeur de la scintigraphie au 99m Tc-MIBI. Rev Med Interne 18:21–25

Kilgore EJ, Teigne EL, Cowan RJ (1996) Imaging of transplanted parathyroid tissue in a patient with recurrent hyperparathyroidism. Clin Nucl Med 21:383–386

Kipper MS, LaBarbera JJ, Krohn LD, Marcou LM (1997) Localization of a parathyroid adenoma by the addition of pinhole imaging to Tc-99m sestamibi dual-phase scintigraphy. Report of a case and review of experience. Clin Nucl Med 22 :73–75

Kitaoka M, Fukagawa M, Ogata E et al (1994) Reduction of functioning parathyroid cell mass by ethanol injection in chronic dialysis patients. Kidney Int 46:1110–1117

Lee VS, Wilkinson RH Jr, Leight GS Jr, Coogan AC, Coleman RE (1995) Hyperparathyroidism in high-risk surgical patients: evaluation with double-phase technetium-99m sestamibi imaging. Radiology 197:627–633

Legmann P, Fayet P, Fulla Y, Hoeffel C, Bonnin A et al (1995) Imagerie de l'hyperparathyroidie primaire. Feuil Radiol 35:260–271

Liehn JC, Amico S, Delisle MJ, Flament JB (1988) Improvement of parathyroid T1-Tc scintigraphy by using a new image subtraction method. Eur J Nucl Med 14:184–189

Livolsi VA, Hamilton R (1994) Intraoperative assessment of parathyroid gland pathology. A common view from the surgeon and the pathologist. Am J Clin Pathol 102:365–373

Loevner LA (1996) Imaging of the parathyroid glands. Semin Ultrasound CT MR 17:563–575

Lossef SV, Ziessman HA, Alijani MR, Gomes MN, Barth KH (1993) Multiple hyperfunctioning mediastinal parathyroid glands in a patient with tertiary hyperparathyroidism. AJR 161:285–286

Lu G, Shih WJ, Xiu JY (1995) Technetium-99m MIBI uptake in recurrent parathyroid carcinoma and brown tumors. J Nucl Med 236:811–813

McDermott VG, Mendez Fernandez RJ, Meakem III TJ, Stolpen AH, Spritzer CE, Gefter WB (1996) Preoperative MR imaging in hyperparathyroidism: results and factors affecting parathyroid detection. AJR 166:705–710

Miller DL (1991) Preoperative localization and interventional treatment of parathyroid tumors: when and how? World J Surg 15:706–715

Miller DL, Doppman JL, Chang R et al (1987a) Angiographic ablation of parathyroid adenomas: lessons from a 10 year experience. Radiology 165:601–607

Miller DL, Doppman JL, Krudy AG et al (1987b) Localization of parathyroid adenomas in patients who have undergone surgery. II. Invasive procedures. Radiology 161:138–141

Miller DL, Doppman JL, Shawker TH et al (1987c) Localization of parathyroid adenomas in patients who have undergone surgery. I. Noninvasive imaging methods. Radiology 162:133–137

Moinuddin M, Whynott C (1996) Ectopic parathyroid adenomas. Multi-imaging modalities and its management. Clin Nucl Med 21:27–32

Nakahara H, Noguchi S, Murakami N et al (1997) Gadolinium-enhanced MR imaging of thyroid and parathyroid masses. Radiology 202:765–772

Neumann DR, Esselstyn CG Jr, Macintyre WJ et al (1994) Primary hyperparathyroidism: preoperative parathyroid imaging with regional body FDG-PET. Radiology 192:509–512

Neumann DR, Esselstyn CG Jr, Go RT, Wong CO, Rice TW, Obuchowski NA (1997) Comparison of double-phase 99mTc-sestamibi with 123I-99mTc-sestamibi subtraction SPECT in hyperparathyroidism. AJR 169:1671–1674

Numerow ŁM, Morita ET, Clark OH, Higgins CB (1995) Persistent/recurrent hyperparathyroidism: a comparison of sestamibi scintigraphy, MRI and ultrasonography. J Magn Reson Imaging 5:702–708

O'Doherty MJ (1997) Radionuclide parathyroid imaging. J Nucl Med 38:840–841

O'Doherty MJ, Kettle AG, Welles PC, Collins REC, Coakley AJ (1992) Parathyroid imaging with technetium-99m-sestamibi: preoperative localization and tissue uptake studies. J Nucl Med 33:313–318

Okada Y, Mizutani Y, Takeuchi H, Shigeno C, Konishi J, Yoshida O (1997) Preoperative imaging for parathyroid localization in primary hyperparathyroidism. Int J Urol 4:338–342

Perkins I (1996) Nuclear medicine: science and safety. Libbey, London

Price DC (1993) Radioisotopic evolution of the thyroid and the parathyroid. Radiol Clin North Am 31:967–989

Proye C, Bizard JP, Carnaille B, Quievreux JL (1994) Hyperparathyroïdie et parathyroïde intrathyroïdienne. 43 observations. Ann Chir 48:501–506

Rauth JD, Sessions RB, Shupe SC, Ziessman HA (1996) Comparison of Tc-99m MIBI and TI-201/Tc-99m pertechnetate for diagnosis of primary hyperparathyroidism. Clin Nucl Med 21:602–608

Rodriquez JM, Tezelman S, Siperstein AE et al (1994) Localization procedures in patients with persistent or recurrent hyperparathyroidism. Arch Surg 129:870–875

Sacks BA, Pallotta JA, Cole A, Hurwitz J (1994) Diagnosis of parathyroid adenomas: efficacy of measuring parathormone levels in needle aspirates of cervical masses. AJR 163:1223–1226

Sadoul JL (1996) Parathyroïdes. Introduction clinique. In: Bruneton JN, Padovani B (eds) Imagerie en endocrinologie. Masson, Paris, pp 81–83

Sandrock D, Merino MJ, Norton JA, Neumann RD (1993) Ultrastructural histology correlates with results of thallium-201/technetium-99m parathyroid subtraction scintigraphy. J Nucl Med 34:24–29

Sarfati E, Casanova D, Dubost CL (1994) Traitement chirurgical de l'hyperparathyroïdie primaire. Ann Endocrinol 55:165–170

Schvartz C, Liehn JC, Delisle MJ, Flament JB, Patey M (1996) Scintigraphie parathyroïdienne au sestamibi: une évaluation des images précoces, tardives ou de soustraction chez 33 patients opérés. Med Nucl 20:425–429

Sfakianakis GN, Irvin GL III, Foss J et al (1996) Efficient parathyroidectomy guided by SPECT-MIBI and hormonal measurements. J Nucl Med 37:798–804

Solbiati L, Giangrande A, De Pra L et al (1985) Percutaneous ethanol injection of parathyroid tumor under US guidance: treatment for secondary hyperparathyroidism. Radiology 155:607–610

Stark DD, Gooding GA, Moss AA, Clark OH, Ovenfors CO (1983) Parathyroid imaging: comparison of high resolution CT and high resolution sonography. AJR 141:633–638

Stevens SK, Chang JM, Clark OH, Chang PJ, Higgins CB (1993) Detection of abnormal parathyroid glands in postoperative patients with recurrent hyperparathyroidism: sensitivity of MR imaging. AJR 160:607–612

Sundin A, Johansson C, Hellman P et al (1996) PET and parathyroid L-11C-methionine accumulation in hyperparathyroidism. J Nucl Med 37:1766–1770

Taillefer R, Boucher Y, Potvin C et al (1992) Detection and localization of parathyroid adenomas in patients with hyperparathyroidism using a single radionuclide imaging procedure with technetium-99m-sestamibi (double-phase study). J Nucl Med 33:1801–1807

Thompson NW (1988) CT localisation studies in patients with hyperparathyroidism. Br J Surg 75:97–98

Verges BL, Cercueil JP, Jacob D, Vaillant G, Brun JM, Putelat R (1993) Results of ultrasonically guided percutaneous ethanol injection into parathyroid adenomas in primary hyperparathyroidism. Acta Endocrinol 129:381–387

Wang C (1976) The anatomic basis of parathyroid surgery. Ann Surg 183:271–275

Wei JP, Burke GJ (1995) Analysis of savings in operative time for primary hyperparathyroidism using localization with technetium-99m-sestamibi scan. Am J Surg 170:488–4911

Winkelbauer F, Ammann ME, Langle F et al (1993) Diagnosis of hyperparathyroidism with US after autotransplantation: results of a prospective study. Radiology 186:255–257

Wolf RJ, Cronan JJ, Monchik JM (1994) Color Doppler sonography: an adjunctive technique in assessment of parathyroid adenomas. J Ultrasound Med 13:303–308

14 Pancreatic Endocrine Tumors

S. Agostini, P. Bret, T. de Baere, O. Durieux, and A. Roche

CONTENTS

14.1 Introduction

Pancreatic endocrine tumors (islet cell tumors) are rare entities that account for 15%–30% of all primary solid tumors of the pancreas. Endocrine tumors are referred to as functioning or nonfunctioning, depending on whether they elaborate a biologically active product. The term “functioning” is preferable to “secretory” because secretion may occur yet have no biological consequences. Functioning pancreatic endocrine tumors predominate; diagnosis is based on clinical features and laboratory findings. Imaging studies are performed for localization of lesions to the pancreas and determination of their number and exact location prior to surgery. The multiplicity of radiological modalities used for this purpose highlights the difficulties in demonstrating these small focal lesions, which are often smaller than 1 cm. Nonfunctioning pancreatic endocrine tumors are much less common (15%–25%), very discrete clinically and biochemically, but have characteristic radiological features. The problem with these lesions is determination of their exact nature.

S. Agostini, O. Durieux, Service de Radiologie, Hôpital Sainte Marguerite, 270 Bd Sainte Marguerite, 13009 Marseille, France
P. Bret, Service de Radiologie, Hôpital Général de Montréal, 1650 avenue Cédar, H3G 1A4 Montreal, Canada
T. de Baere, A. Roche, Service de Radiodiagnostic Interventionelle, Institut Gustave Roussy, 39-53 avenue Camille Desmoulins, 94805 Villejuif, France

14.2 Functioning Tumors

O. Durieux, P. Bret, and S. Agostini

14.2.1 Etiology and Pathogenesis

Pancreatic endocrine tumors arise from pluripotential endocrine cells around the excretory ducts (nesidioblasts). These neuroendocrine cells belong to the amine precursor uptake and decarboxylation (APUD) system. Elaborated by Pearse and Takor (1976), this concept refers to a group of endocrine cells distributed throughout the body that share certain immunohistochemical characteristics; they arise from the neural crest and contain neurosecretory granules corresponding to polypeptide hormones, biogenic amines, or neurotransmitters. The existence of mixed acinar cell and endocrine tumors illustrates the histogenetic similarity between endocrine and exocrine tumors (Klimstra et al. 1994).

Macroscopically, these round, tan or reddish tumors have a firm homogeneous consistency. They are usually well circumscribed, but rarely encapsulated. Eighty percent of functioning pancreatic endocrine tumors develop in the body and tail, but 20% of gastrinomas are extraglandular, with a predilection for the duodenal or gastric wall (Stefanini et al. 1974; Ellison and Wilson 1986) or the greater omentum. Insulinomas, glucagonomas, and vipomas are usually solitary. Gastrinomas are multiple in half of all cases and are generally small (several millimeters to 1–2 cm). Glucagonomas, vipomas, and somatostatinomas may be larger and multifocal.

In contrast, nonfunctioning tumors are usually large, probably because their asymptomatic character delays diagnosis until a later stage. Small nonfunctioning tumors are generally incidental discoveries at laparotomy. These lesions may cause minimal stenosis of the duct of Wirsung responsible for recurrent acute pancreatitis.

Histologically, pancreatic endocrine tumors show a relative regularity of cells within an endocrinoid architecture; vascularity is extensive. The stroma may contain amyloid deposits and/or calcifications. The endocrine origin of these tumors can be confirmed by immunohistochemical techniques using specific antibodies – anti-insulin, antiglucagon, anti-vasoactive intestinal polypeptide (VIP), antigastrin, anti-pancreatic polypeptide (PP) – or stains – peroxidase-antiperoxidase – performed on tissue specimens fixed in formol or Bouin's solution. These methods also allow identification of the peptide secreted.

Many pancreatic endocrine tumors secrete multiple hormones, and affirmation of their benign or malignant nature is difficult solely on the basis of histological features. Intratumoral emboli must always be sought and reported. The larger the tumor, the older it is, and the higher the risk of malignancy. Endocrine tumors do not all have the same malignant potential; insulinomas are nearly always benign, gastrinomas present signs of malignancy in two thirds of cases, and glucagonomas are practically always malignant. The metastases of these tumors do not present histologic criteria of malignancy, and the hormonal secretion of secondary lesions may differ from that (those) of the main tumor. Furthermore, hepatic metastases may respond to chemotherapy even if the primary tumor is refractory to medical therapy.

Endocrine tumors that secrete a clinically detectable product are referred to as functioning. The percentage of true nonfunctioning tumors has declined in recent years owing to progress in assay techniques; they now represent only 15%.

These pancreatic tumors are named after the peptide that produces the clinical endocrine syndrome. The polypeptide hormones secreted are identified by immunohistochemistry or radioimmunoassay (RIA) in blood or tumor tissue. Insulin is secreted by B cells, glucagon by A_2 cells, gastrin by A_1 cells, somatostatin by D cells, VIP by D_1 cells, and PP by D_2, F, or PP cells. Insulinomas that develop from B cells are by far the most frequent; gastrinomas arise from A_1 cells and are less common; glucagonomas, vipomas, and pancreatic polypeptide tumors are exceptional. Certain tumors secrete hormones not normally produced by the pancreas, e.g., serotonin, somatropic hormone (STH), adrenocorticotropic hormone (ACTH), or elaborate multiple hormones.

Pancreatic endocrine tumors may be solitary or multiple. Insulinomas are solitary in 90% of cases, while 50% of gastrinomas are multiple. Glucagonomas, vipomas, and somatostatinomas are usually solitary. Pancreatic endocrine tumors may be associated with other endocrine lesions in the context of multiple endocrine neoplasia syndromes (MEN). Verner-Morrison syndrome is an association of pancreatic, parathyroid, and pituitary tumors; gastrinomas and somatostatinomas are the predominant lesions in these cases.

14.2.2 Biochemical Diagnosis

Assays demonstrate elevated hormone concentrations that are not regulated during dynamic tests, reflecting inappropriate secretion. Owing to the wide variation in normal levels, serial assays are often required, in particular during symptomatic episodes. The normal values for most clinically important hormones are now well established, and radioimmunological and biochemical hormone assay techniques are specific and reliable. Generally speaking, an elevation in pancreatic polypeptide is a marker for pancreatic endocrine tumors, as is neuron-specific enolase (NSE). An elevation in NSE may help confirm the diagnosis.

14.3 Nonvascular Imaging

14.3.1 Ultrasound

14.3.1.1 Abdominal Ultrasound

The sensitivity of ultrasound for the detection of insulinomas is approximately 60% (GORMAN et al. 1986; GALIBER et al. 1988); it is only 20% for gastrinomas owing to their predilection for extrapancreatic sites (GUNTHER 1985). However, the efficacy of ultrasound depends on the equipment used and examiner's expertise. Obesity, previous surgery, and bowel gas can all interfere with the examination. The overall sensitivity of abdominal ultrasound appears lower than that of computed tomography (CT), but sonograms sometimes disclose tumors that escape CT detection (LONDON et al. 1991).

Sonographically, endocrine tumors are usually well-circumscribed round or oval masses that are hypoechoic relative to the normal pancreas (Fig. 14.1). A hyperechoic capsule may be observed. They may be located deep within the gland or on the surface. Certain tumors are isoechoic and can only be detected if they modify pancreatic contours. Hyperechoic tumors and tumors containing calcifications have also been described. Color Doppler (CD) occasionally demonstrates vascular flow reflecting hypervascularity (NAMIENO et al. 1995). Doppler studies have limited value for hemodynamic analysis of vessels with slow flow, and their reliability for assessment of lesion vascularity is thus limited. Use of an ultrasound contrast agent may reinforce the Doppler signal (UENO et al. 1996).

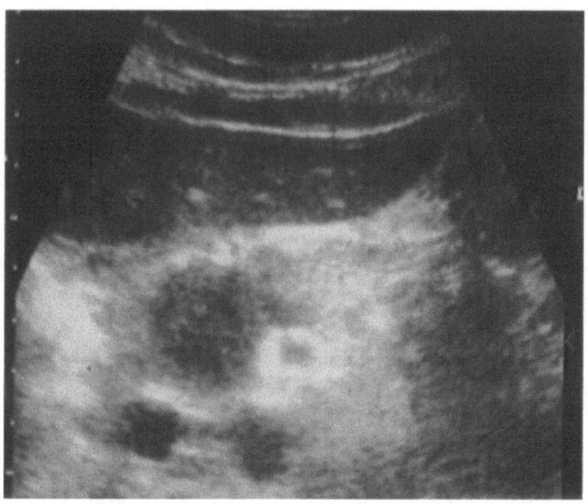

Fig. 14.1. Sonogram of a well-circumscribed hypoechoic nodule: insulinoma

In addition to its role for tumor localization, ultrasound can demonstrate metastases and nodal or vascular invasion.

14.3.1.2 Endoscopic Ultrasonography

The most sensitive technique for detection of small pancreatic endocrine tumors is endoscopic ultrasonography (EUS) (PALAZZO and ROSEAU 1992), which is gradually becoming the method of reference for topographic localization of small endocrine tumors. Examiner experience is indispensable to guarantee the result. By providing very high resolution images of the pancreas, EUS can depict structures as small as 2–3 mm (ROSCH et al. 1992). EUS detects approximately 80% of all small endocrine tumors not detected by abdominal ultrasound or CT and thus appears superior to angiography (LIGHTDALE et al. 1991). All portions of the pancreas can be effectively evaluated by EUS, but results for extrapancreatic tumors are not as good.

The tumor appears as a sharply marginated, relatively homogeneous hypoechoic round mass. Posterior reinforcement is frequent due to lesion hypervascularity (Fig. 14.2). Intratumoral calcifications may be observed. A cystic component occasionally predominates. A careful search must be made for a small tissue mass adjacent to the cystic lesion. The tumor occasionally appears hyperechoic to the adjacent parenchyma. CD may demonstrate increased flow in the tumor reflecting hypervascularity.

14.3.1.3 Intraoperative Ultrasound

Intraoperative ultrasound and direct palpation are complementary techniques for tumor localization and selection of the most appropriate treatment. Intraoperative ultrasound has a sensitivity of 84% for the detection of insulinomas; this figure rises to 100% when associated with palpation (NORTON et al. 1988). The caudal region of the pancreas is the most

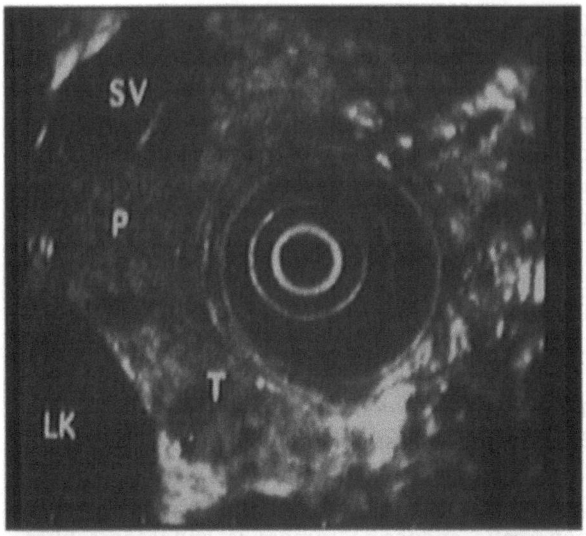

a

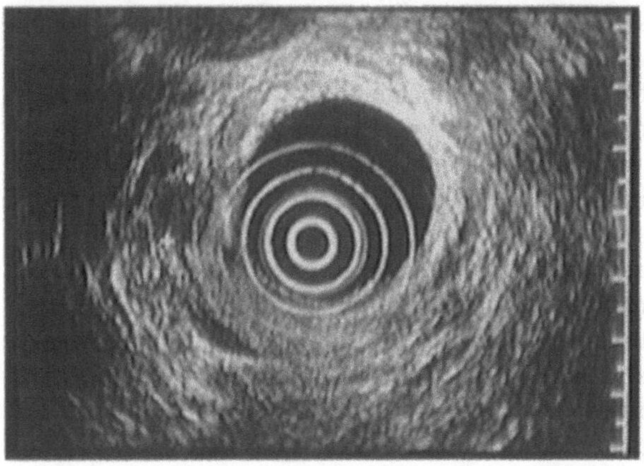

b

Fig. 14.2a,b. Endoscopic ultrasonography. **a** 8-mm insulinoma in the tail of the pancreas. *T*, tumor; *P*, pancreas; *SV*, splenic vein; *LK*, left kidney. **b** 20-mm insulinoma

difficult to examine. The sensitivity of intraoperative ultrasound for the detection of multiple tumors is lower (36%). Palpation is superior to ultrasound for detection of extrapancreatic gastrinomas. Intraoperative ultrasound can evaluate tumor relations with the pancreatic and biliary ducts, which is important when deciding whether to perform simple enucleation or segmental pancreatectomy.

Endocrine tumors appear hypoechoic within the hyperechoic pancreas in 90% of patients, and isoechoic or hypoechoic in 10% (Agostini 1993). The variability in nodule echogenicity appears related to the normal age-related increase in echogenicity. Isoechoic tumors can be detected due to their hyperechoic rim or the presence of focal calcification; peripheral tumors may distort gland contours. Hyperechoic tumors may show posterior shadowing.

14.3.2 Computed Tomography

Various CT studies have reported a sensitivity of approximately 66%, which is slightly better than ultrasound (Galiber et al. 1988). Meticulous methodology is indispensable, using thin sections (2–5 mm), small acquisition fields to increase spatial resolution, short acquisition times to reduce respiratory artifacts, and large bolus injections to obtain sufficient contrast between the tumor and the parenchyma on the arterial, parenchymal, and venous phases (Rossi et al. 1989). Use of an oral contrast agent for intestinal opacification is a source of artifacts and should be avoided. Optimum CT detection of endocrine tumors is achieved with helical acquisition, which associates volumetric acquisition (thus free from respiratory artifacts) and maximum vascular enhancement during acquisition (Fishman et al. 1992). The liver and the retroperitoneum should be examined during the same session to search for metastases.

On noncontrast scans, pancreatic endocrine tumors are usually isodense to the normal parenchyma. Tumors smaller than 15 mm do not modify gland dimensions. Only peripheral tumors that obliterate the lobulus can be detected; these lesions are often solid and homogeneous. Fine linear or nodular calcifications are sometimes observed (Fig. 14.3). Cystic lesions with thick, irregular walls (Takeshita et al. 1994) and spontaneously hyperdense lesions without calcification have been described (Kurosaki et al. 1996). Finally, even tumors outside of the preferential caudal location have

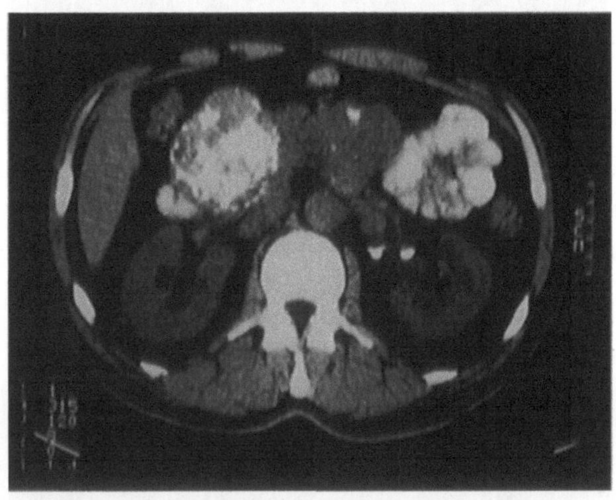

Fig. 14.3. Noncontrast CT scan: tumor calcifications (somatostatinoma)

no impact on the ducts (Rossi et al. 1989). The main bile duct is not dilated.

Functioning pancreatic endocrine tumors have characteristic appearances on postcontrast scans. Enhancement is early, intense, and transient; annular enhancement may be seen for lesions with central necrosis. Such typical enhancement behavior is actually observed in only 50%–80% of patients (Smith and Koenigsberg 1990). From 20% to 50% of all functioning endocrine tumors enhance in the same manner as the normal pancreatic parenchyma; they can be detected by demonstration of a contour abnormality or by the use of special injection techniques.

CT angiography consists in injection of dilute quantities of contrast material through a catheter placed directly in the celiac axis or the superior mesenteric artery. However, the diagnostic accuracy of this technique is not superior to that of angiography.

CT determination of the benign or malignant nature of pancreatic endocrine tumors is difficult in the absence of signs of local invasion or metastasis. Local spread occurs to the pancreatic ducts and combines dilatation of the main duct and the peripancreatic spaces with celiomesenteric nodal metastases. The appearance of these metastatic nodes is similar to that of the main tumor (hyperdense with strong enhancement after contrast injection). Metastases of pancreatic endocrine tumors are essentially hepatic and also appear hyperdense after contrast injection.

True multiple localizations (adenomatosis) are exceptional. Microadenomatosis (diffuse tumors measuring a few millimeters throughout the gland) and nontumoral hyperplasia cannot be detected by CT.

14.3.3 Magnetic Resonance Imaging

Magnetic resonance imaging (MRI) was initially of limited value for pancreatic studies due to extensive artifacts (particularly respiratory motion) and mediocre spatial and contrast resolution (Tscholakoff et al. 1987; Frucht et al. 1989; Steiner et al. 1989). The introduction of new sequences and contrast agents has improved MRI assessment of the pancreas, and results appear promising for investigation of endocrine tumors (Gehl et al. 1991,1993; Semelka et al. 1991; Mitchell et al. 1992; Moore et al. 1995).

Spin-echo (SE) sequences with respiratory compensation and gradient-echo sequences during suspended respiration reduce respiratory artifacts. Fat signal suppression decreases artifacts due to intestinal motility and thus limits image degradation due to respiratory motion. Used in combination, sequences with fat suppression and reduction of respiratory artifacts results in enhancement of the signal of the normal pancreas and higher resolution (Moore et al. 1995; Mori et al. 1996).

Satisfactory MRI demonstration of endocrine tumors (Semelka and Ascher 1993; Moore et al. 1995) is attributable to the existence of good contrast between the tumor and the normal pancreas and to tumor enhancement after gadolinium administration.

MRI appears to be more sensitive than CT (Kraus and Ros 1994; Semelka et al. 1993; Mori et al. 1996) or angiography (Eshkar et al. 1995; Moore et al. 1995) for the detection of pancreatic endocrine tumors. Moore et al. (1995) reported MRI depiction of a 5-mm insulinoma that was not detected by either CT or angiography.

MRI is also helpful for detection of hepatic metastases, which are of uniform size and possess a peripheral ring of enhancement on postcontrast scans (Fig. 14.4). Differential diagnosis from an angioma is sometimes difficult. For angiomas larger than 2 cm, dynamic sequences obtained after gadolinium administration reveal patchy enhancement and complete or partial centripetal filling. These enhancement characteristics are less constant for smaller angiomas. For Berger and Stephens (1996), T_1-weighted sequences obtained 5 min after gadolinium administration allow differentiation of angiomas and hypervascular metastases: angiomas are hyperintense, whereas metastases become isodense. MRI appears more sensitive than CT with an iodinated contrast material for the detection of these hypervascular metastases. Like the primary tumors, these metastases are readily depicted on T_2-weighted sequences as hyperintense lesions (Semelka and Asher 1993).

14.3.4 Scintigraphy

Somatostatin receptors are present on the surface of numerous cells in the body. The tumors with the highest density of these receptors are neuroendocrine tumors, including pancreatic endocrine tumors. This property is exploited in scintigraphy by intravenous administration of a radiolabeled somatostatin analogue. The most widely used product is

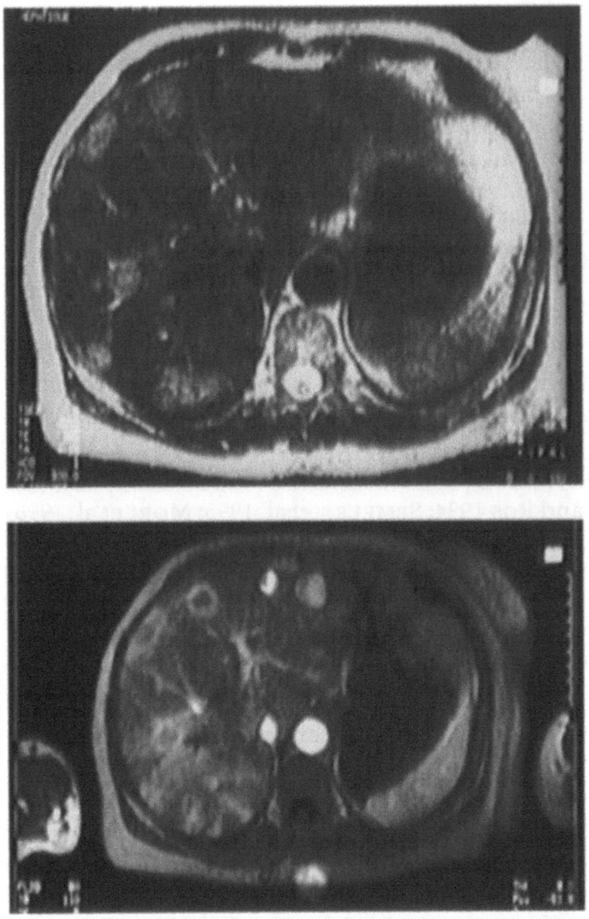

a

b

Fig. 14.4a,b. MRI of the liver. **a** T_2-weighted short-echo (SE) sequence: disseminated hyperintense nodules. **b** Gadolinium-enhanced T_1-weighted SE sequence: multiple hypervascular nodules

iodine-125–tyr-3-octreotide; utilization of iodine-111 pentreotide is more recent. Scintigraphic detection of these tumors depends on their density in somatostatin receptors, which also determines the therapeutic efficacy of somatostatin analogues.

A good correlation has been observed between the results of octreotide suppression tests and scintigraphic results, suggesting that this test may be useful to judge the diagnostic utility of octreoscanning (Nocaudie-Calzada et al. 1994).

Gastrinomas are particularly rich in somatostatin receptors. McCown et al. (1995) reported scintigraphic detection of a gastrinoma that had not been found by CT, angiography, or MRI. Few studies have compared the sensitivity of scintigraphy with that of other imaging modalities.

The site of radioactive tracer uptake can be observed in situ, intraoperatively, using a manual gamma camera (Schirmer et al. 1993).

The second property that can be exploited for scintigraphic evaluation of endocrine tumors is the capacity of endocrine cells to take up and decarboxylate L-dopa. Endocrine tumors can be visualized by positron emission tomography (PET) after administration of [^{11}C]-L-dopa. Prior treatment by a somatostatin analogue increases tumoral tracer uptake by inhibiting cellular secretion (Bergstrom et al. 1996).

14.4 Vascular Imaging

A. Roche and T. de Baere

14.4.1 Transhepatic Venous Sampling

14.4.1.1 General Features

The techniques for entry and catheterization of the portal system were fine-tuned by Swedish investigators in the 1970s (Ingemansson et al. 1975, 1976, 1977; Lunderquist et al. 1978; Reichardt and Ingemansson 1980). These techniques allow morphological study of the pancreatic veins in patients with a tumor or inflammatory disease and collection of venous blood samples from pancreatic efferent veins, enabling hormone-secreting tumors to be localized. This latter application has benefited from improvements in RIA techniques, which now provide extremely accurate results even for very small blood samples.

14.4.1.2 Rationale

Transhepatic venous sampling (TVS), also referred to as pancreatic or portal venous sampling, was developed essentially for two reasons:

- The small size of the most frequent pancreatic endocrine tumors (insulinomas, gastrinomas) that often elude detection by morphological localization techniques
- The possibility of micropolyadenomatosis or hyperplasia, which cannot be detected by morphological examination

TVS circumvents these difficulties by localizing the tumor, not because of its space-occupying effects, but rather by detection of the abnormal secretions that it releases into its venous drainage system. The intensity of hormone secretion is independent of tumor size, and pancreatic venous mapping must be as complete as possible so that hormone assays can be plotted accurately. Familiarity with the anatomy of the pancreatic and peripancreatic veins is indispensable for effective TVS and interpretation of results.

14.4.1.3 Anatomy of the Pancreatic Veins

As is the case for all venous systems, individual variations in the anatomy of the pancreatic veins (Keller et al. 1980; Reichardt and Cameron 1980) are frequent, and personalized interpretation is required for each examination. A general approach dividing the pancreatic veins into three systems (head, body, and tail) plus the neck is useful for descriptive purposes (Fig. 14.5).

Veins of the Head of the Pancreas. This venous system is composed of three superficial arcades (posterior, anterior, and inferior) and an intraglandular arcade. It has three principal efferent veins: the posterior superior, anterior inferior, and posterior inferior pancreaticoduodenal veins.

- The *posterior superior pancreaticoduodenal vein* is the major drainage vessel of the head in 94% of cases. This vein drains into the right posterior aspect of the inferior two thirds of the portal vein and, much more rarely, into the angle it forms with the superior mesenteric vein and, exceptionally, into the superior mesenteric vein. Given the functional importance of this vein in drainage of the pancreatic head, functioning cephalic tumors, regardless of their location, drain predominantly into the posterior superior pancreaticoduodenal vein in over 75% of patients. Catheterization of this vein is thus indispensable.
- The *anterior inferior pancreaticoduodenal vein* generally empties into the gastrocolic venous trunk. The latter is not constant, and the branches that form it may end either singly or after partial junction in the superior mesenteric vein.
- The *posterior inferior pancreaticoduodenal vein* usually empties into the first jejunal vein. In some cases, its anastomosis joins with the second jejunal vein.

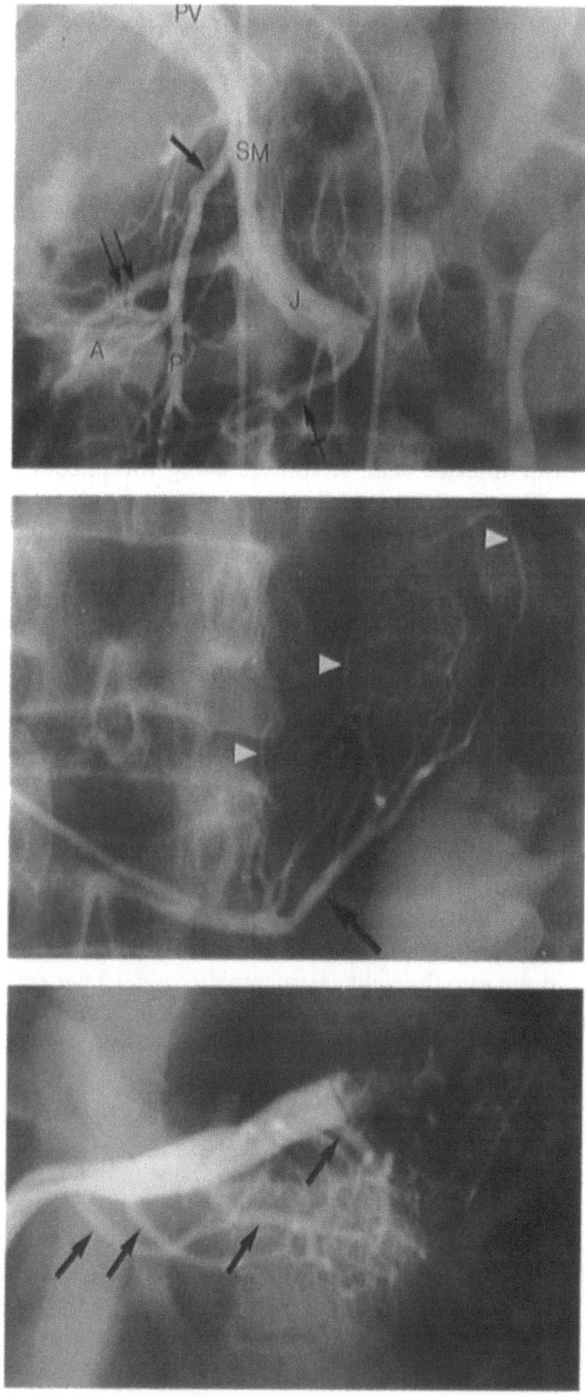

a

b

c

Fig. 14.5a–c. Radiological anatomy of the pancreatic veins. **a** Injection into the posterior superior pancreaticoduodenal vein (*dark arrow*) with opacification of the cephalic arcades (*A*, anterior; *P*, posterior) and the anterior inferior (*double arrow*) and posterior inferior (*crossed arrow*) pancreaticoduodenal veins (*SM*, superior mesenteric vein; *PV*, portal vein; *J*, first jejunal vein). **b** Injection into the transverse pancreatic vein (*arrow*) with opacification of numerous dorsal pancreatic veins (*arrowheads*) draining into the splenic vein. **c** Injection into a dorsal pancreatic vein draining into the splenic vein; opacification of several contiguous dorsal pancreatic veins (*arrows*) via their intrapancreatic anastomoses

- The *posterior cephalic venous arcade* extends between the medial branch of the posterior superior vein and the superior branch of the posterior inferior vein. This arcade is located on the posterior surface of the gland and the superior mesenteric vessels. Identification of this arcade is generally easy because it lies clearly inside the other arcades of the head. However, unlike the other arcades, it is often straight or only slightly concave above and to the left. Compared to the anterior arcade, it receives few duodenal veins.
- The *inferior cephalic venous arcade* lies suspended between the medial branch of the anterior inferior vein and the inferior branch of the posterior inferior vein. It courses along the uncinate process of the pancreas and ascending duodenum, from which it receives the respective branches, and passes behind the superior mesenteric vessels. This arcade is readily identified owing to its very inferior location running closely alongside the duodenum, showing a very pronounced superior concavity.
- The *anterior cephalic venous arcade* lies between the lateral branch of the posterior superior vein and the lateral branch of the anterior inferior vein. This arcade goes around the common bile duct on the outside. This cephalic arcade is the most difficult to identify clearly on venography because of the many superimposed large duodenal vessels it receives, as well as antral and pyloric veins, which drain into the right gastroepiploic vein. Its general position is somewhat vertical and slightly concave on the left. It is usually the most lateral arcade throughout almost its entire course.
- The *intrapancreatic cephalic venous arcade* lies suspended between the medial branch of the posterior superior vein and the medial branch of the anterior inferior vein. It descends between the common bile duct and the major pancreatic duct and then between the two pancreatic ducts. It then projects vertically between the anterior arcades (more lateral) and posterior arcades (more medial). It is seldom clearly identifiable on angiography.
- *Anastomoses:* In addition to anastomoses with veins of the neck and body, the cephalic veins are anastomosed with the medial colic veins, the gastric veins, the biliary veins, and the intrahepatic portal system.

*Veins of the Body and Tail of the Pancreas.*Two venous systems drain the body and tail of the pancreas: (1) multiple relatively vertical veins that drain into the splenic vein, homologous to the pancreatic corporeal arteries, and (2) a horizontal venous axis, homologous to the transverse pancreatic artery.

- The *pancreatic corporeal veins* are consistently found to empty into the splenic vein. The left gastric vein occasionally receives, at its end, a large pancreatic vein that drains the right side of the body. The left gastroepiploic vein receives one or more small veins that drain the left extremity of the tail, homologous to the caudal pancreatic arteries. Depending on their relations to the splenic and pancreatic veins, they may follow a descending or ascending course. In the right part of the body, they usually follow an ascending, almost vertical course because the splenic vein generally lies above the pancreas. In the medial and left part of the pancreatic body, their course usually slants toward the left and is almost horizontal.
- The *transverse pancreatic vein* represents the longitudinal drainage axis of the body and tail of the pancreas. This vein empties into the inferior mesenteric vein half of the time but only, it would seem, when the latter drains markedly to the right, into the superior mesenteric vein or at the angle it forms with the splenic vein. In other cases, it tends to drain into the end of the splenic vein. We found one or more well-defined transverse pancreatic veins in 56 of 100 complete venographies. In three patients, two transverse veins of equal size were present.
- *Anastomoses:* The corporeal veins are extensively anastomosed to one another and to the transverse pancreatic vein. When the latter vein is not clearly individualized, the longitudinal anastomoses between the corporeal veins are the equivalent. Both venous systems form anastomoses with the other veins of the neck and the head. Like their homologous arteries, they are anastomosed to the middle colic veins, the veins of the left colic angle, and to the gastric and epiploic veins, following a course similar to the arterial anastomoses.

Veins of the Neck of the Pancreas.</phead1> These veins form an anastomotic bridge between the cephalic and corporeal systems. Often, however, drainage of the neck is very individualized, and there are two separate veins. On pancreatic venography, these veins are identified by their median position and by their anastomoses with the cephalic arcades and the corporeal venous system.

- The *superior vein of the neck* empties into the end of the splenic vein, generally on its upper surface.

It may also drain into the left gastric vein or the superior mesenteric vein.

- The *posterior vein of the neck* empties into the inferior mesenteric vein, generally close to its end. It sometimes empties into the superior mesenteric vein, just beneath the angle it forms with the splenic vein, into an accessory middle colic vein that drains into the superior mesenteric vein, or even into the splenic vein.

14.4.1.4 Technique and Methodology

(Roche et al. 1982, 1983)

The technique of entry into the portal system has been extensively described in the literature (Hoevels et al. 1978; Doyon et al. 1979). For patient comfort, the examination is usually conducted under general anesthesia. In such cases, care must be taken to ensure that the drugs used do not interfere with the metabolism of the hormones to be assayed.

TVS requires a number of precautions to limit artifacts and errors in interpretation:

- Given the systematically laminar blood flow into the large trunks, selective pancreatic samples must be collected to avoid serious misinterpretation of assay results.
- The small size of the veins used for blood sampling may require wedge catheterization; this may artificially increase the hormone concentration in the blood sample by stopping the flow upstream. Errors in interpretation can be avoided by comparing simultaneous assay of another substance independent of the pathology being investigated.
- The iodinated contrast medium in the blood sample may interfere with RIA over a certain threshold (30% in a sample collected for gastrin assay). This can be prevented by collecting blood samples before local contrast injection or after careful aspiration of the contrast agent. As demonstrated for parathyroid adenomas (Doppman et al. 1981), contrast medium can have a toxic effect on pancreatic endocrine tumor cells, leading to an inordinate release of hormones. However, the risk of interference seems to be fairly low given the numerous anastomoses in pancreatic vascularity.
- Simultaneous stimulation tests do not appear to improve localization of insulinomas or gastrinomas. For insulinomas, however, the patient's glycemia should be kept low and stable by close monitoring during the examination. The aim is to preferentially lower physiological secretion, because tumoral secretion is not very sensitive to the glucose stimulus. Hyperglycemic medications should be stopped at least 2 days before the examination. Anti-H_2 treatment can be continued in patients being examined for gastrinoma because such therapy does not alter gastrin secretion, and interruption may exacerbate symptoms.

Persistent errors in interpretation despite these precautions are attributable to anatomic variants and insufficient familiarity with normal secretory mapping.

14.4.1.5 Indications

TVS is indicated for tumor localization only after the diagnosis has been formally established by other means. Pancreatic secretion of gastrin is in itself abnormal (even though it is practically impossible to differentiate between duodenal and cephalic pancreatic secretion). By contrast, physiological secretion of insulin is normally asymmetrical and is higher in the tail. Patients with insulin-secreting tumors exhibit high peripheral levels during examination (systematically carried out at a low blood sugar level), unlike normal subjects. Conversely, some patients with an insulinoma have a lower insulin level in the tumor drainage vein than that encountered at the same site in certain normal individuals.

14.4.1.6 Overall Findings

Depending on the series, the effectiveness of TVS for tumor localization ranges from 90% to 100% (Passariello et al. 1978; Turner et al. 1978; Burcharth et al. 1979; Kallio and Suoranta 1979; Millan et al. 1979; Mitty et al. 1979; Passaro 1979; Doppman et al. 1981; Roche et al. 1982). Only one series, limited to eight patients, reported very poor results (62.5% localization errors; Daggett et al. 1981). We currently adapt investigations to the type of functioning tumor to be localized.

14.4.1.7 Value of Transhepatic Venous Sampling by Tumor Type

Insulinomas. Results from several large series are summarized in Table 14.1. TVS gives excellent re-

Table 14.1. Sensitivity of localization procedures and transhepatic venous sampling (TVS) for insulinomas (including hyperplasia)

Imaging modality	Sensitivity (%)
Ultrasound	20.2
CT	24.1
MRI	20.0
Arteriography	86.2
EUS	88.8
TVS	91.2
Intraoperative ultrasound	6.4

Personal series of 118 surgically treated patients; minimum preoperative workup consisted in ultrasound, arteriography, and TVS.
CT, computed tomography; MRI, magnetic resonance imaging; EUS, endoscopic ultrasound; TVS, transhepatic venous sampling.

Table 14.2. Location of insulinomas

Tumor site	Tumors (*n*)	(%)
Head	45	34
Neck	14	11
Body	38	29
Tail	34	26
Total	131	100

Personal series of 131 proven tumors.

sults for insulinomas and appears indispensable for definitive preoperative localization (Houlbert et al. 1984). Indeed, this pathology is so rare, with almost no recurrences, and the course is so benign after complete exeresis, yet so serious after inappropriate pancreatic exeresis, that it seems futile to discuss an imaging algorithm when all available means should be used to ensure accurate localization. In a series of 1067 patients collected by Stefanini et al. (1974), 76% of tumors were found at initial laparotomy and 11% at repeat laparotomy; 7% were never found. When aware of preoperative radiological findings, the surgeon sees or palpates the lesion in 80%–90% of cases. Thus, in at least one out of ten cases, resection must be performed solely on the basis of imaging data.

Functional localization by selective venous sampling appears indispensable, not only because of the technique's higher sensitivity for localization of solitary and multiple lesions, but also, and especially, because TVS is the sole diagnostic method for hyperplasia (6.7% of cases), even when associated with one or more macroscopic tumors (4.2%); it can localize occult tumors (2.5% of cases) and can identify one or more insulinomas within multiple tumors (6.8% of cases). Restriction of TVS to patients with MEN type I syndromes is unjustifiable because 62.5% of all cases of hyperplasia and 72% of all multiple tumors (with or without hyperplasia) occur in patients without MEN (Tables 14.2, 14.3).

Zollinger-Ellison Syndrome. The results of TVS and surgical exploration are summarized in Table 14.4. Mignon et al. (1987) found a gross lesion at surgery in 77% of patients despite negative preoperative imaging. However, 75% of the tumors were ectopic (usually duodenal). The indication for TVS remains questionable in Zollinger-Ellison syndrome (ZES) (Bonfils 1983). Preoperative lesion localization is important for some authors (Vinik and Thompson 1986), while others claim that such information does not change the surgical results (Cherner et al. 1986) because most patients have multiple more or less functioning tumors (McCarthy 1980). Only tumors that are secreting sufficient amounts of hormone when blood samples are collected can be localized. Almost 90% of tumors localized by hormone assays are in the head of the pancreas or the duodenum. This means that, nine times out of ten, cephalic duodenopancreatectomy would probably be proposed because these tumors are too small and cannot

Table 14.3. Tumor presentation in 110 surgically treated patients with hyperinsulinemia

Presentation	Patients without MEN (%)	Patients with MEN (%)	Total of surgically treated patients (%)
Solitary tumor	88	28	85
Multiple tumors	7	29	8
Hyperplasia	3	0	3
Hyperplasia + tumor	2	43	4

Patients without MEN, 94%; patients with MEN, 6%.
MEN, multiple endocrine neoplasia.

Table 14.4. Comparison of transhepatic venous sampling (TVS) and surgical exploration in Zollinger-Ellison syndrome

	Type of lesion (% of patients)			Location of lesion (% of patients)		
	Solitary lesion	Multiple lesions	Not found	Head or duodenum	Body or tail	Head and/or duodenum + body and/or tail
TVS	92.5	7.5	–	86.8	5.6	7.6
Surgery	28.3	28.3	43.4	50.0	6.7	43.3

Personal series of 53 surgically treated patients.

be found preoperatively in 40% of patients. However, authentic cases of complete cure have been reported after TVS-guided cephalic pancreatectomy (Hautefeuille et al. 1979). Nonetheless, this procedure seems all the more aggressive because over half of all nonfunctioning corporeal lesions are not invasive (Deveney et al. 1978) and 25% of all cases of ZES develop in patients with MEN type I.

Glucagonomas. Localization is usually no problem because these tumors are large at initial diagnosis. TVS is indicated in those rare cases where the diagnosis seems sufficiently probable, but localization procedures are negative or contradictory. In one of our own series of six patients, TVS permitted localization of three glucagonomas, two of which were smaller than 5 mm. In all known cases of glucagonoma, the hormone gradient in the pathological area was more than ten times the peripheral value. Nevertheless, caution is required when interpreting results, because functioning regional or nodal metastases are frequent and complicate analysis of hormone mapping.

Vipomas and Other Rare Functional Tumors. The remarks concerning glucagonomas also apply to vipomas. Although venography does not seem to play a major role for diagnosis, it remains the only technique that provides any hope of localization or early diagnosis of these tumors before they reach a size where malignancy is the rule.

14.4.2 Arterial Stimulation and Venous Sampling

14.4.2.1 *Principle*

Localization of a functioning tumor is based on identification of the arterial pedicle in which the hormone concentration increases significantly when infused with a secretagogue, a product that stimulates hormone secretion by the tumor.

14.4.2.2 *Technique*

The secretagogue is injected successively into the major arteries supplying the potentially tumoral areas, i.e., the splenic, gastroduodenal, and pancreatic arteries for the pancreas and the hepatic artery if liver metastases are suspected. Secretin (20–30 IU in 5 ml saline) is rapidly injected when searching for a gastrinoma (Imamura et al. 1989; Doppman et al. 1990). Selection of the stimulant is more controversial for insulinomas. Calcium has been used because intravenous injection stimulates tumoral insulin secretion (Brunt et al. 1986) without risk of severe hyperglycemia (Doppman et al. 1991). Doses range from 0.01 (in obese patients) to 0.025 mEq Ca^{2+}/kg (recommended dose for nonobese patients) as a rapid injection of calcium gluconate.

Venous samples are obtained in the right hepatic vein before and 30, 60, 120, and 210 s after injection. Sampling in both the right and left hepatic veins was initially recommended (Doppman et al. 1990) because the splenic portal flow may drain preferentially into the left liver and the mesenteric flow into the right liver. Placement of a single catheter in the right hepatic vein is currently considered sufficient (Doppman et al. 1995). Elevation in hormone levels has a localizing value only in early samples, because they are the only ones that are affected by the first-pass effect before systemic redistribution of the secretagogue.

14.4.2.3 *Results*

Few teams have experience with the technique, but for those that do the results are encouraging.

In ZES, Imamura et al. (1989) reported an accuracy of 100% for tumor localization in 11 patients. These authors considered the test positive if the gastrin level rose by more than 80 pg/ml (corresponding to a 120% elevation above baseline) after 40 s. For Doppman et al. (1991), a postinjection to preinjection secretin gradient over 50% after 30 s was considered positive. These latter authors successfully localized seven of 13 lesions and, in one case, were able to differentiate between a hemangioma and a hepatic metastasis. In their study, arteriography was positive in 38% of the patients, the intra-arterial stimulation test in 54%, and TVS in 46%. The overall efficacy of arteriography combined with the intra-arterial stimulation test was 77%; this is noteworthy in light of the mildly invasive nature of the exploratory method. The arterial stimulation test has also been proposed for the detection of liver metastases, especially in patients in whom imaging findings are contradictory. In a series of 22 patients with hepatic metastases (Gibril et al. 1996), the intra-arterial secretin test improved clinical management in 22% due to its high specificity. In that study, a 50% increase in venous gastrin 30 s after injection was considered significant.

For insulinomas, the intra-arterial calcium test allowed accurate tumor localization in the first four patients reported by Doppman et al. (1991). Using the doubling of the insulin level at 30 or 60 s as a criterion (Fig. 14.6), these authors were able to differentiate between the multiple tumors in a patient with MEN type I. The sensitivity of the method seems highest for tumors in the head of the pancreas. In a subsequent series limited to solitary tumors (Doppman et al. 1995), 22 of 25 insulinomas (88%) were successfully localized using the calcium test. In the nine patients explored using both the intra-arterial calcium test and TVS, results were 78% and 67%, respectively. Our experience with 15 patients explored by these two methods (including two cases of hyperplasia) currently remains in favor of TVS (74% and 88%, respectively).

If these findings are confirmed in larger series, TVS would be a valuable addition to our arsenal of methods for localization of insulinomas, especially since it is only mildly invasive.

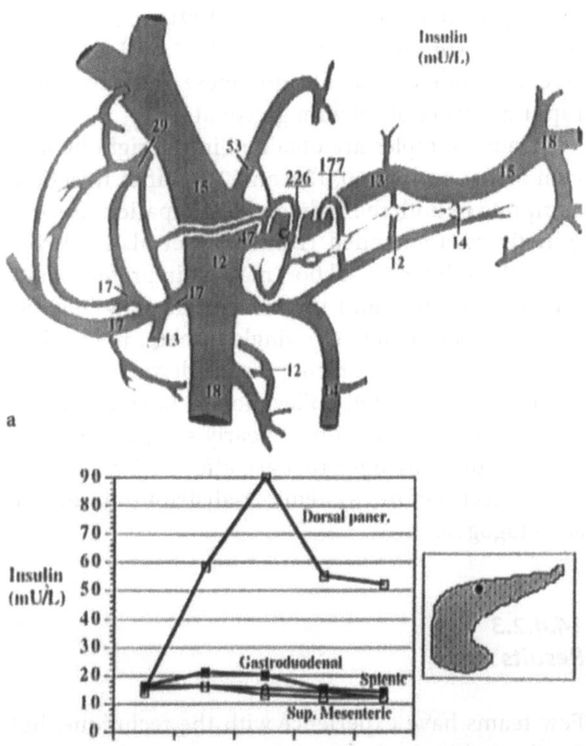

Fig. 14.6a,b. Localization of a paramedial insulinoma in the body of the pancreas by transhepatic venous sampling (TVS) and selective intra-arterial calcium infusion. **a** Abnormal insulin secretion into two right-sided dorsal pancreatic veins allowed localization of the adenoma. Other pancreatic veins contained a normal concentration, which ruled out hyperplasia and multiple tumors. **b** The dorsal pancreatic artery is clearly identified as the main feeding vessel of the insulinoma. No significant elevation was observed in insulin secretion after infusions of the splenic, gastroduodenal, and superior mesenteric arteries

14.5 Clinical Syndromes

O. Durieux, P. Bret, and S. Agostini

14.5.1 Insulinomas

Insulinomas are by far the most frequent pancreatic endocrine tumor. Women are affected most often. Age at diagnosis is usually between 50 and 60 years, but is earlier in patients with MEN type I. These lesions tend to be solitary (92%), intrapancreatic (99%), and benign (90%). They are also typically small: 70% are smaller than 1.5 cm, 5% are smaller than 0.5 cm, and only 8% are larger than 5 cm.

Hypoglycemia is the major symptom. Hypoglycemic manifestations (central nerve system or vasomotor symptoms) occur with fasting or exercise (postprandial symptoms are rare), but are relieved by glucose administration. These latter two clinical features, together with low blood sugar levels, constitute Whipple's triad.

Although imaging studies are not always positive, a number of typical features are encountered. Sonography depicts a well-delimited hypoechoic nodule. On CT, these very hypervascular tumors are typically hypodense on noncontrast scans and enhance intensely on the arterial phase, as in arteriography (Fig. 14.7). On MRI, insulinomas are hypointense on T_1-weighted sequences with fat suppression (KRAUS and ROS 1994); contrast administration reveals diffuse or annular (complete or partial) enhancement. The T_2-weighted signal is variable (iso- or hyperintense). Intratumoral calcifications are possible. Atypical cases corresponding to nonenhancing iso- or hypovascular tumors (25% of insulinomas are not hypervascular) (SMITH and KOENIGSBERG 1990) and cystic lesions have been reported.

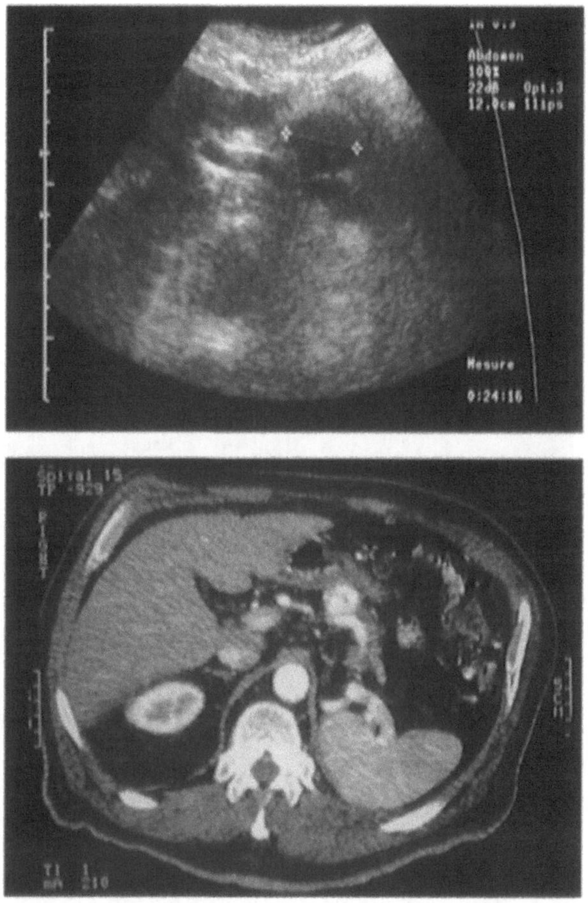

Fig. 14.7a,b. Benign insulinoma. **a** Sonogram: hypoechoic nodule in the tail of the pancreas. **b** Arterial-phase helical CT: located anterior to the splenic artery, this tumor was hyperdense during the early phase

14.5.2 Gastrinomas

Gastrinomas differ in numerous ways from insulinomas; 60% are malignant, with no correlation to size, 50% are metastatic at initial diagnosis, surgery is possible for only 20%–40%, 60% are multiple, and 30% are extrapancreatic (usually duodenal lesions less than 1 cm in diameter). These tumors are typically small (1–2 mm in diameter); up to 40% are occult and are not demonstrable by imaging. Approximately 25% are associated with MEN type I. Peak incidence is in the 40- to 50-year age-group.

Pancreatic gastrinomas cause intractable peptic ulcer disease, often with diarrhea (ZES) due to gastric acid hypersecretion, which leads to inactivation of digestive juices and malabsorption. Gastrin levels are elevated despite the high gastric acidity. Severe prolonged hypergastrinemia may result in development of a gastric carcinoid. Compared to sporadic cases, these carcinoids are typically small, multiple, and less aggressive (BERGER et al. 1996). This association of lesions is usually encountered in patients with MEN.

Gastrinomas tend to be hypervascular, although less so than insulinomas. However, the existence of numerous hypovascular lesions renders diagnosis difficult. The only suggestive imaging feature is tumor heterogeneity, which is rare in insulinomas. Gastrinomas are frequently located outside the pancreas in the duodenal wall, gastric wall, or greater omentum and are typically small (38% are smaller than 10 mm) (ELLISON and WILSON 1986).

Sonographically, gastrinomas image as heterogeneous solid tumors. At CT, their less extensive vascularity renders them less characteristic than insulinomas. Hypervascularity often occurs late in their course owing to tumor fibrosis (Fig. 14.8). At MRI, they appear hypointense on T_1-weighted sequences with fat suppression and are less enhanced after gadolinium (ESHKAR et al. 1995). On T_2-weighted sequences, gastrinomas often appear hyperintense.

14.5.3 Glucagonomas

Approximately 150 cases were published worldwide up until 1990. These essentially corporocaudal

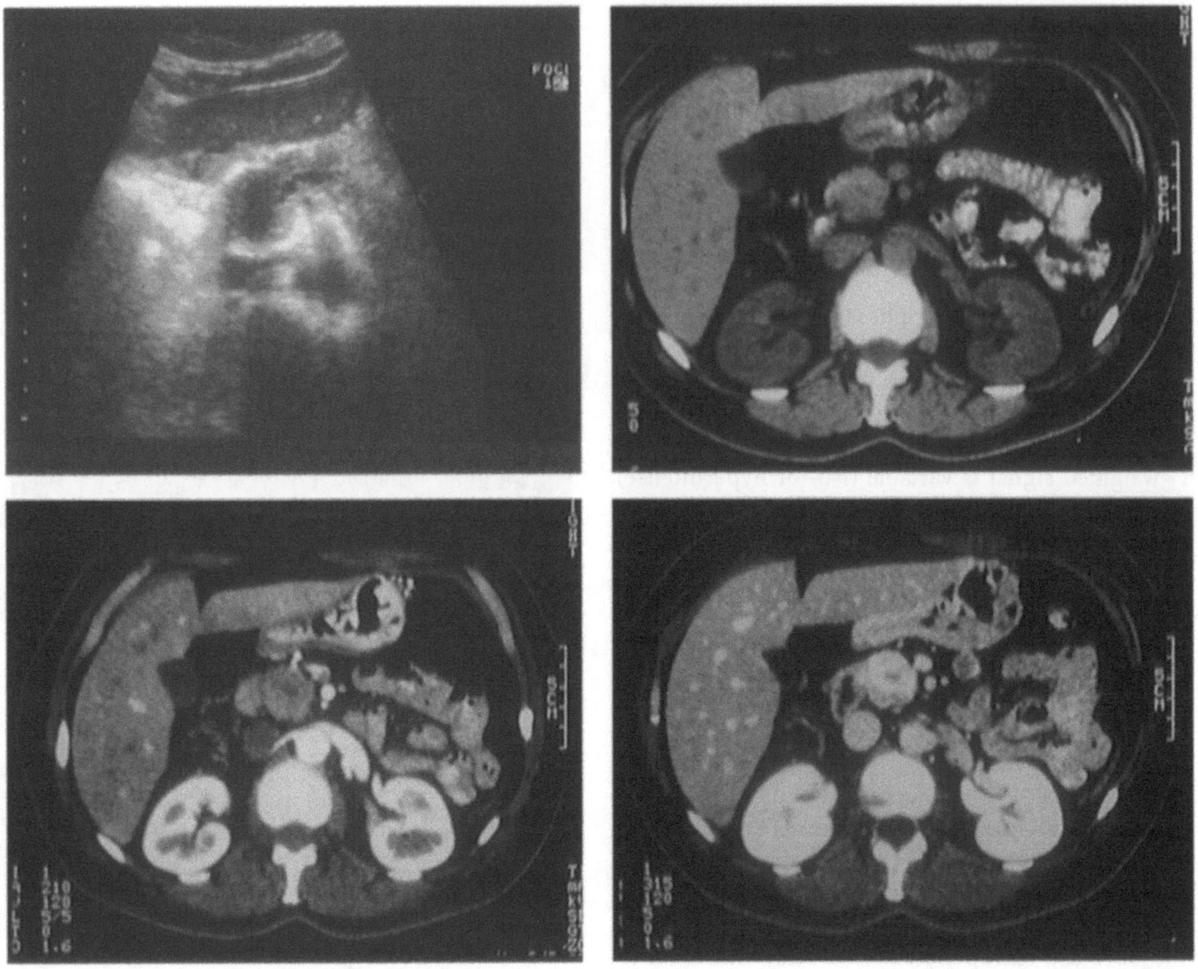

a b c d

Fig. 14.8a–d. Malignant gastrinoma. **a** Sonogram: hypoechoic nodule with dilatation of the pancreatic duct. **b** Precontrast CT: no obvious tumor. **c** Contrast-enhanced helical CT in the arterial phase: nonenhancing heterogeneous solid nodule. **d** Contrast-enhanced CT in the venous phase revealed late tumor enhancement

intrapancreatic tumors (75%) are malignant in at least 60% of cases and are usually large (over 5 cm). The mean age at diagnosis is 55 years, and there is a slight predilection for women. Glucagonomas cause distinctive, but inconsistent dermatological manifestations, i.e., a migrating skin rash over the buttocks, perineum, and lower extremities (necrolytic migratory erythema) associated with diabetes mellitus. An elevated plasma glucagon level confirms the diagnosis. On imaging studies, these large and fairly hypervascular tumors are often heterogeneous due to intratumoral necrosis.

14.5.4 Vipomas

Vipomas are very rare. Hypersecretion of VIP and its precursors causes profuse watery diarrhea resulting in hypokalemia and gastric achlorhydria (not always found). This association is referred to as Verner-Morrison syndrome or WDHA syndrome (watery diarrhea, hypokalemia, achlorhydria). Hypercalcemia may also be caused by the direct action of VIP on bone.

These solitary intrapancreatic tumors generally occur in the pancreatic head and tend to be malignant. They are intermediate in size (3 cm) between insulinomas and glucagonomas. Adrenal, pulmonary, and gastrointestinal localizations have been described. Vipomas are often hypervascular and may be revealed by metastatic disease.

14.5.5
Somatostatinomas

Approximately half of all patients with a somatostatinoma have diabetes mellitus, cholelithiasis, and weight loss. Duodenal localizations are possible, especially in the ampullary region. Somatostatinomas are the pancreatic endocrine tumor with the slowest growth rate. Cure of long-standing diabetes (25 years) following resection of a somatostatinoma has been reported. These tumors are sometimes associated with von Recklinghausen's disease.

14.5.6
Other Functioning Tumors

Certain rare endocrine tumors that develop from pluripotential cells secrete substances that are not normally produced by the pancreas (serotonin, STH, ACTH). Clinical manifestations associated with aberrant secretion include carcinoid syndrome, cushingoid syndrome, and acromegaly. Clinical and biological findings are not always as suggestive of disease, however, especially when secretion is minimal or when multiple products are elaborated. Diagnosis may thus be delayed for several months or even several years.

14.6
Imaging Strategies for Functioning Tumors

When clinical features and laboratory findings suggest an endocrine tumor and a pancreatic site is suspected, localization procedures and disease staging are required. Among the noninvasive techniques, ultrasound has a sensitivity of approximately 60% when performed under good conditions. Ultrasound is the initial imaging modality for disease staging, in particular for detection of metastases. CT, optimized by the helical acquisition technique, has better sensitivity than ultrasound; it can refine the local and regional disease workup and should be performed in a second stage. If ultrasound and CT do not yield useful results, EUS appears advisable (PALAZZO et al. 1990). If EUS proves negative or if the method is not available, the need for additional preoperative investigations is debatable in light of the sensitivity of intraoperative ultrasound combined with palpation (HEERDEN et al. 1992; MOORE et al. 1995). MRI seem promising, with studies announcing higher localization rates than with CT (KRAUS and ROS 1993; SEMELKA et al. 1993; ESHKAR et al. 1995; MOORE et al. 1995; MORI et al. 1996). The utility of MRI at this stage of investigations is increasingly apparent.

The indications for arteriography, alone or combined with arterial stimulation using secretin or calcium, remain controversial. TVS can be reserved for suspected cases of micropolyadenomatosis or hyperplasia.

14.7
Nonfunctioning Tumors

14.7.1
General Features

Nonfunctioning pancreatic endocrine tumors occur at all ages, but predominate in the fifth decade of life. The sexes are affected equally. These tumors are discovered at a late stage following investigations for nonspecific symptoms caused by the tumor mass and/or prevalent metastases. At diagnosis, 75% are already larger than 5 cm.

A mass in the epigastric region or left lower quadrant may be palpated during routine physical examination or workup for nonspecific gastrointestinal symptoms (epigastric pain, anorexia, weight loss, asthenia, fever). Once the tumor reaches a sufficient size, compression of adjacent organs may cause mid-epigastric pain, symptoms related to biliary or pancreatic obstruction, or vascular or digestive symptoms. Metastasis occurs predominantly to the liver and the peritoneum. Bone, renal, cardiac, pulmonary, adrenal, mediastinal, and brain metastases may occur at a later stage. Small tumors are usually incidental findings at surgery.

Laboratory findings are nonspecific and include hypochromic anemia during gastrointestinal hemorrhage, accelerated sedimentation rate, and hepatic function tests revealing cholestasis. Glycemia and pancreatic enzymes are normal.

The results of clinical and laboratory workup are similar to those for adenocarcinoma, which is much more frequent and has a much more somber prognosis.

14.7.2
Imaging

Ultrasound readily demonstrates these often large, inhomogeneously hypoechoic pancreatic tumors and signs of disease extension reflecting their malignant nature. Doppler ultrasound can reveal tumor hypervascularity, a feature which is itself suggestive of the diagnosis.

CT depicts 95% of all nonfunctioning endocrine tumors and allows optimal disease staging (Fugazzola et al. 1990). Morphological modifications caused by the tumor (increased gland thickness, obliteration of peripheral lobulation) are visible on noncontrast scans. Tumors larger than 10 cm are not uncommon. They are usually well limited, solid, homogeneous, and isodense to the parenchyma. Tumors containing areas of necrosis may be slightly hypodense and inhomogeneous. Coarse nodular calcifications are seen in 20% of patients. Cystic lesions are not infrequent; they may correspond to extensively necrotic tumors or to true retention cysts distal to an obstruction of the duct of Wirsung.

The marked enhancement behavior of nonfunctioning tumors on contrast-enhanced CT scans reveals their endocrine nature in 80% of patients. However, enhancement is not as intense as with functioning endocrine tumors (Figs. 14.9, 14.10). Twenty percent of all nonfunctioning endocrine tumors have scant vascularity and remain hypodense after injection; these lesions are difficult to distinguish from solid exocrine tumors. Nonfunctioning cystic endocrine tumors have occasionally been described and show an annular enhancement pattern after contrast injection.

In contrast to functioning endocrine tumors, signs of duct compression are frequent, with dilatation of the bile ducts and pancreatic ducts. Nonfunctioning pancreatic endocrine tumors may also compress adjacent organs (digestive compression, ureteral stenosis, renal or splenic displacement). As for functioning endocrine tumors,

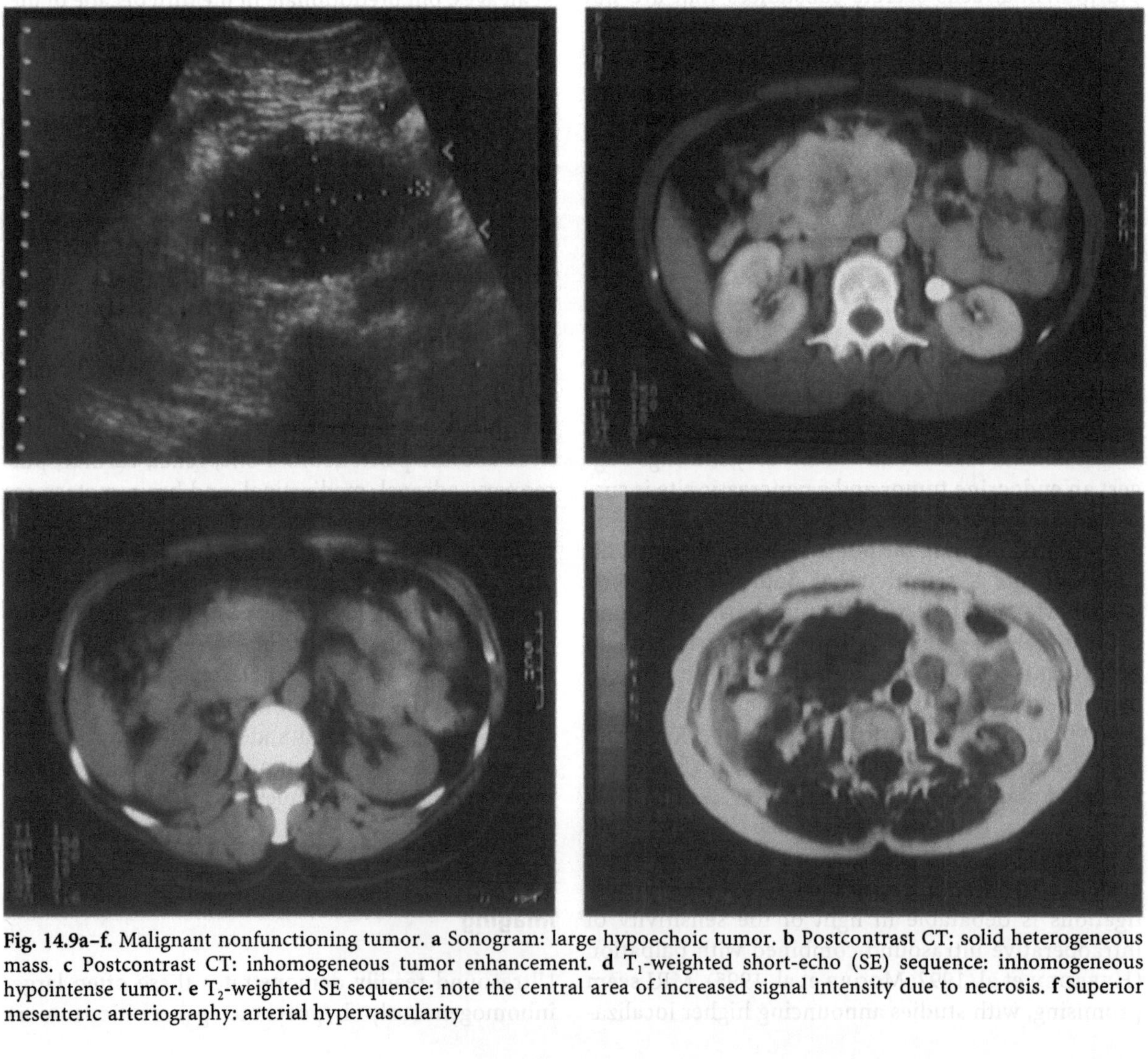

a c b d

Fig. 14.9a–f. Malignant nonfunctioning tumor. **a** Sonogram: large hypoechoic tumor. **b** Postcontrast CT: solid heterogeneous mass. **c** Postcontrast CT: inhomogeneous tumor enhancement. **d** T_1-weighted short-echo (SE) sequence: inhomogeneous hypointense tumor. **e** T_2-weighted SE sequence: note the central area of increased signal intensity due to necrosis. **f** Superior mesenteric arteriography: arterial hypervascularity malignancy can be affirmed only if there are signs of disease spread or presence of a metastasis.

Arteriography often allows tumor characterization by demonstrating hypervascularity and can demonstrate spread to the liver.

Wirsungography can demonstrate the ductal impact of tumors but cannot specify their nature.

CT appears the best technique for assessment of nonfunctioning pancreatic endocrine tumors, as it allows both accurate diagnosis and comprehensive workup.

The major differential diagnosis is an exocrine adenocarcinoma, which has a much poorer prognosis. Certain imaging features allow differentiation, but diagnosis of nonenhancing, nonfunctioning endocrine tumors remains difficult. The existence of nonfunctioning endocrine tumors mimicking adenocarcinoma justifies systematic aspiration biopsy of solid pancreatic tumors when surgery is not envisaged.

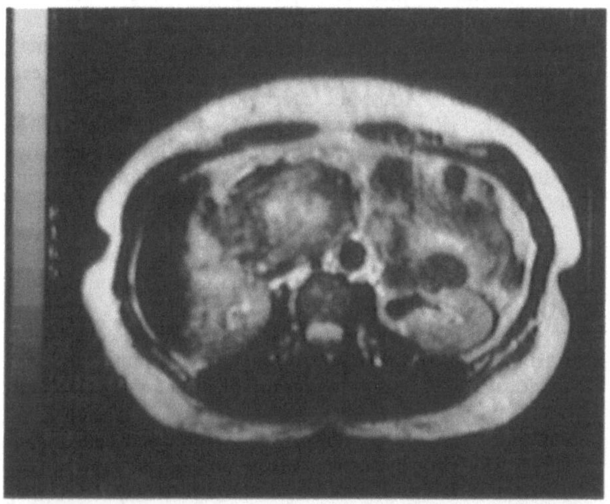
e

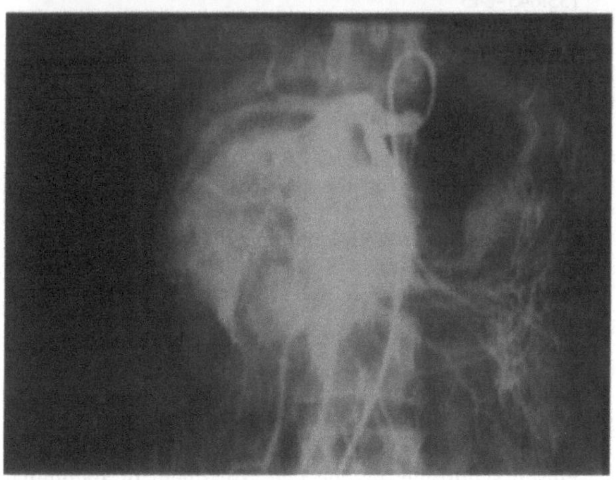
f

Fig. 14.9e,f

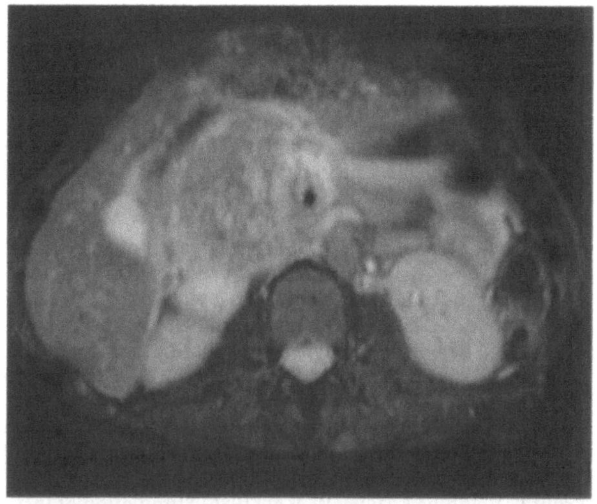
a

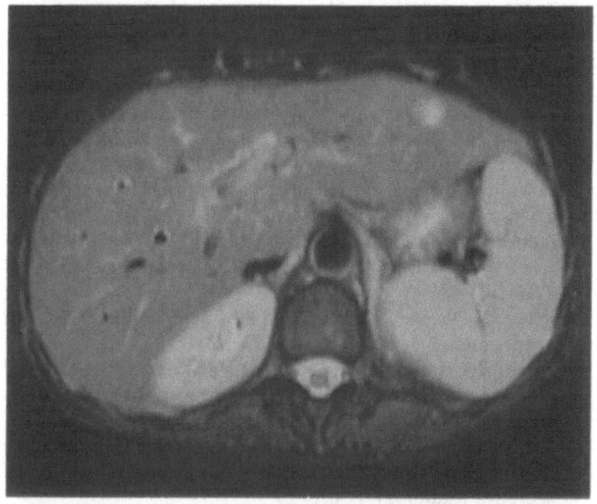
b

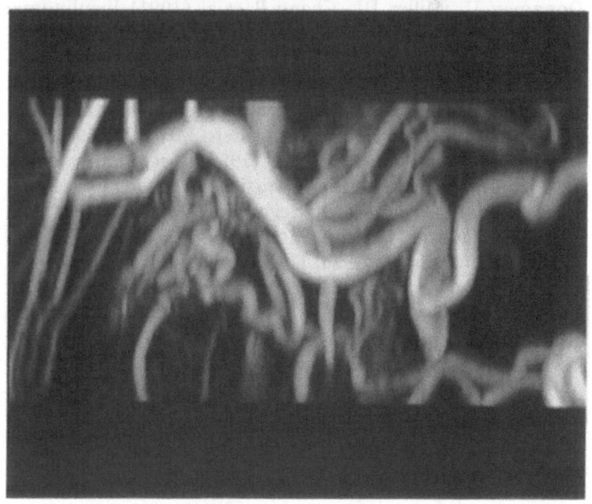
c

Fig. 14.10a–c. Malignant nonfunctioning pancreatic endocrine tumor. **a** T_2-weighted short tau inversion recovery (SPIR) sequence: heterogeneous tumor in the head of the pancreas with venous collaterals. **b** Same sequence as in Fig. 14.10a: hepatic metastasis and dilatation of the intrahepatic bile ducts. **c** Portal MR angiography: multiple pericephalic pancreatic venous collaterals

References

Agostini S (1993) Pancréas. In: Jouve P (ed) Manuel d'echographie. Masson, Paris, pp 73–79

Berger FJ, Laissy JP, Limot O et al (1996) Differentiation between multiple liver hemangiomas and liver metastases of gastrinomas: value of enhanced MRI. J Comput Assist Tomogr 20:349–355

Berger MW, Stephens DH (1996) Gastric carcinoid associated with chronic hypergastrinemia in a patient with Zollinger-Ellison syndrome. Radiology 201:371–373

Bergstrom M, Eriksson B, Oberg K et al (1996) In vivo demonstration of enzyme activity in endocrine pancreatic tumors: decarboxylation of carbon-11-DOPA to carbon-11-dopamine. J Nucl Med 37:32–37

Bonfils S (1983) Les difficultés de la localisation topographique du gastrinome. Gastroenterol Clin Biol 7:639

Brunt L, Veldhuis J, Dilley W et al (1986) Stimulation of insulin secretion by a rapid intravenous calcium infusion in patients with b-cell neoplasms of the pancreas. J Clin Endocrinol Metab 62:210–216

Burcharth F, Stage J, Stadil F, Jensen, Fischermann K (1979) Localization of gastrinomas by transhepatic portal catheterization and gastrin assay. Gastroenterology 77:444–450

Cherner RJ, Doppman J, Norton J et al (1986) Selective venous sampling for gastrin to localize gastrinomas: a prospective assessment. Ann Intern Med 105:841–847

Daggett PR, Goodburn EA, Kurtz AB et al (1981) Is preoperative localisation of insulinomas necessary? Lancet 8218:483–486

Deveney C, Deveney K, Way L (1978) The Zollinger-Ellison syndrome. 23 years later. Ann Surg 188:384–391

Doppman JL, Brennan MF, Dunnick NR, Kahn CR, Gorden P (1981) The role of pancreatic venous sampling in the localization of occult insulinomas. Radiology 138:557–562

Doppman JL, Miller DL, Chang R et al (1990) Gastrinomas: localization by means of selective intraarterial injection of secretin. Radiology 174:25–29

Doppman JL, Miller DL, Chang R et al (1991) Insulinoma: Localization with selective intraarterial injection of calcium. Radiology 178:237–241

Doppman JL, Chang R, Fraker D et al (1995) Localization of insulinomas to regions of the pancreas by intraarterial stimulation with calcium. Ann Intern Med 123:269–273

Doyon D, Harry G, Roche A (1979) Techniques de la portographie. In: Ecoiffier J, Tessier JP, Roche A, Fischgold H (eds) Précis de techniques spécialisées en radiodiagnositc. Masson, Paris, pp 518–520

Ellison EH, Wilson SD (1986) The Zollinger-Ellison syndrome: re-appraisal and evaluation of 260 registered cases. Ann Surg 204:468–479

Eshkar NS, Shapiro RS, Shafir M, Sung M (1995) Case report: MRI of extrapancreatic gastrinoma. Comput Med Imaging Graph 19:447–449

Fishman EK, Wyatt SH, Ney DR, Kuhlman JE, Siegelmann SS (1992) Spiral CT of the pancreas with multiplanar display. AJR 159:1209–1215

Frucht H, Doppman JL, Norton JA et al (1989) Gastrinomas: comparison of MR imaging with CT, angiography, and US. Radiology 171:713–717

Fugazzola C, Procacci C, Andreis I et al (1990) The contribution of ultrasonography and computed tomography in the diagnosis of nonfunctioning islet cell tumors of the pancreas. Gastrointest Radiol 15:139–144

Galiber AK, Reading CC, Charbonneau JW et al (1988) Localization of pancreatic insulinoma: comparison of pre and intraoperative ultrasound with CT and angiography. Radiology 166:405–408

Gehl HB, Vorwerk D, Lose KC, Guenther RW (1991) Pancreatic enhancement after low-dose infusion of Mn-DPDP. Radiology 180:337–339

Gehl HB, Urhahn R, Bohndorf K et al (1993) Mn-DPDP in MR imaging of pancreatic adenocarcinoma: initial clinical experience. Radiology 186:795–798

Gibril F, Doppmann J, Chang R, Weber H, Termanini B, Jensen R (1996) Metastatic gastrinomas: localization with selective arterial injection of secretin. Radiology 198:77–84

Gorman B, Charbonneau JW, James EM (1986) Benign pancreatic insulinoma: preoperative and intraoperative sonographic localization. AJR 147:929–934

Gunther RW (1985) Ultrasound and CT in the assessment of suspected islet-cell tumors of the pancreas. Semin Ultrasound CT MR 6:261

Hautefeuille P, Valeur P, Roche A et al (1979) Surgical cure of malignant microscopic gastrinoma. Lancet 8109:222

Heerden JAV, Grant CS, Czako PF (1992) Occult functioning insulinomas: which localizing studies are indicated? Surgery 112:1005–1010

Hoevels J, Lunderquist A, Tylen U (1978) Percutaneous transhepatic portography. Acta Radiol 19:643–655

Houlbert D, Roche A, Dorf G, Gardies A, Roche D, Segrestaa J (1984) La localisation préopératoire des insulinomes estelle nécessaire? Ann Med Interne (Paris) 13:16–20

Imamura M, Takahashi K, Isobe Y, Hattori Y, Satomura K, Tobe T (1989) Curative resection of multiple gastrinomas aided by selective arterial injection test and intraoperative secretin test. Ann Surg 210:710–718

Ingemansson S, Lunderquist A, Lundquist I, Lovdahl R, Tibblin S (1975) Portal and pancreatic vein catheterization with radioimmunologic determination of insulin. Surg Gynecol Obstet 141:705–711

Ingemansson S, Lunderquist A, Holst J (1976) Selective catheterization of the pancreatic veins for radioimmunoassay in glucagon-secreting carcinoma of the pancreas. Radiology 119:555–556

Ingemansson S, Kuhl C, Larsson L, Lunderquist A, Nobin A (1977) Islet cell hyperplasia localized by pancreatic vein catheterization and insulin radioimmunoassay. Am J Surg 133:643–645

Kallio H, Suoranta H (1979) Localization of occult insulin secreting tumors of the pancreas. Ann Surg 133:643–645

Keller F, Niles N, Rosch J, Dotter C, Stenzel-Poore M (1980) Retrograde pancreatic venography: autopsy study. Radiology 135:285–293

Klimstra DS, Rosai J, Heffess CS (1994) Mixed acinar-endocrine carcinomas of the pancreas. Am J Surg Pathol 18:765–778

Kraus BB, Ros PR (1994) Insulinoma: diagnosis with fat-suppressed MR imaging. AJR 162:69–70

Kurosaki Y, Kuramoto K, Itai Y (1996) Hyperattenuating insulinoma at unenhanced CT. Abdom Imaging 21:334–336

Lightdale CJ, Botet JF, Woodruff JM (1991) Localization of endocrine tumors of the pancreas with endoscopic ultrasonography. Cancer 68:1815–1820

London JR, Shawker TH, Doppman JL et al (1991) Zollinger-Ellison syndrome: prospective assessment of abdominal US in the localization of gastrinomas. Radiology 178:763–767

Lunderquist A, Eriksson M, Ingemansson S, Larsson L, Reichardt W (1978) Selective pancreatic vein catheterization for hormone assay in endocrine tumors of the pancreas. Cardiovasc Radiol 1:117–124
McCarthy D (1980) The place of surgery in the Zollinger-Ellison syndrome. N Engl J Med 302:1344–1347
McCown JS, Gordon L, Uflacker RP (1995) In-111 pentetreotide. Superior imaging agent for gastrinomas. Clin Nucl Med 20:896–898
Mignon M, Rigaud D, Ruszniewski P, Vallot T, Rene E, Bonfils S (1987) Le syndrome de Zollinger-Ellison. Stratégie diagnostique et thérapeutique actuelle. In: Bonfils S, Mignon M (eds) Tumeurs endocrines du pancréas. Doin, Paris, pp 37–66
Millan V, Urosa C, Militch M, Miller H, Jackson I (1979) Localization of occult insulinoma by superselective pancreatic venous sampling for insulin assay through percutaneous transhepatic catheterization. Diabetes 28:249–251
Mitchell DG, Cruvella M, Eschelman DJ, Miettinen MM, Vernick JJ (1992) MRI of pancreatic gastrinomas. J Comput Assist Tomogr 16:583–585
Mitty H, Efremidis S, Wertkin M, Dreiling D, Rayfield E (1979) Localization in insulinomas by radio-immunoassay of blood obtained by the transportal route. J Clin Endocrinol Metab 48:1035–1037
Moore NR, Rogers CE, Britton BJ (1995) Magnetic resonance imaging of endocrine tumours of the pancreas. Br J Radiol 68:341–347
Mori M, Fukuda T, Nagayoshi K et al (1996) Insulinoma: correlation of short-TI inversion-recovery (STIR) imaging and histopathologic findings. Abdom Imaging 21:337–341
Namieno T, Koito K, Uchino J (1995) Doppler color flow imaging for assessment and localization of pancreatic insulinoma. Eur J Radiol 20:208–209
Nocaudie-Calzada M, Huglo D, Deveaux M, Carnaille B, Proye C, Marchandise X (1994) Iodine-123-Tyr-3-octreotide uptake in pancreatic endocrine tumors and in carcinoids in relation to hormonal inhibition by octreotide. J Nucl Med 35:57–62
Norton JA, Cromack DT, Shawker TH (1988) Intraoperative ultrasonographic localization of islet cell tumors: a prospective comparison to palpation. Ann Surg 207:160–168
Palazzo L, Roseau G (1992) Echoendoscopie digestive. Masson, Paris
Palazzo L, Chigot JP, De Gennes JL, Paolaggi JA (1990) Apport de l'écho-endoscopie dans la localisation pré-opératoire d'un insulinome de petite taille. Presse Med 42:1947–1948
Passariello R, Rossi P, Simonetti G, Di Paolo A (1978) Cathétérisme portal transhépatique pour la localisation des tumeurs sécrétantes du pancréas. Ann Radiol 21:485–490
Passaro E (1979) Localization of pancreatic endocrine tumors by selective portal vein catheterization and radioimmunoassay. Gastroenterology 77:806–807
Pearse AGE, Takor T (1976) Neuroendocrine embryology and the APUD concept. Clin Endocrinol 5:229
Reichardt W, Cameron R (1980) Anatomy of the pancreatic veins. A post mortem and clinical phlebographic investigation. Acta Radiol 21:33–41
Reichardt W, Ingemansson S (1980) Selective vein catheterization for hormone assay in endocrine tumours of the pancreas: technique and results. Acta Radiol 21:177–187
Roche A, Raisonnier A, Gillon-Savouret M (1982) Pancreatic venous sampling and arteriography in localizing insulinomas and gastrinomas: procedure and results in 55 cases. Radiology 145:621–627
Roche A, Capeau J, Halimi P (1983) Méthodes radiologiques de localisation des tumeurs endocrines du pancréas. Gastroenterol Clin Biol 7:49–58
Rosch T, Lightdale CJ, Botet JF et al (1992) Localization of pancreatic endocrine tumors by endoscopic ultrasonography. New Engl J Med 326:1721–1726
Rossi P, Allison DJ, Bezzi M (1989) Endocrine tumors of the pancreas. Radiol Clin North Am 27:129–160
Schirmer WJ, O'Dorisio TM, Schirmer TP, Mojzisik CM, Hinkle GH, Martin EW (1993) Intraoperative localization of neuroendocrine tumors with 125I-TYR (3)-octreotiode and a hand-held gamma-detecting probe. Surgery 114:745–752
Semelka RC, Ascher SM (1993) MR imaging of the pancreas. Radiology 188:593–602
Semelka RC, Simm FC, Recht MP, Deimling M, Lenz G, Laub GA (1991) MR imaging of the pancreas at high field strength: comparison of six sequences. J Comput Assist Tomogr 15:966–971
Semelka RC, Cumming MJ, Shoenut JP et al (1993) Islet cell tumors: comparison of dynamic contrast-enhanced CT and MR imaging with dynamic gadolinium enhancement and fat suppression. Radiology 189:799–802
Smith TR, Koenigsberg M (1990) Low-density insulinoma on dynamic CT. AJR 155:995–996
Stefanini P, Carbonni M, Patrassi N, Basoli A (1974) Beta-islet cell tumors of the pancreas: results of a study on 1067 cases. Surgery 75:597–609
Steiner E, Stark DD, Hahn PF (1989) Imaging of pancreatic neoplasms: comparison of MR and CT. AJR 152:487–491
Takeshita K, Furui S, Makita K et al (1994) Cystic islet cell tumors: radiologic findings in three cases. Abdom Imaging 19:225–228
Tscholakoff D, Hricak H, Thoeni R, Winkler ML, Margulis AR (1987) MR imaging in the diagnosis of pancreatic disease. AJR 148:703–709
Turner RC, Lee EC, Morris PJ, Harris E A(1978) Localization of insulinomas. Lancet 8063:515–518
Ueno N, Tomiyama T, Tano S, Miyata T, Kimura K (1996) Contrast-enhanced color Doppler ultrasonography in diagnosis of pancreatic tumor: two case reports. J Ultrasound Med 15:527–530
Vinik A, Thompson N (1986) Controversies in the management of Zollinger-Ellison syndrome. Ann Intern Med 105:956–959

15 Adrenal Glands

M. Belaidi, J.-M. Bruel, C. Calvet, P. Chevallier, B. Padovani, J. Pradel, and J.L. Sadoul

CONTENTS

15.1 Introduction

Computed tomography (CT) currently plays a major role in assessment of the adrenal glands and related pathologies. Due to its high spatial resolution, CT can demonstrate adrenals of normal size and detect tumors as small as 1 cm. CT characterization of adrenal tumors is more difficult, however, and differentiation of malignant tumors from benign lesions remains a challenge. As a result of the development of new imaging sequences, magnetic resonance imaging (MRI) has become an increasingly valuable modality for both the detection and characterization of adrenal masses. Advances have also been made in other diagnostic techniques, in particular adrenal scintigraphy.

In addition to imaging data, establishment of the etiology of adrenal tumors requires integration of clinical data and hormone assays. Certain masses, however, are incidental findings in patients without any clinical signs of an adrenal lesion at CT performed for an unrelated condition. These "incidentalomas" involve considerable clinical problems requiring a rational diagnostic strategy for determination of their benign or malignant nature.

15.2 Hyperfunctioning Adrenal Tumors

B. Padovani, M. Belaidi, P. Chevallier, and J.L. Sadoul

15.2.1 Tumors of the Adrenal Medulla

15.2.1.1 Pheochromocytoma

The most frequent tumors of the adrenal medulla are pheochromocytomas, which arise from chromaffin cells and elaborate catecholamines. Extra-adrenal lesions along the sympathetic chain (paragangliomas) account for 10% of cases; abdominal and thoracic localizations predominate. The majority of pheochromocytomas (90%) are sporadic, but they are also encountered in endocrine disorders such as multiple endocrine neoplasia (MEN) type II and neurofibromatosis. Multiple tumors are found in 10% of patients, and between 3% and 13% are malignant. Malignant tumors are reportedly more frequent in patients with MEN, as are multicentric

M. Belaidi, B. Padovani, Service de Radiodiagnostic, Hôpital Pasteur, 30 avenue de la Voie Romaine, BP 69, 06002 Nice, France
J. M. Bruel, C. Calvet, Service d'Imagerie Médicale, Hôpital Saint-Eloi, Avenue Bertin Sans, 34295 Monpellier, France
P. Chevallier, Service de Radiodiagnostic, Hôpital de l'Archet, 151 chemin de St. Antoine de Ginestière, 06200 Nice, France
J. Pradel, Service de Radiologie, Centre Hospitalier, BP 718, 10000 Troyes, France
J. L. Sadoul, Service de Diabétologie et d'Ondocrinologie, Hôpital Pasteur, 30 avenue de la Voie Romaine, BP 69, 06002 Nice, France

and bilateral lesions (SHEPS et al. 1990). Diagnosis of malignant pheochromocytomas is difficult owing to the absence of specific criteria; diagnosis thus relies essentially on demonstration of related metastases.

The clinical manifestations of pheochromocytomas reflect raised catecholamine secretion and are identical for benign and malignant lesions. Persistent or intermittent hypertension is almost constant and may be associated with cardiac shock, which explains the severity of these tumors. Biochemical assays of serum catecholamines and their urinary metabolites (vanillylmandelic acid, metanephrines) allow diagnosis. Imaging studies are performed to localize the tumor and search for metastases. The difficulties encountered are related to the possibility of extra-adrenal and multiple tumors. Several imaging modalities, e.g., CT, MRI, iodine-131 meta-iodobenzylguanidine (MIBG) scintigraphy, may thus be required to assess the entire abdominal and pelvic cavity (as well as other sites if initial studies are negative) (VELCHIK et al. 1989; PRADEL et al. 1990). Imaging may be prompted by symptoms related to excessive catecholamine secretion or be performed during systematic workup of patients with MEN type II.

Ultrasonography may demonstrate large pheochromocytomas, but remains less effective than CT for evaluation of the adrenal glands. The sonographic features of pheochromocytomas are highly variable; solid, cystic, and mixed tumors have all been described (SCHWERK et al. 1994). Ultrasound is helpful primarily for hepatic examination in search of metastases when a malignant pheochromocytoma is suspected.

CT readily demonstrates adrenal pheochromocytomas (WELCH et al. 1983), which are typically larger than 3 cm and sometimes reach 20 cm in diameter. The CT appearance varies considerably, but is often a well-delimited mass with a cystic component or a necrotic center that enhances intensely after intravenous iodinated contrast administration (WELCH et al. 1983; FRANCIS et al. 1992; Fig. 15.1). More homogeneous patterns and moderate contrast enhancement are also seen. Intravenous contrast injection occasionally triggers a hypertensive crisis; use of a nonionic contrast medium appears to significantly reduce this risk (MUCKERJEE et al. 1997). Signs of malignancy include invasion of a renal vascular pedicle and the presence of satellite nodal or regional metastases (especially hepatic metastases). If adrenal studies are negative, the entire abdominal and pelvic cavity should be scanned to search for an extra-adrenal pheochromocytoma.

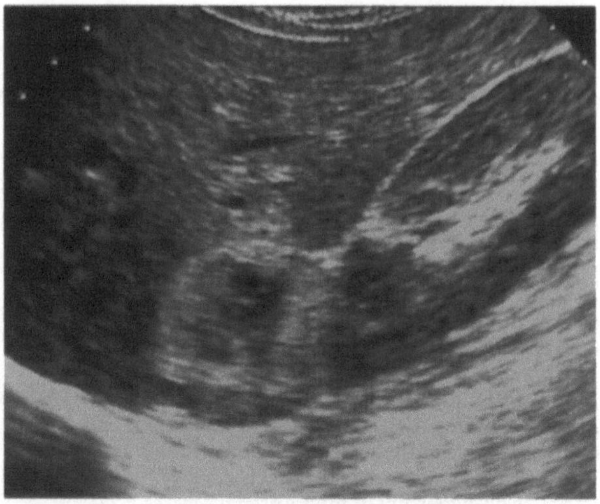

a

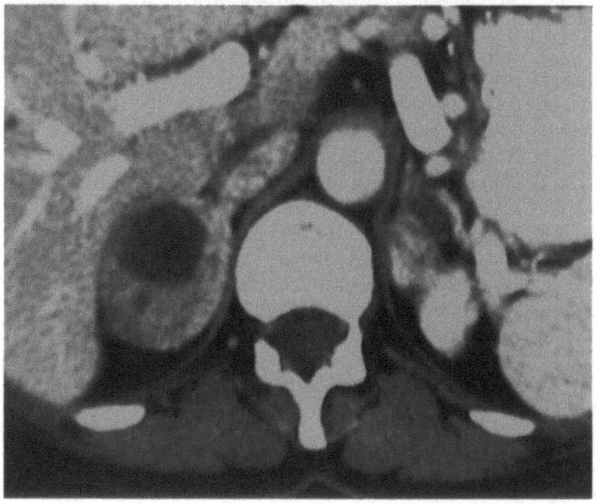

b

Fig. 15.1a,b. Right adrenal pheochromocytoma. **a** Longitudinal sonogram: heterogeneous adrenal mass (hyperechoic periphery, cystic center). **b** Contrast-enhanced CT revealed peripheral enhancement and confirmed the cystic nature of the central zone

Magnetic resonance imaging has acquired an important role for assessment of pheochromocytomas. Along with a sensitivity for their detection comparable to that of CT (QUINT et al. 1987; VELCHIK et al. 1989; VAN GILS et al. 1991), MRI has two advantages: (1) it does not require injection of an iodinated contrast material, which may precipitate a hypertensive crisis, and (2) it provides better tissue characterization. On T_1-weighted short-echo (SE) sequences, pheochromocytomas have a low-intensity signal that is slightly lower than that of the liver. On T_2-weighted SE sequences, these lesions typically have an extremely intense signal that allows differentiation from other adrenal masses (FINK et al. 1985; VAN GILS et al. 1991; LEE et al. 1994a; Fig. 15.2). However,

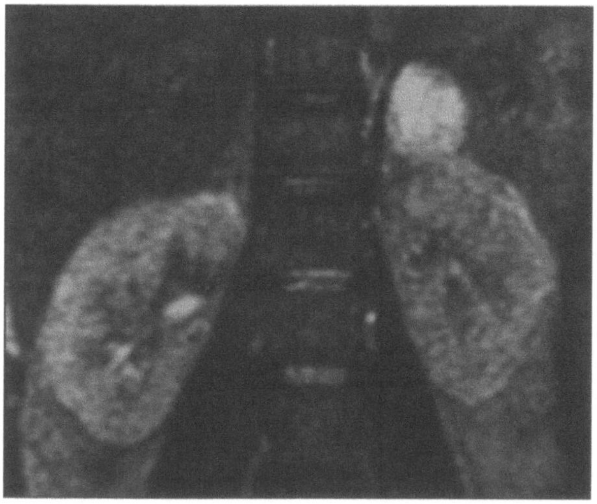

Fig. 15.2. Coronal T_2-weighted sequence (TR, 2000; TE, 80) depicted an extremely hyperintense mass corresponding to a left adrenal pheochromocytoma

there have been several reports of pheochromocytomas with an atypical signal (LEE et al. 1994a,b). As with CT, gadolinium administration produces marked, rapid, and transient enhancement (FRESTIN et al. 1991; VAN GILS et al. 1991; FRANCIS et al. 1992; LEE et al. 1994b). When CT is negative, coronal T_2-weighted SE sequences are particularly interesting to search for extra-adrenal localizations in the abdominopelvic cavity or the thorax, especially in the paravertebral and paracardiac regions (PEPPERCORN and REZNEK 1997). Hepatic and bone metastases are also reliably depicted by MRI.

MIBG scintigraphy also has a high sensitivity for the demonstration of extra-adrenal and/or multiple pheochromocytomas that are difficult to detect by CT. Radionuclide scanning is particularly useful for detection of secondary malignant localizations and recurrence after surgical resection (SISSON et al. 1981; SHAPIRO et al. 1984).

15.2.1.2 Neuroblastoma

Most prevalent in children from 1 to 6 years of age, neuroblastomas are rare in adults. Seventy percent arise in the adrenal medulla; those involving the paravertebral sympathetic chain are referred to as sympathicoblastomas. Clinical manifestations may consist in an abdominal mass, an alteration in general condition, or symptoms of metastatic disease that can delay the diagnosis. These frequently large tumors infiltrate the retroperitoneum, encase the vessels, and often penetrate the extradural space of the spinal canal through the intervertebral formina. Intracanal extension is more frequent with sympathicoblastomas than with adrenal neuroblastomas. Metastases are frequent, essentially to bone, the bone marrow, and occasionally the liver. Hepatomegaly due to metastatic spread from the adrenal medulla to the liver is referred to as Pepper's syndrome.

Neuroblastomas nearly always secrete catecholamines; this allows diagnosis by serum and urinary assays of their catabolites and by MIBG scintigraphy. The prognosis depends on tumor stage and histologic type. Most neuroblastomas are metastatic from the outset. Survival at 3 years is 40%–60% for tumors with metastases or distant nodal extension. Treatment (surgery, chemotherapy) depends on the tumor stage defined by imaging. Stage I is confined to the organ of origin. Stage II extends into adjacent structures but does not extend beyond the midline; ipsilateral nodes are invaded. Stage III crosses the midline and/or involves the contralateral nodes. Stage IV is a tumor with distant metastasis. Imaging thus has a dual role: localization of the tumor and comprehensive disease staging.

Abdominal plain films may demonstrate a large retroperitoneal mass. Half of all cases contain calcifications. Displacement of the paravertebral line reflects nodal spread towards the posterior inframediastinal space.

Ultrasound demonstrates a relatively well-circumscribed mass at the upper pole of the kidney that may infiltrate the medial retroperitoneum by encasing the vascular structures (aorta and inferior vena cava). The echotexture is inhomogeneous, containing hyperechoic zones and occasionally calcifications. When the mass cannot be distinguished from the upper pole of the kidney, differential diagnosis from nephroblastoma is difficult. Ultrasound is also extremely helpful for demonstration of hepatic metastases.

MRI has acquired an important role for the diagnosis and staging of neuroblastomas (DIETRICH et al. 1987; WESTRA et al. 1994), as it allows comprehensive evaluation of lymphadenopathy, tumor relations with the retroperitoneal vessels, possible intraspinal extension, and any bone or hepatic metastases. CT is currently less useful. Post-therapy surveillance is performed by ultrasound and MRI.

15.2.2
Tumors of the Adrenal Cortex

15.2.2.1
Primary Aldosteronism (Conn's Syndrome)

Excessive aldosterone secretion may be due to a benign aldosterone-secreting adrenal adenoma (70%–80% of patients) or bilateral adrenal hyperplasia. Differentiation of these two etiologies is essential because functioning adenomas can be cured surgically, whereas bilateral adrenal hyperplasia is managed medically. Primary aldosteronism manifests as hypertension associated with hypokalemia and metabolic alkalosis. Diagnosis is made by plasma aldosterone assays.

Ultrasound is of little benefit because lesions are usually smaller than 30 mm (mean, 15 mm), and 15%–20% of adrenal adenomas are smaller than 10 mm (Ikeda et al. 1989; Young et al. 1990). CT provides excellent delineation of adrenal morphology even though it is much less effective for the detection of adenomas than for pheochromocytomas. Its sensitivity is satisfactory, however, ranging from 82% to 88% (Ikeda et al. 1989; Dunnick et al. 1993). Aldosteronomas are usually small nodules of low attenuation that enhance discretely after contrast administration.

CT of bilateral adrenal hyperplasia may reveal normal-appearing glands, increased thickness of both glands, or deformation of gland contours by multiple small nodules varying in size from several millimeters to 2 cm (Fig. 15.3). Differentation of an aldosteronoma from bilateral adrenal hyperplasia can be difficult; for example, a macronodule within an enlarged adrenal gland may be confused with an adrenal adenoma. Similarly, etiologic diagnosis may be difficult when a functioning adrenal adenoma is associated with a nonfunctioning adenoma in the contralateral gland.

Although less sensitive than CT, MRI is reportedly more specific for differentiation of a unilateral adenoma from bilateral adrenal hyperplasia (Rossi et al. 1993).

When findings are equivocal, other examinations may prove helpful to distinguish between an adrenal adenoma and bilateral adrenal hyperplasia. Iodine-131-6-iodomethyl-19-norcholesterol (NP-59) scintigraphy reveals unilateral uptake by adenomas and bilateral uptake in the case of hyperplasia. Adrenal venous sampling of aldosterone in the right and left adrenal veins may assist diagnosis of indeterminate lesions (Doppman and Gill 1996).

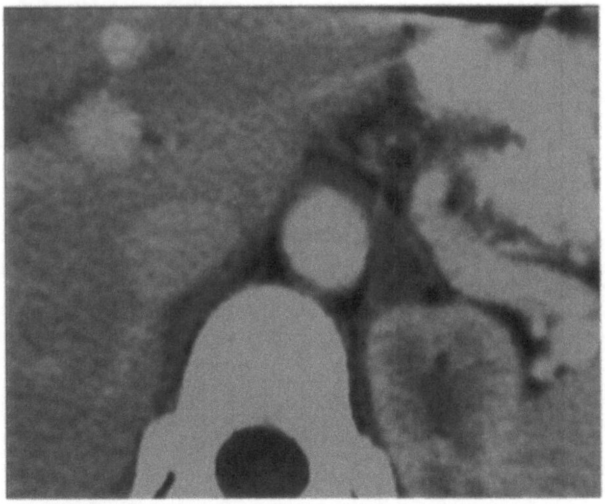

Fig. 15.3. Contrast-enhanced CT revealed a discretely enhancing 15-mm nodule in the left adrenal gland: Conn adenoma

15.2.2.2
Hypercortisolism (Cushing's Syndrome)

Only 30% of all cases of Cushing's syndrome are related to an adrenal tumor. Iatrogenic (corticosteroid therapy) and endogenous causes (excessive adrenocorticotropic hormone (ACTH) secretion by a pituitary adenoma or ectopic secretion) are much more frequent. Bronchial and thymic carcinoids, pancreatic endocrine tumors, and medullary thyroid carcinoma are the main sources of ectopic ACTH secretion. Adrenal anomalies such as bilateral macronodular hyperplasia are present in 15% of patients with ACTH-dependent Cushing's syndrome (Doppman et al. 1988). Cortical macronodular hyperplasia may be confused with true adrenal adenomas, especially if macronodules predominate in one of the glands.

Two primary adrenal tumors can cause ACTH-independent Cushing's syndrome: adrenocortical adenoma and adrenocortical carcinoma.

Adrenocortical adenomas are responsible for 10%–20% of all cases of Cushing's syndrome. These benign tumors are typically smaller than 5 cm (mean, 2.5 cm) and have a wide variety of nonspecific features on CT and MRI (Lee et al. 1994b). Large adenomas may involve problems for differential diagnosis from carcinoma.

Primary adrenocortical carcinomas are rare entities that account for only 0.02% of all malignant tumors. There is a slight female predominance, and peak incidence for diagnosis is in the 40- to 50-year age-group. Excessive hormone secretion occurs in

50%–75% of patients. Functioning tumors are more frequent in women and in young patients (SAMAAN and HICKEY 1987); most secrete excessive cortisol responsible for Cushing's syndrome, but others secrete androgens (in particular in children), estrogens, or even aldosterone. Nonfunctioning adrenocortical carcinomas usually manifest at a later stage as weight loss, asthenia, and a palpable abdominal mass in 50% of cases. These tumors are serious owing to their propensity for local invasion and metastatic spread (liver, lungs, bone, brain). After surgical resection, survival rates at 5 and 10 years are 30% and 10%, respectively (DUNNICK 1994). Characterization on the basis of cytologic features is often difficult, making diagnosis by percutaneous aspiration biopsy illusory. Capsular or venous invasion is the principal sign of malignancy. One of the aims of imaging is to predict the malignant nature of an adrenal mass by searching for signs of invasion of adjacent organs.

Ultrasound readily visualizes these large adrenal tumors, which image as an inhomogeneous mass containing hypoechoic areas of necrosis or hemorrhagic foci. A tumoral capsule is sometimes visible as a hyperechoic peripheral rim (HAMPER et al. 1987). Ultrasound can helpfully demonstrate the mass's relations with the kidney and adjacent structures. The absence of invasion can be predicted when a peritumoral fat plane persists, especially when the adrenal mass moves independently of the adjacent organs during respiration (DUNNICK 1994).

CT easily detects these tumors, which are usually larger than 6 cm in diameter (FISHMAN et al. 1987). Large lesions can reach up to 25 cm and involve problems for localization to the adrenal gland. These well-delimited, heterogeneous masses may have a peripheral capsule that enhances after contrast injection. Nonenhancing areas of hemorrhage or necrosis are common (DUNNICK et al. 1982). Microcalcifications are observed in 30% of patients. Certain lesions are homogeneous, however, and mimic an adenoma (FISHMAN et al. 1987); this is particularly true for small tumors between 3 and 6 cm in diameter. In practice, this is not very important, because all adrenal masses in patients with ACTH-independent Cushing's syndrome are managed surgically (Fig. 15.4).

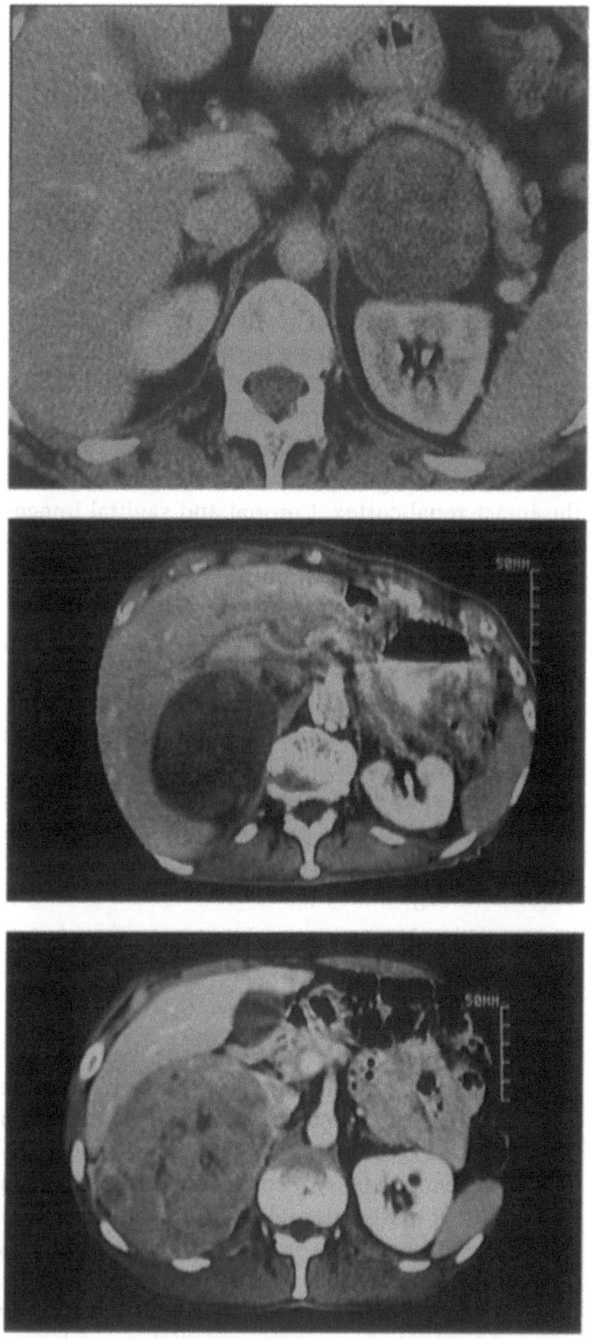

a b c

Fig. 15.4a–c. CT appearances in Cushing's syndrome. a Large, discretely heterogeneous mass in the left adrenal gland without invasion of adjacent structures: an adrenal adenoma was found at surgery. b Large right adrenal mass displacing the adjacent organs: an adrenal carcinoma was found at surgery. c Extremely heterogeneous mass in the right adrenal gland invading the inferior vena cava: adrenal carcinoma

CT can also readily demonstrate invasion of adjacent organs. The persistence of peritumoral fat planes permits affirmation of the absence of extension, but disappearance of these planes does not affirm local invasion. Tumor spread to the renal vein or the inferior vena cava manifests as tumor thrombus or vascular wall enhancement. Accurate depiction of the upper limit of intracaval extension (which may extend to the right atrium) can be difficult (DUNNICK 1994). Retroperitoneal lymphadenopathy and distant metastases should be sought systematically, particularly in the liver and lungs.

MRI is useful when a doubt persists after CT concerning disease spread to adjacent organs. Adrenocortical carcinomas are hypointense on T_1-weighted sequences and are often extremely hyperintense on T_2-weighted sequences; this may cause problems for differential diagnosis from a pheochromocytoma (Smith et al. 1989). Schlund et al. (1995) defined the major MRI features of these tumors as being central necrosis, enhancing peripheral nodules, and central areas of hemorrhage that are readily detected on T_1-weighted fat suppression sequences. Sagittal scans are more useful than coronal views to affirm the extrarenal origin of the tumor by demonstrating the intact renal cortex. Coronal and sagittal images can accurately demonstrate contiguous spread to the liver and the kidney and into the vena cava. MRI is more effective than CT for demonstration of the upper limit of tumor thrombus (Francis et al. 1992; Dunnick 1994), but complementary venacavography may be useful for accurate determination when surgery is indicated. T_2-weighted sequences are helpful for detection of hepatic metastases.

Arteriography no longer has many indications, but may be helpful for preoperative vascular mapping or when difficulties occur in determining the origin of a large tumor (Kolmannskog et al. 1992).

15.2.2.3
Excessive Androgen Secretion

Excessive androgen secretion is rare and may be due to congenital adrenal hyperplasia or hypersecretion by an adrenal carcinoma. Congenital adrenal hyperplasia (adrenogenital syndrome) is a rare entity seen essentially in newborns and children. An inborn error in the enzyme 11b- or 22-hydroxylase, which is responsible for cortisol and aldosterone production, leads to excessive ACTH secretion and secondarily adrenal hyperplasia, causing a virilizing syndrome. Sonography reveals bilateral symmetrical enlargement and thickening of the adrenal glands. Transformation into adenoma may occur if the diagnosis is not made early enough.

15.3
Non-hyperfunctioning Adrenal Masses

Adenomas and metastases account for the majority of non-hyperfunctioning adrenal masses.

15.3.1
Non-hyperfunctioning Adenomas

Non-hyperfunctioning adenomas are common benign tumors that are found in 2%–3% of autopsies and 0.5%–1% of all patients examined by abdominal CT (Glazer et al. 1982). This discrepancy is explained by the low spatial resolution of CT for detection of nodules less than 1 cm in diameter. Most non-hyperfunctioning adrenal adenomas are asymptomatic and are incidental discoveries during CT performed for another reason. The diagnostic difficulties with these "incidentalomas" are discussed at the end of this chapter.

At CT, non-hyperfunctioning adrenal adenomas are small (usually less than 3 cm), sharply marginated, rounded homogeneous masses (Dunnick 1990). Their CT density is often less than 10 HU and sometimes below 0 HU. In the study by Lee et al. (1991), the mean unenhanced CT density of adrenal adenomas was −2.2 HU±16.0. Low lesion density has been attributed to a high lipid content (Fig. 15.5). Miyake et al. (1995) compared adenomas with nonadenomatous tumors; in their study, all asymptomatic homogeneous adrenal masses less than 4 cm with a low density (less than 15 HU) were nonfunctioning adenomas. These tumors enhance little, if at all, after injection of iodinated contrast medium.

At MRI, these adenomas have a weak signal similar to the liver on T_2-weighted SE sequences (Lee et al. 1994b). However, certain non-hyperfunctioning adenomas have a higher signal. Gadolinium-enhanced dynamic T_1-weighted fast gradient-echo

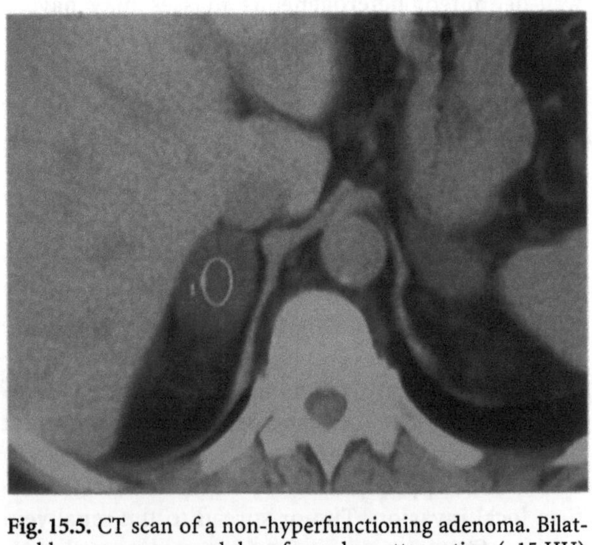

Fig. 15.5. CT scan of a non-hyperfunctioning adenoma. Bilateral homogeneous nodules of very low attenuation (−15 HU)

sequences typically demonstrate minimal enhancement (KRESTIN et al. 1989). New sequences capable of characterizing adenomas by demonstrating their lipid content (chemical-shift MRI) have shown excellent specificity (MITCHELL et al. 1992; TSUSHIMA et al. 1993; BILBEY et al. 1995; MAYO-SMITH et al. 1995; OUTWATER et al. 1995; KOROBKIN et al. 1996b). The major aim of these new sequences is to differentiate nonfunctioning adenomas from adrenal metastases.

15.3.2 Adrenal Metastases

The adrenal glands are one of the most common sites of metastatic disease after the lungs, the liver, and bone. Lung, kidney, and breast carcinomas and melanoma are the most common primaries. Adrenal metastases of bronchial cancers have been found in 35%–38% of autopsy series. Bilateral involvement occurs in 30% of patients. Adrenal metastases are usually asymptomatic and are discovered during disease staging for a primary neoplasm. However, nearly 50% of all adrenal tumors discovered in patients with a primary cancer are benign (OLIVER et al. 1984; KATZ and SHIRKHODA1985). Imaging is thus performed not only to detect the adrenal mass, but also to determine its benign or malignant nature.

Ultrasound can detect metastases that are at least 3 cm in diameter. However, the often hypoechoic ultrasound pattern is not very specific and depends on both lesion size and any associated necrosis or hemorrhage.

CT is the technique of choice for detection of adrenal metastases (GLAZER et al. 1988; DUNNICK 1990; FRANCIS et al. 1992). CT features suggestive of metastasis include size greater than 5 cm, inhomogeneous attenuation, irregular margins, and an irregular enhancing rim with a hypodense center (HUSSAIN et al. 1985). Small, sharply marginated homogeneous metastases may mimic a nonfunctioning adenoma. Nevertheless, size remains an interesting diagnostic criterion. In the study by CANDEL et al. (1993), 87% of the adrenal masses smaller than 3 cm were benign, while 95% of those larger than 3 cm were malignant. LEE et al. (1991) proposed use of the mean unenhanced CT attenuation value to distinguish a metastasis from a nonfunctioning adenoma. In their study, the mean CT attenuation of malignant lesions was 28.9 HU±10.6, whereas adenomas are usually between 0 and 10 HU. The presence of coexistent metastases in other sites also suggests the metastatic nature of an adrenal nodule. The benign or malignant nature of the adrenal mass is of little importance in such cases because the lesion does not modify the therapeutic approach (Fig. 15.6).

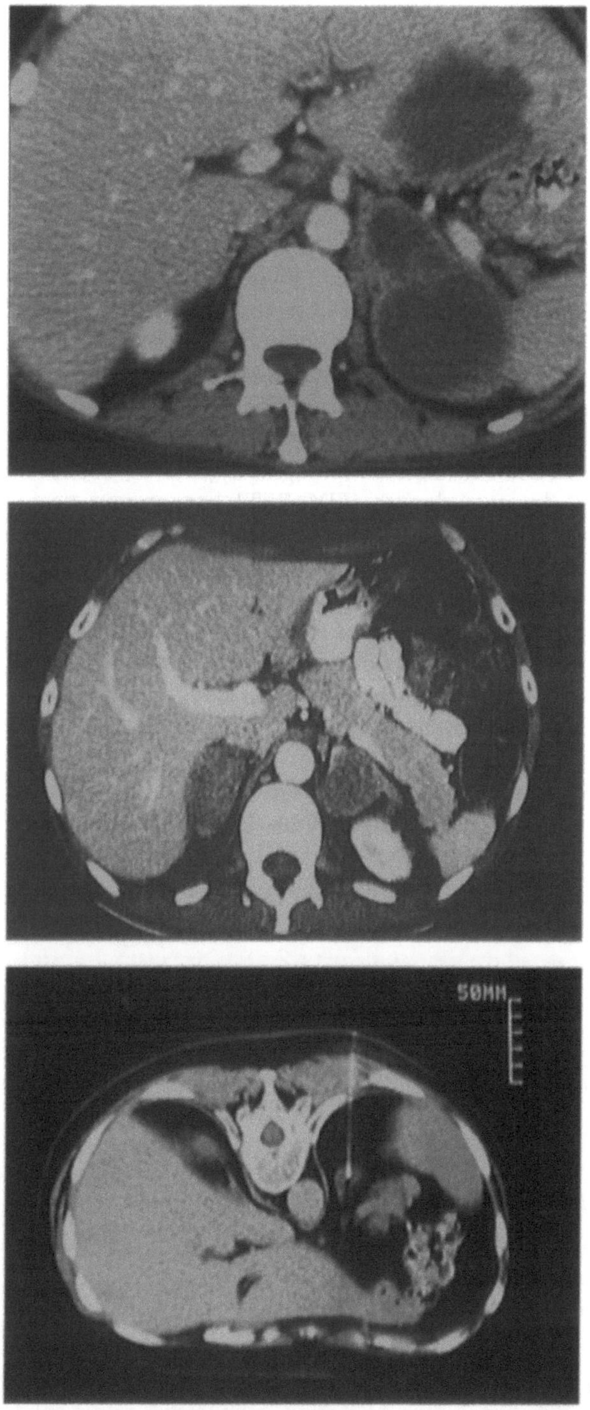

a

b

c

Fig. 15.6a–c. CT appearances of adrenal metastases. **a** Large necrotic mass in the left adrenal gland associated with hepatic metastases. **b** Bilateral adrenal metastases of bronchial cancer. **c** Percutaneous biopsy of a small adrenal nodule in a patient with bronchial cancer: adrenal metastasis

MRI can refine tissue characterization of adrenal metastases (Glazer et al. 1986; Reinig et al. 1986; Chezmar et al. 1988; Kier and McCarthy 1989). These lesions have a low-intensity signal similar to the liver or muscle on T_1-weighted sequences and a high-intensity signal greater than that of the liver on T_2-weighted sequences (Fig. 15.7). However, 20%–30% of all adrenal metastases have a lower signal intensity close to that of nonfunctioning adenomas on T_2-weighted sequences. Gadolinium injection during fast gradient-echo sequences typically demonstrates strong signal enhancement (Krestin et al. 1989). Variations in contrast uptake are common, however, and enhancement of adrenal lesions during contrast injection does not allow differentiation of benign and malignant tumors (Semelka et al. 1993; Reinig et al. 1994). Chemical-shift MRI appears more specific for differentiation of metastases from adenomas.

Positron emission tomography with 2-[^{F}18]fluoro-2-deoxy-D-glucose (FDG-PET) has proven useful for workup of adrenal masses in cancer patients (Boland et al. 1995).

CT-guided percutaneous biopsy of adrenal nodules remains indicated in numerous circumstances to confirm or rule out a metastatic nature. Material obtained with narrow needles (19–21 gauge) is usually sufficient (diagnostic accuracy, 85%–93%) (Welch et al. 1994). However, a negative biopsy does not exclude a metastasis and may justify repeat biopsy. Major complications (pneumothorax, hemorrhage) occur in 2.8%–3.6% of patients and are essentially related to the approach (transhepatic, anterior, posterior transpleural). The main indication for percutaneous adrenal biopsy is a mass discovered during initial workup of a primary malignancy that remains indeterminate after imaging studies, because the nature of the adrenal mass may modify the therapeutic approach in such cases (Robert et al. 1994).

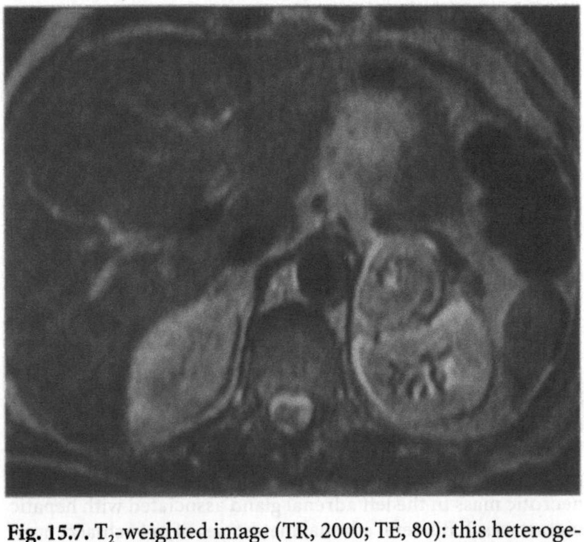

Fig. 15.7. T_2-weighted image (TR, 2000; TE, 80): this heterogeneous mass in the left adrenal gland hyperintense to the liver corresponds to a metastasis

15.3.3 Adrenocortical Carcinomas

The appearance of malignant adrenal cortex tumors has already been discussed in connection with functioning tumors. Nearly one third of adrenocortical carcinomas are nonfunctioning. Their morphologic features are comparable to those of functioning tumors, but they are often larger at diagnosis owing to their asymptomatic nature, which delays discovery until a later stage.

15.3.4 Myelolipomas

Myelolipomas are uncommon benign tumors arising from the adrenal cortex that are composed of variable proportions of mature fat and myeloid tissue. The majority are asymptomatic and are discovered during CT performed for another purpose. Large lesions may cause pain, however, or be associated with retroperitoneal hemorrhage.

Sonographically, these lesions are highly echogenic if the fat component predominates (Musante et al. 1988). Hypoechoic myeloid zones and areas of hyperechoic fat are frequent (Cyran et al. 1996).

CT diagnosis of myelolipomas is based on demonstration of areas of fat attenuation within an adrenal mass. These regions of fat may be difficult to demonstrate if the myeloid component predominates or if intratumoral hemorrhage is present. These tumors often have a peritumoral capsule and may contain calcification (Cyran et al. 1996). Small regions of fat are not pathognomonic for myelolipoma, however, as they have also been described for certain rare adenomas (Sato et al. 1995) and adenocarcinomas (Ferrozzi and Bova 1995). Localization of large myelolipomas to the adrenal gland can involve problems for differential diagnosis from other fat-containing retroperitoneal tumors (lipoma, liposarcoma, renal angiomyolipoma) (Fig. 15.8).

At MRI, the fatty tissue is easily recognized by its high signal intensity on T_1-weighted images, compa-

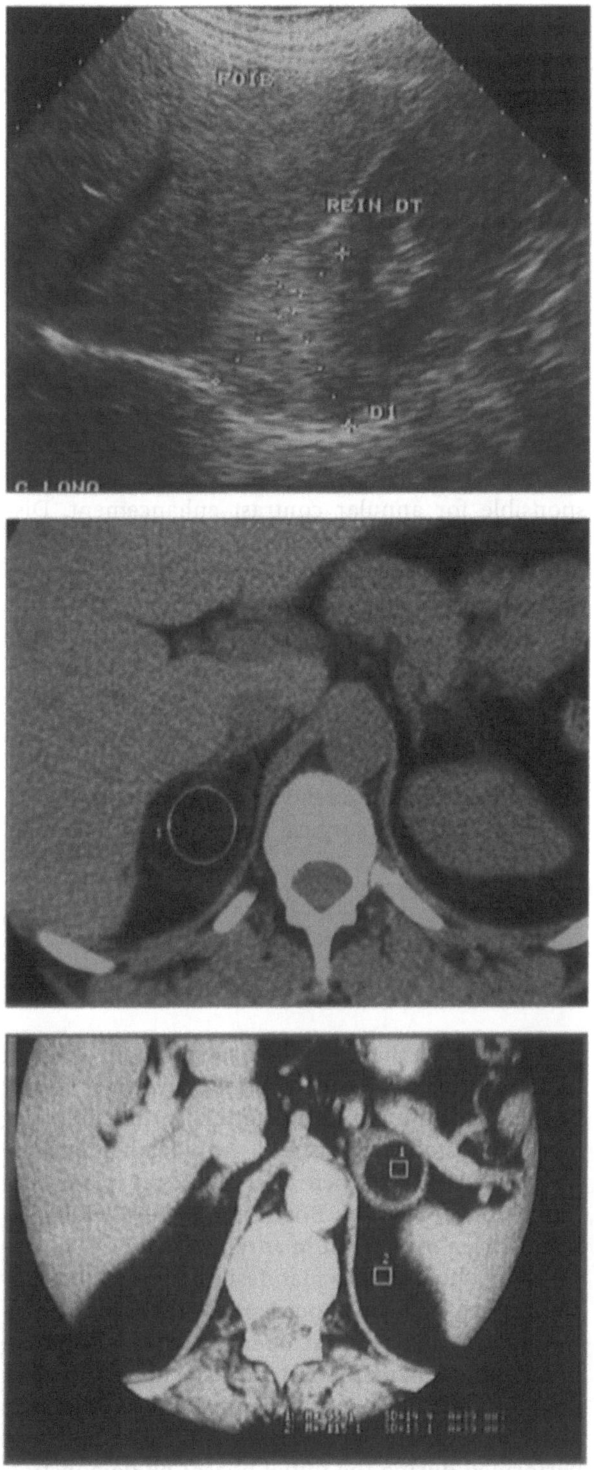

a

b

c

Fig. 15.8a–c. Adrenal myelolipoma. **a** Longitudinal sonogram: homogeneously hyperechoic mass in the right adrenal gland. **b** CT (same patient as Fig. 15.8a): the right adrenal mass has a predominant fat density (–78 HU). **c** CT depiction of a large, central fat component in the tumor of another patient

rable to that of the subcutaneous or retroperitoneal fat (Cyran et al. 1996). Fat suppression sequences can confirm the presence of fat by demonstrating a signal loss in the mass. Tumors with a high fat component can be difficult to distinguish from the adjacent retroperitoneal fat by either CT or MRI, because they have the same CT attenuation and signal intensity.

15.3.5 Adrenal Cysts

Cystic adrenal lesions are uncommon entities with a predilection for females. Size varies from several millimeters to over 20 cm; bilateral cysts occur in 8%–10% of patients. Four histologic types have been described: endothelial cysts (lymphangiomas or, more rarely, hemangiomas), which predominate, epithelial cysts, parasitic cysts, and pseudocysts. Pseudocysts are considered secondary to adrenal hemorrhage. Adrenal cysts are usually asymptomatic.

Ultrasound demonstrates a thin-walled cystic mass with a fluid echotexture. CT characteristically demonstrates a nonenhancing water-density mass. Peripheral calcification may be present, particularly in pseudocysts; wall calcification was observed in 69% of the lesions examined by Rozenblit et al. (1996). Central calcification is less common (19% of cases). Rim-like enhancement of the cyst wall is frequent. The cyst wall may be very thin or up to 3 mm thick. Intracystic hemorrhage may modify the CT pattern and justify surgery (Fig. 15.9).

MRI is of little interest for these cystic lesions, but can confirm their fluid nature by demonstrating a low signal intensity mass on T_1-weighted sequences and a hyperintense mass on T_2-weighted images. Atypical cystic lesions with thick or irregular walls and cysts containing nodular zones can involve diagnostic problems, in particular for differentiation from cystic adrenal carcinoma. Like symptomatic and hemorrhagic adrenal cysts, these atypical lesions warrant surgical resection.

Percutaneous fluid aspiration has been advocated for indeterminate cystic lesions to allow cytologic analysis (Rozenblit et al. 1996). However, the possibility of a cystic pheochromocytoma should be ruled out first by hormone assays.

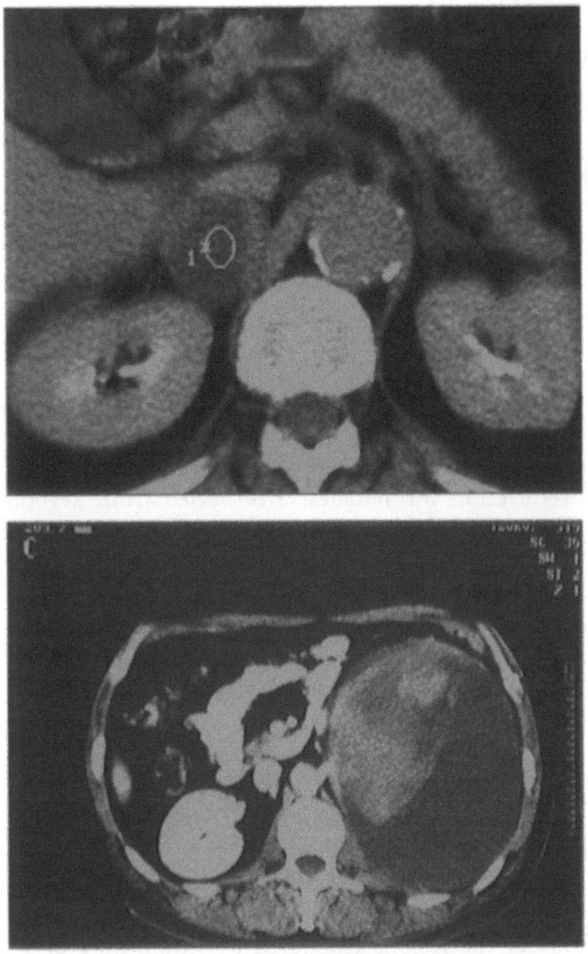

a

b

Fig. 15.9a,b. Adrenal cysts. **a** Contrast-enhanced CT revealed a thick-walled right adrenal mass with a fluid-density center: adrenal pseudocyst. **b** CT scan of a large heterogeneous retroperitoneal mass with a large cystic component: cystic adrenal lymphangioma

15.3.6
Adrenal Lymphomas

Involvement of the adrenal glands in Non-Hodgkin lymphoma (NHL) is frequent (of the order of 25% in autopsy series) (Alvarez-Castells et al. 1993). Contiguous spread from retroperitoneal nodes is the predominant mode, but specific involvement of the adrenal gland is also possible. Adrenal involvement by Hodgkin's disease is very rare. Primary adrenal lymphomas corresponding to isolated adrenal disease are exceptional. A solitary lesion may also represent a post-therapy recurrence of NHL. Imaging features are nonspecific. Ultrasound usually reveals a hypoechoic tissue mass (Vicks et al. 1987). On CT (Paling and Williamson 1983), the mass is typically homogeneous, well circumscribed, often hypodense, and enhances discretely after contrast injection. During chemotherapy, a zone of necrosis may rapidly appear within the adrenal mass. MRI features are similar to those for adrenal metastases. An adrenal mass that does not respond to treatment for an otherwise chemosensitive NHL requires imaging-guided aspiration biopsy to rule out another adrenal pathology.

15.3.7
Rare Adrenal Tumors

Cavernous hemangiomas of the adrenal gland (Boraschi et al. 1995) are often large, asymptomatic lesions. CT depicts peripheral hypervascularity responsible for annular contrast enhancement. Disseminated calcifications have been described in some patients and are linked to the presence of phlebolytes.

Adrenocortical oncocytoma is extremely rare (Gandras et al. 1996). The literature contains only eight cases of these large tumors (over 5 cm) without necrosis or hemorrhage. They have no specific features allowing differentiation from other adrenal tumors (adenoma, adenocarcinoma, metastasis). Diagnosis requires surgical resection and histologic analysis.

15.3.8
Hemorrhagic Adrenal Masses

Adrenal hemorrhage may occur spontaneously in infants during the perinatal period; in adults, it may be related to trauma, hemostatic disorders, septicemia, or postoperative stress. Adrenal hemorrhage has also been described after liver transplantation (Solomon et al. 1988; Bowen et al. 1990). Bilateral hemorrhage may result in adrenal failure.

At CT, these lesions manifest as a poorly marginated, spontaneously hyperdense adrenal mass infiltrating the adjacent retroperitoneal fat. After an initial period, hematomas tend to be hypodense and then disappear or persist as a pseudocyst. MRI may assist diagnosis (especially when CT has not been performed during the initial phase) by demonstrating diffuse or annular hyperintensity on T_1-weighted sequences. This high signal intensity is related to the paramagnetic effect of methemoglobin. This feature may be absent in very early (presence of oxyhemoglobin) or very late phases (when hemosiderin deposits are present).

15.4 Adrenal Incidentalomas

Adrenal masses may be fortuitous findings during examinations performed in patients without any clinical evidence of an adrenal lesion. The increasingly frequent indications for abdominal CT and the elevated number of asymptomatic adrenal lesions explain the frequency of such incidentalomas. The diagnostic strategy must be aimed at determining whether the tumor is benign or malignant, keeping in mind the fact that most adrenal incidentalomas are nonfunctioning adenomas.

In the absence of any known malignancy, the first step after incidental discovery of an adrenal mass consists in clinical investigations to confirm the absence of a neoplastic process and biochemical profiles in search of excess hormone secretion. If these studies do not provide useful information, diagnosis relies on imaging findings. Infrequent tumors such as myelolipomas and cysts can be characterized by CT densitometry. The diagnostic problem in most cases is to distinguish a nonfunctioning adenoma from a malignant tumor (especially a prevalent metastasis) or, on occasion, a nonfunctioning adrenocortical adenoma.

At CT, two essential criteria must be analyzed: tumor size and density. Lesions smaller than 3 cm with a low density (less than 10 HU on unenhanced CT) in all likelihood correspond to a nonfunctioning adenoma and may merely be kept under surveillance. Lesions larger than 6 cm have a much greater risk of malignancy and warrant surgical resection. The imaging strategy for lesions between 3 and 6 cm depends on clinical data (age, general condition), CT densitometry (unenhanced CT attenuation value, homogeneity), and chemical-shift MRI. Comparison of clinical data and imaging findings should facilitate decisions on whether to orient the patient toward mere surveillance, percutaneous aspiration biopsy, or surgical resection. McNicholas et al. (1995) developed an imaging algorithm for differential diagnosis of adrenal adenomas and metastases based solely on the noncontrast CT density: lesions below 0 HU were considered benign, while tumors over 20 HU were considered malignant and biopsy was proposed. Lesions with a noncontrast CT density between 0 and 20 HU were considered indeterminate and were referred for chemical-shift MRI.

15.5 Diagnostic Value of Computed Tomography and Magnetic Resonance Imaging

J.M. Bruel, C. Calvet, and J. Pradel

Noninvasive characterization of adrenal tumors has been one of the major aims of clinical research in medical imaging over the past 15 years. Such intensive interest can be explained primarily by the elevated frequency of these lesions. In a Mayo Clinic review of over 60,000 consecutive CT examinations, an adrenal mass was found in 3.4% of all patients (Herrera et al. 1991). In hospital populations, this high percentage is explained essentially by the frequency of adrenal metastases, because the adrenal glands are one of the main sites of metastatic disease, in particular from bronchial, renal, breast, and digestive cancers. Confirmation of the metastatic nature of an adrenal mass in an oncologic patient does not always have an impact on management, especially in cases of multiorgan metastatic disease. Confirmation may be crucial, however, when the therapeutic approach, and namely the decision to perform surgical resection, depends on whether the adrenal mass is really a metastasis. This is the case when no other secondary localization is found and when there are no local or systemic contraindications for surgery.

Nonhyperfunctioning adenomas are the most prevalent adrenal tumor in the general population, occurring in 0.6% of all individuals examined by abdominal CT (Glazer et al. 1982). The frequency increases regularly with age. Like other less common benign, non-hyperfunctioning tumors (myelolipomas and occasionally adrenal cysts), non-hyperfunctioning adenomas do not require treatment if their nature can be established with certainty. Primary malignant non-hyperfunctioning tumors are very rare: malignant non-hyperfunctioning adrenocortical tumors (which account for one third of all malignant tumors of the adrenal cortex) (Copeland 1983), ganglioneuroblastomas, primary adrenal NHL. Benign hyperfunctioning adrenal tumors include aldosterone-secreting adenomas (Conn adenomas), cortisol-secreting adenomas (Cushing's adenomas), and pheochromocytomas. Malignant hyperfunctioning adrenal tumors include malignant hyperfunctioning adrenocortical tumors, which account for two thirds of all malignant tumors of the adrenal cortex, and malignant aldosteronomas and pheochromocytomas, which are exceptional. Hyperfunctioning tumors and primary malignant non-hyperfunctioning adrenal tumors are much less frequent than non-hyperfunctioning adenomas, but determination of their functioning and/or malignant nature is crucial for effective management.

In practice, investigations following discovery of an adrenal mass must address two questions (HERRERA et al. 1991):

1. Is the tumor functioning? If so, surgical resection is the rule, independent of the lesion's benign or malignant nature.
2. If the tumor is not hyperfunctioning, it is benign or malignant?

Neither CT nor MRI can determine whether an adrenal mass is hyperfunctioning or not. This information is provided by biochemical tests and radionuclide studies. The primary purpose of cross-sectional imaging for adrenal masses is determination of their benign or malignant nature as accurately, noninvasively, and inexpensively as possible.

Two different situations can be defined:

1. If an adrenal mass is discovered during disease staging in a cancer patient, the main problem is differentiation between metastases (as this might modify the therapeutic approach) and non-hyperfunctioning adenomas (which occur at a similar frequency in the general population).
2. If an adrenal mass is an incidental imaging finding in an individual without a recognized cancer or adrenal hyperfunction, the major problem is differential diagnosis of a non-hyperfunctioning adenoma from a malignant non-hyperfunctioning adrenocortical tumor, keeping in mind the exceptional character of the latter compared to the former.

15.5.1 Common Diagnostic Criteria

Tumor size is one of the most important diagnostic parameters. Non-hyperfunctioning adenomas are typically small and only rarely exceed 6 cm (GLAZER et al. 1982; COPELAND 1983; MITNICK et al. 1983); 85%–90% are smaller than 3 cm (OLIVER et al. 1984; LEE et al. 1991; VAN ERKEL et al. 1994). Inversely, non-hyperfunctioning adrenocortical tumors are usually already large (greater than 6 cm) when diagnosed. CT can demonstrate malignant adrenocortical tumors between 3 and 6 cm, e.g., five patients (16%) in the series of 31 adult patients studied by FISHMAN et al. (1987), but CT depiction of non-hyperfunctioning adrenocortical tumors smaller than 3 cm is exceptional. By contrast, the size of adrenal metastases is quite variable, even though their mean size is larger than that of adenomas (OLIVER et al. 1984; LEE et al. 1991, 1994). Because of this, if the cutoff for benignity is set at 2.5 cm, the specificity is only 79% and the sensitivity 84%. If the threshold is lowered to 1.5 cm in order to obtain a specificity of 93%, the sensitivity drops to 16% (LEE et al. 1991).

Bilateral involvement is common with adrenal metastases, but is also observed with adenomas, regardless of their functional status (bilateral nodular hyperplasia), and in familial forms of pheochromocytoma (Sipple syndrome).

Contiguous spread to the left renal vein or the inferior vena cava is highly suggestive of a malignant adrenocortical tumor. However, this feature was seen in only two of the 31 lesions (6%) examined by FISHMAN et al. (1987).

Coexistence of a primary tumor in another organ or other secondary sites (e.g., nodal, hepatic, pulmonary) is not synonymous with malignancy, because the frequency of non-hyperfunctioning adenomas in these patients is the same as in the general population. In the series studied by OLIVER et al. (1984), for example, over two thirds of the adrenal masses detected by CT in patients with a bronchial neoplasm were actually adenomas.

15.5.2 Computed Tomography

Demonstration of zones of pure fat density (less than –40 HU) within an adrenal mass is pathognomonic for myelolipoma (MUSANTE et al. 1988) and formally establishes the diagnosis (Fig. 15.10).

The mean attenuation value on unenhanced CT scans is an effective parameter for characterization of adenomas compared to other adrenal masses. Histologically, adenomas are composed of cells with an elevated lipid content. They thus have a relatively low spontaneous density (water or near-water density) that is significantly lower than that of malignant adrenal tumors and pheochromocytomas. A number of studies have attempted to determine the optimum CT attenuation value, allowing differential diagnosis of adenomas from malignant tumors. This threshold was set at 10 HU (LEE et al. 1991), 13 HU (BOLAND et al. 1997), 15 HU (MIYAKE et al. 1995), 16.5 HU (VAN ERKEL et al. 1994), and 18 HU (BRODEUR et al. 1994). The sensitivities were 79%, 100%, 64%, 100%, and

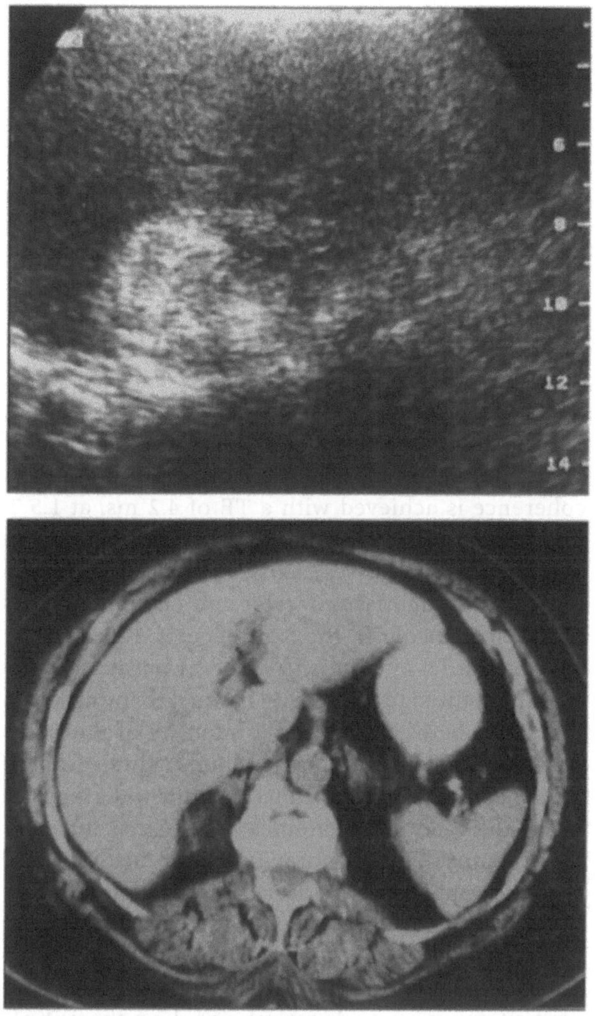

Fig. 15.10a,b. Right adrenal myelolipoma. **a** Ultrasound: the highly hyperechoic pattern is due to the presence of intratumoral fat. **b** The extremely low CT density (–44 HU) is pathognomonic for myelolipoma

88% and the specificities 96%, 100%, 100%, 95%, and 100%, respectively. Based on these five series, a mean spontaneous density under 10 HU rules out a malignant lesion. However, this feature is present in only 70%–80% of adenomas.

Measurement of mean tumor density immediately after contrast administration is generally considered of little benefit (Berland et al. 1988; Korobkin et al. 1996c). Although the postcontrast density of adenomas is lower than that of malignant tumors, considerable overlap in values exists between the two groups, namely due to the existence of strongly enhancing adenomas. Korobkin et al. (1996a) reported a specificity of 100% for diagnosis of benignity using a postcontrast CT threshold of 38 HU, but only 15 out of 41 (37%) of the benign lesions had a density under this threshold. The efficacy of enhanced CT densitometry is improved by use of delayed scans. Using CT scans obtained 1 h after iodine injection, Korobkin et al. (1996a) demonstrated that a mean density threshold of 30 HU had a sensitivity of 95% and a specificity of 100% for the diagnosis of adenoma. Boland et al. (1997) obtained scans 15 min after injection; using an optimum threshold of 24 HU, benign masses were diagnosed with a sensitivity of 96% and a specificity of 96%. Compared to unenhanced CT, delayed CT scans permit immediate diagnosis of incidentalomas without additional cost when initial CT is performed with contrast administration and when unenhanced scans are not available.

15.5.3 Magnetic Resonance Imaging

MRI characterization of adrenal tumors has been the subject of numerous investigations using a variety of techniques.

15.5.3.1 Standard Spin-Echo Sequences

T_2-weighted SE sequences with long repetition (TR) and echo times (TE) allow classification of adrenal tumors in three groups depending on their signal intensity relative to the liver (Glazer et al. 1986; Reinig et al. 1986) or fat (Chang et al. 1987): (1) hypointense tumors corresponding to adenomas, (2) hyperintense tumors corresponding to pheochromocytomas and cysts, and (3) tumors with an intermediate signal intensity, including malignant adrenocortical tumors and metastases. However, considerable overlap exists between the maximum and minimum values for these groups (Kier and McCarthy 1989; Lee et al. 1994; Reinig et al. 1994). In practice, T_2-weighted SE sequences have little value for characterization of adrenal tumors. The calculated T2 relaxation time is more discriminant according to some authors (Kier and McCarthy 1989), but is not useful according to others (Reinig et al. 1994). On T_1-weighted SE sequences with short TR and TE times, adenomas have a significantly higher signal intensity than malignant tumors (Chezmar et al. 1988), although considerable overlap exists here as well between the two groups (Chezmar et al. 1988; Reinig et al. 1994).

15.5.3.2
Contrast-Enhanced Magnetic Resonance Imaging

Gadolinium-enhanced dynamic MRI using gradient-echo sequences has a reported accuracy of 91% for differential diagnosis of adenomas (which feature weak and transient enhancement) from malignant tumors and pheochromocytomas (which show strong prolonged enhancement) (KRESTIN et al. 1989). ICHIKAWA et al. (1995) described five enhancement patterns after gadolinium injection: (1) early enhancement with rapid washout (adenomas), (2) progressive enhancement with slow washout (metastases), (3) rapid enhancement with slow washout (pheochromocytomas), (4) progressively increasing and persistent enhancement (neurogenic tumors), and (5) weak enhancement (tuberculous granulomas). These authors correctly classified 56 of 65 lesions (86%) using these five patterns. For other authors, however, the discriminant value of this technique for differentiation of adenomas from malignant tumors is low (REINIG et al. 1994).

MITCHELL et al. (1995) described the MRI appearance of the normal adrenal glands and a small series of adrenal tumors (three nonhyperfunctioning adenomas and two metastases) after intravenous injection of manganese dipyridoxyl diphosphate (Mn DPDP). Owing to this contrast agent's high affinity for hepatocytes, trials are in progress to evaluate its utility in liver disease. However, Mn DPDP is also taken up by the kidney, pancreas, and, in a general manner, by all abundantly vascularized organs rich in mitochondria. This is the case for the adrenals, where the mitochondria are implicated in the synthesis of catecholamines and steroids. Uptake is seen as a high-intensity signal on T_1-weighted sequences; visualization of uptake is improved on sequences performed with saturation of the periadrenal fat signal. Mn DPDP is reportedly taken up not only by the normal adrenal parenchyma, but also by adenomas, which are composed of functioning tissue (hyperfunctioning or not). By contrast, it is apparently not taken up by metastases, which correspond to totally nonfunctioning tissue. Despite the preliminary nature of research to date, it opens new perspectives by offering radiologic imaging a means for functional characterization of adrenal tumors. The information obtained with post-Mn DPDP MRI for differential diagnosis of metastases and adenomas will probably be similar to that currently provided by scintigraphy using iodine-cholesterol derivatives (NP-59). In this latter technique, the tracer is taken up by adenomas (reflecting their functioning character), but not by metastases (FRANCIS et al. 1988).

15.5.3.3
Sequences for Evaluation of Intratumoral Fat

MRI sequences for evaluation of intratumoral fat have the same purpose as measurement of the mean tumor CT density, i.e., characterization of adenomas compared to primary and secondary malignant tumors by demonstration of their elevated fat content.

Chemical-shift MRI, the most widely used method (MITCHELL et al. 1992; TSUSHIMA et al. 1993; BILBEY et al. 1995; MAYO-SMITH et al. 1995), is based on the difference in precession frequencies between water and lipid protons. When the echo time is varied, protons resonate alternatively "in phase" and "out of phase" following a cycle of 2.1 ms. Optimum phase coherence is achieved with a TE of 4.2 ms. at 1.5 T (MITCHELL et al. 1992) and 6.3 ms at 0.5 T (BILBEY et al. 1995). In such cases, signal intensity is maximal regardless of the tissue's water and fat contents (in-phase sequence). If the sequence is repeated by shifting the TE by 2.1 ms (a TE of 2.1 ms at 1.5 T, for example), the signal intensity is equal to the absolute difference between the signal intensity of the water protons and that of the lipids (out-of-phase sequence). If the tissue contains both water and fat (as is the case for adenomas), the signal intensity drops considerably compared to the in-phase sequence; the closer the lesion's lipid content to its water content, the greater the loss of signal (MITCHELL et al. 1992). Inversely, tissues with a very low fat content and those with a nearly exclusive fat content conserve an identical signal on the out-of-phase sequence. More useful than SE sequences, chemical-shift MRI is performed with a gradient-echo sequence without a 180° refocalization pulse, with the shortest possible TE, and without a presaturation pulse to suppress the fat signal (Figs. 15.11–15.13).

The loss of signal in an adrenal mass between the in-phase and out-of-phase sequences can be evaluated quantitatively, using the spleen as the internal standard (BILBEY et al. 1995; MAYO-SMITH et al. 1995). The spleen is preferable to the liver because the hepatic signal also drops in the case of hepatic steatosis. However, qualitative visual analysis of the signal loss appears to be just as accurate (MITCHELL et al. 1992; MAYO-SMITH et al. 1995). Remarkable results have been reported (MITCHELL et al. 1992; TSUSHIMA et al. 1993; BILBEY et al. 1995) for distinction between adenomas (20% signal loss compared to the spleen) (BILBEY et al. 1995) and other malignant adrenal masses whose signal is not modified. According to other authors (REINIG et al.

a
b
c
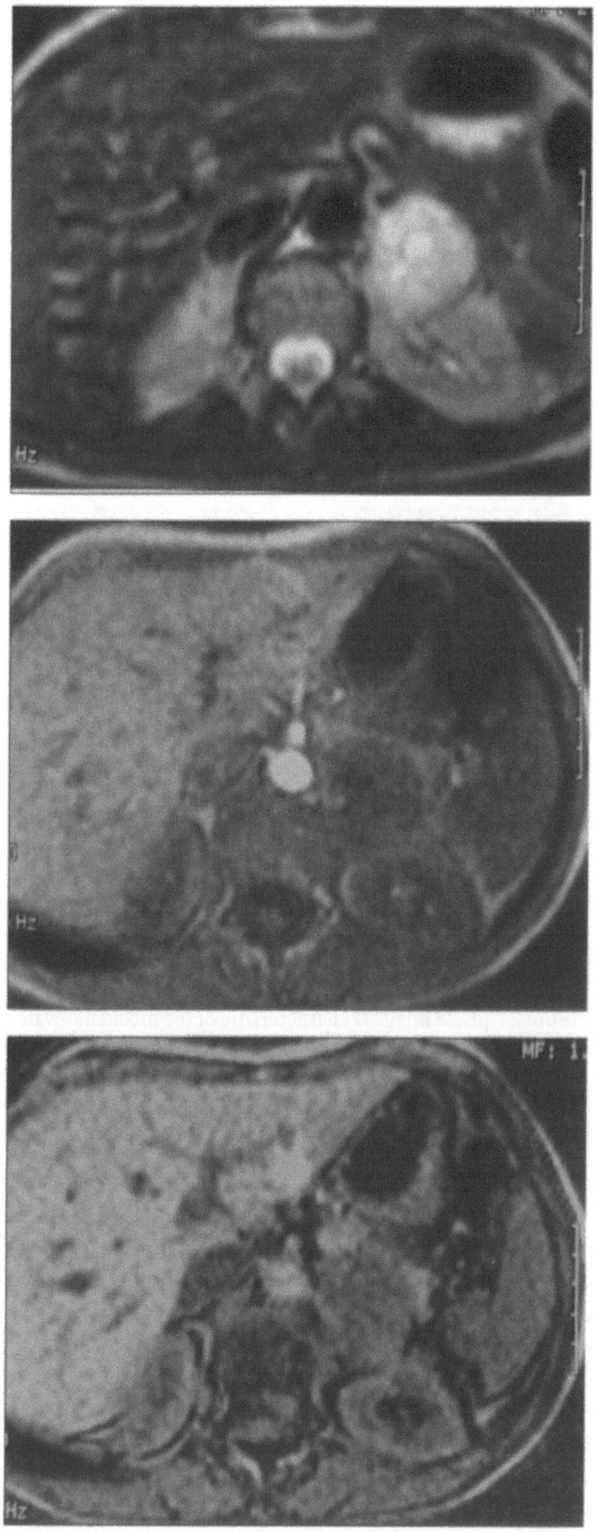

Fig. 15.11a–c. This 5-cm left adrenal pheochromocytoma was strongly hyperintense on T_2-weighted sequences. No evidence of signal loss on the out-of-phase image. **a** T_2-weighted short-echo (SE) image. **b** T_1-weighted in-phase fast multiplanar spoiled gradient echo (FMSPGR) image. **c** T_1-weighted out-of-phase FMPSPGR image

1994; Mayo-Smith et al. 1995), an overlap persists between the two groups. In the study by Mayo-Smith et al. (1995), use of an adrenal lesion to spleen ratio of –25 as the threshold had a sensitivity of 100% for diagnosis of adenoma, but a specificity of only 82%.

T_1-weighted (Mitchell et al. 1992; Ichikawa et al. 1994) and T_2-weighted (Schwartz et al. 1995) sequences with fat suppression both appear less discriminant than previously mentioned sequences. Although its histopathologic significance remains unclear, the presence of a hyperintense peripheral ring around adrenal masses reportedly has a sensitivity of 92% and a specificity of 95% for diagnosis of adenoma (Ichikawa et al. 1994).

Finally, MR spectroscopy using the Dixon method (SE in-phase and opposed-phase imaging) is reportedly highly reliable (sensitivity, 93%; specificity, 100%) for differentiation of adenomas from primary malignant adrenocortical tumors (Leroy-Willig et al. 1989).

15.5.3.4
Echo Planar Magnetic Resonance Imaging

In the only report to date on the recent technique of echo planar MRI (Schwartz et al. 1995), the T_2-weighted relaxation time was used for diagnostic purposes. The results for 68 adrenal lesions (sensitivity 82% and specificity 96% for the diagnosis of benignity) were practically identical to those obtained with chemical-shift MRI.

15.6
Conclusion

Despite extensive research in recent years, noninvasive characterization of adrenal tumors by CT and MRI aimed at differentiation of adenomas from primary and secondary tumors remains a challenge. Most initially promising criteria for characterization (especially in MRI) have proved unreliable in subsequent studies.

Until recently, measurement of the mean CT attenuation value on unenhanced CT scans using a threshold 10–18 HU, depending on the author, appeared the most cost-effective technique for diagnosis of adenomas, with a specificity of nearly 100%. However, up to 36% of adenomas in the various literature reports had a density over the selected threshold. Enhanced CT densitometry may prove

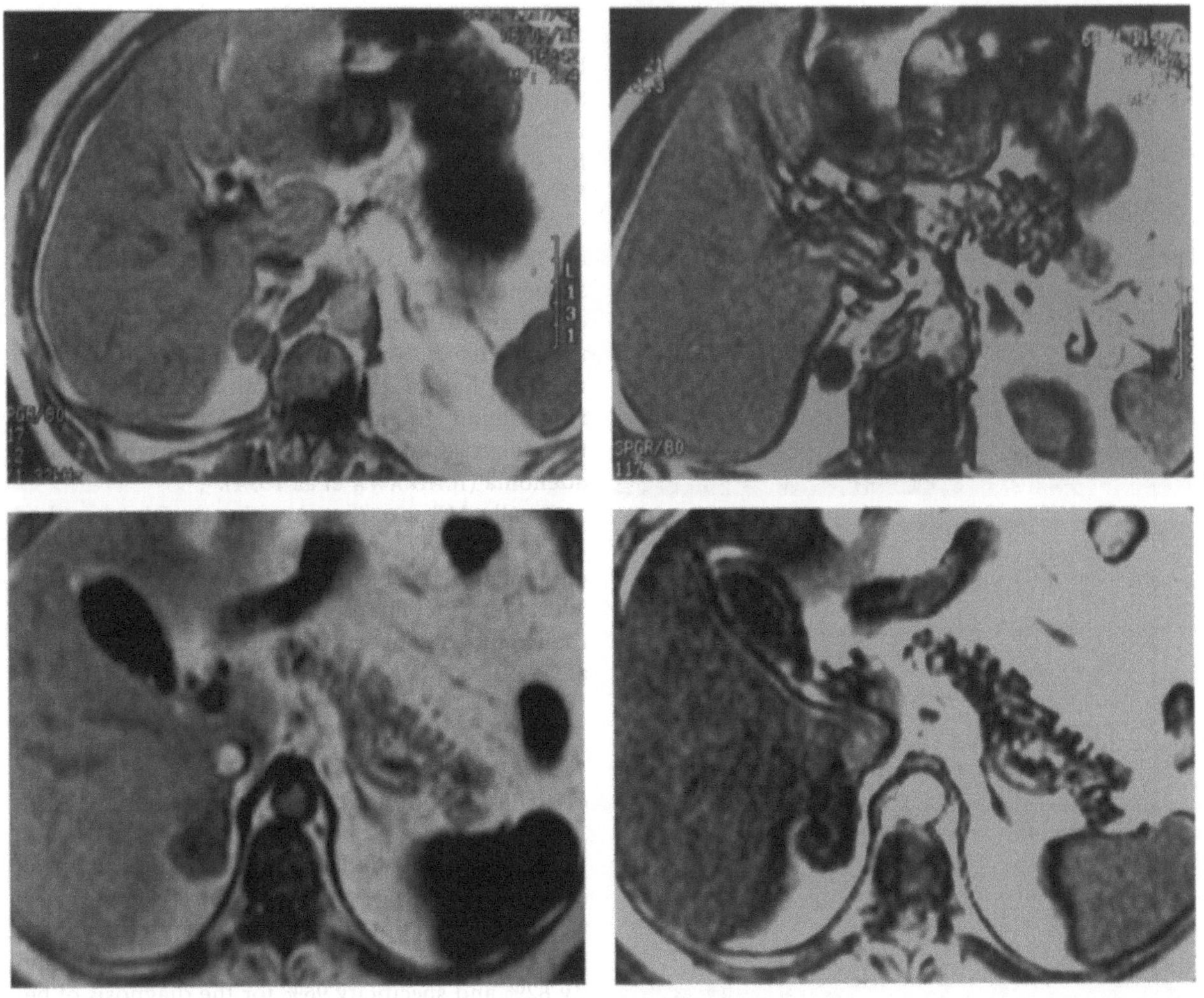

Fig. 15.12a–d. Right adrenal adenoma: the strong loss of signal on the out-of-phase image is characteristic of the mixed fat–water content of these lesions. On three-dimensional imaging, note the signal loss in the liver due to steatosis. **a.b** T_1-weighted in-phase images. **c,d** T_1-weighted out-of-phase image

more practical, less expensive, and more effective if the encouraging results of the two studies published to date are confirmed.

Compared to unenhanced CT, chemical-shift MRI has comparable efficacy for demonstration of intratumoral fat (Korobkin et al. 1996b), although at higher cost. This technique can be proposed for CT-indeterminate lesions with calculated densities close to the CT threshold value. CT-guided percutaneous adrenal biopsy is currently the examination of choice for differentiation between benign and malignant lesions in oncologic patients; the procedure has a diagnostic accuracy of 93%–96%, even though complications occur in 2.8%–9% of patients (Silverman et al. 1993; Welch et al. 1994).

The efficacy of noninvasive imaging procedures should considerably reduce the indications for percutaneous adrenal biopsy by identifying of over 80% of adenomas (although adenomas represent 44%–68% of all adrenal masses in cancer patients) (Oliver et al. 1984; Katz and Shirkhoda 1985).

The imaging strategy for adrenal tumors in patients without any known neoplasm or signs of adrenal hyperfunction (incidentalomas) must take lesion size into account. Surgical resection remains indicated for lesions larger than 5 cm owing to the high risk of a malignant adrenocortical tumor. Inversely, lesions smaller than 3 cm are unlikely to be malignant adrenocortical tumors. The literature recommends serial CT studies to monitor these latter lesions; this is a costly solution for the improbable

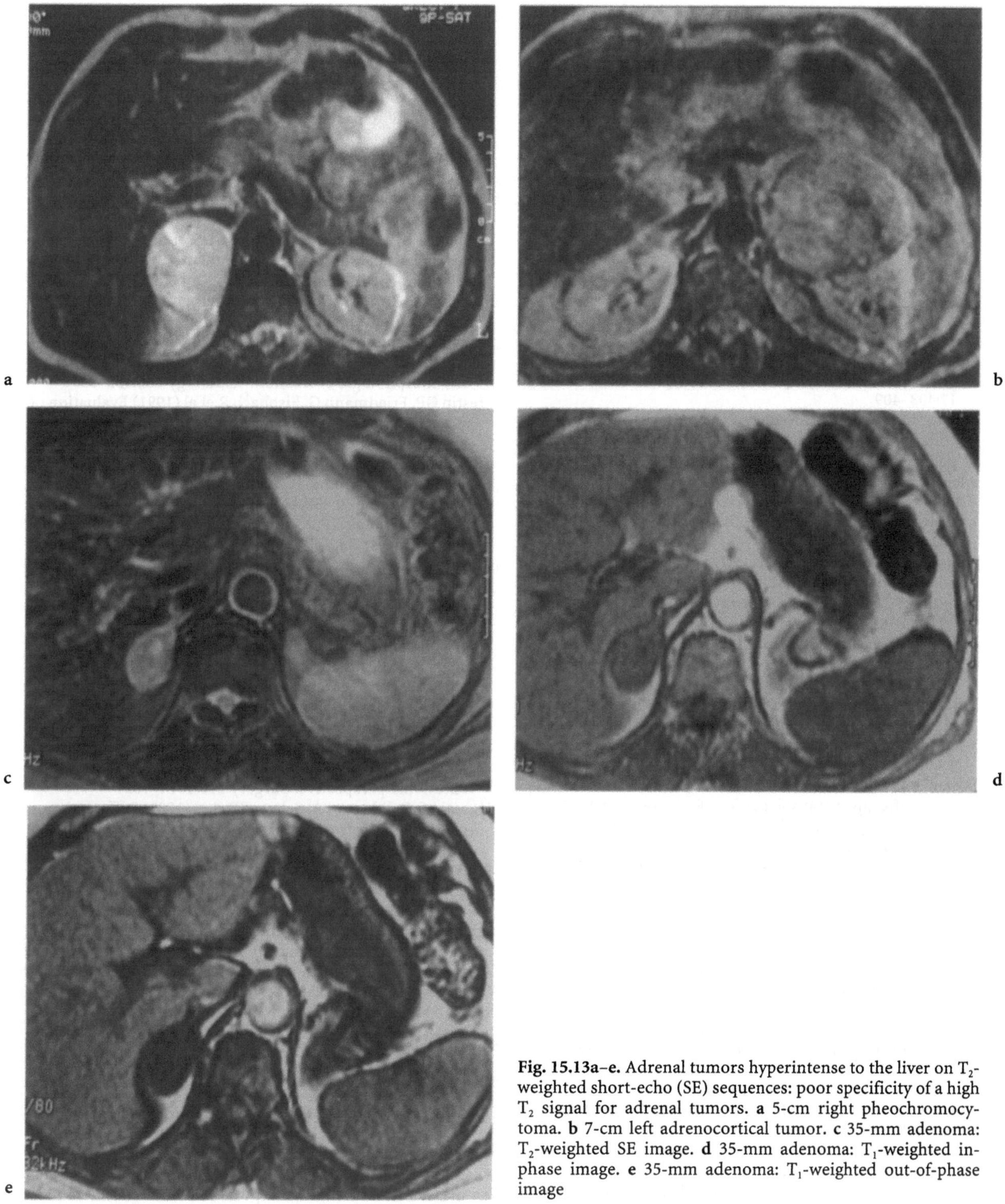

Fig. 15.13a–e. Adrenal tumors hyperintense to the liver on T_2-weighted short-echo (SE) sequences: poor specificity of a high T_2 signal for adrenal tumors. **a** 5-cm right pheochromocytoma. **b** 7-cm left adrenocortical tumor. **c** 35-mm adenoma: T_2-weighted SE image. **d** 35-mm adenoma: T_1-weighted in-phase image. **e** 35-mm adenoma: T_1-weighted out-of-phase image

diagnosis of a small, progressive, malignant adrenocortical tumor. For example, no malignant adrenocortical tumor was detected in over 150 incidentalomas followed up at the Mayo Clinic (Herrera et al. 1991).

Follow-up is thus probably unnecessary, at least for lesions with a mean unenhanced CT attenuation value under 10 HU. Lesions between 3 and 5 cm involve the greatest problems; the majority are adenomas, but malignant adrenocortical tumors account for a non-negligible percentage. Tissue samples obtained by guided percutaneous biopsy are insufficient for histologic differentiation of adenoma from malignant adrenocortical tumor (COPELAND 1983), and most authors recommend surgical resection. The data provided by CT densitometry and/or chemical-shift MRI should permit accurate diagnosis of at least 80% of all adenomas in this group and thus avoid many unnecessary adrenalectomies.

References

Alvarez-Castells A, Pedraza S, Tallada N (1993) CT of primary bilateral adrenal lymphoma. J Comput Assist Tomogr 17:408–409

Berland LL, Koslin DB, Kenney PJ, Stanley RJ, Lee JY (1988) Differentiation between small benign and malignant adrenal masses with dynamic incremented CT. AJR 151:95–101

Bilbey JH, McLoughlin RF, Kurkjian PS et al (1995) MR imaging of adrenal masses: value of chemical-shift imaging for distinguishing adenomas from other tumors. AJR 164:637–642

Boland GW, Goldberg MA, Lee MJ et al (1995) Indeterminate adrenal mass in patients with cancer: evaluation at PET with 2-[F-18]-fluoro-2-deoxy-D-glucose. Radiology 194:131–134

Boland GW, Hahn PF, Pena C, Mueller PR (1997) Adrenal masses: characterization with delayed contrast-enhanced CT. Radiology 202:693–696

Boraschi P, Campatelli A, Di Vito A, Perri G (1995) Hemorrhage in cavernous hemangioma of the adrenal gland: US, CT and MRI appearances with pathologic correlation. Eur J Radiol 21:41–43

Bowen A, Keslar PJ, Newman B et al (1990) Adrenal hemorrhage after liver transplantation. Radiology 176:85–88

Brodeur FJ, Korobkin MT, Yutzy GG, Francis IR, Quint LE (1994) Differentiation of adrenal adenomas from nonadenomas by using CT attenuation numbers. Radiology 193(P):195

Candel AG, Gattuso P, Reyes CV et al (1993) Fine needle aspiration biopsy of adrenal masses in patients with extraadrenal malignancy. Surgery 114:1132–1137

Chang A, Glazer HS, Lee JKT, Ling D, Heiken JP (1987) Adrenal gland: MR imaging. Radiology 163:123–128

Chezmar JL, Robbins SM, Nelson RC, Steinberg HV, Torres WE, Bernardino ME (1988) Adrenal masses: characterization with T1-weighted MR imaging. Radiology 166:357–359

Copeland PM (1983) The incidentally discovered adrenal mass. Ann Intern Med 98:940–945

Cyran KM, Kenney PJ, Memel DS, Yacoub I (1996) Adrenal myelolipoma. AJR 166:395–400

Dietrich RB, Kangarloo H, Lenarsky C, Feig SA (1987) Neuroblastoma: the role of MR imaging. AJR 148:937–942

Doppman JL, Gill JR Jr (1996) Hyperaldosteronism: sampling the adrenal veins. Radiology 198:309–312

Doppman JL, Miller DL, Dwyer AJ et al (1988) Macronodular adrenal hyperplasia in Cushing disease. Radiology 166:347–352

Dunnick NR (1990) Adrenal imaging: current status. AJR 154: 927–936

Dunnick NR (1994) Adrenal carcinoma. Radiol Clin North Am 32:99–108

Dunnick NR, Heaston D, Halvorsen R et al (1982) CT appearance of adrenal cortical carcinoma. J Comput Assist Tomogr 6:978–982

Dunnick NR, Leight GS, Roubidoux MA et al (1993) CT in the diagnosis of primary aldosteronism: sensitivity in 29 patients. AJR 160:321–324

Ferrozzi F, Bova D (1995) CT and MR demonstration of fat within an adrenal cortical carcinoma. Abdom Imaging 20:272–274

Fink IJ, Reinig JW, Dwyer AJ et al (1985) MR imaging of pheochromocytomas. J Comput Assist Tomogr 9:454–458

Fishman EK, Deutch BM, Hartman DS et al (1987) Primary adrenocortical carcinoma: CT evaluation with clinical correlation. AJR 148:531–535

Francis B, Gross MD, Shapiro B et al (1992) Integrated imaging of adrenal disease. Radiology 184:1–13

Francis IR, Smid A, Gross MD, Shapiro B, Naylor B, Glazer GM (1988) Adrenal masses in oncologic patients: functional and morphologic evaluation. Radiology 166:353–356

Frestin GP, Friedmann G, Fishbach R et al (1991) Evaluation of adrenal masses in oncological patients: dynamic contrast-enhanced MR vs CT. J Comput Assist Tomogr 15:104–110

Gandras EJ, Schwartz LH, Panicek DM, Levi G (1996) Adrenocortical oncocytoma: CT and MRI findings. J Comput Assist Tomogr 20:407–409

Glazer GM, Francis IR, Quint E (1988) Imaging the adrenal glands. Invest Radiol 23:3–11

Glazer GM, Woolsey EJ, Borrello J et al (1986) Adrenal tissue characterization using MR imaging. Radiology 158:73–79

Glazer HS, Weyman PJ, Sagel SS, Levitt RG, McLennan BL (1982) Non-functioning adrenal masses: incidental discovery on computed tomography. AJR 139:81–85

Hamper UM, Fishman EK, Hartman DS et al (1987) Primary adrenocortical carcinoma: sonographic evaluation with clinical and pathologic correlation in 26 patients. AJR 148:915–919

Herrera MF, Grant CS, Van Heerden JA, Sheedy PF, Ilstrup DM (1991) Incidentally discovered adrenal tumors: an institutional perspective. Surgery 110:1014–1021

Hussain S, Belldegrun A, Seltzer SE et al (1985) Differentiation of malignant from benign adrenal masses: predictive indices on computed tomography. AJR 144:61–65

Ichikawa T, Ohtomo K, Uchiyama G et al (1994) Adrenal adenomas: characterization hyperintense rim sign on fat-saturated spin-echo MR images. Radiology 193:247–250

Ichikawa T, Ohtomo K, Uchiyama G, Fujimoto H, Nasu K (1995) Contrast-enhanced dynamic MRI of adrenal masses: classification of characteristic enhancement patterns. Clin Radiol 50:295–300

Ikeda DM, Francis IR, Glazer GM, Amendola MA, Gross MD, Aisen AM (1989) The detection of adrenal tumors and hyperplasia in patients with primary aldosteronism: comparison of scintigraphy, CT and MR imaging. AJR 153:301–306

Katz RL, Shirkhoda A (1985) Diagnostic approach of incidental adrenal nodules in the cancer patient. Cancer 55:1995–2000

Kier R, McCarthy S (1989) MR characterization of adrenal masses: field strength and pulse sequence considerations. Radiology 171:671–674

Kolmannskog F, Kolbenstvedt A, Brekke IB (1992) CT and angiography in adrenocortical carcinoma. Acta Radiol. 33:45–49

Korobkin M, Brodeur FJ, Francis IR, Quint LE, Reed Dunnick N, Goodsitt M (1996a) Delayed enhanced CT for differentiation of benign from malignant adrenal masses. Radiology 200:737–742

Korobkin M, Giordano TJ, Brodeur FJ et al (1996b) Adrenal adenomas: relationship between histologic lipid and CT and MR findings. Radiology 200:743–747

Korobkin M, Brodeur FJ, Yutzy GG et al (1996c) Differentiation of adrenal adenomas from non adenomas using CT attenuation values. AJR 166:531–536

Krestin GP, Steinbrich W, Friedman G (1989) Adrenal masses: evaluation with fast gradient-echo MR imaging and Gd-DTPA-enhanced dynamic studies. Radiology 171:675–680

Lee MJ, Hahn PF, Papanicolaou N et al (1991) Benign and malignant adrenal masses: CT distinction with attenuation coefficients, size, and observer analysis. Radiology 179:415–418

Lee MJ, Hahn PF, Mayo Smith WW, Gaa J, Papanicolaou N, Saini S (1994a) Characterization of adrenal pheochromocytoma at T2-weighted MR imaging: is lesion hyperintensity specific for diagnosis? Radiology 193(P):195

Lee MJ, Mayo-Smith WW, Hahn PF et al (1994b) State-of-the-art MR imaging of the adrenal gland. Radiographics 14:1015–1029

Leroy-Willig A, Bittoun J, Luton JP et al (1989) In vivo MR spectroscopic imaging of the adrenal glands: distinction between adenomas and carcinomas larger than 15 mm based on lipid content. AJR 153:771–773

Mayo-Smith WW, Lee MJ, McNicholas MMJ, Hahn PF, Boland GW, Saini S (1995) Characterization of adrenal masses (<5 cm) by use of chemical shift MR imaging: observer performance versus quantitative measures. AJR 165:91–95

McNicholas MM, Lee MJ, Mayo-Smith WW, Hahn PF, Boland GM, Mueller PR (1995) An imaging algorithm for the differential diagnosis of adrenal adenomas and metastases. AJR 165:1453–1459

Mitchell DG, Crovello M, Matteucci T, Petersen RO, Miettinen MM (1992) Benign adrenocortical masses: diagnosis with chemical shift MR imaging. Radiology 185:345–351

Mitchell DG, Outwater EK, Matteucci T, Rubin DL, Chezmar JL, Saini S (1995) Adrenal gland enhancement at MR imaging with Mn-DPDP. Radiology 194:783–787

Mitnick JS, Bosniak MA, Megibow AJ, Naidich DP (1983) Nonfunctioning adrenal adenomas discovered incidentally on computed tomography. Radiology 148:495–499

Miyake H, Takaki H, Matsumoto S, Yoshida S, Maeda T, Mori H (1995) Adrenal nonhyperfunctioning adenoma and nonadenoma: CT attenuation value as discriminative index. Abdom Imaging 20:559–562

Muckerjee JJ, Peppercorn PD, Reznek RH et al (1997) Pheochromocytomas: effect of nonionic contrast medium in CT on circulating catecholamine levels. Radiology 202:227–231

Musante F, Derchi LE, Zappasodi F et al (1988) Myelolipoma of the adrenal gland: sonographic and CT features. AJR 151:961–964

Oliver TW, Bernardino ME, Miller JL, Mansour K, Greene D, Davis WA (1984) Isolated adrenal masses in nonsmall-cell bronchogenic carcinoma. Radiology 153:217–218

Outwater EK, Siegelman ES, Radeski PF, Piccoli CW, Mitchell DG (1995) Distinction between benign and malignant adrenal masses: value of T1-weighted chemical-shift MR imaging. AJR 165:579–583

Paling MR, Williamson BRJ (1983) Adrenal involvement in non-Hodgkin's lymphoma. AJR 141:303–305

Peppercorn PD, Reznek RH (1997) State-of-art CT and MRI of the adrenal gland. Eur Radiol 7:822–836

Pradel J, Bruel JM, Cyteval C et al (1990) Exploration radiologique des glandes surrénales. Feuil Radiol 30:323–346

Quint LE, Glazer GM, Francis IR et al (1987) Pheochromocytoma and paraganglioma: comparison of MR imaging with CT and I-131 MIBG scintigraphy. Radiology 165:89–93

Reinig JW, Doppman JL, Dwyer AJ et al (1986) Adrenal masses differentiated by MR. Radiology 158:81–84

Reinig JW, Stutley JE, Leonhardt CM, Spicer KM, Margolis M, Caldwell CB (1994) Differentiation of adrenal masses with MR imaging: comparison of techniques. Radiology 192:41–46

Robert Y, Wurtz A, Taieb S, Lemaitre L (1994) CT-guided biopsy of adrenal masses in preoperative management of bronchogenic carcinoma. Eur Radiol 4:221–224

Rossi GP, Chiesura-Corona M, Tregnaghi A et al (1993) Imaging of aldosterone-secreting adenomas: a prospective comparison of computed tomography and magnetic resonance imaging in 27 patients with suspected primary aldosteronism. J Hum Hypertens 7:357–363

Rozenblit A, Morehous HT, Amis ES Jr (1996) Cystic adrenal lesions: CT features. Radiology 201:541–548

Samaan NA, Hickey RC (1987) Adrenal cortical carcinoma. Semin Oncol 14:292–296

Sato N, Watanabe Y, Saga T, Mitsudo K, Dohke M, Minami K (1995) Adrenocortical adenoma containing a fat component: CT and MR image evaluation. Abdom Imaging 20:489–490

Schlund JF, Kenney PJ, Brown ED, Ascher SM, Brown JJ, Semelka RC (1995) Adrenocortical carcinoma: MR imaging appearance with current techniques. J Magn Reson Imaging 5:171–174

Schwartz LH, Panicek DM, Koutcher JA et al (1995) Echoplanar MR imaging for characterization of adrenal masses in patients with malignant neoplasms: preliminary evaluation of calculated T2 relaxation values. AJR 164:911–915

Schwerk WB, Gorg C, Gorg K, Restrepo IK (1994) Adrenal pheochromocytomas: a broad spectrum of sonographic presentation. J Ultrasound Med 13:517–521

Semelka RC, Shoenut JP, Lawrence PH et al (1993) Evaluation of adrenal masses with gadolinium enhancement and fat-suppressed MR imaging. J Magn Reson Imaging 3:337–343

Shapiro B, Sisson JC, Lloyd R et al (1984) Malignant pheochromocytoma: clinical, biochemical, and scintigraphic characterization. Clin Endocrinol 20:189–203

Sheps SG, Jiang NS, Klee GG et al (1990) Recent developments in the diagnosis and manaagement of pheochromocytoma. Mayo Clin Proc 65:88–95

Silverman SG, Mueller PR, Pinkney LP, Koenker PM, Seltzer SE (1993) Predictive value of image guided adrenal biopsy; analysis of results of 101 biopsies. Radiology 187:715–718

Sisson JC, Frager MS, Valk TW et al (1981) Scintigraphic localization of pheochromocytoma. N Engl J Med 305:12–17

Smith SM, Patel SK, Turner DA et al (1989) Magnetic resonance imaging of adrenal cortical carcinoma. Urol Radiol 11:1–6

Solomon N, Sumkin J (1988) Right adrenal gland hemorrhage as a complication of liver transplantation: CT appearance. J Comput Assist Tomogr 12 95–97

Tshushima Y, Ishizaka H, Matsumoto M (1993) Adrenal masses: differentiation with chemical shift, fast low angle shot MR imaging. Radiology 186:705–709

Van Erkel AR, Van Gils APG, Lequin M, Kruitwagen C, Bloem JL, Falke THM (1994) CT and MR distinction of adenomas and nonadenomas of the adrenal gland. J Comput Assist Tomogr 18:432–438

Van Gils APG, Falke THM, Van Erkel AR et al (1991) MR imaging and MIBG scintigraphy of pheochromocytomas

and extraadrenal functioning paragangliomas. Radiographics 11:37–57
Velchik MG, Alavi A, Kressel HY et al (1989) Localization of pheochromocytoma: MIBG, CT and MRI correlation. J Nucl Med 30:328–336
Vicks BS, Perusek M, Johnson J et al (1987) Primary adrenal lymphoma. CT and sonography appearances. J Clin Ultrasound 15:135–137
Welch TJ, Sheedy PF, Van Heerden JA et al (1983) Pheochromocytoma: value of computed tomography. Radiology 148:501–503
Welch TJ, Sheedy PF, Stephens DH et al (1994) Percutaneous adrenal biopsy : review of a 10-year experience. Radiology 193:341–344
Westra SJ, Zaninovic AC, Hall Tr, Kangarloo H, Boechat MI (1994) Imaging of the adrenal gland in children. Radiographics 14:1323–1340
Young WF Jr, Hogan MJ, Klee GG, Grant CS, Van Heerden JA (1990) Primary aldosteronism: diagnosis and treatment. Mayo Clin Proc 65:96–99

16 Carcinoid Tumors

P. CHEVALLIER, T. DE BAERE, B. PADOVANI, C. RAFFAELLI, and A. ROCHE

CONTENTS

16.1 Introduction

B. PADOVANI, P. CHEVALLIER, AND C. RAFFAELLI

Carcinoid tumors are rare tumors arising from the endocrine system; they develop from Kulchitsky cells and are classed among the apudomas. The majority develop from the embryologic midgut (jejunum, ileum, right colon). Carcinoids that develop from the hindgut (left colon, rectum) or the foregut (stomach, lung, duodenum, pancreas) are less common. Gastrointestinal carcinoids are by far the most prevalent (90%). Bronchial localizations are the second most common site, while ovarian, pancreatic, thymic, and renal carcinoids are extremely rare.

The highly variable clinical course of these tumors depends essentially on their size and location. Clinical manifestations are often nonspecific or absent, in particular for tumors of the hindgut. Certain carcinoids (especially tumors of the midgut) produce a carcinoid syndrome; symptoms related to ectopic hormone production are most frequent with foregut tumors. The frequency of asymptomatic and nonspecific carcinoids explains the difficulties for early diagnosis. The role of imaging studies varies with the clinical presentation: asymptomatic tumors may be incidental findings, and workup of nonspecific symptoms may reveal a tumor. In patients with the carcinoid syndrome, imaging studies should initially be concentrated on the gastrointestinal tract; other localizations can be sought secondarily if gastrointestinal studies are negative. In patients with ectopic hormone production, imaging serves primarily to rule out a pathologic process involving the organ responsible for physiologic secretion and to localize the ectopic secretion. Finally, imaging plays an essential role in disease staging and therapeutic surveillance.

16.2 Carcinoid Tumors of the Gastrointestinal Tract

16.2.1 Introduction

Carcinoids account for 1.5% of all gastrointestinal tumors and 55% of all gastrointestinal endocrine tumors. The sexes are affected equally by these tumors, except for appendiceal carcinoids, which are more

P. CHEVALLIER, Service de Radiodiagnostic, Hôpital de l'Archet, 151 chemin de St. Antoine Ginestière, 06200 Nice, France
T. DE BAERE, A. ROCHE, Service de Radiodiagnostic Interventionelle, Institut Gustave Roussy, 39-53 avenue Camille Desmoulins, 94805 Villejuif, France
B. PADOVANI, C. RAFFAELLI, Service de Radiodiagnostic, Hôpital Pasteur, 30 avenue de la Voie Romaine, BP 69, 06002 Nice, France

frequent in women. The mean age at diagnosis is 35 years. All parts of the gastrointestinal tract can be affected, with a predilection for the appendix (40%–50%), the ileum (20%–25%), and the colon and rectum (15%). Multiple lesions are not infrequent, especially in the ileum (30%). The circumstances of discovery of gastrointestinal carcinoids vary with lesion size and location. Clinical symptoms (gastrointestinal bleeding, pain due to obstruction, carcinoid syndrome) are often indicative of an advanced tumor. Approximately 50% of gastrointestinal carcinoids are asymptomatic (especially appendiceal and rectal carcinoids). The carcinoid syndrome manifests as vasomotor instability, including cutaneous flushing, diarrhea, bronchospasm, and cardiac valvular lesions. Due to excessive serotonin production, this syndrome is particularly frequent with jejunoileal carcinoids and is often associated with large hepatic metastases.

Histologically, gastrointestinal carcinoids develop deep within the mucosa and the submucosa. Metastatic spread is closely related to invasion of the musculosa and tumor size; metastases are rare with carcinoids smaller than 1 cm (2% of cases), but occur with 80% of tumors larger than 2 cm (Godwin 1975; Buck and Sobin 1990).

The prognosis also depends on the site of the tumor. Primary carcinoids of the appendix often have a benign course, whereas ileal carcinoids have a propensity for metastasis. Generally speaking, carcinoids have a slow rate of growth, and long-term survival has often been reported, even in patients with nodal or liver metastases. However, 30%–35% of patients with a carcinoid tumor have a second malignancy that aggravates the prognosis (Beaton 1982).

The role of imaging modalities varies with tumor location. Imaging studies are essential for detection of lesions not accessible to endoscopy (ileum, jejunum) and, more generally, for disease staging (Chopier-Richaud et al. 1993).

16.2.2 Carcinoids of the Small Intestine

Small intestinal carcinoids account for 20%–25% of carcinoid tumors. Ileal lesions are eight times more common than lesions in the jejunum. The distal ileum is the site of predilection. These tumors are difficult to detect at an early stage owing to their small dimensions; this explains the frequency of mesenteric involvement at initial diagnosis (40%–80% of patients) (Picus et al. 1984; Cockey et al. 1985; Gould and Johnson 1986). A variety of patterns are seen on barium studies. Opacification by the enteroclysis technique is more effective than standard examinations (Jeffree et al. 1984). Early lesions appear as small submucosal nodules in the distal ileum. Anomalies are usually more extensive, however, reflecting invasion of the small intestine and the mesentery. The various radiologic features reflect contiguous spread to the ileum and the mesentery and local hormone secretion, causing retractile fibrosis of the adjacent mesentery. Imaging studies may reveal multiple intramural nodules, hypertrophic thickening of the folds, focal fixation of bowel loops or even luminal narrowing (of neoplastic origin or secondary to ischemia). Mesenteric sclerosis produces images of small-bowel angulation and rigidity. Mesenteric lymphadenopathy may cause displacement of the intestinal loops. Ileal carcinoids do not cause linear ulcerations or fistulae (Buck and Sobin 1990), in contrast to Crohn's disease, which may have similar features.

Computed tomography (CT) plays an important role in the diagnosis and staging of small-bowel carcinoids (Picus et al. 1984; Gould and Johnson 1986; Woodard et al. 1995). Although the primary ileal tumor is rarely visualized, mesenteric spread and nodal and hepatic metastases are frequently seen. Mesenteric involvement is depicted as an irregular mass that may contain calcifications (Picus et al. 1984; Gould and Johnson 1986; Panton-Grag-Brown et al. 1995; Woodard et al. 1995) surrounded by fine, linear densities radiating toward the adjacent bowel loops (Figs. 16.1, 16.2). The mass may lie in contact with the intestinal wall, indicating the site of the primary tumor, or may be located more centrally, near the root of the mesentery. Radiating densities in the mesenteric fat reflect fibrosis and may be accompanied by retraction and dilatation of the adjacent bowel loops. Fibrosis may extend to the mesenteric vessels and cause vascular occlusion responsible for bowel wall thickening. Retroperitoneal nodal metastases are readily demonstrated by CT and may be solitary or associated with hepatic metastases.

Ultrasound, although rarely performed in routine practice, may demonstrate small tumors in the distal ileum as homogeneously hypoechoic oval masses interrupting the submucosa (Rioux et al. 1995).

Scintigraphy has proven beneficial for detection of both the tumor and metastases (Adolf et al. 1987). Metaiodobenzylguanidine (MIBG) scintigraphy reveals high uptake in 59%–73% of in-

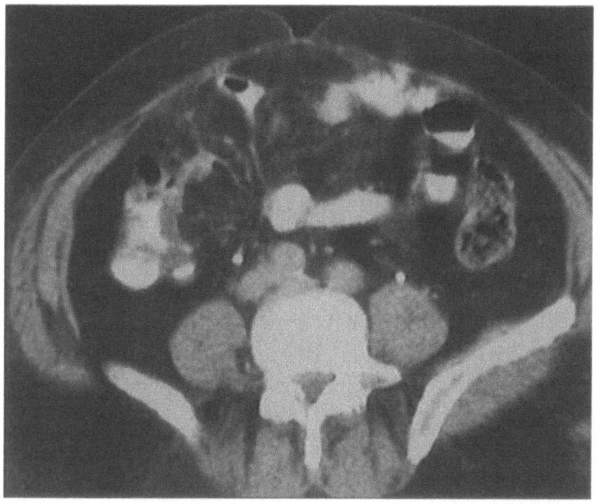

Fig. 16.1. Carcinoid tumor of the small bowel: parietal thickening of an intestinal loop and thin stellate infiltration of mesentery

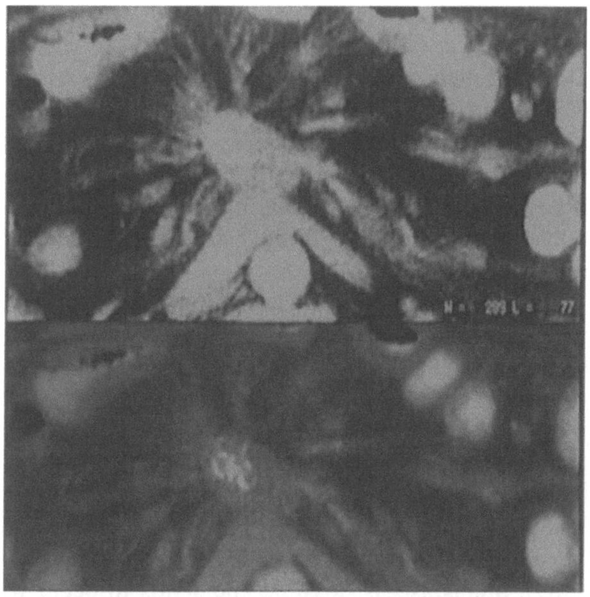

Fig. 16.2. Calcified mesenteric mass surrounded by stellate infiltration of the mesenteric fat

testinal carcinoids. Tracer uptake is reportedly correlated with circulating serotonin levels (Hanson et al. 1989). However, uptake also occurs in individuals with normal serotonin concentrations (Watanabe et al. 1995). High uptake is not specific to carcinoids; pheochromocytomas and medullary carcinoma of the thyroid also take up MIBG. Scintigraphy with octreotide, based on the presence of somatostatin receptors in certain carcinoid tumors, is currently under investigation. This technique can reportedly demonstrate small tumors (<15 mm), improves detection of hepatic and especially bone metastases and aids post-therapy follow-up (Kvols and Reubi 1993; Schillaci et al. 1996). Its therapeutic value for metabolic irradiation is currently under evaluation.

16.2.3 Appendiceal Carcinoids

Carcinoids of the appendix represent 40%–50% of all gastrointestinal carcinoid tumors. The distal appendix is the site of predilection (Rioux et al. 1994). Ultrasound may demonstrate nonspecific features of appendicitis or an appendiceal mucocele (Buck and Sobin 1990). These typically small lesions confined to the appendix are usually discovered at surgery for appendicitis (Hermans et al. 1993). In a study at the Mayo Clinic (Moertel et al. 1987), appendectomy was considered curative for tumors smaller than 2 cm, whereas right hemicolectomy was performed for larger lesions.

16.2.4 Colorectal Carcinoids

Colorectal carcinoids account for 15% of all gastrointestinal carcinoids. Rectal sites predominate. Barium enema studies demonstrate a nonspecific small sessile polyp. Endoscopic ultrasonography (EUS) depicts a small (<2 cm in diameter), well-delimited, homogeneously hypoechoic mass in the second and third coats (Kawamoto et al. 1994). Colon carcinoids are very rare; they may manifest as bulky stenotic or polypoid lesions mimicking a colon adenocarcinoma and are often accompanied by hepatic metastases.

16.2.5 Gastric Carcinoids

Gastric carcinoids are much rarer. Barium studies typically show a nonspecific, well-delimited intramural mass measuring 1–3 cm in diameter. Central mucosal ulceration is common. Polypoid lesions (Berger and Stephens 1996) and large, ulcerated masses mimicking gastric adenocarcinoma are also encountered. Multiple lesions are possible, particularly in association with atrophic gastritis (Borch 1989).

16.2.6 Duodenal Carcinoids

On barium transit examinations, duodenal carcinoids image as small (1 cm), sessile polyps in the duodenal bulb. Localizations in the first portion of the duodenum predominate (Clements and Roche 1984). These lesions sometimes image as a submucosal intramural mass in the region of the ampulla, responsible for dilatation of the common bile duct (Buck and Sobin 1990).

16.2.7 Hepatic Metastases of Gastrointestinal Carcinoids

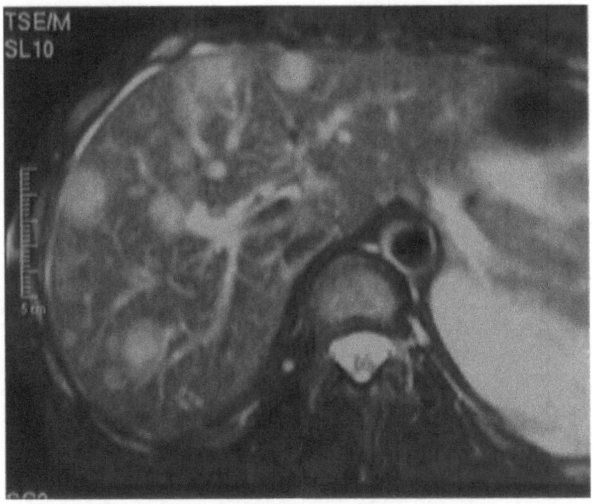

Fig. 16.3. T_2-weighted sequence; repetition time (TR), 1800 ms; echo time (TE), 80 ms: these hepatic metastases of a carcinoid tumor are visible as multiple, extremely hyperintense nodules

The frequency of hepatic metastases justifies systematic examination of the liver during workup of gastrointestinal carcinoids (Smevic et al. 1983; Andersson et al. 1987; Woodard et al. 1995). In a series of 52 midgut carcinoids (including 43 in the ileum) published by Woodard et al. (1995), hepatic metastases were found in 34 patients. Hepatic metastases are often multiple and affect both lobes (Picus et al. 1984). CT visualization is sometimes difficult because they are practically isodense to the normal liver parenchyma. Both pre- and postcontrast CT scans using narrow windows are required. The benefits of spiral CT are currently under evaluation. Abdominal ultrasound may demonstrate metastases undetected by CT. Magnetic resonance imaging (MRI) appears slightly superior to CT for the detection of hepatic nodules, which appear strongly hyperintense on T_2-weighted sequences (Fig. 16.3).

16.3 Bronchial Carcinoids

16.3.1 General Features

Bronchial carcinoids represent 1%–2% of all primary bronchial cancers. These tumors arising from the bronchial submucosa are considered neuroendocrine tumors because of their ability to secrete chemical substances. The "typical" highly differentiated carcinoids seen in 75%–90% of patients must be differentiated from "atypical" carcinoids, which have a much greater malignant potential (Davila et al. 1993; Marty-Ane et al. 1995). These two types of tumors are distinguished by cytological criteria, i.e., hypercellularity, nuclear polymorphism, prominent nucleolus, mitotic activity, areas of necrosis (Ranfaing 1993).

Bronchial carcinoids are slow-growing tumors with a favorable prognosis after resection. Overall survival is 78% at 5 years and 71% at 10 years (Harpole et al. 1992). Survival is even better for tumors resected at an early stage: 95% and 93% at 5 and 10 years, respectively (Harpole et al. 1992).

The main prognostic factors are tumor stage and histology (Okike et al. 1976). Atypical carcinoids have a 5-year survival rate of 57% (Forster et al. 1989). Metastasis is possible and tends to occur to regional nodes (intrathoracic lymphadenopathy). Other potential sites of metastasis include the liver, the adrenal glands, the brain and bone. Bone metastases are often osteosclerotic (Toomey and Felson 1960). Bronchial carcinoid tumors are classically centrally located (85% of cases: 75% in a lobar bronchus and 10% in a principal bronchus). Peripheral sites generally represent only 15% of cases (Davila et al. 1993), although several reports cite higher frequencies (Beaton 1982; McCaughan et al. 1985; Choplin et al. 1986; Buck and Sobin 1990). These variations depend at least partially on whether or not the segmental bronchi are considered central. Zwiebel et al. (1991) defined peripheral tumors as lesions located more than 2 cm downstream from the origin of the appropriate segmental bronchus.

At gross examination, central bronchial carcinoids comprise a smooth, bosselated exophytic component projecting into the bronchial lumen and an infiltrating component that extends into the bronchial wall, sometimes beyond the cartilage (RANFAING 1993). Clinical manifestations are variable. Peripheral bronchial tumors are usually asymptomatic, whereas central lesions may be revealed by symptoms of airway obstruction, such as cough, hemoptysis, or recurrent pneumonitis. Asymptomatic bronchial carcinoids may be discovered on routine chest radiographs. The rare bronchial carcinoids revealed by a carcinoid syndrome (BEATON 1982; CLEMENTS and ROCHE 1984) are centrally located tumors that have metastasized. A paraneoplastic Cushing syndome related to ectopic adrenocorticotropic hormone (ACTH) production occasionally reveals the tumor.

16.3.2 Imaging

Over 75% of all bronchial carcinoids are visible on chest radiographs. Peripheral tumors image as solitary, well-delimited round or lobulated nodules, without spiculations (Fig. 16.4). Central tumors corresponding to a hilar mass, an endoluminal nodule, atelectasis, or obstructive pneumonitis can be more difficult to visualize (HURT and BATES 1984). Intratumoral calcifications are seen in up to 8% of patients. CT plays an essential role for detection and staging (FORSTER et al. 1989; MAGID et al. 1989; MULLER and MILLER 1990; ZWIEBEL et al. 1991; DAVILA et al. 1993). Along with better detection of hilar masses, endoluminal lesions, and intratumoral calcifications, CT can accurately evaluate spread beyond the bronchial wall and allows both hilar and mediastinal nodal metastases and distant metastases to be searched for (MULLER and MILLER 1990).

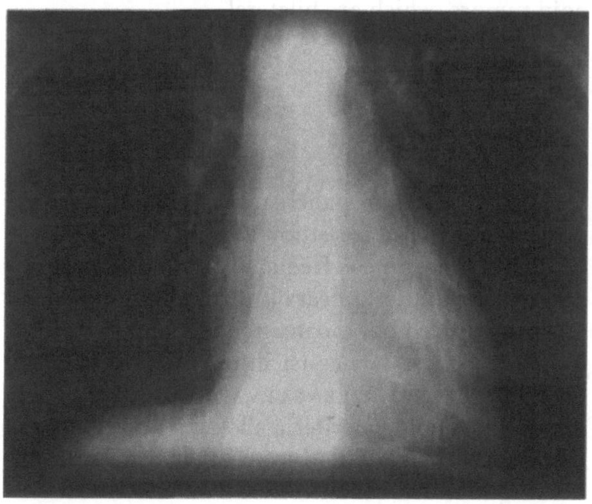

Fig. 16.4. Round retrocardiac nodule corresponding to a bronchial carcinoid

CT can also accurately determine tumor shape and density. Most bronchial carcinoids are smoothly marginated round, ovoid, or occasionally lobulated nodules less than 2.5 cm in diameter. The usual absence of spicules (MAGID et al. 1989) is explained by the low grade of malignancy of these tumors. Certain authors advocate measurement of the axis of oval tumors (FORSTER et al. 1989; ZWIEBEL et al. 1991) because numerous carcinoids are specifically oriented with their long axis parallel to the nearest major bronchus or pulmonary arterial division. This "parallel sign" was found in 87% of patients by ZWIEBEL et al. (1991). Seen essentially with peripheral carcinoids, this parallel sign is easier to analyze on plain chest radiographs than on CT scans. Thin-section CT scans allow identification of endobronchial tumors (Fig. 16.5) and determination of their exact location and disease spread or coexistent respiratory pathologies that may go unnoticed on standard radiographs. Helical CT should improve the assessment of these carcinoid tumors.

Calcification and ossification have both been described in bronchial carcinoids (TROUPIN 1968; MAGID et al. 1989; ZWIEBEL et al. 1991; MCADAMS et al. 1995). These features (26% of patients; ZWIEBEL et al. 1991) are seen more often on CT scans than on standard radiographs. They are more frequent in central tumors than in peripheral tumors (10%) (MAGID et al. 1989; ZWIEBEL et al. 1991) and appear more prevalent in tumors larger than 2 cm.

The enhancement observed after iodine injection (Fig. 16.6; ARONCHICK et al. 1986) is a diagnostic CT feature reflecting extensive tumor hypervascularity (RANFAING 1993). Such contrast enhancement is frequently but not always observed and may be confused with an arteriovenous malformation or a varicose pulmonary vein.

Few studies have described the MRI features of bronchial carcinoids (DOPPMAN et al. 1991; DOUEK et al. 1994). Their characteristic high-intensity signal on T_2-weighted short-echo (SE) sequences allows differentiation from perihilar vessels (Fig. 16.7). After gadolinium injection, MRI, like CT, may reveal pronounced signal enhancement on T_1-weighted sequences (DOUEK et al. 1994).

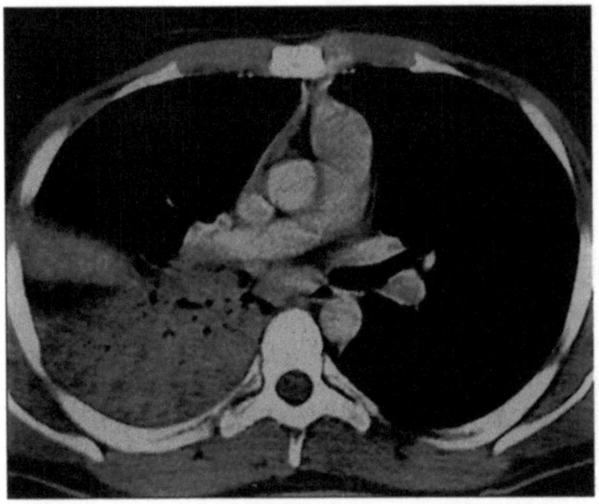

Fig. 16.5. CT of an endobronchial carcinoid tumor: retention pneumonitis of the right inferior lobe

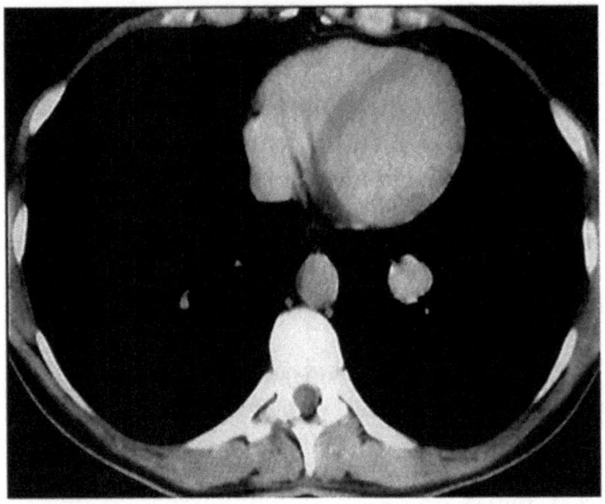

Fig. 16.6. Contrast-enhanced CT of the thorax: this nodule in the left lower lobe enhanced after iodinated contrast administration and corresponded to a carcinoid

As for other neuroendocrine tumors, scintigraphy with iodine-131 MIBG or somatostatin analogues (octreotide, pentetreotide) can detect small bronchial carcinoids and associated metastases (O'Byrne et al. 1994).

16.4 Rare Carcinoid Tumors

Rare carcinoid tumors represent less than 5% of all carcinoid tumors.

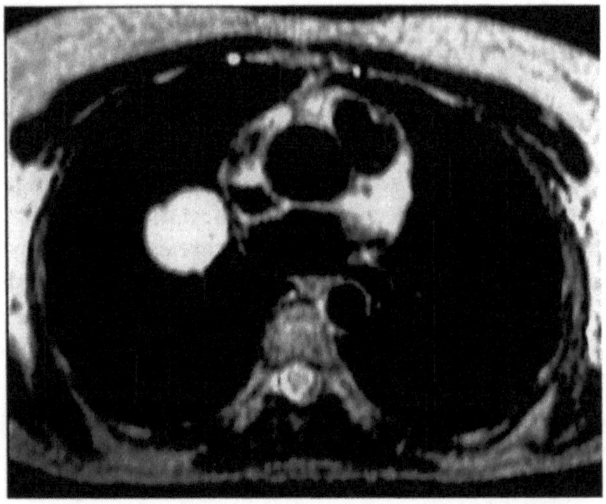

Fig. 16.7. MRI of the thorax. T_2-weighted sequence; repetition time, (TR), 1600 ms; echo time (TE), 80 ms: hyperintense nodule corresponding to a carcinoid tumor

16.4.1 Ovarian Carcinoids

Ovarian carcinoids account for less than 1% of all carcinoid tumors and are usually diagnosed in patients older than 50 years (Erhan et al. 1992). These solid encapsulated lesions vary in size from 1 to 25 cm; large tumors may produce a carcinoid syndrome. Histologically, these tumors are often mixed and associated with a teratoid component (cystic zones are frequent when a teratoid component is present). Ovarian carcinoids are nearly always unilateral, as opposed to ovarian metastases of carcinoid tumors, which are bilateral.

16.4.2 Pancreatic Carcinoids

In 1993, 23 cases of pancreatic carcinoids were reported in a literature study (Taidi et al. 1993). A carcinoid syndrome is frequently but not always observed. The tumor appears isodense on noncontrast CT; pronounced but inconsistent enhancement after iodine injection can assist differentiation from an adenocarcinoma (Villanueva et al. 1994). There are no morphologic criteria allowing differentiation of a pancreatic carcinoid from other pancreatic endocrine tumors (Villanueva et al. 1994). All four tumors described by this author contained calcification. Pancreatic carcinoids vary in size and may be quite small; endoscopic ultrasonography is helpful for detection in such cases.

16.4.3 Primary Carcinoids of the Liver

In 1992, 27 cases of primary carcinoids of the liver were reported in a literature review (Takayasu et al. 1992). Sonographically, the mass is often hyperechoic, mimicking a hemangioma. The first CT description is credited to Takayahu et al. (1992), who described multiple small, intratumoral cystic images corresponding to small thrombosed vascular lakes. Early and transient enhancement was observed on postcontrast CT. On MRI, primary liver carcinoids have a nonspecific high-intensity signal on T_2-weighted sequences; the small cystic images appear very hyperintense.

16.4.4 Primary Renal Carcinoids

Twenty-eight cases of primary renal carcinoids have been reported in the literature (Kurl et al. 1996). These tumors may be asymptomatic or may cause symptoms identical to those for other renal tumors (deterioration in general health, hematuria, fever) or, less often, a carcinoid syndrome. There are no specific imaging findings allowing differentiation from renal adenocarcinoma, although several features have been described. At ultrasonography, primary renal carcinoids are often hyperechoic, sometimes with a hypoechoic halo. On CT and angiography, these tumors are hypo- or avascular (McKeown et al. 1988; Moulopoulos et al. 1991). Cystic tumors have also been described, which creates problems for diagnosis.

16.4.5 Carcinoids of the Thymus

Approximately 100 thymic carcinoids have been reported since the first description by Rosai and Higa (1972). These tumors produce a clinical endocrine syndrome in 20%–50% of patients, in particular Cushing's syndrome (Herbst et al. 1987; Economopoulos et al. 1990), due to ectopic ACTH production. Thymic carcinoids characteristically cause extrathoracic metastases (Economopoulos et al. 1990) of bone, skin, or the adrenal glands. They also have a propensity for local and metastatic recurrence several years after initial diagnosis and treatment (Wang et al. 1994). These often large, invasive tumors may take up MIBG (Hirano et al. 1995). Microscopic lesions not detectable by CT have also been described and may be revealed by a Cushing syndrome. Thymic venous sampling of ACTH may allow tumor localization in such cases (Doppman et al. 1992).

16.5 Diagnostic and Therapeutic Arteriography of Gastrointestinal Carcinoid Tumors

T. de Baere and A. Roche

16.5.1 Diagnostic Angiography

Although digital subtraction angiography, by replacing conventional angiography, has lowered the rate of complications, essentially through reduction of the contrast dose and the examination duration (Waugh and Sacharias 1992), this technique has few remaining indications for the localization of primary carcinoids. This is due to the much higher efficacy of less invasive techniques, namely CT (Gould and Johnson 1986). The imaging features of small-bowel carcinoids are related more to the associated reactive fibrosis and mesenteric nodal metastases than to the tumors themselves. CT typically demonstrates a mesenteric mass with a more or less stellate appearance (Cockey et al. 1985; Gould and Johnson 1986). Angiography depicts hypervascularity in only 15% of patients. The most consistently observed angiographic feature is the stellate appearance of the ileal vasa recta, which are deformed and retracted as the result of fibrous changes in the mesentery (Reuter and Redman 1977; Bigot and Roche 1981). Stenosis or obstruction of mesenteric arterial branches and/or veins occurs in around one third of patients; in these patients, retractile mesenteritis is accompanied by the development of arterial or venous collaterals (Fig. 16.8). Somatostatin receptor scintigraphy is proving increasingly helpful for localization of carcinoid tumors (Kvols et al. 1993). This noninvasive technique is much more sensitive than other imaging modalities for extrahepatic sites, but appears less ef-

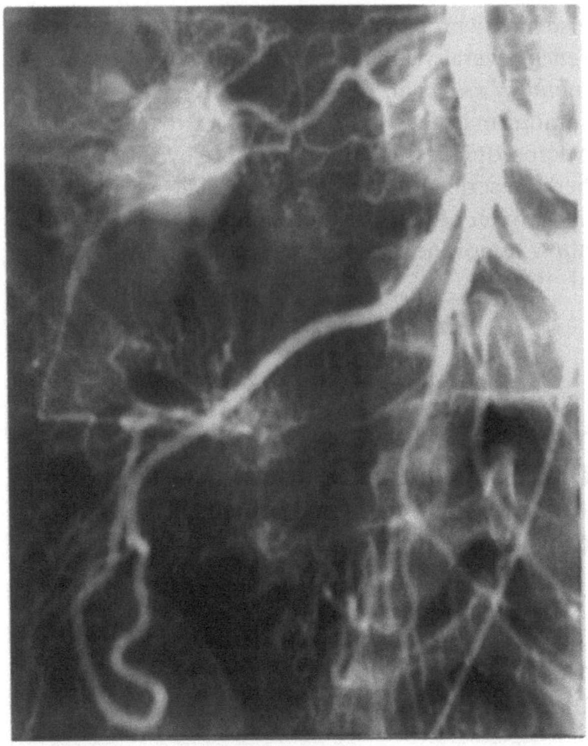

a

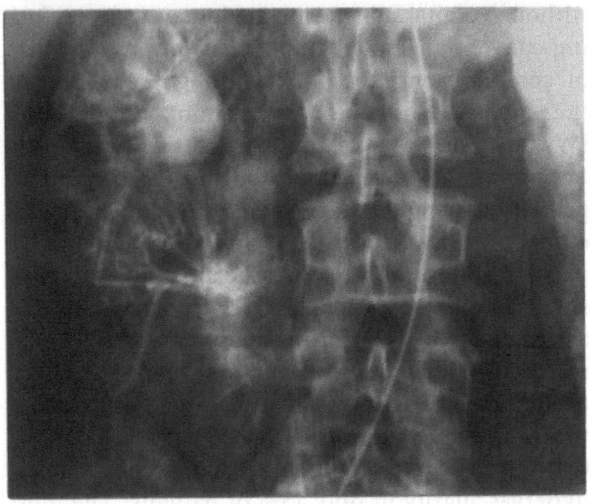

b

Fig. 16.8a,b. Superior mesenteric arteriogram in a patient with an ileal carcinoid tumor. **a** Early arterial phase: nearly complete occlusion of the thinned ileocolic artery, with a change in caliber at the end of the superior mesenteric artery, reflecting distant mesenteric invasion. **b** Late arterial phase: note the retractile stellate appearance of the arteries around the weakly hypervascular tumor

fective for detection of hepatic metastases (Krenning et al. 1993; Lamberts et al. 1993). EUS appears extremely promising for the localization of foregut tumors (Zimmer et al. 1994).

Hepatic angiography has a high sensitivity for the localization of hepatic metastases of carcinoids, which appear as hypervascular, often multiple round nodules. For the staging of hepatic metastases of carcinoid origin, however, angiography has been replaced by combinations of angiography and CT, i.e., CT arterial portography (CTAP) and CT hepatic angiography. These relatively invasive techniques are indicated only when other examinations are negative and/or when the presence or absence of metastases and their location may modify treatment planning. Ultrasound, the most reliable noninvasive technique for the diagnosis of hepatic metastases of carcinoid tumors (Andersson et al. 1987), should remain the initial morphologic examination for diagnosis and surveillance. Sonography is often associated with urinary assays of 5-hydroxy-indoleacetic acid (5-HIAA), a serotonin metabolite.

16.5.1.1 Computed Tomography Arterial Portography

Indirect CTAP, performed by injection into the mesenteric artery, is currently the most sensitive imaging modality (after intraoperative ultrasound) for the detection of hepatic metastases of colorectal origin. Sensitivity ranges from 85% to 91%, depending on the series (Nelson et al. 1989; Soyer et al. 1992). CTAP is also highly sensitive for the detection of metastases of carcinoid origin (McGrath and Malone 1993). CTAP should thus be performed as part of preoperative workup of metastatic liver disease, not only to determine the number and location of metastases, but also to make sure that at least 30% of the liver volume will be functional after resection. If there is a risk that the residual liver volume will be insufficient, and in the absence of other contraindications for surgery, preoperative portal vein embolization of the sectors to be resected permits redistribution of the portal blood flow toward the future hepatic remnant; subsequent hypertrophy of this segment is an indication for hepatectomy in the month following embolization (de Baere et al. 1996b).

CTAP is based on the fact that most hepatic metastases have a nearly exclusive arterial blood supply, whereas the portal vein ensures 70% of the supply to the healthy liver parenchyma. Metastases thus become hypodense within the liver parenchyma enhanced by the opacified portal blood (the liver enhances by approximately 100 HU). While CTAP is highly sensitive, its specificity is reduced by numerous false-positive results corresponding to focal portal perfusion abnormalities. The most frequent perfusion abnormalities are recognized by their shape (rectilinear or angular contours, sometimes triangular at the periphery of the liver) and their location (umbilical fissure, fossa of gallbladder, hepatic segment IV in contact with the origin of the right portal branch) (NELSON et al. 1992; PETERSON et al. 1992). Delayed scans obtained 4–6 h after injection increase the specificity of CTAP because the healthy parenchyma enhances following hepatocytic excretion of 1%–2% of the contrast medium (BRUNETON et al. 1990; NAZARIAN et al. 1992).

The tip of the catheter is selectively placed in the initial portion of the superior mesenteric artery under fluoroscopic control. If a right hepatic artery originates from the superior mesenteric artery, the tip of the catheter must be advanced beyond the origin to avoid opacification of the arterial hepatic blood. The catheter is secured in place, with continuous drip infusion of the lumen with saline, and the patient is transferred to the CT scanner. CT acquisition is initiated 10–12 s after the start of mesenteric injection (2 ml/s) to ensure that satisfactory portal opacification of the hepatic parenchyma is obtained from the outset. An iodine concentration of 15–18 mg/100 ml suffices. Injection can be stopped 10–12 s before the end of acquisition. Injection of 40 mg papaverine hydrochloride immediately before contrast administration increases enhancement of the liver parenchyma, which rises from 91±19 HU to 123±25 HU (SOYER et al. 1993). As injection of contrast material may trigger a carcinoid syndrome (MCGRATH and MALONE 1993), arteriographic procedures should be performed under the cover of prophylaxis by somatostatin analogues (Sandostatin, Sandoz, Basel; 100–400 μg subcutaneously 20 min before the procedure).

16.5.1.2
Computed Tomography Hepatic Angiography

CT hepatic angiography is based on the purely arterial vascularity of metastases, which renders them hyperdense to the normal parenchyma (only 30% arterial supply) on CT scans obtained during contrast injection into the hepatic artery. The main technical problem, which reduces the method's reproducibility, is the high frequency of anomalous hepatic artery branching patterns; 15%–20% of individuals have more than one hepatic artery, and even in individuals with a single hepatic artery, hepatic perfusion abnormalities are often seen on CT hepatic angiography (FREENY and MARKS 1986). Although CT angiography occasionally improves the specificity of CTAP, assessment of the entire liver is not possible in 20% of patients (CHEZMAR et al. 1993). It is thus difficult to use this examination in routine clinical practice.

Following arteriography to assess hepatic arterial vascularity, the distal tip of the catheter is placed in the common hepatic artery; two catheters may be required to evaluate the entire liver. The catheter is secured in place, continuous drip infusion of saline is initiated, and the patient is moved to the CT scanner. Acquisition can be begun 4–6 s after the start of injection (2 ml/s). An iodine concentration of 15–18 mg/100 ml suffices.

16.5.2
Therapeutic Angiography

Treatment of carcinoid tumors actually has two distinct targets: (1) the tumor and (2) the carcinoid syndrome. Owing to the usually slow growth rate of these tumors, the carcinoid syndrome is sometimes the major therapeutic preoccupation. Most treatments are therefore evaluated in terms of both morphological tumor response and symptomatic response.

16.5.2.1
Indications and Results

Surgery should obviously be proposed to all patients, regardless of whether metastases are present or not, provided all lesions are totally resectable. Recourse to hepatic intra-arterial therapies has been proposed to palliate the low efficacy of systemic chemotherapy and is based on the preferential arterial supply of hepatic metastases. Multiagent systemic chemotherapy regimens produce objective response rates of up to 40% for periods of 4–7 months (KVOLS and REUBI 1993; NORTON et al. 1993; MOERTEL et al. 1994). Intra-arterial chemotherapy has not proven superior to systemic chemotherapy (MATON and HODGSON 1984).

In contrast, surgical or radiological hepatic dearterialization has shown an antitumoral effect. Embolization and dearterialization produce equivalent response rates estimated at 40%–56%, with a response duration of 6–12 months (NOBIN et al. 1989; MOERTEL et al. 1994). The frequency and the duration of responses achieved by dearterialization are clearly improved by combination with systemic or intra-arterial chemotherapy. No guidelines currently exist for selection between surgical and radiological dearterialization. Two of the largest published series (Nobin et al. 1989; Moertel et al. 1994) are not able to conclude for benefit of a technique over the other. However, in the series presented by Moertel et al. (1994), the elevated frequency of vesicular necrosis and liver abscess was probably due to use of small-caliber and thus highly aggressive emboli.

In a personal series of 23 patients with invasive advanced tumors (hepatic invasion greater than 60% in 15 patients, another treatment ineffective in 16 patients), iodized oil chemoembolization plus Adriamycin (doxorubicin hydrochloride) produced a morphological response in 60% and disease stabilization in 28%. All 23 patients achieved a symptomatic response (70% complete response, 30% partial response) for a mean duration of 22 months.

A study of nine patients treated by iodized oil chemoembolization plus streptozocin reported a morphological response rate of 44% over 19 months. Despite its reported efficacy when administered by a systemic route, streptozocin has a major drawback: general anesthesia is necessary because of the intense pain caused by its very acid pH during hepatic intra-arterial injection. The morphological responses obtained with chemoembolization appear superior to those achieved with other medical treatments, i.e., systemic chemotherapy (11%–40% for 4–7 months), interferon (28%–50% for 2–11 months), and somatostatin analogues (77%–89% for 9–12 months).

Outside of surgery, only patients with symptomatic and/or progressive disease require treatment. However, somatostatin analogues provide excellent symptomatic relief (although without any true antineoplastic effect proven to date) and can be administered alone or in combination with another treatment. Use of somatostatin analogues requires particular caution in patients with biliary dysfunction because of the frequency of iatrogenic lithiasis. Supplementation with pancreatic hormones is usually indicated to prevent digestive malabsorption with steatorrhea.

16.5.2.2 Principle

For iodized oil hepatic chemoembolization, Lipiodol Ultra-fluide (Laboratoires Guerbet, Aulnay sous Bois, France) is mixed with Adriamycin (50 mg/m^2) by means of a three-way stopcock connecting the two syringes. Lipiodol acts as a plastic embolizing agent that temporarily reduces or stops the arterial circulation. Fragmentation of the lipid globules occurs at each successive arterial division as the product adapts to the increasingly smaller size of the vessels, until finally it is distributed in both the arterial circulation and the portal circulation due to the presinusoidal anastomoses between the two systems (Kan et al. 1989). During endovascular transit, Lipiodol passes preferentially into tumoral vessels (De Baere et al. 1995), is transported across the vascular wall, and becomes selectively and durably fixed in the hepatic tumor or tumors (Miller et al. 1987; Venook et al. 1990).

For hepatocellular carcinoma, the ratio of intratumoral to healthy liver Lipiodol reported in the literature varies from 4.7 to 15, depending on the author and injection parameters (Iwai et al. 1987; Raoul et al. 1988; Yoo et al. 1994). The ratio is approximately twofold lower for hepatic metastases of colorectal origin (Miller et al. 1987; Raoul et al. 1988). No study has investigated carcinoids in particular. Mixed with and administered at the same time as Lipiodol, the chemotherapeutic agent theoretically benefits from two effects: (1) the reduction of the flow rate, which increases the duration of exposure, and (2) vectorization (if the selectivity of Lipiodol for the tumor also applies to the drug). This mode of administration has a widely documented pharmacokinetic advantage (Zhao et al. 1993) and increases the response rate for hepatocellular carcinoma (Wakasa et al. 1990).

The rationale for locoregional drug administration by chemoembolization is the increase in tumor exposure associated with reduced systemic exposure. The pharmadynamic advantage (A) of this technique compared to systemic injection is expressed by the formula: $A = C/Q_a(1-E)$, where C is the total body clearance of the drug, Q_a is the flow in the perfused artery, and E is the coefficient of drug extraction. Embolization diminishes or even annuls the arterial flow and thus increases this advantage; it also has an inherent antitumoral action related to lesion ischemia. The aggressivity of the procedure can be modulated by varying the size of the particles used. Resorbable particulate embolizing agents are used for hepatic chemoembolization in order to preserve the vascular route for subsequent therapy.

16.5.2.3
Technique

Iodized oil chemoembolization is always preceded by arteriography; this allows evaluation of portal venous drainage (in search of abnormalities) and hepatic arterial anatomy (anatomic variants are frequent) and determination of the location and type of vascularity of hepatic or distant metastases (especially nodal metastases), which are often hypervascular. The tip of the catheter must be positioned in the hepatic artery or arteries distal to the origin of any branch to the gastrointestinal tract. In general, a mixture of 50 mg Adriamycin (m^2) and 10 ml Lipiodol Ultra-fluide is distributed throughout the entire liver. Embolization is achieved by injecting 2–3 mm gelatin sponge dedglets until arterial stagnation is obtained. Resorbable gelatin sponge is recommended because it permits repeat treatment through the same arterial vessels. Except for hyperselective embolizations, fine particles or powders should be avoided because of their high aggressivity (SONOMURA et al. 1997), which is a source of complications. The arteries of patients with carcinoid tumors appear much more reactive in terms of vascular spasm and dissection and much more fragile than in other patients. This is probably due to the vascular effects (flushing) induced by hormones (especially serotonin). Catheterization must thus be as atraumatic as possible. Despite precautions, arterial occlusion occurred in nearly 60% of patients in a personal series of patients who underwent chemoembolization for a carcinoid tumor; the rate is usually only 30% in patients treated for other pathologies. The only consequence of occlusion is the need to halt treatment using the damaged vessel.

In patients with proximal occlusion of the hepatic artery, chemoembolization can be performed through the collateral circulation: pancreaticoduodenal arcades arising from the superior mesenteric artery, gastric arteries, inferior phrenic arteries, internal mammary arteries (ANDREWS et al. 1989; MACAULAY and CODWELL 1995). If the occlusion is recent, several months must be allowed to elapse so that sufficient collateral circulation can develop, thereby facilitating ulterior catheterization. Extensive distal occlusion is often due to vasculitis caused by the direct toxicity of the products injected. Collateral flow suitable for ulterior intra-arterial treatment rarely develops in these patients.

16.5.2.4
Number of Embolization Sessions

The rhythm of embolization sessions is relatively slow for carcinoid tumors, mainly because of their indolent course, but also to preserve hepatic vessels. As for most tumors treated by chemoembolization, the first two sessions are routinely given at a 2-month interval; clinical, morphological, and biological evaluation is performed 1 month after the second session. Assessment of response is facilitated by comparison with the pretherapy tumor growth rate determined by initial morphologic studies. Therapy sessions are scheduled as a function of the response, patient tolerance, evolution of the residual tumor mass, and tumor markers (urinary 5-HIAA). In our experience, the interval between sessions ranged from 2 to 12 months (Fig. 16.9).

16.5.2.5
Contraindications

Whether due to complete portal thrombosis, tumor obliteration, tumor compression, or reversal of the portal flow, absence of portal perfusion of the liver is always a formal contraindication for embolization.

Partial portal thrombosis, in contrast, is not a formal contraindication. Postembolization ischemia is the sum of preexistent portal ischemia and arterial ischemia induced and modulated by the operator. In practice, complete portal occlusion of three major segments appears a reasonable limit. However, when possible, the extent and the aggressiveness of embolization should be adapted to portal status and tumor location; a vessel that vascularizes a tumor exclusively or nearly exclusively can be embolized, even with powder, if adequate portal perfusion is preserved.

Retention jaundice is a potential source of infectious complications (DOPPMAN et al. 1979) due to necrosis of the gallbladder walls by stagnant and thus possibly infected bile. This is a formal contraindication, and chemoembolization can be envisaged only after gallbladder drainage. Keeping this in mind, patients with biliary–digestive anastomoses account for the only severe necrotic–infectious complications with chemoembolization that we have encountered since the introduction of systematic antibiotic prophylaxis (DE BAERE et al. 1996a). These complications are unpredictable because they do not always occur during the first session. Furthermore, they have also been described after chemotherapy/

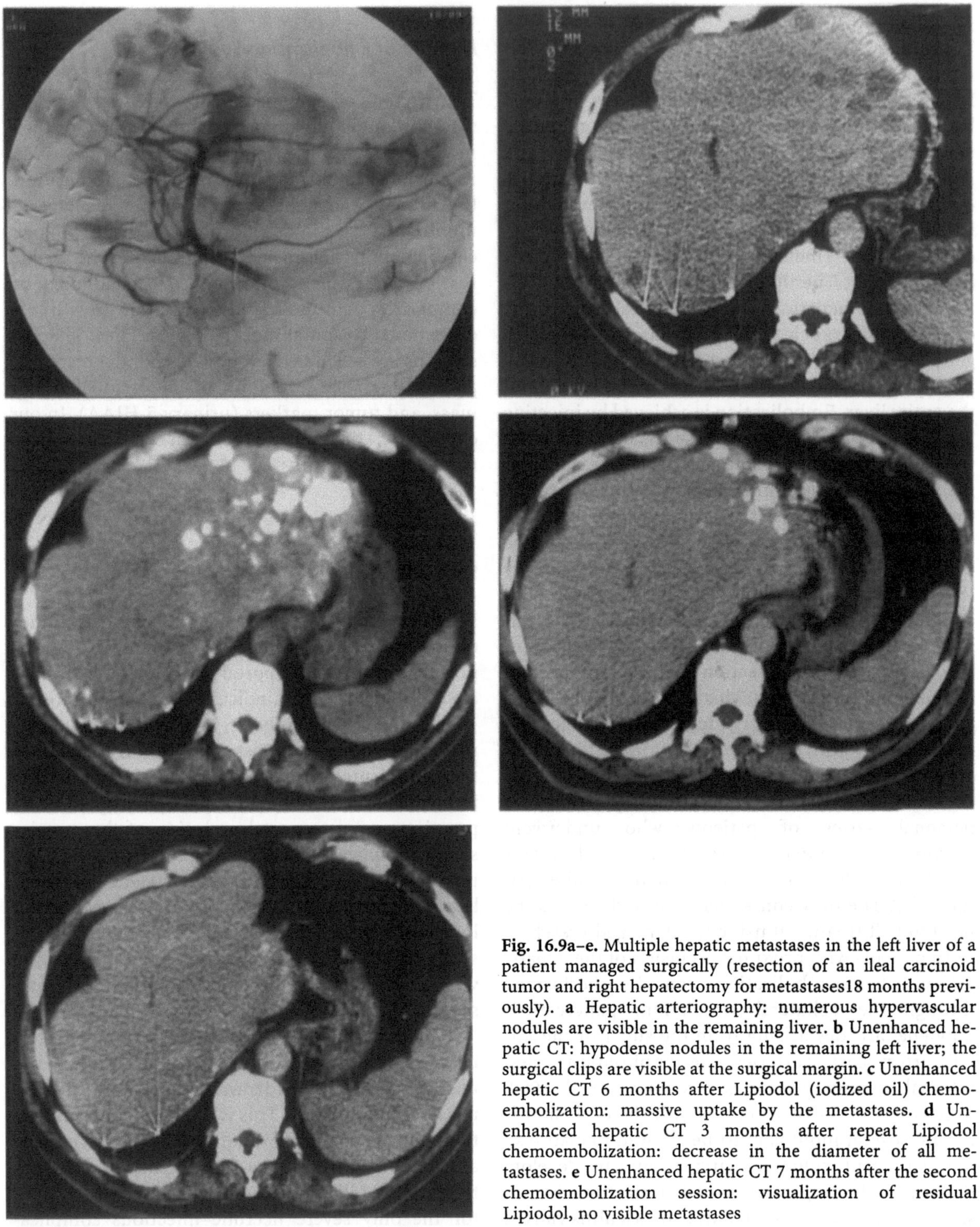

Fig. 16.9a–e. Multiple hepatic metastases in the left liver of a patient managed surgically (resection of an ileal carcinoid tumor and right hepatectomy for metastases18 months previously). **a** Hepatic arteriography: numerous hypervascular nodules are visible in the remaining liver. **b** Unenhanced hepatic CT: hypodense nodules in the remaining left liver; the surgical clips are visible at the surgical margin. **c** Unenhanced hepatic CT 6 months after Lipiodol (iodized oil) chemoembolization: massive uptake by the metastases. **d** Unenhanced hepatic CT 3 months after repeat Lipiodol chemoembolization: decrease in the diameter of all metastases. **e** Unenhanced hepatic CT 7 months after the second chemoembolization session: visualization of residual Lipiodol, no visible metastases

Lipiodol injection without complementary embolization. These infectious complications might be explained by the toxicity of Lipiodol and the antineoplastic drug on the peribiliary capillary plexus, associated with retrograde bacterial bile infection favored by the absence of a sphincter (during stagnation in the hepatic artery, Lipiodol reaches the portal system through small collaterals forming the peribiliary capillary plexus) (KAN et al. 1994; DE BAERE et al. 1995). Biliary–digestive anastomoses are not uncommon after resection of primary neuroendocrine or carcinoid tumors in or near the head of the pancreas. In our experience, these patients should not be treated by iodized oil chemoembolization.

Even minimal liver failure is a formal contraindication, because it usually reflects massive invasion that is much more extensive than suggested by imaging studies. Embolization is not justified, as it would only aggravate liver function in patients with end-stage disease.

16.5.2.6
Normal Postembolization Course

Inflammatory responses such as fever, pain, nausea, and vomiting comprise the postembolization syndrome, which is accompanied by hyperleukocytosis and hyperthrombocytosis. Tumor necrosis is the origin of this syndrome, probably due to release of cytokines such as interleukin-6, which is markedly elevated 24 h after transcatheter arterial embolization (TAE) and peaks at eight times the pretreatment level 4 days later (MATSUDA et al. 1994). Preventive measures should be taken, accompanied when necessary by symptomatic treatment, to reduce patient discomfort during the postoperative period. Morphine or meperidine hydrochloride is often required for pain relief during the first 48 h. Prochlorperazine is indicated for nausea and vomiting. Fever is generally rapidly jugulated by naproxen or indomethacin.

16.5.2.7
Complications

Any procedure in a patient with a carcinoid tumor may trigger an acute carcinoid crisis, and prophylaxis with somatostatin analogues should thus be instituted before chemoembolization.

Embolization always causes cytolysis of the normal hepatic parenchyma, which is reflected by an elevation in transaminases. Consequences are minimal in the absence of preexistent hepatic failure. The main periprocedural risk is renal failure, which is favored by acidosis secondary to tumor necrosis, preexistent renal failure, and the inherent effects of the contrast medium. Certain ongoing studies, for example, use streptozocin, which has high renal toxicity. This complication can be prevented by adequate pre- and postembolization hydration.

Infection of the embolized segment can be prevented by antibiotic prophylaxis for 3–5 days; the risk of infection is especially high in the case of bile retention or biliary–digestive anastomosis. Hyperleukocytosis is frequent and sometimes severe, but is usually noninfectious and purely inflammatory. The presence of gas in the embolized tumor tissue has no particular significance, i.e., does not mean that there is infection (MARKS and FILLY 1979; SIIM and FLECKENSTEIN 1982).

Ischemic cholecystitis may occur if hepatic embolization is not sufficiently selective, if the gastroduodenal artery has been partially embolized, or if very fine particles (which can migrate distally) have been injected upstream of the origin of the cystic artery. Systematic ultrasound follow-up often demonstrates transient gallbladder wall thickening (BOTET et al. 1985), but most patients are asymptomatic, and cholecystectomy is rarely indicated.

The complications of local chemotherapy vary with the drug and the cumulative dose. Depending on the clinical situation, certain drugs must be avoided because of their major toxicity: Adriamycin should be avoided because of its cardiac toxicity and the risk of alopecia, while cisplatin and streptozocin should be avoided because of their renal toxicity. Certain drug combinations also have deleterious effects. SOULEN et al. (1996) described severe complications in four patients who underwent iodized oil chemoembolization with a triple-agent chemotherapy combination (cisplatin, Adriamycin, mitomycin-C) and polyvinyl alcohol particles; in contrast, no complications were observed when embolization was performed with the same particles, but without chemotherapy.

Overall, except for CTAP with mesenteric injection, which is extremely helpful for preoperative workup of hepatic metastases, arteriography has few remaining indications for diagnosis of carcinoid tumors. Embolization and chemoembolization play major roles in the treatment of progressive and/or symptomatic hepatic metastases.

References

Adolf JMG, Kimmig BN, Georgi P et al (1987) Carcinoid tumors: CT and I-131 meta-iodo-benzylguanidine scintigraphy. Radiology 164:199–203

Andersson T, Eriksson B, Hemmingsson A, Lindgren PG, Oberg K (1987) Angiography, computed tomography, magnetic resonance imaging and ultrasonography in detection of liver metastases from endocrine gastrointestinal tumours. Acta Radiol 28:535–539

Andrews J, Guy G, Walker-Andrews S (1989) Treatment of hepatic cancer through arterial collaterals – a simple cost-effective technique. J Intervent Radiol 4:127–129

Aronchick JM, Wexler JA, Christen B et al (1986) Computed tomography of bronchial carcinoid. J Comput Assist Tomogr 10:71–74

Beaton HL (1982) Carcinoid tumors of the alimentary tract. CA Cancer J Clin 32:92–97

Berger MW, Stephens DH (1996) Gastric carcinoid tumors associated with chronic hypergastrinemia in a patient with Zollinger-Ellison syndrome. Radiology 201:371–373

Bigot J, Roche A (1981) Possibilités diagnostiques et thérapeutiques dans les tumeurs carcinoïdes du tube digestif. Acta Gastroenterol Belg 44:120–140

Borch K (1989) Atrophic gastritis and gastric carcinoid tumors. Ann Med 21:291–297

Botet JF, Watson RC, Kemeny N et al (1985) Cholangitis complicating intra-arterial chemotherapy in liver metastasis. Radiology 156:335–337

Bruneton JN, Rogopoulos A, Merran D et al (1990) Scanographie hépatique: utilité des coupes tardives (6 heures) chez des patients ayant une fonction biliaire normale. J Radiol 71:271–277

Buck JL, Sobin LH (1990) Carcinoids of the gastrointestinal tract. Radiographics 10:1081–1095

Chezmar JL, Bernardino ME, Kaufman SH, Nelson RC (1993) Combined CT arterial portography and CT hepatic angiography for evaluation of the hepatic resection candidate. Work in progress. Radiology 189:407–410

Chopier-Richaud J, Ouahes N, Breittmayer F (1993) Tumeurs carcinoïdes digestives. J Radiol 74:279–282

Choplin RH, Kawamoto EH, Dyer RB et al (1986) Atypical carcinoid of the lung: radiographic features. AJR 146:665–668

Clements JL, Roche RR (1984) Carcinoid of the duodenum: a report of six cases. Gastrointest Radiol 9:17

Cockey B, Fishman E, Jones B, Siegelman S (1985) Computed tomography of abdominal carcinoid tumor. J Comp Assist Tomogr 9:38–42

Davila DG, Dunn WF, Tazelaar HD et al (1993) Bronchial carcinoid tumors. Mayo Clin Proc 68:795–803

de Baere T, Dufaux J, Roche A et al (1995) Circulatory alterations induced by intra-arterial injection of iodized oil and emulsions of iodized oil and doxorubicin: experimental study. Radiology 194:165–170

de Baere T, Roche A, Amenabar J et al (1996a) Liver abscess formation after local treatment of liver tumors. Hepatology 23:1436–1440

de Baere T, Roche A, Elias D et al (1996b) Preoperative portal vein embolization for extension of hepatectomy indications. Hepatology 24:1386–1391

Doppman JL, Pass HI, Nieman LK et al (1991) Detection of ACTH-producing bronchial carcinoid tumors: MR imaging vs CT. AJR 156:39–43

Doppman JL, Pass HI, Nieman LK et al (1992) Corticopin-secretin carcinoid tumors of the thymus: diagnostic unreliability of thymic venous sampling. Radiology 184:71–74

Doppman L, Dunnick NR, Girton RT et al (1979) Bile duct cysts secondary to liver infarcts: report of case and experimental production by small vessel hepatic artery occlusion. Radiology 130:1–5

Douek PC, Simoni L, Revel D, Cordier JF, Amiel M (1994) Diagnosis of bronchial carcinoid tumor by ultrafast contrast-enhanced MR imaging. AJR 163:563–564

Economopoulos GC, Lewis JW Jr, Lee MW et al (1990) Carcinoid tumors of the thymus. Ann Thorac Surg 50:58–61

Erhan Y, Dikicioglu E, Alkanat MB et al (1992) Primary carcinoid tumor of the ovary. A case report. Acta Oncol 31:790–792

Forster BB, Muller NL, Miller RR et al (1989) Neuroendocrine carcinomas of the lung: clinical, radiologic, and pathologic correlation. Radiology 170:441–445

Freeny P, Marks W (1986) Hepatic perfusion abnormalities during CT angiography: detection and interpretation. Radiology 159:685–691

Godwin JD (1975) Carcinoid tumors: an analysis of 2837 cases. Cancer 36:560–569

Gould M, Johnson RJ (1986) Computed tomography of abdominal carcinoid tumor. Br J Radiol 59:881–885

Hanson MW, Feldman JM, Blinder RA et al (1989) Carcinoid tumors: iodine-131 MIBG scintigraphy. Radiology 170:699–703

Harpole DH, Feldman JM, Buchanan S et al (1992) Bronchial carcinoid tumors: A retrospective analysis of 126 patients. Ann Thorac Surg 54:50–55

Herbst WM, Kummer W, Hofmann WJ et al (1987) Carcinoid tumors of the thymus: an immunohistochemical study. Cancer 60:2465–2470

Hermans JJ, Hermans AL, Risseuw GA et al (1993) Appendicitis caused by carcinoid tumor. Radiology 188:71–72

Hirano T, Otake H, Watanabe N et al (1995) Presurgical diagnosis of a primary carcinoid tumor of the thymus with MIBG. J Nucl Med 36:2243–2245

Hurt R, Bates M (1984) Carcinoid tumors of the bronchus: a 33-year experience. Thorax 39:617–623

Iwai K, Maeda H, Konno T et al (1987) Tumor targeting by arterial administration of lipids: rabbit model with VX 2 carcinoma in the liver. Anticancer Res 7:321–328

Jeffree MA, Barter SJ, Hemingway AP et al (1984) Primary carcinoid tumor of the ileum. Clin Radiol 35:451–455

Kan K, Ivancev I, Hägerstrand CV, Lunderquist A (1989) In vivo microscopy of the liver after injection of lipiodol into the hepatic artery and portal vein in the rat. Acta Radiol 30:419–425

Kan Z, Ivancev K, Lunderquist A (1994) Peribiliary plexa – important pathways for shunting of iodized oil and silicon rubber solution from the hepatic artery to the portal vein: an experimental study in rats. Invest Radiol 29:671–676

Kawamoto K, Heyama T, Iwashita I et al (1994) Colonic submucosal tumors: comparison of endoscopic US and target air-enema CT with barium enema study and colonoscopy. Radiology 192:697–702

Krenning E, Kwekkeboom D, Bakker W et al (1993) Somatostatin receptor scintigraphy with (111In-DTPA-d-Phe1)- and (123I-Tyr3)-octreotide: the Rotterdam experience with more than 1000 patients. Eur J Nucl Med 20:716–731

Kurl S, Rytkonen H, Farin P, Ala-Opas M, Soimakallio S (1996) Primary carcinoid tumor of the kidney: case report and review of the literature. Abdom Imaging 21:464–467

Kvols L, Reubi J (1993) Metastatic carcinoid tumors and the malignant carcinoid syndrome. Acta Oncol 32:197–201

Kvols LK, Brown ML, O'Connor MK et al (1993) Evaluation of

a radiolabeled somatostatin analog (I-123 octreotide) in the detection and localization of carcinoid and islet cell tumors. Radiology 187:129–133
Lamberts S, Reubi J, Krenning E (1993) Validation of somatostatin receptor scintigraphy in the localization of neuroendocrine tumors. Acta Oncol 32:167–170
Lawson RM, Ramanathan L, Hurley G et al (1976) Bronchial adenoma: review of an 18-year experience at the Brompton Hospital. Thorax 31:245–253
Macaulay S, Codwell D (1995) Internal mammary artery embolization for hepatic tumors. Cardiovasc Intervent Radiol 18:20–24
Magid D, Siegelman SS, Eggleston JC, Fishman EK, Zerhouni EA (1989) Pulmonary carcinoid tumors: CT assessment. J Comput Assist Tomogr 13:244–247
Marks WM, Filly RA (1979) Computed tomographic demonstration of intra-arterial air following hepatic artery ligation. Radiology 132:665–666
Marty-Ane CH, Costes V, Pujol JL et al (1995) Carcinoid tumors of the lung: Do atypical features require aggressive management ? Ann Thorac Surg 59:78–83
Maton P, Hodgson H (1984) Carcinoid tumors and the carcinoid syndrome. In: Bouchier IAD, Allan RN, Hodgson HJF, Keighly MRB (eds) Textbook of gastroenterology. Bailliere-Tindall, Ville, pp 620–648
Matsuda Y, Kawata S, Nagase T et al (1994) Interleukine-6 in transcatheter arterial embolization for patients with hepatocellular carcinoma. Cancer 73:53–57
McAdams HP, Mc Elaney B, Erasmus J (1995) Chest case of the day. Case 1: metastatic bronchial carcinoid. AJR 165:186–191
McCaughan BC, Martini N, Bains MS (1985) Bronchial carcinoids: review of 124 cases. J Cardiovasc Surg 89:8–17
McGrath FP, Malone DE (1993) Computed tomography during arterial portography in malignant carcinoid syndrome: a report of two patients. Can Assoc Radiol J 44:117–120
McKeown DK, Nguyen GK, Rudrick B, Johnson MA (1988) Carcinoid of the kidney: radiologic findings. AJR 150:143–144
Miller L, Oleary T, Girton M (1987) Distribution of iodized oil within the liver after hepatic arterial injection. Radiology 162:849–852
Moertel CG, Weiland LH, Nagorney DM, Dockerty MD (1987) Carcinoid tumor of the appendix: treatment and prognosis. N Engl J Med 317:1699–1701
Moertel CG, Johnson CM, McKusick MA et al (1994) The management of patients with advanced carcinoid tumors and islet cell carcinomas. Ann Intern Med 120:302–309
Moulopoulos A, Dubrow R, Davd C, Dimopoulos MA (1991) Primary renal carcinoid: computed tomography, ultrasound, and angiographic findings. J Comput Assist Tomogr 15:323–325
Muller NL, Miller RR (1990) Neuroendocrine carcinomas of the lung. Semin Roentgenol 25:96–104
Nazarian L, Wechsler R, Grady C et al (1992) CT done 4–6 hr after CT arterial portography: value of detecting hepatic tumors and differentiating from other hepatic function perfusion defects. AJR 163:851–855
Nelson C, Chezmar J, Sugarbaker P, Bernardino M (1989) Hepatic tumors: comparison of CT during arterial portography, delayed CT, and MR imaging for preoperative evaluation. Radiology 172:27–34
Nelson R, Thompson G, Chezmar J, Harned R, Fernandez M (1992) CT during arterial portography: diagnostic pitfalls. Radiographics 12:705–719
Nobin A, Mansson B, Lunderquist A (1989) Evaluation of temporary liver dearterialization and embolization in patients with metastatic carcinoid tumour. Acta Oncol 28:419–424
Norton A, Levin B, Jensen R (1993) Cancer of the endocrine system. In: DeVita VT Jr, Hellman S, Rosenberg SA (eds) Cancer: principles and practice of oncology, 4th edn. Lippincott, Philadelphia, pp 1333–1435
O'Byrne KJ, O'Hare NJ, Freyne PJ et al (1994) Imaging of bronchial carcinoid tumors with indium-111 pentetreotide. Thorax 49:284–286
Okike N, Bernatz PE, Woolner LB (1976) Carcinoid tumors of the lung. Ann Thorac Surg 22:270–275
Pantongrad-Brown L, Buetow PC, Carr NJ et al (1995) Calcification and fibrosis in mesenteric carcinoid tumor: CT findings and pathologic correlation. AJR 164: 387–391
Peterson M, Baron R, Dodd G et al (1992) Hepatic parenchymal perfusion defects detected with CTAP: imaging-pathologic correlation. Radiology 185:149–155
Picus D, Glazer HS, Levitt RG (1984) Computed tomography of abdominal carcinoid tumors. AJR 143:581–584
Ranfaing E (1993) Tumeurs neuro-endocrines pulmonaires. Ann Pathol 13:414–421
Raoul JL, Bourguet P, Bretagne JF et al (1988) Hepatic artery injection of I-131-labeled lipiodol. Biodistribution study results in patients with hepatocellular carcinoma and liver metastases. Radiology 168:541–545
Reuter SR, Redman HC (1977) Tumors. In: Reuter SR, Redman HC (eds) Gastrointestinal angiography, 2nd edn. Saunders, Philadelphia, pp 106–188
Rioux M, Duchesne N, Langis P (1994) Carcinoid tumor of the appendix: ultrasound findings in two cases. J Clin Ultrasound 22:129–133
Rioux M, Langis P, Naud F (1995) Sonographic appearance of primary small bowel carcinoid tumor. Abdom Imaging 20:37–43
Rosai T, Higa E (1972) Mediastinal endocrine neoplasm of probably thymic origin, related to carcinoid tumor: clinico-pathologic study of 8 cases. Cancer 29:1061–1074
Schillaci O, Scopinaro F, Angeletti A et al (1996) SPECT improves accuracy of somatostatin receptor scintigraphy in abdominal carcinoid tumors. J Nucl Med 37:1452–1456
Siim E, Fleckenstein P (1982) Gas formation following hepatic tumour embolisation. Br J Radiol 55:926–928
Smevic B, Kolmannskog F, Aakhus T (1983) Computed tomography and angiography in carcinoid liver metastases. Acta Radiol 24:189–193
Sonomura T, Yamada R, Kishi K et al (1997) Dependence of tissue necrosis on gelatine sponge particule size after canine hepatic artery embolisation. Cardiovasc Intervent Radiol 20:50–53
Soulen MC, Pentecost MJ, Baum RA, Shlansky-Goldberg RD, Haskal ZJ (1996) CAM/oil/polyvinyl alcohol chemoembolization: life-threatening complications with metastatic carcinoid. J Vasc Intervent Radiol [Suppl] 7:148 (abstr)
Soyer P, Levesque M, Elias D, Zeitoun G, Roche A (1992) Detection of liver metastases from colorectal cancer: comparison of intraoperative US and CT during arterial portography. Radiology 183:541–544
Soyer P, Lacheheb D, Levesque M (1993) CT arterial portography of the abdomen: effect of injecting papaverine into the mesenteric artery on hepatic contrast enhancement. AJR 160:1213–1215
Taidi C, Soyer P, Barge J et al (1993) Tumeur carcinoïde primitive du pancréas. Aspects tomodensitométriques et écho-endoscopiques. J Radiol 74:347–350
Takayasu K, Muramatsu Y, Sakamoto M et al (1992) Findings in primary hepatic carcinoid tumor: US, CT, MRI, and angiography. J Comput Assist Tomogr 16:99–102

Toomey FB, Felson B (1960) Osteoblastic bone metastasis in gastrointestinal and bronchial carcinoids. AJR 83:709–715
Troupin RH (1968) Ossifying bronchial carcinoid: a case report. AJR 104:808–809
Venook P, Stagg RJ, Lewis BJ et al (1990) Chemoembolization for hepatocellular carcinoma. J Clin Oncol 8:1108–1114
Villanueva A, Perez C, Llauger J, Traid C, Parellada JA, Puig P (1994) Carcinoid tumors of the pancreas: CT findings. Abdom Imaging 19:221–224
Wakasa K, Sakurai M, Kuroda C et al (1990) Effect of transcatheter embolization on the boundary architecture of hepatocellular carcinoma. Cancer 65:913–919
Wang DY, Chang DB, Kuo SH et al (1994) Carcinoid tumors of the thymus. Thorax 49:357–360
Watanabe N, Seto H, Ishiki M et al (1995) I-123 MIBG imaging of metastatic carcinoid tumor from the rectum. Clin Nucl Med 20:357–360
Waugh J, Sacharias N (1992) Arteriographic complications in the DSA era. Radiology 182:243–246
Woodard PK, Feldman JM, Paine SS, Baker ME (1995) Midgut carcinoid tumors: CT findings and biochemical profiles. J Comput Assist Tomogr 19:400–405
Yoo HS, Park CH, Lee JT et al (1994) Small hepatocellular carcinoma: high dose internal radiation therapy with superselective intra-arterial injection of I-131-labeled lipiodol. Cancer Chemother Pharmacol 33:128–133
Zhao Z, Ramirez L, Ardouin P et al (1993) Intra hepatic arterial chemotherapy using pirarubicin combined with lipiodol in rabbits bearing VX2 tumors. Reg Cancer Treat 4:213–217
Zimmer T, Ziegler K, Bader M et al (1994) Localisation of neuroendocrine tumours of the upper gastrointestinal tract. Gut 35:471–475
Zwiebel BR, Austin JHM, Grimes MM (1991) Bronchial carcinoid tumors: assessment with CT of location and intratumoral calcification in 31 patients. Radiology 179:483–486

17 Multiple Endocrine Neoplasia Syndromes

B. PADOVANI and P. CHEVALLIER

CONTENTS

17.1 Introduction

The multiple endocrine neoplasia (MEN) syndromes are inherited disorders of the neuroendocrine system and are characterized by a predisposition to simultaneous or successive development of neoplasia and/or hyperplasia of several endocrine glands. Transmitted as an autosomal dominant disorder, the endocrine abnormalities in MEN reflect involvement of the amine precursor uptake and decarboxylation (APUD) system.

Three genetically distinct MEN syndromes are distinguished according to the sites of endocrine gland involvement. MEN type I (Wermer's syndrome) comprises involvement of the anterior pituitary gland, the parathyroids, and the endocrine pancreas. MEN type II (Sipple's syndrome) is an association of medullary carcinoma of the thyroid, pheochromocytoma, and hyperparathyroidism. In MEN type IIb or III (Gorlin's syndrome, mucosal neuroma syndrome), medullary thyroid carcinoma and pheochromocytoma are accompanied by dysmorphic features, multiple neuromas, and intestinal ganglioneuromatosis.

The lesions of MEN type I syndrome are usually diagnosed in patients around 40 years of age and can correspond to hyperplasia or carcinoma (BONE 1990; SKOGSEID et al. 1991). Hyperparathyroidism is the most frequent manifestation, occurring in 90% of patients. Clinical symptoms include hypercalcemia with hypophosphatemia and elevated parathyroid hormone (PTH) production due to hyperplasia or, less often, an adenoma. In 50% of patients, the anterior pituitary lobe is the site of a prolactin-secreting adenoma (prolactinoma); adenomas secreting growth hormone (GH) are also encountered. Macroadenomas account for 73% of these lesions. Clinical symptoms depend on the size of the adenoma and the intensity of hormone secretion. Nonfunctioning chromophobe adenomas are also possible. Pancreatic involvement, present in 70%–80% of patients, dominates the prognosis for MEN type I; multiple lesions are frequent and can correspond to hyperplasia, adenoma, or even carcinoma. Their clinical endocrine symptoms depend on hormone production. The most frequent tumors are gastrinomas (75% of patients), which are responsible for Zollinger-Ellison syndrome (peptic ulcer disease and gastritis). These lesions are usually discovered in patients older than 25 years and are always multifocal. Gastrinomas occur in the duodenal wall and the pancreas and cause considerable diagnostic and therapeutic problems owing to their dissemination and small size (PIPELEERS-MARICHAL et al. 1990; AKERSTRÖM et al. 1991). Diagnosis is based on demonstration of hypergastrinemia with hypersecretion of gastric acid. Insulinomas are less frequent than gastrinomas and are often discovered in younger patients (around 18 years). These tumors are responsible for hypoglycemic episodes due to insulin secretion. Functioning tumors of the endocrine pancreas secreting vasoactive intestinal peptide (VIP), somatostatin, or gluca-

B. PADOVANI, Service de Radiodiagnostic, Hôpital Pasteur, 30 avenue de la Voie Romaine, BP 69, 06002 Nice, France
P. CHEVALLIER, Service de Radiodiagnostic, Hôpital de l'Archet, 151 chemin de St. Antoine de Ginestière, 06200 Nice, France

gon and nonfunctioning tumors are much less common. Infrequent types of glandular involvement include often latent adrenal lesions (hyperplasia or nonfunctioning adenoma) present in 20%–40% of patients, carcinoids (10% of patients), thyroid lesions (colloid goiter, thyroiditis or adenoma) thymomas, and schwannomas.

The most consistently observed feature of MEN type IIa is medullary carcinoma of the thyroid, a tumor of the parafollicular C cells (Saad et al. 1984). Clinical manifestations are variable, and some patients are even asymptomatic. Systematic search for thyroid disease is thus mandatory in patients with involvement of the other endocrine glands and during family screening studies. Medullary thyroid cancer is sometimes revealed by symptoms related to excessive calcitonin secretion, i.e., diarrhea, flush, peptic ulcer. Ectopic secretion of adrenocorticotropic hormone (ACTH), VIP, somatostatin and serotonin has also been described. Frequently multifocal and bilateral, medullary thyroid cancer is commonly accompanied by cervicomediastinal lymphadenopathy and occasionally by bone, liver, or lung metastases. The prognosis depends on the quality of surgical resection and the degree of disease spread. This explains the value of early diagnosis in families at risk. Biochemical diagnosis by calcitonin assays is sometimes associated with stimulation tests (pentagastrin). Pheochromocytomas occur in 50%–60% of patients. These lesions should be sought systematically by urinary catecholamine assays in patients with other forms of endocrine dysfunction. Ectopic lesions are possible. Bilateral tumors are more frequent in MEN IIa than sporadic cases (Gagel et al. 1988). Hyperparathyroidism, which is very often latent, occurs in 40% of patients; the clinical manifestations are similar to those in MEN type I (Öberg 1994).

MEN type IIb is a much rarer entity characterized by marfanoid dysmorphic features, medullary thyroid carcinoma (which often occurs earlier than in MEN IIa), and pheochromocytoma (frequently bilateral). Cutaneous or mucosal neuromatosis and intestinal ganglioneuromatosis are common.

The diagnosis of MEN syndromes is established by family screening, clinical data, and appropriate laboratory tests (hormone assays, stimulation tests). Preoperative imaging studies play an essential role in tumor localization, disease staging, and searches for any occult coexistent lesions.

17.2 Multiple Endocrine Neoplasia Type I

17.2.1 Parathyroids

Workup for MEN-related parathyroid lesions is similar to that for sporadic parathyroid tumors and is based essentially on cervical ultrasound. If cervical sonography is negative, computed tomography (CT) or magnetic resonance imaging (MRI) is indicated to demonstrate ectopic localizations in the anterior mediastinum.

17.2.2 Pituitary Gland

Examination of the pituitary is also identical to that for sporadic pituitary tumors. MRI is currently the technique of choice; it can readily demonstrate macroadenomas and has satisfactory sensitivity for the detection of microadenomas smaller than 10 mm (Kucharczy 1986).

17.2.3 Pancreas

Examination of the pancreas involves particular difficulties owing to the small size of most tumors (usually less than 15 mm) and the frequency of multiple lesions. Imaging modalities play a critical role in tumor localization when the tumor is still small, as early diagnosis can improve the prognosis.

Pancreatic ultrasound is insufficient for pancreatic assessment; sensitivity is only 60% for insulinomas (Gorman et al. 1986; Galiber 1988) and 20%–30% for gastrinomas (Frucht et al. 1989; London et al. 1991). Although a recent report described the utility of sonography for detection of insulinomas, which image as small, hypoechoic nodules (Angeli et al. 1997), ultrasound is essentially beneficial for detection of liver metastases (Andersson et al. 1987; London et al. 1991).

Endoscopic ultrasonography (EUS) has improved the rate of detection of small tumors (lower limit of detectability, 5 mm) in the pancreas and the duodenal wall (Bolondi et al. 1990; Lightdale et al. 1991; Yamada et al. 1991). These small, hypoechoic nodules occasionally contain a central area of increased echogenicity.

CT has an overall sensitivity of 50% for the detection of pancreatic endocrine tumors. Sensitivity ranges from 30% to 60% for gastrinomas (Norton et al. 1986; Wank et al. 1987; Frucht et al. 1989; Wise et al. 1989) and from 11% to 73% for insulinomas (Stark et al. 1984; Galiber et al. 1988; Gianello et al. 1988). Pancreatic endocrine lesions image as small, round masses that are often isodense on unenhanced scans and may contains small calcifications. These lesions constantly enhance after contrast injection, sometimes very intensely, which makes them more conspicuous. The CT examination technique is an essential factor influencing tumor detection. Several recent studies have emphasized the value of spiral CT for pancreatic studies during both the arterial and parenchymal phases (Van Hoe et al. 1995; Chung et al. 1997). Van Hoe et al. (1995) accurately localized nine of 11 tumors by spiral CT, including one gastrinoma 4 mm in diameter. The two lesions that escaped detection were both smaller than 5 mm. Only one patient in their series had MEN type I; CT correctly detected both of his pancreatic tumors (a 2.8-cm gastrinoma and a 3-mm cystic insulinoma).

As gastrinomas are frequently located in the duodenal wall, water should be used as an oral contrast agent (Winter et al. 1996) to avoid masking a small tumor by a hyperdense contrast agent.

In addition to locoregional disease staging, CT is particulárly indicated for liver examination, which is indispensable before any surgical decision is made. The sensitivity of CT for the detection of hepatic metastases and pancreatic endocrine tumors is 75%–85% (Fig. 17.1).

Initial studies evaluating the efficacy of MRI for detection of endocrine tumors of the pancreas reported a sensitivity of only 20% (Frucht et al. 1989). On standard T_2-weighted sequences, these lesions manifest as an extremely hyperintense nodule. More recently, T_1-weighted sequences with fat suppression and fast gradient-echo sequences with gadolinium enhancement have significantly improved the sensitivity of MRI (Semelca et al. 1993; Kraus and Ros 1994; Angeli et al. 1997). In the study by Semelca et al. (1993), MRI had a sensitivity of 100% for detection of endocrine tumors, and lesions as small as 6 mm were accurately localized. According to Angeli et al. (1997), MRI has a sensitivity of 65.5% for the detection of insulinomas (Figs. 17.2, 17.3). These lesions are depicted as hypointense nodules on fat suppression sequences. MRI also appears effective for detection and characterization of hepatic metastases of pancreatic endocrine tumors (Semelca et al. 1993; Soyer et al. 1995).

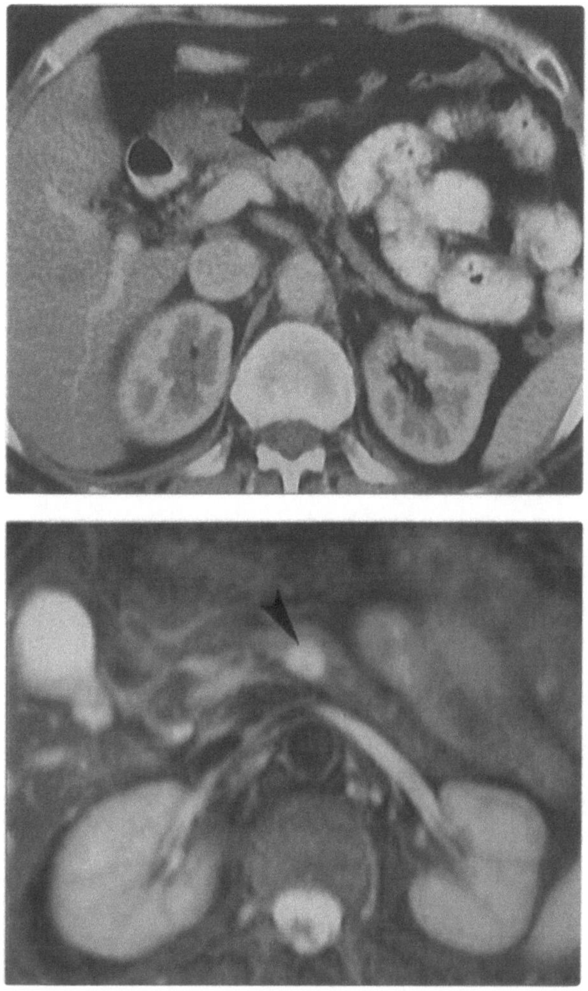

a

b

Fig. 17.1a,b. Insulinoma in a patient with MEN type I. **a** Contrast-enhanced CT of the pancreas. This small nodule in the body of the pancreas enhanced moderately after iodinated contrast injection (*arrowhead*). **b** T_2-weighted sequence; repetition time (TR), 2425 ms; echo time (TE), 80 ms. The insulinoma is more conspicuous due to its strong hypersignal (*arrowhead*)

Arteriography has a sensitivity of 65% for the detection of small pancreatic endocrine tumors provided injections are sufficiently selective (into the hepatic artery, gastroduodenal artery, splenic artery, superior mesenteric artery) (Maton et al. 1987; Galiber et al. 1988; Frucht et al. 1989; Wise et al. 1989). Lesions as small as 5 mm can be detected owing to their hypervascularity. In MEN type I, however, the value of arteriography is decreased because of the multicentric nature of the lesions. On arteriograms, these tumors present as a small, well-delimited, round mass that enhances intensely and remains opacified on late films. Arteriography also has good sensitivity for detection of hypervascular hepatic metastases.

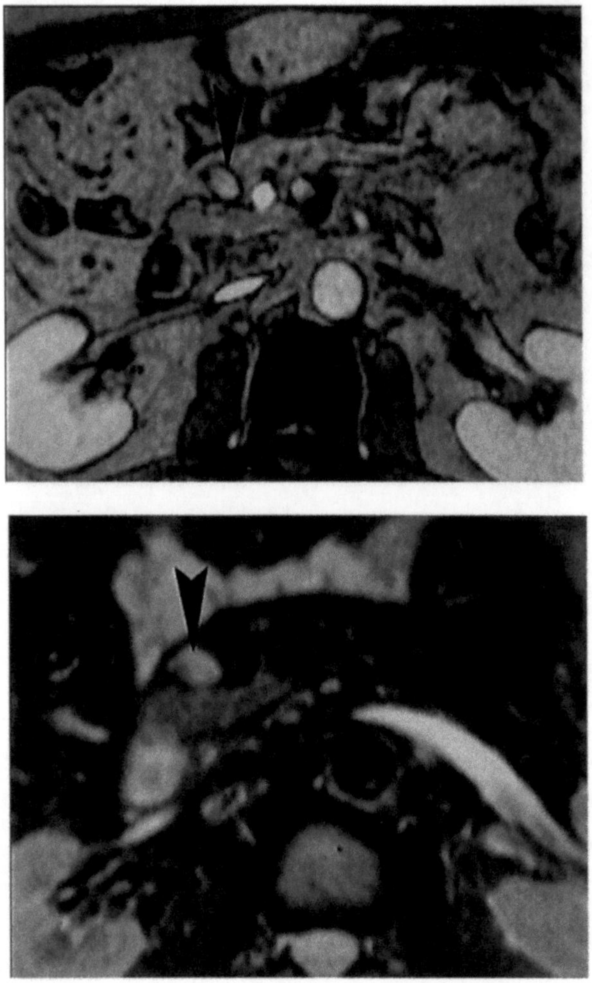

a

b

Fig. 17.2a,b. Extrapancreatic gastrinoma in a patient with MEN type I. **a** T_1-weighted gradient-echo sequence with gadolinium enhancement; repetition time (TR), 139 ms; echo time (TE), 4.5 ms; flip angle, 80°. Small, contrast-enhanced nodule located to the right of the superior mesenteric vein (*arrowhead*). **b** T_2-weighted sequence; repetition time (TR), 1800 ms; echo time (TE), 80 ms. The gastrinoma is extremely hyperintense (*arrowhead*)

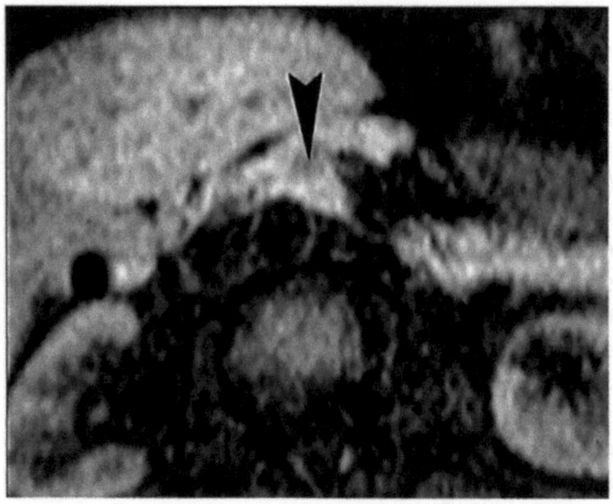

Fig. 17.3. Fat-suppression T_1-weighted sequence; repetition time (TR), 550 ms; echo time (TE), 18 ms. Small hypointense nodule in the head of the pancreas (*arrowhead*) corresponding to a pancreatic insulinoma

Tumor localization is facilitated by pancreatic venous sampling (PVS). Following transhepatic portal vein catheterization, the hormone concentrations in the pancreatic veins are assayed. The hormone concentration gradients determined in each vein are then plotted to localize functioning tumors. This time-consuming technique must be performed by an experienced team and should be reserved for the localization of small secretory lesions. Its sensitivity ranges from 80% to 95% (Roche et al. 1982; Gunther et al. 1985). PVS is primarily useful for preoperative workup of insulinomas, which require surgical resection. The value of PVS is more controversial for gastrinomas; these lesions tend to be multiple, and the frequency of small ectopic lesions renders surgery more problematic.

Several authors have proposed hormone sampling in the suprahepatic veins after selective intra-arterial stimulation by appropriate secretagogues, i.e., secretin for gastrinomas and calcium for insulinomas (Imamura et al. 1987; Doppman et al. 1990,1991). Arterial stimulation and venous sampling appears superior to PVS for the localization of gastrinomas and insulinomas and is easier to perform. This technique reportedly has a high specificity for localization of occult hepatic metastases in gastrinomas, although its sensitivity is low (Gibril et al. 1996).

Scintigraphy performed after administration of somatostatin analogues (octreotide) is a more recent technique based on the presence of somatostatin receptors in endocrine tumors (Lamberts et al. 1990; Krenning et al. 1993; Weinel et al. 1993; Modelin et al. 1995). This technique's main advantage is that it allows evaluation of the entire pancreas and detection of metastases not seen by other methods. Although it is not very sensitive for small intrapancreatic tumors, association of octreotide injection with single photon emission CT (SPECT) may improve scintigraphic localization of small tumors (Bajc et al. 1995). Intracellular radiotherapy of pancreatic endocrine tumors is a potential application of octreotide scintigraphy.

Intraoperative ultrasound combined with surgical palpation is currently the best method for detection of pancreatic endocrine tumors (GORMAN et al. 1986; GRANT et al. 1988; NORTON et al. 1990). The lower limit of detectability is a diameter of 3 mm. False-negative results do occur, however, namely for gastrinomas, owing to the frequency of extra-pancreatic localizations.

The multiplicity of imaging methods used reflects the difficulties in localization of pancreatic endocrine tumors diagnosed by endocrinologic studies. No consensus has been reached on the indications for the different techniques, and selection of one or another generally depends on the preference of the medical team. Gastrinomas are more difficult to identify than insulinomas because multicentric and extrapancreatic lesions are common. This also explains the surgical difficulties for gastrinomas. The surgical indications for MEN type I-related gastrinomas remain highly controversial, especially because these patients can benefit from medical therapy (NORTON et al. 1986, VAN HEERDEN et al. 1986; FRAKER and NORTON 1989). In contrast, localization of insulinomas is essential because surgery is the sole possibility for cure. New imaging modalities such as spiral CT, MRI with fat suppression sequences, and endosonography are proving increasingly useful. More invasive techniques such as PVS should be reserved as second-line methods following assessment by the endocrinologist, surgeon, and radiologist. PVS may provide useful information concerning gastrinomas in MEN type I by allowing identification of the gastrin-secreting tumor (VINIK et al. 1990). Scintigraphy with somatostatin analogues is still under evaluation, but has the capability to examine the entire pancreas and thus detect multiple lesions or occult metastases.

17.2.4 Other Manifestations of Multiple Endocrine Neoplasia Type I

Adrenal adenomas, thyroid nodules, carcinoid tumors, and thymomas are also encountered in MEN type I. Evaluation of these lesions does not involve any specific problems and is safely managed by standard techniques.

17.3 Multiple Endocrine Neoplasia Type II

17.3.1 Medullary Carcinoma of the Thyroid

First-line imaging assessment of medullary carcinoma of the thyroid is performed by cervical ultrasound, which can also detect nodal metastases or an associated parathyroid adenoma (GORMAN et al. 1987). Sonographically, medullary thyroid carcinoma images as a hypoechoic mass that may contain irregular clusters of calcifications (GORMAN et al. 1987). In MEN type II, medullary thyroid carcinoma is often bilateral and multicentric (McCOOK et al. 1982). In contrast, sporadic cases tend to be large, solitary masses that invade a single lobe. Metastatic cervical nodes may contain calcifications that are easily visualized by ultrasound. Owing to its low specificity, thyroid scintigraphy has limited value for examination of patients with MEN type II.

CT plays an important role, permitting assessment of the tumor, evaluation of locoregional spread, and detection of any metastases, particularly in the mediastinum. Medullary thyroid cancer presents as a hypodense and often multicentric lesion. Contiguous spread may manifest as an intense fibrous reaction in the cervical and superior mediastinal regions. Systematic search is necessary for mediastinal lymphadenopathy and pulmonary metastases, which may contain calcifications (McCOOK et al. 1982). Abdominal CT is indicated for detection of hepatic metastases, which may be calcified (McDONNELL et al. 1986). Abdominal CT scans occasionally reveal a coexistent pheochromocytoma.

Little documentation exists concerning the efficacy of MRI for initial workup of medullary thyroid carcinomas. However, MRI appears to be of use during postoperative follow-up for detection of local or mediastinal recurrence (CROW et al. 1989; DORR et al. 1993).

Other techniques have also been proposed for postoperative surveillance. Persistence of an elevated calcitonin concentration, for example, suggests metastatic spread. In such patients, octreotide or metaiodobenzylguanidine (MIBG) scintigraphy may help detect small metastases not seen by imaging techniques (LUPOLI et al. 1991; DORR et al. 1993; THOMAS et al. 1994; BAUDIN et al. 1996). Postoperatively, selective venous sampling for calcitonin assays can help localize residual tumor or distant metastases (ABDELMOUMENE et al. 1994).

17.3.2 Pheochromocytoma

Pheochromocystomas should be sought systematically in patients with medullary thyroid cancer because they are asymptomatic in half of all individuals with MEN type II. Adrenal involvement is readily demonstrated by CT, even though MEN-associated lesions are usually smaller than sporadic pheochromocytomas (Francis et al. 1992). Pheochromocytomas are bilateral in 70% of patients and may contain calcifications. MIBG scintigraphy has a sensitivity of 90% and a specificity of 95% for the detection of pheochromocytomas. Scintiscanning may also be used as the initial postoperative procedure if recurrence or metastases are suspected (Quint et al. 1987).

17.3.3 Parathyroid Involvement

The parathyroids are involved in 20% of patients with MEN type II. Assessment of the parathyroids is similar to evaluation of patients with a sporadic tumor.

17.3.4 Other Manifestations of Multiple Endocrine Neoplasia Type II

Multiple endocrine gland lesions may be accompanied by bone involvement. Metastases of thyroid cancer may cause sclerotic or mixed bone lesions at any skeletal site (McCook et al. 1982). Chondrocalcinosis secondary to hyperparathyroidism is also encountered.

Possible intestinal abnormalities include accelerated transit during barium studies performed to determine the cause of severe diarrhea. Colon lesions (megacolon, thickening of the mucosal folds, haustral anomalies, diverticulosis) reflecting intestinal ganglioneuromatosis or mucosal neuromatosis are less frequent.

17.4 Conclusion

Imaging plays an essential role for patients with MEN syndromes. In addition to localization of tumors diagnosed by endocrinologic studies, imaging helps detect metastases or latent associated tumors and allows satisfactory post-therapy follow-up.

References

Abdelmoumene N, Schlumberger M, Gardet P et al (1994) Selective venous sampling for localization of persisting medullary thyroid carcinoma. Br J Cancer 69:1141–1144

Akerström G, Johansson H, Grama D (1991) Surgical treatment of endocrine pancreatic lesions in NEM-1. Acta Oncol 30:541–545

Andersson T, Eriksson B, Hemmingsson A et al (1987) Angiography, computed tomography, magnetic resonance imaging and ultrasonography in detection of liver metastases from endocrine gastrointestinal tumors. Acta Radiol 28:535–539

Angeli E, Vanzulli A, Castrucci M et al. (1997) Value of abdominal sonography and MR imaging at O.ST in preoperative detection of pancreatic insulinoma: a comparison with dynamic CT and angiography. Abdom Imag 22:295–303

Angemoe E, Vanzulli A, Castrucci M et al (1997) Value of abdominal sonography and MR imaging at 0.5T in preoperative detection of pancreatic insulinoma: a comparison with dynamic CT and angiography. Abdom Imaging 22:295–303

Bajc M, Ingvar C, Persson B et al (1995) Dynamic octreotide scintigraphy in neuroendocrine tumours. Acta Radiol 36:474–477

Baudin E, Lumbroso J, Schlumberger M et al (1996) Comparison of octreotide scintigraphy and conventional imaging in medullary thyroid carcinoma. J Nucl Med 37:912–916

Bolondi L, Li Bassi S, Gaiani S et al (1990) Diagnosis of islet cell tumor by means of endoscopic ultrasonography. J Clin Gastroenterol 12:218–221

Bone HG III (1990) Diagnosis of the multiglandular endocrine neoplasias. Clin Chem 36:711–716

Chung MJ, Choi BI, Han JK, Chung JW, Han MC, Bae SH (1997) Functioning islet cell tumor of the pancreas. Localization with dynamic spiral CT. Acta Radiol 38:135–138

Crow JP, Azar-Kia B, Prinz RA (1989) Recurrent occult medullary thyroid carcinoma detected by MR imaging. AJR 152:1255–1256

Doppman JL, Miller DL, Chang R et al (1990) Gastrinomas: localization by means of selective intra-arterial injection of secretin. Radiology 174:25–29

Doppman JL, Miller DL, Chang R et al (1991) Insulinomas: localization with selective intra-arterial injection of calcium. Radiology 178:237–241

Dorr U, Wurstlin S, Frank-Ralle K et al (1993) Somatostatin receptor scintigraphy (SRS) and MRI in recurrent medullary thyroid carcinoma: a comparative study. Horm Metab Res 27:48–55

Fraker DL, Norton JA (1989) The role of surgery in the management of islet cell tumors. Gastroenterol Clin North Am 18:805–830

Francis IR, Gross MD, Shapiro B, Korobkin M, Quint LE (1992) Integrated imaging of adrenal disease. Radiology 184:1–13

Frucht H, Doppman JL, Norton JA et al (1989) Gastrinomas: comparison of MR imaging with CT, angiography, and US. Radiology 171:713–717

Gagel RF, Tashjan AH Jr, Cummings T et al (1988) The clinical outcome of prospective screening for multiple endocrine neoplasia type 2a. N Engl J Med 318:478–484

Galiber AK, Reading CC, Charboneau JW et al (1988) Localization of pancreatic insulinoma: comparison of pre and intraoperative US with CT and angiography. Radiology 166:405–408

Gianello P, Gigot JF, Berthet F et al (1988) Pre and intraoperative localization of insulinomas: report of 22 observations. World J Surg 12:389–395

Gibril F, Doppman JL, Chang R, Weiber HC, Termanini B, Jensen RT (1996) Metastatic gastrinomas: localization with selective arterial injection of secretin. Radiology 198:77–84

Gorman B, Charboneau JW, James EM et al (1986) Benign pancreatic insulinoma: preoperative and intraoperative sonographic localization. AJR 147:929–934

Gorman B, Charboneau JW, James EM et al (1987) Medullary thyroid carcinoma: role of high-resolution US. Radiology 162:147–150

Grant CS, Van Heerden J, Charboneau JW et al (1988) Insulinoma: the value of intraoperative ultrasonography. Arch Surg 123:843–848

Gunther RW, Klose KJ, Rucker TK et al (1985) Localization of small islet-cell tumors. Preoperative and intraoperative ultrasound, computed tomography, arteriography, digital subtraction angiography, and pancreatic venous sampling. Gastrointest Radiol 10:145–152

Imamura M, Takahashi K, Adachi H et al (1987) Usefulness of selective arterial secretin injection test for localization of gastrinoma in the Zollinger-Ellison Syndrome. Ann Surg 205:230–239

Kraus BB, Ros PR (1994) Insulinoma: diagnosis with fat-suppressed MR imaging. AJR 162:69–70

Krenning EP, Kwekkeboom DJ, Bakker WH et al (1993) Somatostatin receptor scintigraphy (SRS) with octreotide : the Rotterdam experience with more than 1000 patients. Eur J Nucl Med 20:716–731

Kucharczy KW, Davis DO, Kelly WM et al (1986) Pituitary adenoma: high-Resolution MRI at 1.5T. Radiology 161:761–765

Lamberts SJ, Hofland LJ, Van Koetsveld PM et al (1990) Parallel in vivo and in vitro detection of functional somatostatin receptors in human endocrine pancreatic tumors: consequences with regard to diagnosis, localization and therapy. J Clin Endocrinol Metab 71:566–574

Lightdale CJ, Botet JF, Woodruff JM (1991) Localization of endocrine tumors of the pancreas with endoscopic ultrasonography. Cancer 68:1815–1820

London JF, Shawker TH, Doppman JL et al (1991) Zollinger-Ellison Syndrome: prospective assessment of abdominal US in the localization of gastrinomas. Radiology 178:763–767

Lupoli G, Lombardi G, Panza N et al (1991) MIBI scintigraphy and selective venous catheterization (SVC) after thyroidectomy for medullary thyroid carcinoma. Med Oncol Tumor Pharmacother 8:7–13

Maton PN, Miller DL, Doppman JL et al (1987) Role of selective angiography in the management of patients with Zollinger-Ellison syndrome. Gastroenterology 92:913–918

McCook TA, Putman CE, Dale JK et al (1982) Medullary carcinoma of the thyroid: radiographic features of unique tumor. AJR 139:149–155

McDonnell CH III, Fishman EK, Zerhouni EA (1986) CT demonstration of calcified liver metastases in medullary thyroid carcinoma. J Comput Assist Tomogr 10:976–978

Modelin IM, Cornelius E, Lawton G (1995) Use of an isotopic somatostin receptor probe to image gut endocrine tumors. Arch Surg 130:367–374

Norton JA, Doppman JL, Collen MJ et al (1986) Prospective study of gastrinoma localization and resection in patients with Zollinger-Ellison Syndrome. Ann Surg 204:468–479

Norton JA, Cromack DT, Shawker TH et al (1990) Localization and surgical treatment of occult insulinomas. Ann Surg 212:615–620

Öberg K (1994) Multiple endocrine neoplasia. In: Higgins CB, Auffermann W (eds) Endrocrine imaging. Thieme, Stuttgart, pp 235–245

Pipeleers-Marichal M, Somers G, Willems G et al (1990) Gastrinomas in the duodenums of patients with multiple endocrine neoplasia type 1 and the Zollinger-Ellison syndrome. N Engl J Med 322:723–727

Quint LE, Glazer GM, Francis PR et al (1987) Pheochromocytoma and paraganglioma: comparison of MRI with CT and I-131 MIBG scintigraphy. Radiology 165:89–93

Roche A, Raisonnier A, Gillon-Savouret MC et al (1982) Pancreatic venous sampling and arteriography in localizing insulinomas and gastrinomas: procedure and results in 55 cases. Radiology 145:621–627

Saad RK, Ordonez NG, Rashid RK et al (1984) Medullary carcinoma of the thyroid. A study of the clinical features and prognostic factors in 161 patients. Medicine 63:319–342

Semelca RC, Cumming MJ, Shoenut JP et al (1993) Islet cell tumors: comparison of dynamic contrast-enhanced CT and MR imaging with dynamic gadolinium enhancement and fat suppression. Radiology 186:799–802

Skogseid B, Larsson C, Öberg K (1991) Genetic and clinical characteristics of multiple endocrine neoplasia type I. Acta Oncol 30:485–488

Soyer P, Gueye C, Somveille E, Laissy JP, Scherrer A (1995) MR diagnosis of hepatic metastases from neuroendocrine tumors versus hemangiomas: relative merits of dynamic gadolinium chelate-enhanced gradient-recalled echo and unenhanced spin-echo images. AJR 165:1407–1413

Stark DD, Moss AA, Goldberg HI (1984) CT of pancreatic islet cell tumors. Radiology 150: 491–494

Thomas CC, Cowan RJ, Albertson DA, Cooper R (1994) Detection of medullary carcinoma of the thyroid with I-131 MIBG. Clin Nucl Med 19:1066–1068

Van Heerden JA, Smith SL, Miller LJ (1986) Management of the Zollinger-Ellison syndrome in patients with multiple endocrine neoplasia type I. Surgery 100:971–977

Van Hoe L, Gryspeerdt S, Marchal G, Baert A, Mertens L (1995) Helical CT for the preoperative ocalization of islet cell tumors of the pancreas: value of arterial and parenchymal phase images. AJR 165:1437–1439

Vinik AI, Moattari AR, Cho K et al (1990) Transhepatic portal vein catheterization for localization of sporadic and MEN gastrinomas: a ten-year experience. Surgery 107:246–255

Wank SA, Doppman JL, Miller DL et al (1987) Prospective study of the ability of computerized axial tomography to localize gastrinomas in patients with Zollinger-Ellison syndrome. Gastroenterology 92:905–912

Weinel RJ, Neuhaus C, Stapp J et al (1993) Preoperative localization of gastrointestinal endocrine tumors using somastostin-receptor scintigraphy. Ann Surg 218:640–645

Winter TC III, Freeny PC, Nghiem HV (1996) Extrapancreatic gastrinoma localization: value of arterial-phase helical CT with water as an oral contrast agent. AJR 166:51–52

Wise SR, Johnson J, Sparks J et al (1989) Gastrinoma: the predictive value of preoperative localization. Surgery 106:1087–1093

Yamada M, Komoto E, Naito Y (1991) Endoscopic ultrasonography in the diagnosis of pancreatic islet cell tumors. J Ultrasound Med 10:271–276

18 Complications of Hormone Treatment

J.N. BRUNETON, C. MAESTRO, A. BLEUSE, and A. GRIMAUD

Contents

18.1 Hormone Treatments in Women

18.1.1 Oral Contraceptives

18.1.1.1 Liver

18.1.1.1.1 HEPATIC ADENOMA

Rarely described prior to the introduction of oral contraceptives, hepatic adenoma was long confused with focal nodular hyperplasia (FNH), even though it is five to six times more frequent (Cherqui et al. 1995). Even today, hepatic adenoma can involve problems for differentiation from highly differentiated hepatocellular carcinomas (HCC).

The appearance of oral contraceptives in the early 1960s led to a spectacular rise in the number of hepatic adenomas. Depending on the series, 12- to 100-fold increases were reported. ROOKS et al. (1979) cited an incidence of four cases per 100,000 oral contraceptive users. Studies published at the time all concerned high-dose estrogens and consistently reported a correlation between hepatic adenoma and the dose. However, no recent studies have investigated the relation between low-dose "minipills" and hepatic adenoma (BRUNETON et al. 1993a).

Hepatic adenomas related to the use of oral contraceptives are almost always solitary. Multiple hepatic adenomas (hepatic adenomatosis) are rare and are not linked to oral contraceptives. Hepatic adenomas are often large at diagnosis (GUGENHEIM et al. 1995). In addition to fat, these hypervascular tumors often contain hemorrhagic and necrotic components. Their frequently complex appearance explains difficulties for diagnosis by imaging as well as during surgery (COLAGRANDE et al. 1994). Hepatic adenomas may also exhibit histological features creating confusion with a highly differentiated HCC and malignant transformation (FOSTER and BERMAN 1994).

In addition to being a risk factor for the development of hepatic adenoma, the use of oral contraceptives has been correlated with potential complications of these lesions. The main risk is spontaneous or post-traumatic rupture. Spontaneous hemoperitoneum in a young woman should suggest rupture of a hepatic adenoma. Foster and Berman (1994) reported five cases of malignant transformation in a series of 39 hepatic adenomas. In certain cases, withdrawal of hormone treatment may lead to regression or disappearance of hepatic adenoma. KAWAKATSU et al. (1997), for example, found 11 such cases in the literature.

Along with intraperitoneal hemorrhage, which occurs in one third of patients, hepatomegaly and pain in the right lower quadrant are the main presenting symptoms (ROOKS et al. 1979; COLAGRANDE et al. 1994; GUGENHEIM et al. 1995). Incidental discovery of hepatic adenoma is rare in oral contraceptive users.

Hepatic adenoma is probably the hepatic tumor for which imaging is least useful. The complete spectrum of sonographic patterns is encountered, i.e., hypoechoic, hyperechoic, isoechoic, or complex. A hypoechoic rim may be depicted around encapsu-

J.N. BRUNETON, C. MAESTRO, A. BLEUSE, Centre Antoine-Lacassagne, 33 avenue de Valombrose, 06189 Nice, France
A. GRIMAUD, Service de Radiologic, Hôpital de l'Archet, 151 chemin de St. Antoine de Ginestière, 06200 Nice, France

lated lesions (BRUNETON et al. 1993a). Large adenomas may appear inhomogeneous due to necrotic change. A massive, old hematoma may appear pseudocystic. Intraperitoneal effusion secondary to rupture with hemorrhage may be visualized in patients with severe pain.

GOLLI et al. (1994) performed color Doppler (CD) in eight patients with a total of 11 hepatic adenomas. Central color flow corresponding to intratumoral veins 1–5 mm in diameter was seen in six patients. In another case, the central intratumoral vein measured 10 mm in diameter. These seven hepatic adenomas were all characterized by arterial and venous peritumoral flow that allowed differentiation from FNH. BARTOLOZZI et al. (1997) confirmed these findings and emphasized the superiority of power Doppler (PD) imaging over conventional CD sonography for differentiation between hepatocellular adenoma and FNH (sensitivity, 90% versus 68%). Use of ultrasound contrast agents reportedly improves the sensitivity of CD for demonstration of the central hypervascularity compared to conventional CD (ERNST et al. 1996).

On unenhanced computed tomography (CT), hepatic adenomas usually appear hypodense. Demonstration of a hyperdense center corresponding to recent intratumoral hemorrhage is highly suggestive of the diagnosis. Subcapsular hematoma is occasionally visualized (MATHIEU et al. 1997). On early postcontrast CT scans, the tumor is often inhomogeneously and transiently hyperdense, whereas it appears isodense or hypodense on the portal phase. Contrast-enhanced helical CT improves assessment in the arterial phase and gives a higher percentage of correct diagnoses for hepatic adenoma and FNH (VAN HOE et al. 1997). CT features suggestive of hepatic adenoma include intratumoral hemorrhage or fat, bands of necrosis, inhomogeneous hypervascularity, absence of a stellate scar, and a peripheral capsule (MATHIEU et al. 1986).

On magnetic resonance imaging (MRI), hepatic adenoma may be hypointense or isointense. Enhancement with gadolinium produces an often inhomogeneous, high-intensity signal. The hyperintensity observed on T_2-weighted sequences is not always very strong and is frequently heterogeneous. These signs are inconstant, even though hyperintensity, inhomogeneity, and the presence of a peripheral rim are suggestive of hepatic adenoma (ARRIVE et al. 1994; PAULSON et al. 1994). Endorem (Laboratoires Guerbet, Alunay Sous Bois) enhancement using a proton density-weighted sequence reveals decreased signal intensity in benign hepatic tumors, but this is not specific to hepatic adenomas (Fig. 18.1).

Angiography is nonspecific, but can depict tumor hypervascularity with enlargement of the feeding arteries, centripetal vascularity, and draining veins (BRUNETON et al. 1993a).

Differentiation from other hypervascular lesions can be difficult (ITO et al. 1996; NAKASHIMA and KOJIRO 1996). The diagnosis is actually often made by the association of clinical symptoms, a history of oral contraceptive use, and imaging findings that do not suggest another benign pathology. Although KHIARI et al. 1996) did not encounter any morbidity using guided hepatic biopsy, persistence of indeterminate findings requires surgery for definite diagnosis.

18.1.1.1.2

FOCAL NODULAR HYPERPLASIA

Long confused with hepatic adenoma, FNH has a number of characteristic imaging features that increasingly obviate the need for diagnostic surgery (MATHIEU et al. 1997).

FNH is more frequent than hepatic adenoma, occurring with a female to male sex ratio of 4.5:1. The numerous etiologic factors specific to FNH are still poorly understood. Along with focal agenesis of the intralobular bile ducts, focal arteriovenous malformations may cause ischemia and subsequent atrophy of the parenchyma, resulting in formation of a regenerating nodule. Estrogen, in particular, plays an important role. While it is now generally admitted that estrogen does not provoke the onset of FNH, this hormone has been incriminated in the growth, evolution, and clinical manifestations of these lesions. In the series reported by LANDEN et al. (1993), 64% of the patients with FNH had used oral contraceptives.

FNH nearly always manifests as a solitary nodule. These well-circumscribed lesions are not encapsulated, but sometimes have a pedicle. Histopathologic examination reveals a central stellate scar with fibrous septa in two thirds of patients. The scar is composed of more or less dense collagenous and edematous tissue containing vessels and capillary structures. The septa contain biliary ductules and inflammatory cells (CRAIG and PETERS 1989). There are no necrotic or hemorrhagic foci. These specific morphological features demonstrated by imaging studies permit diagnosis in over 50% of patients (BELGHITI et al. 1993; GUGENHEIM et al. 1995).

Oral contraceptives are responsible for tumor enlargement and clinical manifestations, even though

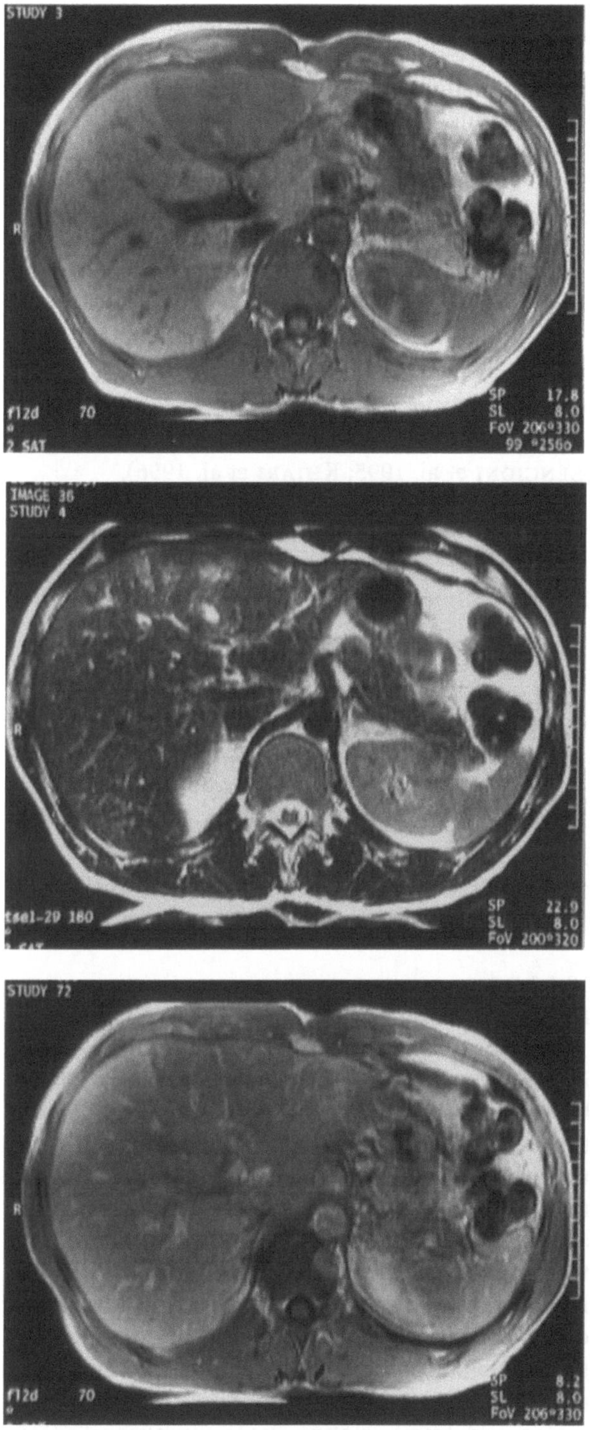

a
b
c

Fig. 18.1a–c. Hepatocellular adenoma. **a** Gradient-echo MRI: this heterogeneous lesion is hypointense relative to the normal parenchyma abd contains a small (1-cm) hyperintense central zone. **b** T_2-weighted turbo spin-echo sequence (same scan level as Fig. 18.1a). The hyperintense focus on T_1 appears hyperintense on T_2. The lesion is practically isointense to the liver. **c** Delayed gradient-echo MRI following i.v. gadolinium administration. The globally hypointense nature of this heterogeneous lesion relative to the liver reflects the existence of intratumoral arteriovenous shunts

FNH was discovered incidentally by ultrasound in 74% of patients by Cherqui et al. (1995). Rupture of FNH is very rare, but the use of oral contraceptives appears to increase the risk (Bruneton et al. 1993b). Surgical resection is thus currently indicated for young women in whom FNH cannot be affirmed by imaging studies (Belghiti et al. 1993; Paineau et al. 1994). Most cases of FNH may simply be kept under surveillance, supplemented, when necessary, by guided biopsy (Mangiante et al. 1994; Khiari et al. 1996).

The sonographic appearance of FNH is variable; hypoechoic, hyperechoic, isoechoic, and complex patterns are all encountered. Homogeneously hypoechoic lesions with a central scar predominate. The central scar is usually less visible with ultrasound than with other imaging techniques (Mathieu et al. 1986). FNH tends to be homogeneous and is not encapsulated. Use of ultrasound contrast agents improves CD detection of tumor vessels by demonstrating signal enhancement in the center of the tumor (Ernst et al. 1996). Three-dimensional ultrasound combined with harmonic imaging may depict the radial pattern of vessels arising from an enlarged feeding artery typical of FNH (Uggowitzer et al. 1997). The resistive index (RI) of 0.51 reflects the presence of arteriovenous shunts. Although currently detectable only for lesions larger than 3 cm, these features are highly suggestive of FNH.

FNH appears hypodense on unenhanced CT scans. Early, massive, and transient hypervascularity is observed following administration of an iodinated contrast agent. The scar has a variable appearance (often hypodense during the early period and then hyperdense on late images) (Fig. 18.2). Late liver scans show tumor isodensity. Demonstration of these CT features usually allows diagnosis of FNH (Shamsi et al. 1993; Mathieu et al. 1997). Arterial-phase, contrast-enhanced helical CT scanning improves characterization of FNH, in particular by demonstrating a spoked-wheel pattern and a central feeding vessel. These features have a positive predictive value of 100% (Van Hoe et al. 1997). Delayed CT scans showing late tumor hyperdensity may also assist diagnosis. CT combined with intravenous cholangiography permits lesion characterization by demonstrating intratumoral biliary ductules (Bruneton et al. 1993b).

MRI features suggestive of FNH include a basket or spoked-wheel pattern, a central scar, and regular contours (Colagrande et al. 1994). These homogeneous lesions appear isointense on T_1- and T_2-

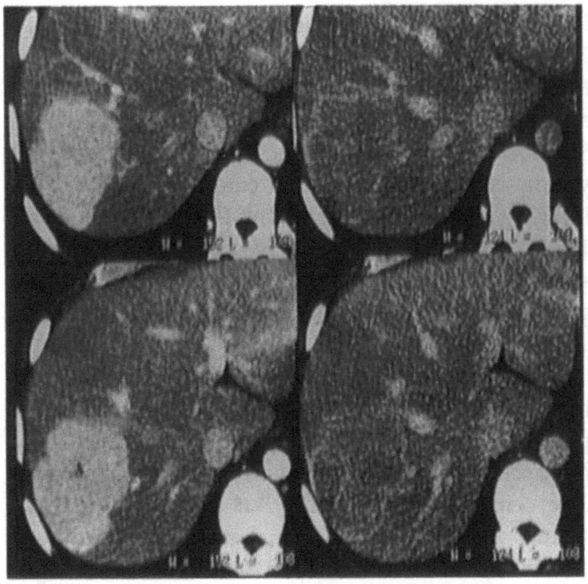

Fig. 18.2. Focal nodular hyperplasia. The hypervascular lesion with a hypodense center visible on the early contrast-enhanced CT scans is isodense relative to the normal parenchyma on the delayed scans

weighted sequences; a hyperintense central scar is visible on T_2-weighted images. These three MRI features were present in only 12% of patients according to SHAMSI et al. (1993), and these authors described two patients in which the scar was hypointense on T_2-weighted images (Fig. 18.3). Gadolinium enhancement improves the diagnostic accuracy of MRI. According to CHERQUI et al. (1995), enhanced MRI has a sensitivity of 70% and a specificity of 98%. AMI-25-enhanced T_2-weighted MRI reveals the significant signal loss specific to benign tumors (DENYS et al. 1994), but it cannot differentiate FNH from hepatic adenoma (GRANDIN et al. 1995; VOGL et al. 1996). Magnetization transfer contrast does not improve MRI characterization of FNH (SCHICK et al. 1997).

Use of angiography for diagnosis of FNH is on the decline. Hypervascularity with a spoked-wheel pattern of centrifugal opacification is observed in over two thirds of patients. One or more draining veins are visible on late scans (ROS 1994).

Despite their high specificity, radionuclide studies are increasingly being abandoned in favor of MRI. In 10% of patients, sulfur colloid scintigraphy reveals a hot spot corresponding to an increase in the number of Kupffer cells (WELCH et al. 1985). Delayed hepatobiliary scans reveal excretion of the isotope in one half of patients, reflecting the presence of bile ductules (DRANE et al. 1987).

In practice, FNH is now often diagnosed by imaging studies, even though differential diagnosis sometimes remains difficult. Central or peripheral calcifications (seen in 1.4% of all FNH patients; CASEIRO-ALVES et al. 1996) can create problems for differentiation from fibrolamellar hepatocellular carcinoma. Concomitant chronic liver disease can also complicate diagnosis (TERADA et al. 1993). Whenever equivocal findings suggest either adenoma or fibrolamellar hepatocellular carcinoma, surgical resection is required for definitive diagnosis (BRADY et al. 1994). Increasing use of ultrasound-guided or CD-guided aspiration biopsy should continue to reduce the indications for diagnostic surgery (LENCIONI et al. 1995; KHIARI et al. 1996).

18.1.1.2 Thromboembolic Complications

Oral contraceptives increase intravascular coagulation by inhibiting the fibrinolytic response. The factor V Leiden mutation is a putative cofactor because it occurs in 5% of all white women and is the most common genetic risk factor for deep vein thrombosis (HIRSCH et al. 1996; VANDENBROUCKE et al. 1996). The pathogenesis of thromboembolic complications related to oral contraceptives probably involves several cofactors (LIDEGAARD 1997).

18.1.1.2.1 DIGESTIVE TRACT

Thrombosis of the superior mesenteric vein causes ischemic and hemorrhagic modifications of the bowel wall (GHAHREMANI 1994). The distal ileum is the site of predilection (LEWIS 1986). Dynamic contrast-enhanced CT has a sensitivity of 64%, a specificity of 92%, and an accuracy of 75% for diagnosis of acute mesenteric ischemia (TAOUREL et al. 1996). CT features include arterial or venous thrombosis, intramural gas, portal vein gas, focal lack of bowel wall enhancement, and liver or spleen infarcts. Barium gastrointestinal studies may demonstrate narrowing and spasticity of the involved loops, mucosal ulcerations, and thumbprinting due to submucosal edema or hemorrhage (GHAHREMANI et al. 1977). These lesions are reversible if diagnosed soon enough (HYSON et al. 1977).

18.1.1.2.2 LIVER

Budd-Chiari syndrome may have an acute or chronic clinical presentation. There are numerous etiologies

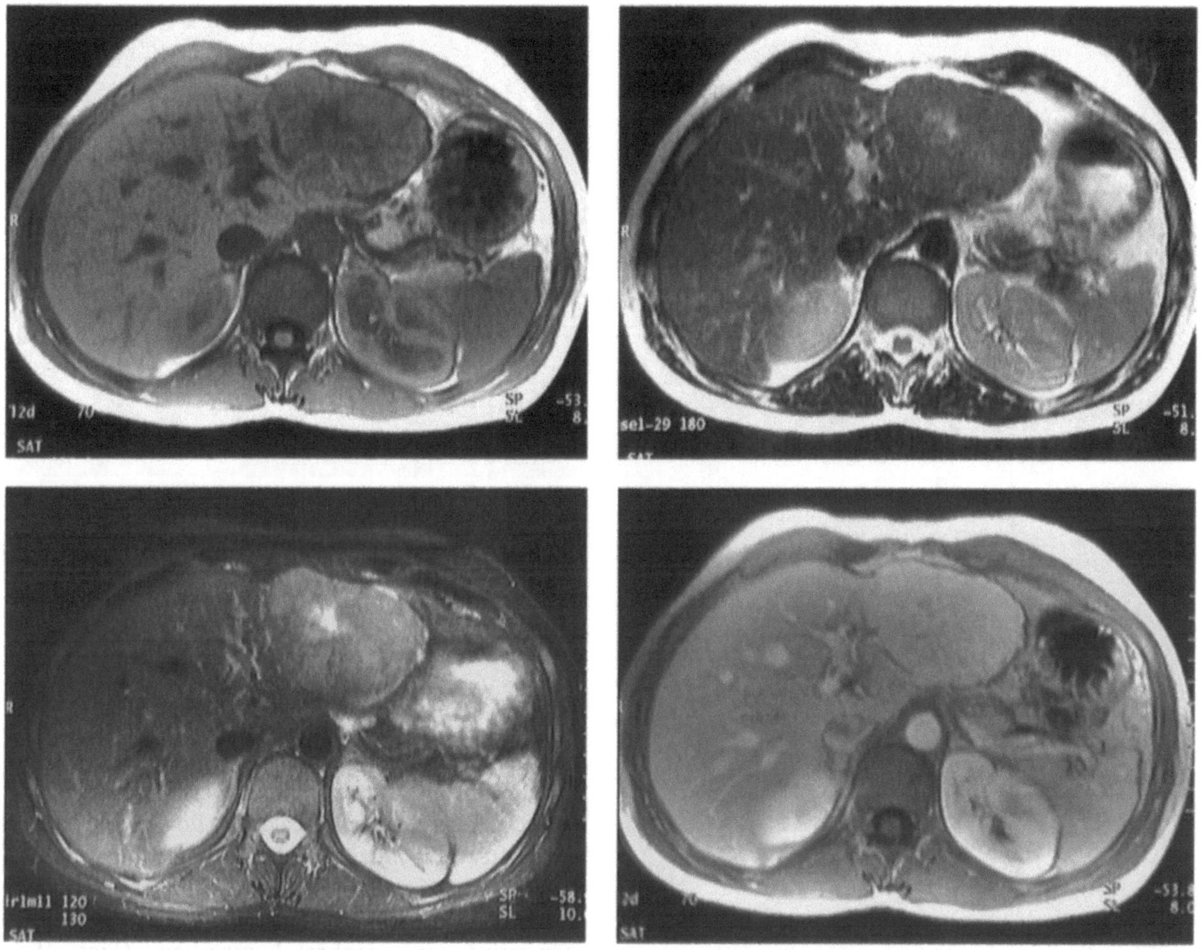

a b c d

Fig. 18.3a–d. Focal nodular hyperplasia in the left liver lobe. **a** T_1-weighted gradient-echo sequence showing a hypointense lesion with a radiating hypointense central component. **b** T_2-weighted turbo spin-echo sequence: this well-delimited lesion is isointense to the liver; the central component is hyperintense. **c** Strongly T_2-weighted short tau inversion recovery (STIR) sequence; echo time (TE), 70 ms; repetition time (TR), 5000 ms. The lesion is hyperintense compared to the liver; the central component appears hyperintense. **d** Delayed T_1-weighted gradient-echo sequence after gadolinium administration. Late enhancement of the central component; the lesion retains the contrast and appears hyperintense relative to the healthy liver

(Zimmerman and Ishak 1987). Oral contraceptives were a predisposing factor in 18 of 45 patients in the series described by Lang et al. (1994). Cavography and hepatic venography are no longer indispensable for diagnosis of Budd-Chiari syndrome (Gore 1994).

Sonographically visible anomalies include stenosis of the suprahepatic veins that have thickened echoic walls and show proximal dilatation, echogenic thrombi, presence of anastomoses and collaterals, narrowing of the inferior vena cava due to liver enlargement, ascites, enlargement of the caudal lobe, and atrophy of the right liver (Baert et al. 1983; Brown et al. 1990). Doppler and CD demonstrate the absence of flow or reversed flow in one or more suprahepatic veins.

The CT appearance of liver involvement depends on the age and extent of lesions. In acute disease, the density of the liver is decreased, and hepatomegaly is accompanied by ascites. Injection of an iodinated contrast material reveals patchy enhancement due to hepatic congestion. The central areas of the liver often appear subnormal, in contrast to the peripheral regions. A "flip-flop" (central hypodensity and peripheral hyperdensity) due to stasis of the contrast agent is apparent on late scans (Baert et al. 1983; Mathieu et al. 1987; Gore 1994).

MRI patterns are comparable to CT findings. Venous thrombi can be demonstrated by standard sequences or gradient-echo sequences (Mitchell and Stark 1992; Fig. 18.4).

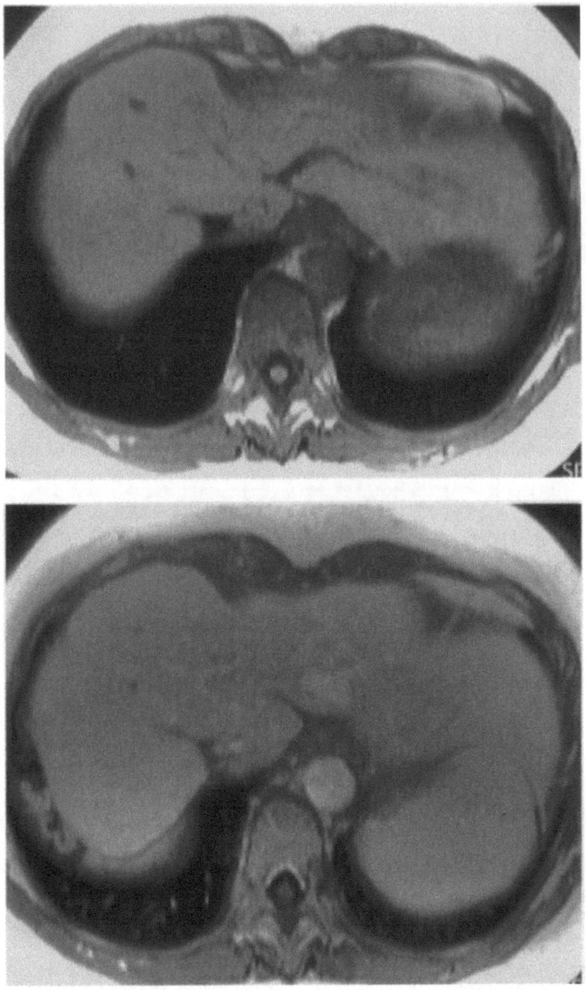

a

b

Fig. 18.4a,b. Chronic Budd-Chiari syndrome with thrombosis of the right and middle suprahepatic veins. **a** T_1-weighted gradient-echo sequence revealing thrombosis of the right and middle suprahepatic veins. **b** Gadolinium-enhanced T_1-weighted gradient-echo sequence

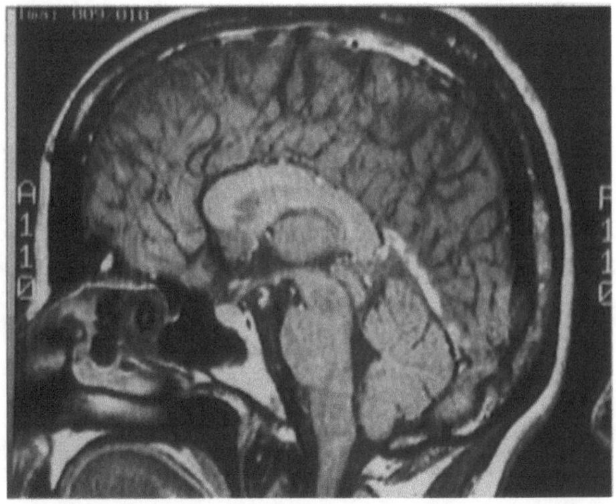

Fig. 18.5. Dural venous thrombosis. MRI reveals thrombosis of the superior longitudinal sinus, the dural sinus, and the internal cerebral veins

Peliosis hepatis (Van Erpecum et al. 1988; Gore 1994) and hepatic infarcts (Adler et al. 1984; Gore 1994) are other potential complications of oral contraceptives.

18.1.1.2.3
Dural Sinus Thrombosis

Oral contraceptives are one of many causes of intracranial vein thrombosis (Malanga and Gangemi 1994). Angiography and CT have now been supplanted by MRI (Goldberg et al.1986). Spin-echo MRI and MR angiography with maximum-intensity projection reconstructions have been advocated for diagnosis and follow-up (Vogl et al. 1994). Direct signs of dural sinus thrombosis on MR angiograms include a lack of typical high flow signal from a sinus that did not previously appear aplastic or hypoplastic and a frayed appearance of the flow signal from a sinus after recanalization. Indirect findings include the presence of collaterals, unusually high flow signal in the deep medullary veins, visualization of emissary veins, and cerebral hemorrhage (Figs. 18.5, 18.6). MRI is the preferred monitoring modality for patients receiving anticoagulant therapy (Wasenko et al. 1995).

18.1.1.2.4
Deep Vein Thrombosis of the Lower Extremities

CD and pulsed Doppler (Fig. 18.7) are the imaging modalities of choice for first-line evaluation of the deep vein system of the lower limbs (Killewich et al. 1993; Lewis et al. 1994; Pezzullo et al. 1996). These techniques, which have replaced venography of the lower extremities for initial studies, may be completed by CT or gradient-recall-echo MR sequences for assessment of deep vein thrombosis (Spritzer et al. 1993).

18.1.1.3
Other Complications of Oral Contraceptives

Additional potential complications (Ansell 1997b) include the following:

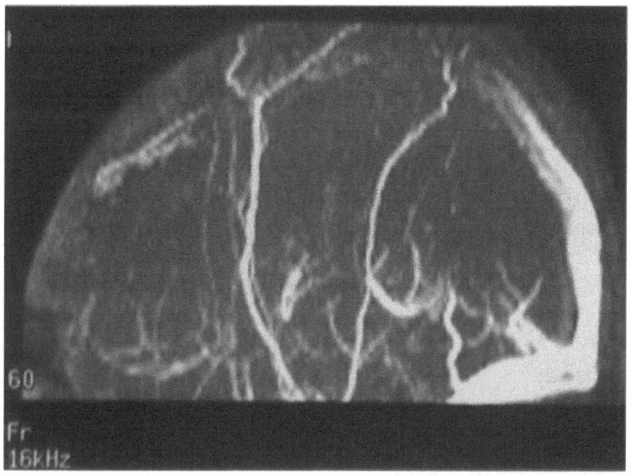

Fig. 18.6. MR angiogram revealing thrombophlebitis of the superior longitudinal sinus

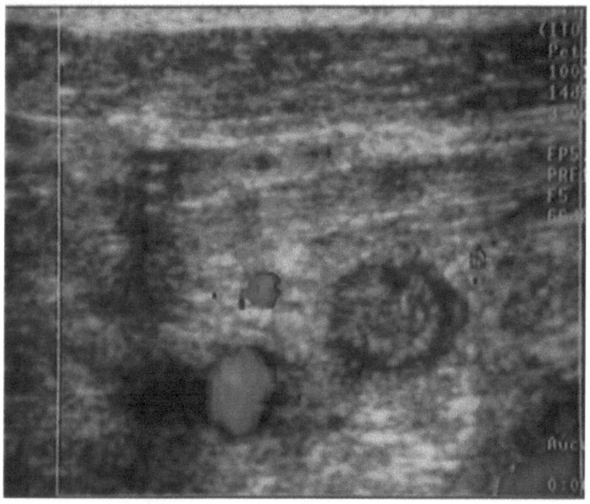

Fig. 18.7. Thrombophlebitis of the left infraclavicular vein (power Doppler, PD). Visualization of the normal adjacent subclavicular vein and small venous collaterals

- Lupus syndrome with patchy peripheral pulmonary infiltrates and a micronodular pattern in the lungs (TROTMAN-DICKENSON et al. 1997)
- Increased frequency of gallbladder stones (ANSELL 1997a)
- Bilateral ureteral dilatation, often more severe on the right than on the left (SIDHU et al. 1997)
- Carotid artery dissection, a rare complication usually associated with other etiologic factors (KLUFAS et al. 1995)

18.1.2 Tamoxifen

Tamoxifen has been prescribed for over 20 years. Initially, this molecule constituted the antiestrogen of reference for adjuvant treatment of metastatic breast cancer in postmenopausal women. Today, nearly 50% of all women with metastatic breast cancer take tamoxifen. The indications for this drug increased rapidly because it reduces by 40% both the risk of developing a new primary cancer in the contralateral breast and the relapse rate, thereby prolonging the disease-free survival and overall survival. Preventive use of tamoxifen for women at risk is currently under evaluation in several countries (United States, Italy, United Kingdom).

Tamoxifen exerts paradoxical estrogen effects that vary with the target tissue, the dosage, and the duration of use. Beneficial effects on bone and the cardiovascular system include maintenance of bone mineral density and reduced mortality from myocardial infarction (reduction of the low-density lipoprotein cholesterol fraction and augmentation of the high-density and ultra-low-density lipoprotein fractions). However, the risk of thromboembolic disease is slightly increased. The adverse effects of tamoxifen therapy are most apparent in the gynecologic sphere and may correspond to the development of lesions or aggravation of an existing pathology (SEOUD et al. 1993):

- Ovaries: development of cysts (KEDAR et al. 1994).
- Vaginal epithelium: tamoxifen exerts a trophic effect, with secretion of mucus.
- Uterus: enlargement in size similar to that observed in women receiving hormone replacement therapy (HRT).
- Myometrium: enlargement of existing fibromas and authentic sarcomas have been described (SILVA et al. 1994; UGWUMADU and HARDING 1994).
- Endometrium: benign modifications predominate (polyps, adenomyosis, endometrial hyperplasia, endometrial atrophy), but there is also a non-negligible risk of tamoxifen-induced malignancy (two- to sixfold increase). Overall, 39% of women receiving tamoxifen develop endometrial abnormalities after 3–6 months of use versus only 10% in controls (KEDAR et al. 1994).

18.1.2.1 *Benign Endometrial Modifications*

Benign endometrial modifications include polyps, adenomyosis, simple hyperplasia, and complex hyperplasia (including cystic – glandular hyperplasia, adenomatous hyperplasia, and proliferative endometrium). When cellular atypia exist, the hyperplastic tissue is less functional owing to a reduction in hormone receptors. Proliferation may persist, even if therapy is interrupted, resulting in malignant transformation. In a group of 111 postmenopausal women treated with tamoxifen, 16% had atypical hyperplasia versus none in the control group (KEDAR et al. 1994). The risk of malignant transformation is estimated at 1% for simple hyperplasia without atypia and 29% for complex atypical hyperplasia (KURMAN et al. 1985). Certain authors consider polyps precancerous, just like atypical hyperplasia.

At low doses, tamoxifen may cause simple or cystic - glandular endometrial atrophy. However, atrophic endometrium is less frequent than in the normal population (61% versus 90%; KEDAR et al. 1994) and decreases with the continuation of tamoxifen.

18.1.2.2 Malignant Endometrial Modifications

The first reports of endometrial cancer in patients treated with tamoxifen were made by KILLACKE et al. (1985). Over 200 cases have been published since then (JORDAN 1995). In one of the largest series to date (2843 patients), the relative risk of developing endometrial cancer was 7.5% in patients receiving tamoxifen; the annual risk was 2 per 1000 patients receiving 20 mg/day (FISHER et al. 1994). In a study by the French National Federation of Cancer Centers concerning 98 endometrial carcinomas in patients receiving tamoxifen, the incidence of cancer was much higher when the drug was used for long periods (over 4 years) and at high doses (BONADONNA et al. 1996).

Endometrioid carcinomas account for 75%–80% of all cases of endometrial carcinoma, followed in frequency by papillary serous carcinoma, clear cell carcinoma, mucinous or undifferentiated carcinoma, and secretory carcinoma. Endometrioid tumors are often surrounded by a hyperplastic or polypoid endometrial mucosa, suggesting that an estrogen mechanism of tamoxifen may be involved in the genesis of these cancers. The mucosa is atrophic in the other histologic types of endometrial carcinoma. Carcinosarcomas are more frequent than in patients who do not receive tamoxifen (10% versus 2.4%). The frequency of endometrial sarcomas does not appear increased.

The prognosis for tamoxifen-induced endometrioid carcinomas is usually favorable. At diagnosis, approximately 80% are grade I or II, and they are usually only slightly invasive, if at all, because patients are often kept under surveillance by ultrasound. Other histologic types, which are less differentiated, have a more somber prognosis. They are usually diagnosed at a more advanced stage when myometrial invasion is more likely (ISMAIL 1996).

18.1.2.3 Imaging

18.1.2.3.1 ULTRASONOGRAPHY

Transvaginal Sonography. In tamoxifen-treated women, the endouterine endometrium is diffusely or focally thickened, echogenic, and microcystic. If the threshold for abnormal thickness is set at 4 or 6 mm, depending on the author, transvaginal sonography has a sensitivity of nearly 100% for detection of endometrial abnormalities (OSMER et al. 1990; HULKA and HALL 1992; WIKLAND et al. 1993; CHAN et al. 1994; HULKA et al. 1994; KARLSSON et al. 1994; WOLMAN et al.1996a–c). Interobserver variations range from 1 to 2 mm (KARLSSON et al. 1994; WOLMAN et al. 1996b). The specificity of the technique ranges from 75% to 83% (KARLSSON et al. 1994; WOLMAN et al. 1996b).

This echogenic, microcystic pattern is seen both in atrophic and in proliferative endometrium. The apparent thickening observed in endometrial atrophy actually corresponds to the sum of the small, dilated cystic glands that are separated by a very low cellularity fibrous chorion, consistent with the paucity of curettage products. This pattern has also been described for solitary simple or complex polyps, especially polyps associated with endometrial hyperplasia or proliferative endometrium (HULKA and HALL 1993; KUPFER et al. 1994). Homogeneous thickening of the endometrial stripe is reportedly more common with endometrial hyperplasia and endometrial atrophy than with polyps. In contrast, a heterogeneously echoic focal or diffuse solid image is suggestive of endometrial neoplasia. Intrauterine fluid collections are associated with malignancy in 25%–94% of patients, even in the absence of abnormal endometrial thickening (KASALES et al. 1996; ZALEL et al. 1996).

Color Doppler Sonography. In a series of 30 tamoxifen-treated patients without any modification in endometrial thickness, ACHIRON et al. (1995a) demonstrated a reduced RI compared to untreated patients. However, the RI of the tamoxifen-treated women was higher than that of postmenopausal women receiving HRT. KEDAR et al. (1994) observed a significant decrease in the pulsatility index (PI) of the uterine artery and an increase in the peak systolic velocities of the subendometrial arteries of women receiving tamoxifen.

In their prospective study of 39 asymptomatic postmenopausal breast cancer patients receiving tamoxifen, TEPPER et al. (1994) evaluated the respective utility of the PI of the uterine artery, endometrial width measured by transvaginal ultrasound, and histological findings. No correlation was found among these three variables, and CD appears nonspecific for diagnosis of endometrial cancer in women on tamoxifen. This contrasts with the generally admitted, although still controversial usefulness of CD for untreated patients (BOURNE et al. 1990; CHAN et al. 1994). Measurement of endometrial blood flow appears more sensitive than uterine artery blood flow analysis (TEPPER et al. 1994). ALEEM et al. (1995) evaluated the density of myometrial and endometrial vessels in a series of untreated patients. CD visualization rates were significantly higher in endometrial cancer than in hyperplasia. In carcinoma, myometrial vessels were visualized in 93% of patients and endometrial vessels in 43% due to intra- and peritumoral neovascularity. In hyperplasia, where vascularity is less extensive, myometrial vessels were visualized in only 43% of patients and endometrial vessels in 12%. Decreased PI and RI values in myometrial vessels are often associated with malignant lesions. Endometrial arterial flow is absent in atrophic endometria (KURJAK et al. 1993). CD and pulsed Doppler might thus help reduce the number of patients referred for curettage on the basis of initial transvaginal ultrasound findings (Figs. 18.8–18.12).

One drawback of transvaginal ultrasound is the fact that it can only provide a global view of the endometrium, because both layers are imaged together. Sonohysterography can detect focal thickening and thus direct more productive guided biopsies because it can analyze each layer separately. In a series of 45 postmenopausal women taking tamoxifen for breast cancer, ACHIRON et al. (1995) observed abnormal endometrial thickening in 20 patients. Endometrial polyps were seen as a free-floating echoic mass in the uterine cavity in eight patients, and irregular cystic thickening was observed in 12 patients (11 due to endometrial atrophy and one due to endometrial hyperplasia). Sonohysterography also appears more effective than transvaginal ultrasound for diagnosis of polyps, although it cannot determine their benign or malignant character (Fig. 18.13). This may prove helpful when deciding whether to refer patients with tamoxifen-associated cystic, thickened endometria for hysteroscopy-guided biopsy or dilatation and curettage (KUPFER et al. 1994; ACHIRON et al. 1995; CULLINAN et al. 1995). Compared with hysteroscopy with biopsy, sonohysterography has a sensitivity of 86% and a specificity of 100% (WOLMAN et al. 1996a).

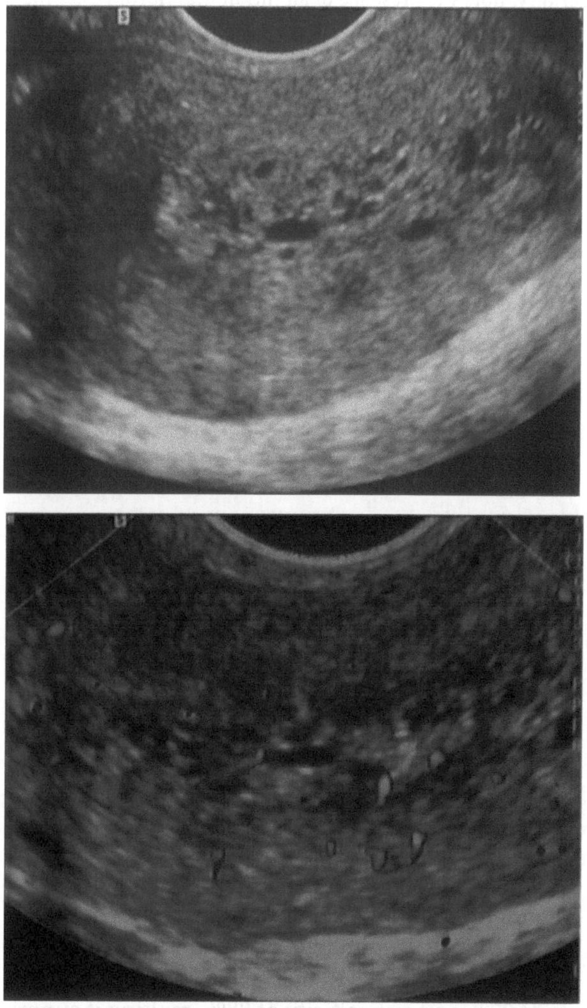

a

b

Fig. 18.8a,b. Patient receiving tamoxifen. **a** Moderate thickening of the endometrium that contains small fluid-like images consistent with endometrial atrophy. **b** Power Doppler (PD) revealed the presence of vessels in the myometrium

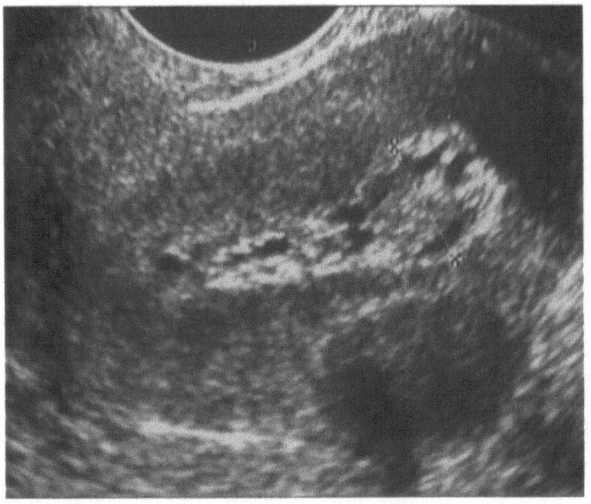

Fig. 18.9. Patient receiving tamoxifen. Transvaginal sonography revealed endometrial thickening (11.1 mm). Posteriorly, note the presence of an intramural fibroid (less than 2 cm in the long axis)

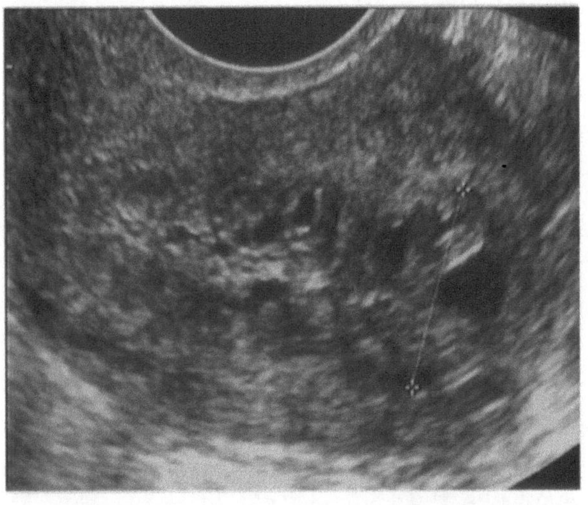

Fig. 18.10. Cystic–glandular atrophy during tamoxifen therapy. Transvaginal sonography revealed endometrial hypertrophy (17 mm between the two *crosses*). Note the presence of small (several millimeters) fluid-like loculi

18.1.2.3.2
Other Diagnostic Methods

Hysteroscopy allows examination of the entire uterine cavity and directed biopsy procedures. It is more effective than dilatation and curettage for diagnosis of endometrial polyps and fibroids and helps eliminate biopsy sampling errors. According to Karlsson et al. (1994), this technique has a sensitivity of 97% and a specificity of 88%, making it superior to transvaginal ultrasound for determination of the cause of postmenopausal bleeding. In patients receiving tamoxifen therapy, hysteroscopy demon-

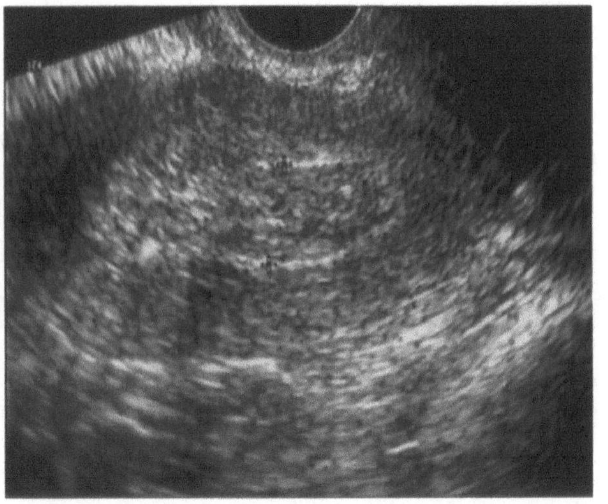

Fig. 18.11. Endometrial polyp (12 mm between the two crosses) in a patient on tamoxifen therapy (transvaginal sonogram)

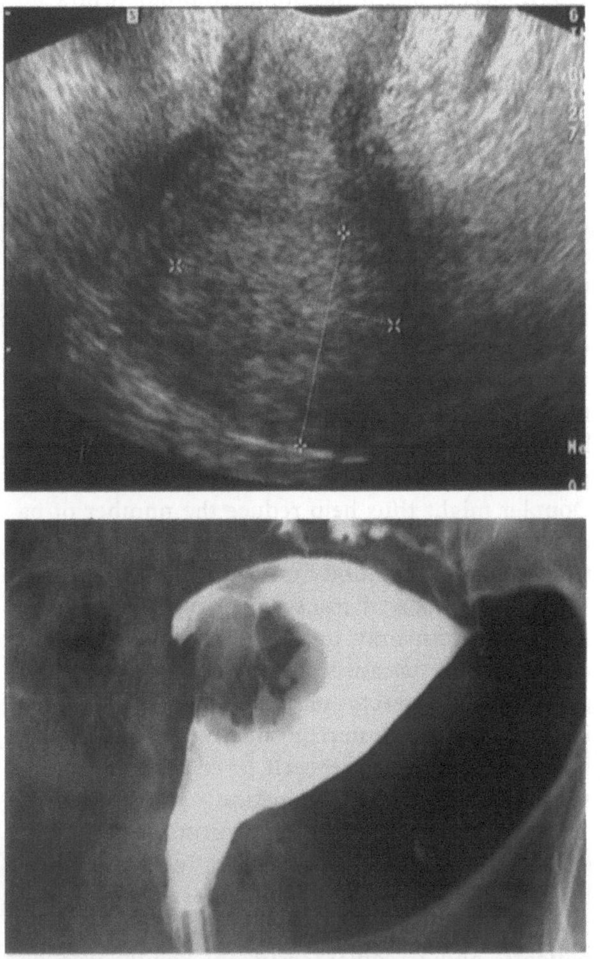

a

b

Fig. 18.12a,b. Endometrial carcinoma. **a** Transvaginal sonogram depicted an echoic lesion (37.5+32.6 mm). **b** Hysterography revealed a heterogeneous filling defect corresponding to the lesion seen at transvaginal sonography

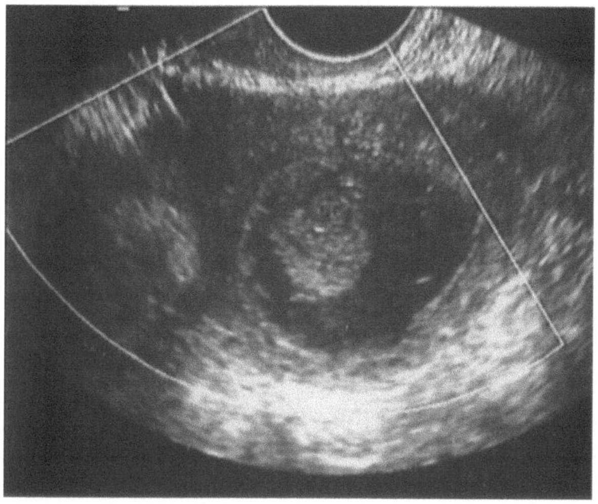

Fig. 18.13. Transvaginal sonography with instillation of fluid into the endometrial cavity. This 12-mm polypoid lesion corresponded to a carcinoma; color Doppler (CD) revealed only weak tumor vascularity

strates the atrophic luminal and glandular epithelium of the endometrium and the presence of dilated cystic glands in the endometrial - myometrial junctional zone.

Following dilatation and curettage, 10% of all women with postmenopausal bleeding are found to have a endometrial cancer; another 20% have other endometrial abnormalities. However, numerous biopsy samples are inadequate or nonspecific. Polyps and submucosal fibroids are often difficult to diagnose, and 2%–6% of all cancers go undetected by dilatation and curettage (KARLSSON et al. 1994). This underscores the value of hysteroscopy-guided endometrial sampling.

Cervical stenosis renders endometrial biopsy difficult in 20% of patients. Furthermore, inadequate tissue sampling precludes interpretation in 20%–25% of patients. Endometrial sampling by aspiration or brush biopsy techniques has a positive rate of 70%–94% and a specificity of approximately 90%, making it a helpful method for endometrial assessment in patients without cervical stenosis.

18.1.2.3.3 MAGNETIC RESONANCE IMAGING

The variety of MR patterns reflects the many endometrial abnormalities related to use of tamoxifen (HRICAK et al. 1992; ASCHER et al. 1996).

Uterine Polyps. On T_2-weighted sequences, the uterine cavity is usually enlarged. The signal of the endometrium is increased and inhomogeneous. Polyps have a low-intensity signal owing to their fibrous component. Pedunculated polyps are easiest to visualize; sessile forms can be difficult to differentiate from submucosal fibroids. The multiplanar imaging capability of MRI is thus particularly helpful. Gadolinium-enhanced MRI improves detection of polyps in 70% of patients by demonstrating lattice-like enhancement that remains hypointense to the endometrium.

Endometrial Atrophy. On T_2-weighted images, the uterine cavity contains hyperintense fluid-like loculi delimited by thin septa (Fig. 18.14). After gadolinium injection, the septa around the hypointense cystic cavities enhance discretely.

Endometrial Hyperplasia. The thickened endometrium has a homogeneous, high-intensity signal; contours appear fringed on T_2-weighted sequences. Postgadolinum enhancement is homogeneous and intense. The junctional zone is always preserved.

Endometrial Carcinoma. The prognosis depends essentially on the depth of myometrial invasion and, to a lesser extent, on involvement of the uterine cervix. The risk of nodal extension is less than 5% when involvement is superficial versus nearly 50% with deep invasion; findings thus significantly affect therapy. On T_2-weighted sequences, the uterine cavity is usually enlarged and inhomogeneously hyperintense. Often difficult to distinguish from the fluid collection, the tumor appears hypointense relative to the intrauterine debris. Gadolinum injection allows

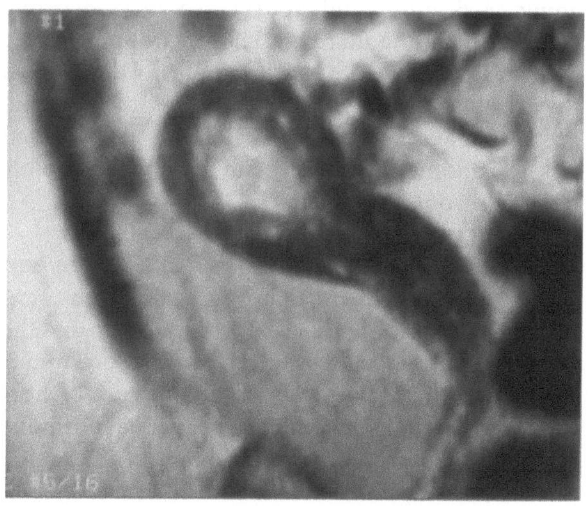

Fig. 18.14. T_2-weighted MRI of cystic–glandular atrophy in a tamoxifen-treated patient

differentiation of the tumor (which displays variable enhancement) from the fluid collection and improves visualization of the junctional zone.

Most recent studies have emphasized the utility of dual-phase dynamic MRI. Early gradient-echo scans, obtained 25 s after injection, correspond to the arterial phase; they reveal enhancement of the internal muscular coat of the myometrium and are thus essential for evaluation of myometrial invasion. Delayed scans, obtained 3 min after injection, correspond to opacification of the parametrial and paravaginal venous plexuses and improve definition of tumor contours. Dynamic MRI of myometrial invasion is superior to T_2-weighted imaging (ITO et al. 1994a,b; SCOUTT et al. 1995). Staging with dynamic sequences is accurate in 84.9%–97% of patients versus only 68%–77% with T_2-weighted sequences. In contrast, there is no significant difference between T_2-weighted images and conventional gadolinium-enhanced T_1-weighted sequences. MRI is more effective than transvaginal pelvic ultrasound for evaluation of myometrial invasion. Ultrasound tends to overestimate disease spread, because echoic intracavitary pseudopolypoid lesions are difficult to differentiate from the uterine muscle (KIM et al. 1995).

18.1.3 Hormone Replacement Therapy

18.1.3.1 *Pelvis*

HRT causes a number of modifications: augmentation of the volume of the uterus, endometrial thickening (4–6 mm), and appearance of a diastolic component in the uterine artery on Doppler study, with a PI of 2 to 3. The ovaries are easily detected as they resume their premenopausal volume. Overall, postmenopausal women on HRT are at increased risk of endometrial cancer, and should thus be offered ultrasound surveillance.

Endometrium. The type of HRT must be taken into account. With sequential hormone regimens, endometrial thickening peaks between the 13th and the 23rd days of the cycle. The mean increase of 8 mm is more than that observed with other types of hormone treatment. For women on segmental hormone regimens who present with endometrial thickening greater than 8 mm, LEVINE et al. (1995) advocate repeat ultrasound earlier or later in the hormone cycle, followed by biopsy if endometrial thickness remains unchanged. For all other hormone replacement regimens, biopsy is required to search for a malignancy whenever endometrial thickness exceeds 8 mm. Doppler findings suggest malignancy when the PI is under 1.5 (BESSIS et al. 1993); this information can also help identify those patients who would benefit from a biopsy.

Myometrium. Fibroids may enlarge and become symptomatic.

Ovaries. Ovarian cysts do not always disappear at menopause, as they are sometimes found during ultrasound screening for ovarian cancer. These cysts, which measure less than 2 cm, may regress (Fig. 18.15). According to LEVINE et al. (1992), simple adnexal cysts smaller than 3 cm with a normal RI in a patient with a normal CA-125 level should be kept under ultrasound surveillance. In women receiving HRT, cysts may merely be monitored by transvaginal ultrasound, pulsed Doppler, and laboratory tests.

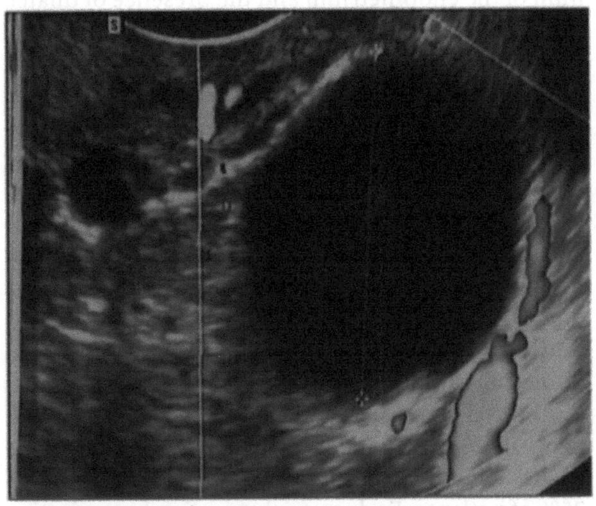

Fig. 18.15. Ovarian cyst (24.9 mm between the two *crosses*) in a postmenopausal woman undergoing hormone replacement therapy (HRT). The patient was monitored by transvaginal sonography (including power Doppler, PD) and CA-125 assays

18.1.3.2 *Breast*

Estrogen induces breast growth by stimulating ductal proliferation and by increasing capillary patency and the vascularity of the connective tissue. Progesterone is the secretory hormone responsible for cellular differentiation in the mammary gland (differentiation into acini, growth of the lobules), in synergy with estrogen. Acting as an antagonist, progesterone converts the proliferative effect of estrogen on ductal cells into cellular differentiation. During the postmenopausal period, long-term exposure to estrogen appears to induce epithelial proliferation and favors the development of cysts (cysts are less frequent when conjugated with progestogens). These histologic modifications explain the various features observed on imaging studies.

18.1.3.2.1 Hormone Replacement Therapy and Risk of Breast Cancer

Although it is widely recognized that oral contraceptives do not increase the risk of breast cancer in the general population, results concerning HRT are contradictory in users with benign breast disease or women with a family risk of the disease. Multiple biases are linked to the indolent course and multifactorial character of breast cancer and to the variety of treatments utilized. Breast cancer is also extremely hormone dependent, and late menopause, like early menses, is a risk factor (Henrich 1992).

In light of the many studies published and meta-analysis of results, if any risk does exist, it is hypothetical, and highly influenced by the dose and the duration of treatment. Half of these studies report an increased risk of breast cancer after prolonged administration (the relative risk is 1.5–2 if the duration of use is over 10 years). The influence of the type of estrogen compound, the dose, and combination with a progestogen (whose protective effect on the endometrium remains to be proven for the breast parenchyma) remain controversial (Nachtigall et al. 1979; Brinton et al. 1986; Gambrell 1986; Bergkvist et al. 1989; Dupont and Page 1990; Gabriel 1992). The meta-analysis carried out by Dupont and Page (1991) covering 28 studies concluded in a relative risk of breast cancer associated with HRT of 1.07. In the study performed by the Collaborative Group on Hormonal Factors in Breast Cancer, which covered 51 studies (1997), the relative risk of developing breast cancer increased by a factor of 1.023 when HRT was used for less than 5 years. The relative risk was 1.35 if the duration of HRT was more than 5 years. This excess risk disappeared 5 years after cessation of treatment. Moreover, cancers occurring after estrogen – progestogen replacement therapy reportedly have a better prognosis than those occurring in untreated women, probably in part because regular mammographic follow-up leads to earlier diagnosis (Magnusson et al. 1996).

18.1.3.2.2 Hormone Replacement Therapy and Benign Breast Disease

Benign Breast Disease and Cancer. The relative risk of developing breast cancer does not increase unless HRT is continued for more than 10 years (Steinberg et al. 1991).

"High-Risk" Benign Breast Disease and Cancer. According to Brinton et al. (1986), the risk of developing cancer is increased if benign breast disease exists prior to initiation of HRT. In contrast, women who develop benign breast disease after initiation of HRT do not seem to have any increase in their relative risk of developing breast cancer in the long term. According to Thomas et al. (1982), the risk is increased in the case of epithelial hyperplasia with microcalcifications. The conclusions of the meta-analysis carried out by Dupont and Page (1989) are particularly interesting. This study covered 3303 women with benign breast disease, including 1716 who took estrogen therapy and were followed up for 17 years. The risk of breast cancer decreased in benign proliferative or nonproliferative breast disease, with or without cellular atypia, unless estrogen therapy had been initiated before the biopsy. Gambrell (1986) and Colditz et al. (1990, 1993) failed to observe any modification in the risk for benign breast disease, but noted an increase in the protective effect conferred by estrogen when conjugated with progestogen. These results conflict with older studies (Rose et al. 1980; Hoover et al. 1981) that reported an increased risk of cancer in women with benign breast disease taking HRT.

Hormone Replacement Therapy and Evolution of Benign Breast Disease. Dose-dependent breast disease develops in 25% of women receiving HRT (Callantine et al. 1975; Rand et al. 1997). Reawakening of the premenstrual mammary syndrome, breast enlargement, and tumefactions are also frequent and can be controlled by modulation of the treatment and surveillance.

Hormone Replacement Therapy in Women with a Personal or Family History of Breast Cancer. The advisability of HRT for patients with a family history of breast cancer (first-degree relatives) remains highly controversial. The risk of breast cancer appears increased, but not significantly (Laforest and Taurelle 1994). With regard to patients who have already been treated for breast cancer, a few teams

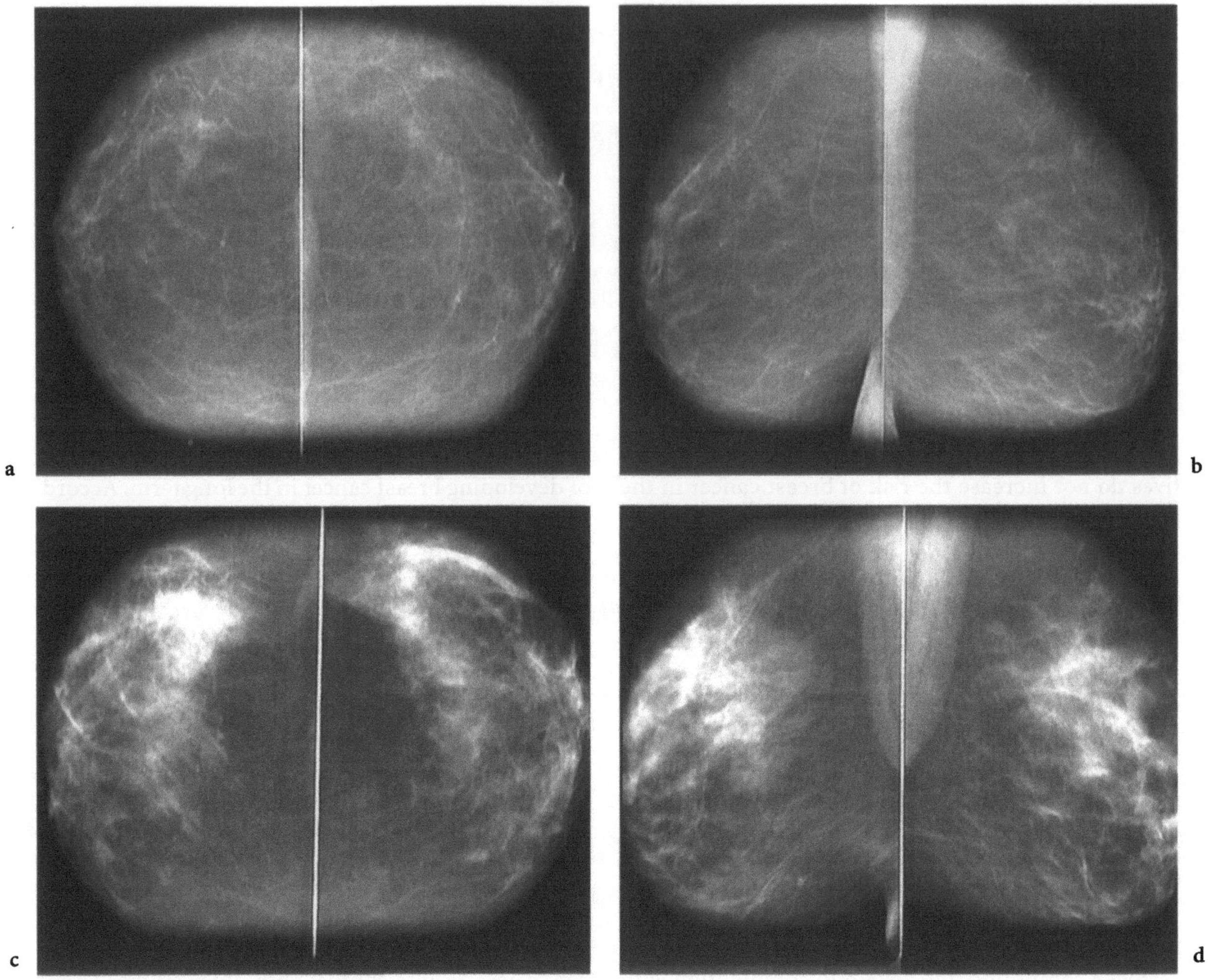

Fig. 18.16a–d. Postmenopausal woman undergoing hormone replacement therapy (HRT). **a** Anteroposterior (AP) and **b** oblique views: nearly complete and symmetrical fatty involution prior to initiation of HRT in this 58-year-old woman. **c** AP and **d** oblique views: global and symmetrical increase in the density of both breasts after 1 year of progestogen therapy

offer HRT to those whose cancer was diagnosed premenopausally. Wile and Disaia (1989) did not find any immediate or short-term effect of HRT on the disease, although their follow-up period was limited to 6 years.

18.1.3.2.3 Hormone Replacement Therapy and Conventional Breast Imaging

Increased Breast Density (Fig. 18.16). HRT inhibits the normal postmenopausal process of fatty involution, especially when associated with low parity (Kaufman et al. 1991), whereas oral contraceptives reduce breast density (Feig 1994; Spicer et al. 1994).

The high risk of breast cancer formerly attributed to dense breasts no longer appears valid (Page and Winfield 1986). Peck and Lowman (1978) were the first to describe benign parenchymal modifications on mammographies that disappeared when HRT was stopped. In contrast, Bland et al. (1980) did not observe any modifications in their analysis of 405 women followed up by xerography.

The few studies on the subject generally report increased breast density in approximately 25% of HRT-managed women. McNicholas et al. (1994) found a subjective increase in breast density in 27% of patients (two blind readings) versus an objective increase in 18% when measured by densitometry (which does not take focal density gradients into account).

Stomper et al. (1990) reported modifications in parenchymal density (without mass effect or architectural distorsion) in 24% of 50 patients; 14% of the changes were diffuse, while 4% were multifocal and asymmetric. In 6% of the patients, these modifications were due to cysts. Such anomalies can appear soon after initiation of HRT; 60% are present at 1 year and 40% at 2 years. Radiologic anomalies are more frequent in symptomatic patients, especially when symptoms are severe; 78% of radiologic anomalies are associated with clinical manifestations (McNicholas et al. 1994). Symptoms are linked to the duration of therapy and are sometimes reversible (Peck et al. 1978). Modifications are more extensive with estrogen - progestogen combinations than with estrogen alone, although the difference is not significant (Berkowitz et al. 1990; Stomper et al. 1990; Rand et al. 1997). Because conjugated regimens lead to hyperproliferation of the ducts, connective tissue, and lobules, the maximum increase in breast density can be expected with estrogen - progestogen therapies (Cyrlak and wong 1993). In one surgically confirmed case, a lesion that appeared during HRT corresponded to moderate hyperplasia (Doyle and McLean 1994).

Increased breast density interferes with early detection of breast cancer, especially because difficulties for breast compression compromise mammographic imaging. This reduction in the sensitivity of mammography for dense breasts is well known in clinical practice; it occurs in 85% of women in the 40- to 49-year age-group and in 93% of those aged 50–70 years (Kopans et al. 1985).

The sensitivity of screening may thus be reduced in a certain percentage of patients on HRT. The risk - benefit ratio must be evaluated for these patients who have the highest prevalence of disease. Ultrasound is disappointing for the detection of subclinical cancers in dense breasts and cannot compensate for the insufficiencies of mammography (Kopans et al. 1985; Basset et al. 1987; Jackson 1990).

Nodular Lesions. Fibroadenomas are a common finding in oral contraceptive users. During the perimenopausal period, lesion cellularity increases in response to the diminution in estrogen (Meyer et al. 1992). The development and growth of fibroadenomas are increased during HRT, but the frequency has not been documented in the literature. Fibroadenomas do not contraindicate HRT providing diagnostic confirmation is obtained first. Any changes on imaging studies should prompt a microbiopsy or surgical resection.

Cysts (Fig. 18.17) are frequent during the premenopausal period. During HRT, they tend to appear or reappear or increase in size. Diagnosis is made by ultrasound. Any modification in echotexture (vegetation, septa) or contours necessitates fine-needle aspiration (FNA).

Microcalcifications During Hormone Replacement Therapy. Resection of microcalcifications is often indispensable prior to initiation of HRT, even if the radiologic appearance is benign. The efficacy of microbiopsies for this purpose is still under evaluation.

Galactorrhea (Fig. 18.18), which reflects proximal or peripheral ductal ectasia, often occurs during HRT (Doyle et al. 1994). It is readily diagnosed by state-of-the-art high-frequency transducers (10–13 MHz). Unilateral serous or bloody nipple discharge should prompt a search for an organic lesion (solitary papilloma or diffuse papillomatosis).

18.1.3.2.4
Color Doppler Ultrasound

In premenopausal women, variations in the frequency and amplitude of mammary blood flows have been correlated with circulatory hormone levels during pregnancy and ovulation (Sambrook et al. 1987). Vascularity increases under estrogen therapy, as demonstrated by thermographic studies. To our knowledge, no studies have been conducted to date concerning potential modifications in vascular flow during HRT. Cosgrove (1993) suggested the use of CD to verify the efficacy of progestogen therapy for benign breast disease. Technical advances have unquestionably increased the sensitivity of CD for demonstration of vascularity in breast lesions, although to the detriment of specificity.

18.1.3.2.5
Magnetic Resonance Imaging

The current value of MRI is relatively satisfactory in terms of sensitivity (90%), but disappointing as concerns specificity (70%–80%). Except for a few specific situations (evaluation of breast implants and/or surveillance of therapy), MRI is not as effective as mammography, which remains the examination of reference for the diagnosis of breast cancer. No study has been published on the MRI patterns of women receiving HRT, but dynamic sequences would probably reveal increased vascularity. A diffuse increase in vascularity is a fairly frequent finding in benign breast disease on late scans (Gilles et al. 1994). No data is currently available on the utility of MRI for overall increases in breast density.

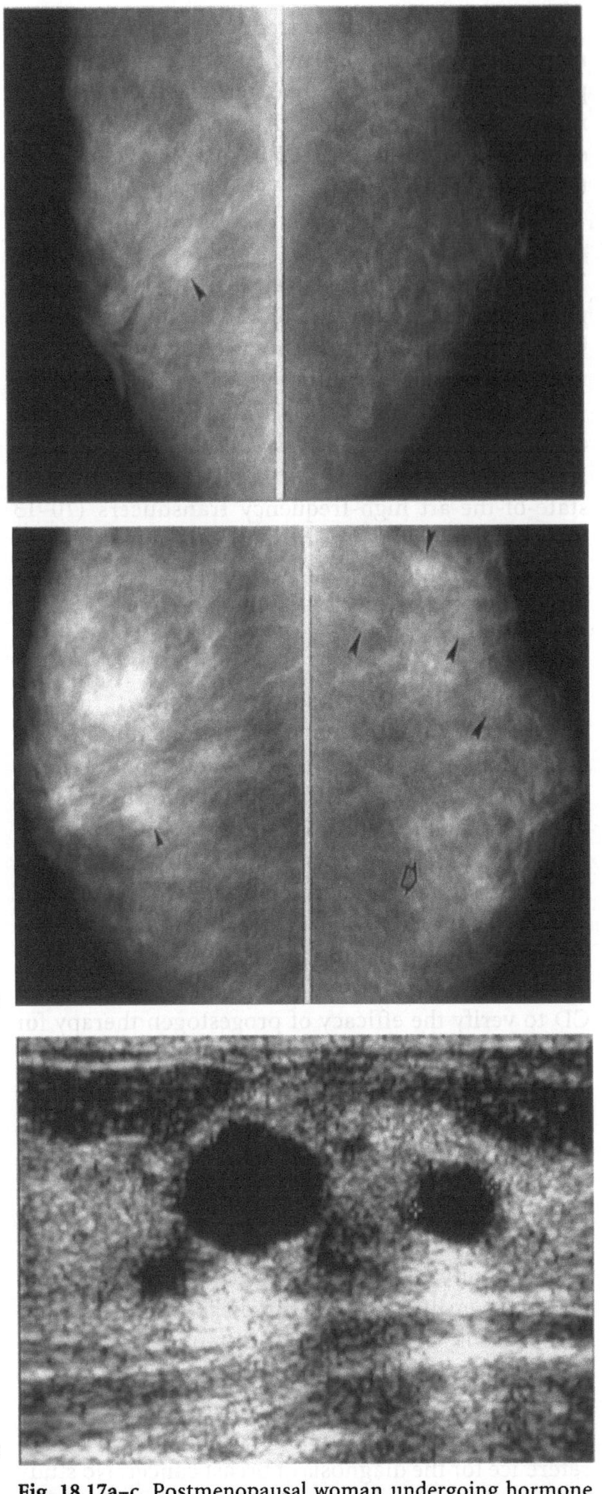

a

b

c

Fig. 18.17a–c. Postmenopausal woman undergoing hormone replacement therapy (HRT). a Oblique view: before HRT, asymmetrical fibrous/fatty involution with a cyst in the right breast (*arrowhead*). b Oblique view: after 8 years of HRT, presence of multiple nodules corresponding to cysts (*arrowheads*). The cyst in the right breast has enlarged; those in the left breast are recent. Note the density gradient in the left breast (*open arrow*). c Sonogram of the right breast revealing multiple simple cysts

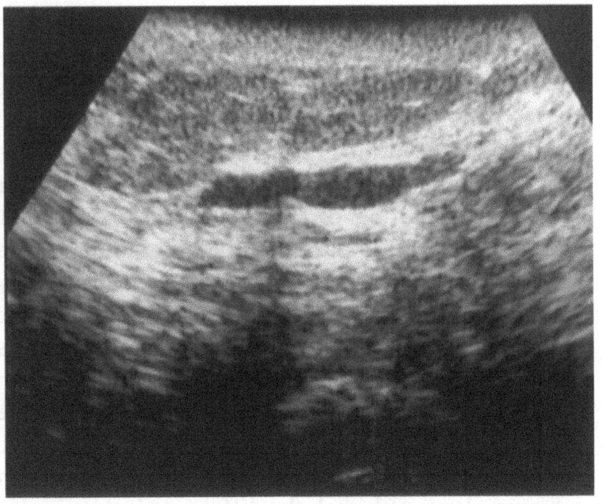

Fig. 18.18. Breast sonogram (13 MHz) demonstrating distal ductal ectasia; the hypoechoic contents correspond to amorphous deposits

In conclusion, HRT can produce particular mammographic features that reduce the technique's sensitivity for early detection of breast cancer. The risk of breast cancer and malignant transformation of high-risk breast disease induced by HRT can probably by avoided using currently recommended doses and durations. Moreover, plasma hormone concentrations in women managed by HRT are much lower than premenopausal levels. In the absence of any clinical abnormality, mammographic surveillance every 2 years appears sufficient.

18.1.4 Stimulation of Ovulation

The use of chorionic gonadotropins to stimulate ovulation requires sonographic monitoring owing to the risks of hyperstimulation, which results in excessive numbers of large follicles that can spontaneously evolve into follicular cysts. Large (up to 15 cm in diameter), painful ovarian cysts may be associated with digestive and systemic complications (ascites, hydrothorax, thromboembolic events). Sonographically, these lesions exhibit the typical features of a cystic structure. Other possible findings include visualization of the cystic ovarian cumulus, parietal changes with thickening, and intraperitoneal fluid effusion or hemorrhage (Besson and Constant 1993).

18.2 Corticosteroids

18.2.1 Osteoarticular Complications

18.2.1.1 Osteoporosis

Corticosteroid therapy is partially responsible for a direct decrease in bone formation and increased bone resorption. Bone resorption induced by the reduction in intestinal calcium absorption leads to an increase in parathyroid hormone secretion, which itself increases bone loss. Biological manifestations include hypercalciuria and a negative calcium balance.

Particularly frequent in elderly women and bedridden individuals, osteoporosis has also been correlated with high cumulative doses of corticosteroids (GLUCK et al. 1981). The sites of predilection are the axial skeleton and the proximal part of the long bones of the appendicular skeleton (RESNICK 1989).

The radiographically visible reduction in bone density is often nonuniform. Biconcave vertebrae (Fig. 18.19) with condensation of the superior and inferior aspects secondary to callus formation are highly suggestive of the diagnosis (LAWSON and ANSELL 1997). Stress fractures with extensive bony callus may be demonstrated (Fig. 18.20). Stress fractures of the ribs are also suggestive of osteoporosis. Diagnosis of sacral fractures can be difficult because the bone is demineralized, and chronic arthropathy (which may have been the original indication for corticosteroid treatment) induces architectural modifications. Bone scintigraphy, CT, or MRI (Figs. 18.21, 18.22) is advisable in such cases (RYAN and FOGELMAN 1994).

Various techniques have been developed for assessment of osteoporosis, including dual X-ray absorptiometry, quantitative CT (GUGLIELMI et al. 1994; DUBOEUF et al. 1995), quantitative ultrasound of the calcaneus (GLUER et al. 1996), and MRI (WEHRLI et al. 1995; LIN et al. 1997).

18.2.1.2 Osteonecrosis

Less frequent than osteoporosis (GENEREAU and CABANE 1992), osteonecrosis is often related to long-term corticosteroid therapy (approximately one third of patients). The risks are increased by long-term (more than 6 months) use of high doses administered in a fractionated manner rather than as a single daily dose. Cofactors have also been incriminated (JONES 1994).

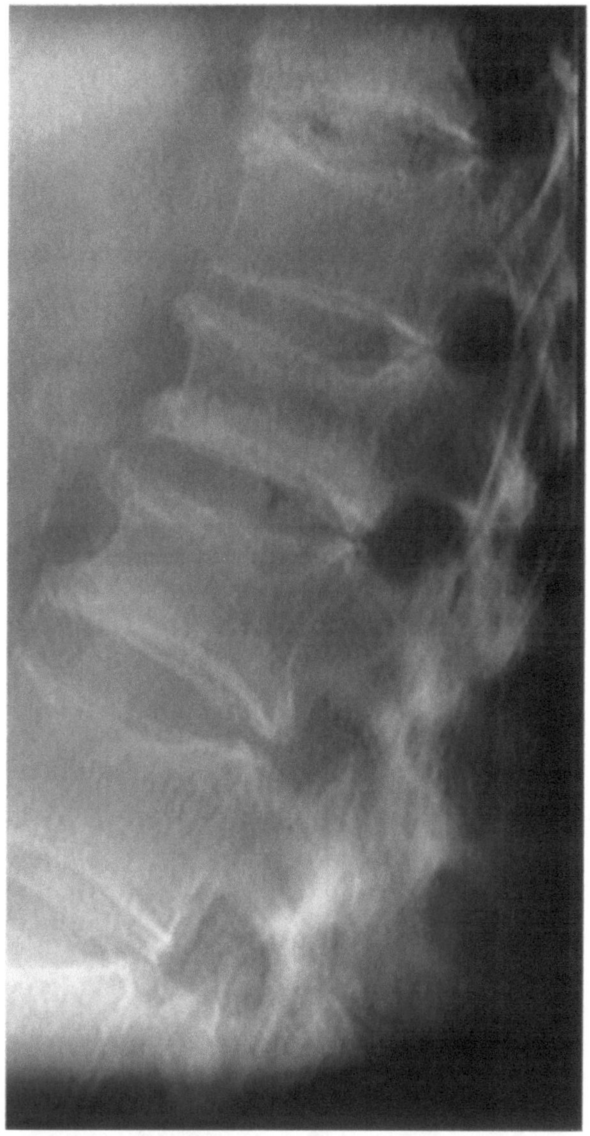

Fig. 18.19. Lateral radiograph of the lumbar spine revealing biconcave vertebrae with condensation of the superior and inferior aspects in a patient receiving long-term corticosteroid therapy

Osteonecrotic lesions generally appear 2–3 years after treatment and have a predilection for the epiphysis at one or more sites, i.e., femoral head, humeral head, distal femur, proximal tibia.

Two mechanisms have been proposed to explain the pathogenesis of osteonecrosis: (1) a vascular

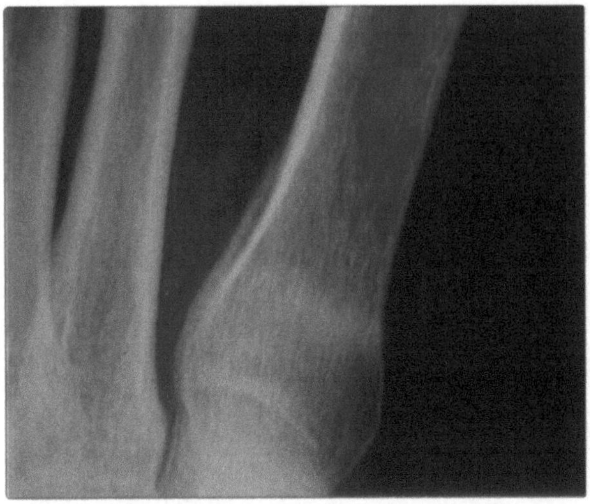

Fig. 18.20. Stress fracture of the first right metatarsus; this old fracture is associated with periosteal thickening

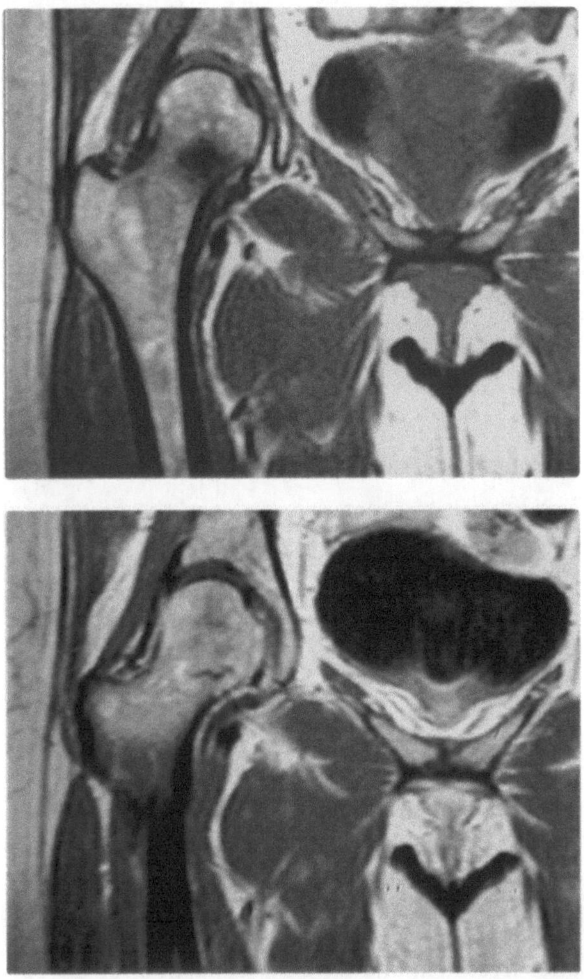

a

b

Fig. 18.21a,b. MRI of the right hip in a patient with Crohn's disease treated by corticosteroids: osteoporotic fracture. **a** T_1-weighted sequence revealing a hypointense zone. **b** Same sequence after gadolinium administration: visualization of the fracture line

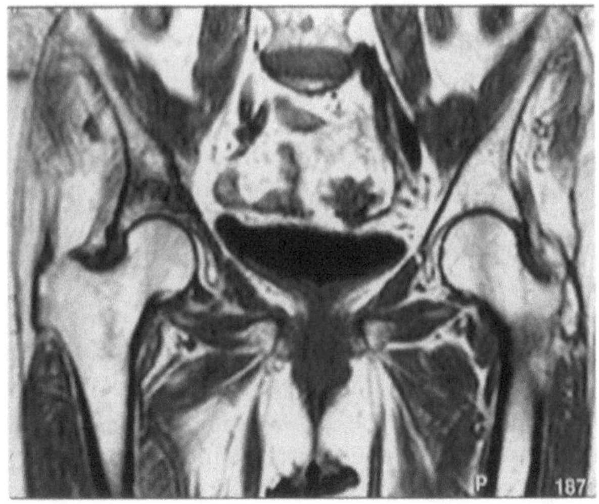

Fig. 18.22. MRI of the right hip in a patient treated by long-term corticosteroids. On this short tau inversion recovery (STIR) sequence, note the hyperintensity of the acetabulum (perifocal edema) with a hypointense fracture line in the center

theory implicating two or more risk factors, including hyperviscosity, vasculitis, vascular compression from marrow accumulation of fat, and fat embolism (Jones et al. 1965), and (2) a mechanical theory inwhich osteonecrosis is secondary to osteoporosis that has caused microfractures and possible bone collapse (Resnick 1989).

Radiologically, osteoporosis is associated with patchy osteosclerosis, subchondral radiolucent lines (crescent sign), bone collapse, fragmentation, and preservation of the joint space during the early phase (Resnick et al. 1989).

MRI is the most effective imaging modality for diagnosis of osteonecrosis, with a sensitivity of nearly 100% (Koo and Kim 1995; Froberg et al. 1996; Figs. 18.23–18.25). MRI features of osteonecrosis include focal subchondral abnormalities that are hypointense on T_1-weighted images and hyperintense on T_2-weighted sequences. Abnormal regions may vary from homogeneous to heretogeneous foci resembling bands, wedges, or rings. A diffuse, low-intensity signal on T_1-weighted images and a diffuse, high-intensity signal on T_2-weighted sequences are nonspecific findings consistent with bone marrow edema. In advanced osteonecrosis, pseudohomogeneous edema may image on T_2-weighted sequences as an inhomogeneous lesion with small, crescent-shaped subchondral marrow areas of low signal intensity. An anatomical MRI staging system for osteonecrosis has been established based on the MRI patterns for fat, blood, fluid, and fibrosis (Mitchell et al. 1987).

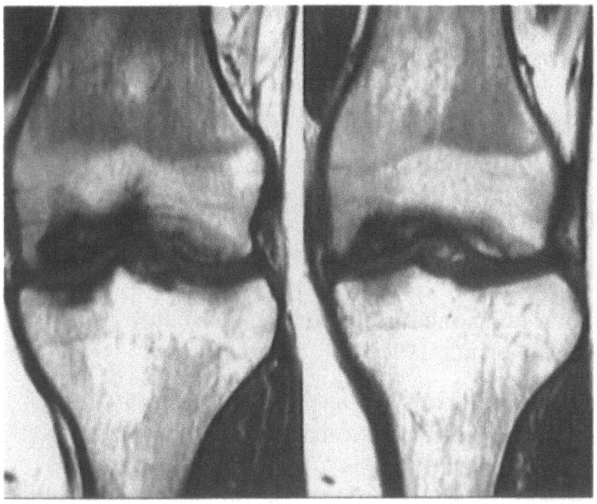

Fig. 18.23. Coronal T_1-weighted MRI revealed osteonecrosis of the left knee in a 26-year-old woman with lupus treated by long-term corticosteroids

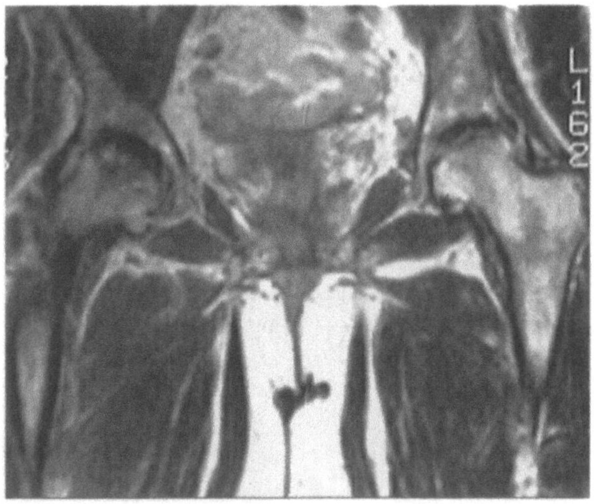

Fig. 18.24. A 51-year-old woman with kidney failure treated by long-term corticosteroids: the heterogeneity of the signal of the hips and the acetabula on the coronal T_2-weighted sequence is due to bilateral osteonecrosis

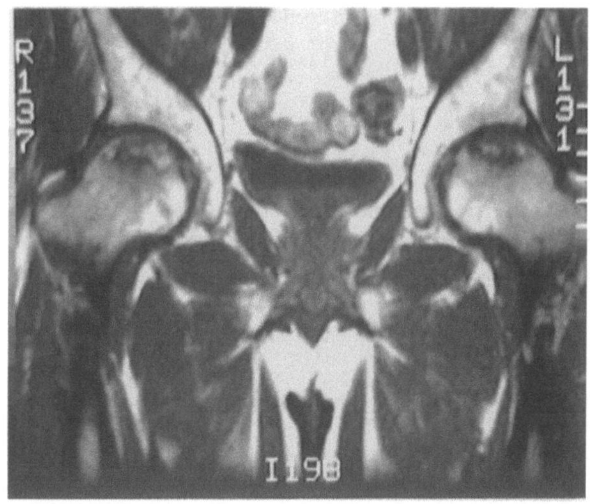

Fig. 18.25. A 28-year-old woman treated by corticosteroids for Crohn's disease: the T_1-weighted sequence reveals extensive architectural changes in the femoral heads secondary to osteonecrosis

18.2.1.3 Other Osteoarticular Complications

Rare complications of corticosteroids include osteomyelitis and infectious arthritis, hemopathy-like articular destruction (hips, knees), intra- and periarticular calcifications, and fat accumulation, particularly in the epidural region (Resnick 1989).

18.2.2 Nonosteoarticular Complications

18.2.2.1 Digestive Tract Complications

Gastroduodenal ulcerations may develop secondary to a reduction in mucosal resistance to peptic digestion (Ghahremani 1994). Lesions are most prevalent in the greater curvature, and large ulcers are common (Hyson et al. 1977). Periulcer edema is minimal because corticosteroid therapy reduces the inflammatory reaction. As these drugs reduce the extent of clinical symptoms, silent perforation may occur. Digestive tract lesions are much larger and more frequent in immunodepressed patients.

Other digestive tract complications include the following (Ansell 1997a): perforation of a colon diverticulum (Munsch et al. 1995), often complicated by an abscess (Fig. 18.26), intestinal pneumatosis, rarely acute pancreatitis. In patients treated using long-term corticosteroid therapy, rapid steroid withdrawal may cause ileus that is reversible with readministration of corticosteroids.

18.2.2.2 Extradigestive Tract Complications

Potential thoracic lesions include edema, lipomatosis, and an increased frequency of infections, especially tuberculosis (Trotman-Dickenson et al. 1997). Central nervous system involvement may

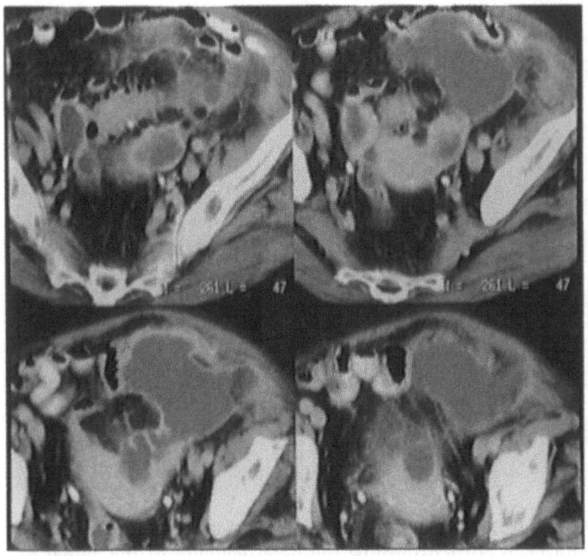

Fig. 18.26. Pelvic CT study (four contiguous scans; slice thickness, 5 mm) after digestive and vascular opacification: presence of an abscess secondary to complicated sigmoiditis in a patient receiving long-term corticosteroid therapy

manifest as mycotic infections (focal or associated with other localizations) or aspergillosis (NENOFF et al. 1995; KENDALL and ANSELL 1997).

18.3 Other Hormone Treatments

18.3.1 Thyroid Treatments

18.3.1.1 Thyrotoxicosis Factitia

Thyrotoxicosis factitia is discussed in Chap. 12.

18.3.1.2 Thyroid Hormones

In adults, thyroid hormones may increase bone resorption and new bone formation, resulting in a decrease in bone mineral density (PAUL et al. 1988). In children, thyroid hormones can produce craniosynostosis.

18.3.1.3 Synthetic Antithyroid Drugs

Rare cases of pericarditis have been described.

18.3.2 Other Hormone Therapies

Other hormone treatments can also cause complications (ANSELL 1997b):

- Growth hormone: necrosis of the femoral head
- ACTH: pancreatic calcifications, duodenal ulceration, renal lithiasis
- Octreotide (treatment of acromegaly): gallbladder stones
- Pituitary extracts: allergic alveolitis (hypersensitivity pneumonitis)
- Androgens: peliosis hepatis
- Megestrol acetate (treatment of prostate cancer): avascular necrosis, cushingoid syndrome

References

Achiron R, Lipitz S, Sivan E, Goldenberg M, Mashiach S (1995) Sonohysterography for ultrasonographic evaluation of tamoxifen-associated cystic thickened endometrium. J Ultrasound Med 14:685–688

Adler DD, Glazer GM, Silver TM (1984) Computed tomography of liver infarction. AJR 142:315–318

Aleem F, Predanic M, Calame R, Moukhtar M, Pennisi J (1995) Transvaginal color and pulsed Doppler sonography of the endometrium: a possible role in reducing the number of dilatation and curettage procedures. J Ultrasound Med 14:139–145

Ansell G (1997a) The gastrointestinal tract. In: Ansell G (ed) Imaging drug reactions and toxic hazards, 3rd edn. Chapman and Hall Medical, London, pp 87–186

Ansell G (1997b) Imaging drug reactions and toxic hazards, 3rd edn. Chapman and Hall Medical, London

Arrive L, Flejou FJ, Vilgrain V et al (1994) Hepatic adenoma: MR findings in 51 pathologically proved lesions. Radiology 193:507–512

Ascher SM, Johnson JC, Barnes WA, Bae CJ, Patt RH, Zeman RK (1996) MR imaging appearance of the uterus in postmenopausal women receiving Tamoxifen therapy for breast cancer: histopatholgoic correlation. Radiology 200:105–110

Baert AL, Fevery J, March G et al (1983) Early diagnosis of Budd-Chiari syndrome by computed tomography and ultrasonography: report of five cases. Gastroenterology 84:587–595

Bartolozzi C, Lencioni R, Paolicchi A, Moretti M, Armillotta N, Pinto F (1997) Differentiation of hepatocellular adenoma and focal nodular hyperplasia of the liver: comparison of power Doppler imaging and conventional color Doppler sonography. Eur Radiol 7:1410–1415

Basset LW, Kimme-Smith C, Sutherland LK, Gold RH, Sarti D, King W III (1987) Automated and hand-held breast US: effect on patient management. Radiology 165:103–108
Belghiti J, Pateron D, Panis Y et al (1993) Resection of presumed benign liver tumours. Br J Surg 80:380–383
Bergkvist L, Adami HO, Persson I, Bergstrom R, Krusemo UB (1989) Prognosis after breast cancer diagnosis in women exposed to estrogen and estrogen-progesteron replacement therapy. Am J Epidemiol 130:221–228
Berkowitz JE, Gatewood OMB, Goldblum LE, Gayler BW (1990) Hormonal replacement therapy: mammographic manifestations. Radiology 174:199–201
Bessis R, Papiernik E, Mergui JL, Monsonego J, Buthiau D, Tristant H (1993) Imagerie de la ménopause. In: Buthiau D, Dargent D (eds) Imagerie clinique en gynécologie. Vigot, Paris, pp 151–164
Besson P, Constant M (1993) Imagerie du pelvis iatrogène. In: Buthiau D, Dargent D (eds) Imagerie clinique en gynécologie. Vigot, Paris, pp 301–312
Bland KI, Buchanan JB, Weisberg, Hagan TA, Gray LA (1980) The effects of exogenous estrogen replacement therapy of the breast: breast cancer risk and mammographic parenchymal patterns. Cancer 45:3027–3033
Bonadona V, Mignotte H, Chauvin F et al (1996) Tamoxifène et cancer de l'endomètre: les résultats d'une étude castémoins multicentrique. Bull Cancer (Paris) 82:507–508
Bourne TH, Campbell S, Whitehead MI et al (1990) Detection of endometrial cancer in postmenopausal women by transvaginal ultrasonography and colour flow imaging. Br Med J 301:369
Brady AP, Malone DE, McGrath FP, Friedman L (1994) Focal nodular hyperplasia of the liver. An imaging conundrum. Can Assoc Radiol J 45:108–116
Brinton LA, Hoover R, Fraumeni JF Jr (1986) Menopausal oestrogens and breast cancer risk: an expanded case-control study. Br J Cancer 54:825–832
Brown BP, Abu-Yousef M, Farner R et al (1990) Doppler sonography: a noninvasive method for evaluation of hepatic venocclusive disease. AJR 154:721–724
Bruneton JN, Falewee MN, Ferrero JM (1993a) Adénome hépatique. In: Bruneton JN (ed) Imagerie des tumeurs du foie. Masson, Paris, pp 129–138
Bruneton JN, Padovani B, Mélia P (1993b) Hyperplasie nodulaire focale. In: Bruneton JN (ed) Imagerie des tumeurs du foie. Masson, Paris, pp139–151
Callantine MR, Martin PL, Bolding OT, Warner PO, Graney MR Jr (1975) Micronized 17 beta-estradiol for oral estrogen therapy in menopausal women. Obstet Gynecol 46:37–41
Caseiro-Alves F, Zins M, Mahfouz AE et al (1996) Calcification in focal nodular hyperplasia: a new problem for differentiation from fibrolamellar hepatocellular carcinoma. Radiology 198:889–892
Chan FY, Chau MT, Pun TC et al (1994) Limitations of transvaginal sonography and color Doppler imaging in the differentiation of endometrial carcinoma from benign lesions. J Ultrasound Med 13:623–628
Cherqui D, Rahmouni A, Charlotte F et al (1995) Management of focal nodular hyperplasia and hepatocellular adenoma in young women: a series of 41 patients with clinical, radiological, and pathological correlations. Hepatology 22:1674–1681
Colagrande S, Barlolozzi A, Tonarelli A (1994) Il ruolo della risonanza magnetica nella caratterizzazione delle lesioni focali epatiche. Radiol Med 87:469–481
Colditz GA, Stampfer MJ, Willet WC, Henneken CH, Rosner B, Speizer FE (1990) Prospective study of oestrogen replacement therapy and risk of breast cancer in post-menopausal women. JAMA 264:2648–2653
Colditz GA, Egan KM, Stampfer MJ (1993) Hormone replacement therapy and risk of breast cancer: results from epidemiologic studies. Am J Obstet Gynecol 168:1473–1480
Collaborative Group on Hormonal Factors in Breast Cancer (1997) Breast cancer and hormone replacement therapy: collaborative reanalysis of data from 51 epidemiological studies of 52 705 women with breast cancer and 108 411 women without breast cancer. Lancet 350:1047–1059
Cosgrove DO, Kedar RP, Bamber JC et al (1993) Breast diseases: color Doppler US in differential diagnosis. Radiology 189:99–104
Craig GR, Peters RL, Edmonson HA (1989) Tumors of the liver and intrahepatic bile ducts. Armed Forces Institute of Pathology, Washington (Atlas of tumor pathology, 2nd series)
Cullinan JA, Fleischer AC, Kepple DM, Arnold AL (1995) Sonohysterography: a technique for endometrial evaluation. Radiographics 15:501–514
Cyrlak D, Wong CH (1993) Mammographic changes in postmenopausal women undergoing hormonal replacement therapy. AJR 161:1177–1183
Denys A, Arrive L, Servois V et al (1994) Hepatic tumors: detection and characterization at 1-T MR imaging enhanced with AMI-25. Radiology 193:665–669
Doyle GJ, McLean L (1994) Unilateral increase in mammographic density with hormone replacement therapy. Clin Radiol 49:50–51
Drane WE, Krasicky GA, Johnson DA (1987) Radionuclide imaging of primary tumors and tumor-like conditions of the liver. Clin Nucl Med 12:569–582
Duboeuf F, Jergas M, Schott AM, Wu CY, Glüer CC, Genant HK (1995) A comparison of bone densitometry measurements of the central skeleton in post-menopausal women with and without vertebral fracture. Br J Radiol 68:747–753
Dupont WD, Page DL (1990) L'estrogénothérapie substitutive accroît-elle le risque de cancer du sein? Contraception Fertil Sexual 18:115–119
Dupont WD, Page DL (1991) Menopausal estrogen replacement therapy and breast cancer. Arch Intern Med 151:67–72
Dupont WD, Page DL, Rogers LW, Parc FF (1989) Influence of exogenous proliferative breast disease and other variables on breast cancer risk. Cancer 63:949–957
Ernst H, Hahn EG, Balzer T, Schlief R, Heyder N (1996) Color Doppler ultrasound of liver lesions: signal enhancement after intravenous injection of the ultrasound contrast agent Levovist. J Clin Ultrasound 24:31–35
Feig SA (1994) Hormonal reduction of mammographic densities: potential effects on breast cancer risk and performance of diagnostic and screening mammography. J Natl Cancer Inst 86:408–409
Fisher B, Costantino JP, Redmond CK et al (1994) Endometrial cancer in tamoxifen-treated breast cancer patients: findings from the National Surgical Adjuvant Breast and Bowel Project (NSABP) B14. J Natl Cancer Inst 86:527–537
Foster JH, Berman MM (1994) The malignant transformation of liver cell adenomas. Arch Surg 129:712–717
Froberg PK, Braunstein EM, Buckwalter KA (1996) Osteonecrosis, transient osteoporosis, and transient bone marrow edema. Current concepts. Radiol Clin North Am 34:273–291

Gabriel R (1992) Contraception orale, estrogénothérapie substitutive et épidémiologie du cancer du sein: données récentes. Reprod Hum Hormon 2: 128–137

Gambrell RD (1986) Cancer and the use of estrogen. Int J Fertil 31: 112–122

Genereau J, Cabane J (1992) Bénéfice des corticoïdes lors du traitement de la maladie de Horton et de la pseudopolyarthérite rhizomélique : avantages et inconvénients. Une méta-analyse. Rev Med Interne 13:387–391

Ghahremani GG (1994) Iatrogenic gastrointestinal disorders. In: Gore RM, Levine M, Laufer I (eds) Textbook of gastrointestinal radiology. Saunders, Philadelphia, pp 2583–2599

Ghahremani GG, Meyers MA, Farman J et al (1977) Ischemic disease of the small bowel and colon associated with oral contraceptives. Gastrointest Radiol 2:221–228

Gilles R, Guinebretière JM, Lucidarme O, Gluzel P, Janaud G, Finet JF et al (1994) Nonpalpable breast tumors: diagnosis with contrast-enhanced subtraction dynamic MR imaging. Radiology 191:625–631

Gluck OS, Murphy WA, Hahn TJ, Hahn BH (1981) Bone loss in adults receiving alternate day glucocorticoid therapy; comparison with daily therapy. Arthritis Rheum 24:892–898

Glüer CC, Cummings SR, Bauer DC et al (1996) Osteoporosis: association of recent fractures with quantitative US findings. Radiology 199:725–732

Goldberg AL, Rosenbaum AE, Wang H, Kim WS, Lewis VL, Hanley DF (1986) Computed tomography of dural sinus thrombosis. J Comput Assist Tomogr 10:16–20

Golli M, Van Nhieu JT, Mathieu D et al (1994) Hepatocellular adenoma: color Doppler US and pathologic correlations. Radiology 190:741–744

Gore RM (1994) Vascular disorders of the liver and the splanchnic circulation. In: Gore RM, Levine MS, Laufer I (eds) Textbook of gastrointestinal radiology. Saunders, Philadelphia, pp 2018–2050

Grandin C, Van Beers BE, Robert A, Gigot JF, Geubel A, Pringot J (1995) Benign hepatocellular tumors: MRI after superparamagnetic iron oxide administrations. J Comput Assist Tomogr 19:412–418

Gugenheim J, Mazza D, Baldini E et al (1995) Il trattamento chirurgico dei tumori epatici benigni. Una sclelta sicura ed efficace. Minerva Chir 50:161–165

Guglielmi G, Grimston SK, Fischer KC, Pacifici R (1994) Osteoporosis: diagnosis with lateral and posteroanterior dual X-ray absorptiometry compared with quantitative CT. Radiology 192: 845–850

Henrich JB (1992) The post-menopausal estrogen/breast cancer controversy. JAMA 268:1900

Hirsch DR, Mikkola KM, Marks PW et al (1996) Pulmonary embolism and deep venous thrombosis during pregnancy or oral contraceptive use: prevalence of factor V Leiden. Am Heart J 131:1145–1148

Hoover R, Gray LA, Cole P, MacMahon B (1981) Menopausal oestrogens and breast cancer. J Natl Cancer Inst 67:815–820

Hricak H, Finck S, Honda G et al (1992) MR imaging in the evaluation of benign uterine masses: value of gadopentetate dimeglumine-enhanced T1-weighted images. AJR 158:1043–1050

Hulka CA, Hall DA (1992) Endometrial abnormalities associated with tamoxifen therapy for breast cancer: sonographic and pathologic correlation. AJR 160:809–812

Hulka CA, Hall DA, McCarthy K, Simeone JF (1994) Endometrial polyps, hyperplasia, and carcinoma in postmenopausal women: differentiation with endovaginal sonography. Radiology 191:755–758

Hyson EA, Burrell M, Toffler R (1977) Drug-induced gastrointestinal disease. Gastrointest Radiol 2:183–212

Ismail SM (1996) The effects of tamoxifen on the uterus. Curr Opin Obstet Gynecol 8:27–31

Ito K, Fujita T, Uchisako H (1994a) MR imaging of the uterus: findings from high-resolution multisection dynamic imaging with a surface coil. AJR 163:873–879

Ito K, Matsumoto T, Nakada T, Nakanishi T, Fujita N, Yamashita H (1994b) Assessing myometrial invasion by endometrial carcinoma with dynamic MRI. J Comput Assist Tomogr 18:77–86

Ito K, Honjo K, Fujika T et al (1996) Liver neoplasms: diagnostic pitfalls in cross-sectional imaging. Radiographics 16:273–293

Jackson VP (1990) The role of US in breast imaging. Radiology 177:305–311

Jones DN (1994) Multifocal osteonecrosis following chemotherapy and short-term corticosteroid therapy in a patient with small-cell bronchogenic carcinoma. J Nucl Med 38:1347–1350

Jones JP, Engelman EP, Najarian JS (1965) Systemic fat embolism after renal homo transplantation and treatment with corticosteroids. New Engl J Med 273:1453–1458

Jordan VC (1995) Long-term tamoxifen treatment for breast cancer. J Natl Cancer Inst 87:1805–1806

Karlsson B, Granberg S, Hellberg P, Wikland M (1994) Comparative study of transvaginal sonography and hysteroscopy for the detection of pathologic endometrial lesions in women with postmenopausal bleeding. J Ultrasound Med 13:757–762

Kasales CJ, Arger PH, Nodine CF, Coleman BG, Langer JE, Jacobs JE (1996) Intrauterine low density in women over 50. Assessment of significance and recommendations for follow-up. Clin Imaging 20:194–198

Kaufman Z, Garstin WIH, Hayes R, Michell MJ, Baum M (1991) The mammographic parenchymal patterns of women on hormonal replacement therapy. Radiology 43:389–392

Kawakatsu M, Vilgrain V, Erling S, Nahum H (1997) Disappearance of liver cell adenoma: CT and MR imaging. Abdom Imaging 22:274–276

Kedar RP, Bourne TH, Powles TJ et al (1994) Effects of tamoxifen on uterus and ovaries of postmenopausal women in a randomised breast cancer prevention trial. Lancet 343:1318–1321

Kendall B, Ansell G (1997) The skull and central nervous system. In: Ansell G (ed) Imaging drug reactions and toxic hazards, 3rd edn. Chapman and Hall Medical, London, pp 323–358

Khiari A, Navarro F, Fabre JM et al (1996) Valeur de la ponction biopsie hépatique percutanée dans le diagnostic des tumeurs présumées bénignes du foie. Ann Chir 50:532–537

Killacke MA, Hakes TB, Pierce UK (1985) Endometrial adenocarcinoma in breast cancer patients receiving anti-estrogens. Cancer Treat Res 69:237–238

Killewich LA, Nunnelee JD, Auer AI (1993) Value of lower extremity venous duplex examination in the diagnosis of pulmonary embolism. J Vasc Surg 17:934–939

Kim SH, Kim HD, Song YS, Kang SB, Lee HP (1995) Detection of deep myometrial invasion in endometrial carcinoma: comparison of transvaginal ultrasound, CT and MRI. J Comput Assist Tomogr 19:766–772

Klufas RA, Hsu L, Barnes PD, Patel MR, Schwartz RB (1995) Dissection of the carotid and vertebral arteries: imaging with MR angiography. AJR 164:673–677
Koo KH, Kim R (1995) Quantifying the extent of osteonecrosis of the femoral head: a new method using MRI. J Bone Joint Surg 77:875–880
Kopans DB, Meyer JE, Lindfors KK (1985) Whole-breast US imaging: four-year follow-up. Radiology 157:505–507
Kupfer MC, Schiller VL, Hansen GC, Tessler FN (1994) Transvaginal sonographic evaluation of endometrial polyps. J Ultrasound Med 13:535–539
Kurjak A, Shalan H, Sosic A et al (1993) Endometrial carcinoma in postmenopausal women: Evaluation by transvaginal color Doppler ultrasonography. Am J Obstet Gynecol 169:1597–1603
Kurman RJ, Raminski F, Norris HJ (1985) The behavior of endometrial hyperplasia. A long-term study of "untreated" hyperplasia in 170 patients. Cancer 56:403–412
Laforest H, Taurelle R (1994) L'hormonothérapie substitutive de la ménopause augmente-t-elle le risque de cancer du sein? Rev Fr Gynécol Obstét 89:181–191
Landen S, Siriser F, Bardaxoglou E et al (1993) Focal nodular hyperplasia of the liver. A retrospective review of 20 patients managed surgically. Acta Chir Bel 93:94–97
Lang H, Oldhafer KJ, Weimann A et al (1994) The Budd-Chiari syndrome: clinical presentation and diagnostic findings in 45 patients treated by surgery. Bildgebung 61:173–181
Lawson JP, Ansell G (1997) The skeletal system and soft tissues. In: Ansell G (ed) Imaging drug reactions and toxic hazards, 3rd edn. Chapman and Hall Medical, London, pp 231–322
Lencioni R, Caramella D, Bartolozzi C (1995) Percutaneous biopsy of liver tumors with color Doppler US guidance. Abdom Imaging 20:206–208
Levine D, Gosink BB, Wolf SI, Feldesman MR, Pretorius DH (1992) Simple adnexal cysts: the natural history in postmenopausal women. Radiology 184:653–659
Levine D, Gosink BB, Johnson LA (1995) Change in endometrial thickness in postmenopausal women undergoing hormone replacement therapy. Radiology 197:603–608
<referenLewis BD, James EM, Welch TJ, Joyce JJ, Hallett JW, Weaver AL (1994) Diagnosis of acute deep venous thrombosis of the lower extremities: prospective evaluation of color Doppler flow imaging versus venography. Radiology 192: 651–655
Lewis JH (1986) Gastrointestinal injury due to medicinal agents. Am J Gastroenterol 81:819–834
Lidegaard O (1997) Thromboembolic complications in the use of oral contraceptives. Ugeskr Laeger 159:1908–1909
Lin JC, Ouyang X, Fan B, Newitt DC, Majumdar S, Genant HK (1997) MR imaging, ultrasound, and bone mineral density in osteoporosis. Radiology 205 (P):259–260
Magnusson C, Holmberg L, Norden T, Lindgren A, Persson I (1996) Prognostic characteristics in breast cancers after hormone replacement therapy. Breast Cancer Res Treat 38:325–334
Malanga GA, Gangemi E (1994) Intracranial venous thrombosis in a patient with multiple sclerosis. A case report and review of contraceptive alternatives in patients with disabilities. Am J Phys Med Rehabil 73:283–285
Mangiante G, Nicoli N, Marchiori L et al (1994) La strategia terapeutica dei tumori epatici benigni: esperienza di 20 anni. Chir Ital 46:50–60
Mathieu D, Bruneton JN, Drouillard J, Caron-Poitreau C, Vasile N (1986) Hepatic adenomas and focal nodular hyperplasia: dynamic CT study. Radiology 160:53–58
Mathieu D, Vasile N, Menu Y et al (1987) Budd-Chiari syndrome: dynamic CT. Radiology 165:409–413
Mathieu D, Vilgrain V, Mahfouz AE, Anglade MC, Vullierme MP, Denys A (1997) Benign liver tumors. Magn Reson Imaging Clin N Am 5:255–288
McNicholas MMJ, Heneghan JP, Milner MH, Tunnery T, Hourihane JB, MacErlaine DP (1994) Pain and increased mammographic density in women receiving hormone replacement therapy: a prospective study. AJR 163:311–315
Meyer JE, Frenna TH, Polger M, Sonnenfeld MR, Shaffer K (1992) Enlarging occult fibroadenomas. Radiology 183:639–641
Mitchell D, Rao B, Dalinka M et al (1987) Femoral head avascular necrosis: correlation of MR imaging, radiographic staging, radionuclide imaging, and clinical findings. Radiology 162:709–715
Mitchell DG, Stark DD (1992) Liver. In: Stark DD, Bradley WG (eds). Magnetic resonance imaging, 2nd edn. Mosby, Chicago, pp 1652–1768
Munsch B, Chauffert B, Cuny C, Lorcerie B, Martin F (1995) Perforation de diverticule colique sous corticoïdes. Rev Med Interne 16:137–140
Nachtigall LE, Nachtigall RH, Nachtigall RD, Beckman EM (1979) Estrogen replacement therapy. II. A prospective study in the relationship to carcinoma and cardiovascular and metabolic problems. Obstet Gynecol 54:74–79
Nakashima O, Kojiro M (1996) Pathomorphologic characteristics and differential diagnosis of small hepatocellular carcinoma. Gan To Kagaku Ryoho 23:827–834
Nenoff P, Horn LC, Mierzwa M et al (1995) Peracute disseminated fatal Aspergillus fumigatus sepsis as a complication of corticoid-treated systemic lupus erythematosus. Mycoses 38:467–471
Osmer R, Völksen M, Schauer A (1990) Vaginosonography for early detection of endometrial carcinoma? Lancet 335:1569–1571
Page DL, Winfield AC (1986) The dense mammogram. AJR 147:487–489
Paineau J, Hamy A, Visset J (1994) Notre expérience chirurgicale d'exérèse des tumeurs hépatiques bénignes. J Chir (Paris) 131:461–465
Paul TL, Kerrigan J, Kelly AM et al (1988) Long-term L-thyroxine therapy is associated with decreased hip bone density in premenopausal women. JAMA 259:3137–3141
Paulson EK, McClellan JS, Washington K, Spritzer CE, Meyers WC, Baker ME (1994) Hepatic adenoma: MR characteristics and correlation with pathologic findings. AJR 163:113–116
Peck DR, Lowman RM (1978) Estrogen and the post-menopausal breast: mammographic considerations. JAMA 240:1733–1735
Pezzullo JA, Perkins AB, Cronan JJ (1996) Symptomatic deep vein thrombosis: diagnosis with limited compression US. Radiology 198:67–70
Rand T, Heytmanek G, Seifert M, Wunderbaldinger P, Kreuzer S, Schneider B, Wolf G (1997) Mammography in women undergoing hormone replacement therapy. Acta Radiol 38:228–231
Resnick D (1989) Disorders caused by medications and other chemical agents. In: Resnick D (ed) Bone and joint imaging. Saunders, Philadelphia, pp 915–956
Resnick D, Niwayama G, Sweet DE, Madewell JE (1989) Osteonecrosis. In: Resnick D (ed) Bone and joint imaging. Saunders, Philadelphia, pp 959–978
Rooks JB, Ory HW, Ishak KG et al (1979) Epidemiology of hepatocellular adenoma: the role of oral contraceptive use. JAMA 242:644–648

Ros RP (1994) Benign liver tumors. In: Gore RM, Levine MS, Laufer I (eds) Textbook of gastrointestinal radiology. Saunders, Philadelphia, pp 1861–1896

Rose RK, Paganini NI, Hill A, Gerlin VB et al (1980) A case control study of menopausal estrogen therapy and breast cancer. JAMA 24:1635–1640

Ryan PJ, Fogelman I (1994) Osteoporotic vertebral fractures: diagnosis with radiography and bone scintigraphy. Radiology 190:669–672

Sambrook M, Bamber JC, Minasian H, Hill CR (1987) Ultrasonic Doppler study of the hormonal response of blood flow in the normal human breast. Ultrasound Med Biol 13:121–129

Schick F, Stern W, Forster J, Laniado M, Lutz O, Claussen CD (1997) Magnetization transfer contrast of hepatic lesions in breath-hold gradient-echo images of different T1 weighting. J Magn Reson Imaging 7:280–285

Scoutt LM, McCarthy SM, Flynn SD et al (1995) Clinical stage I endometrial carcinoma: pitfalls in preoperative assessment with MR imaging. Radiology 194:567–572

Seoud MA, Johnson J, Weed JC Jr (1993) Gynecologic tumors in tamoxifen-treated women with breast cancer. Obstet Gynecol 82:165–169

Shamsi K, De Schepper A, Degryse H, Deckers F (1993) Focal nodular hyperplasia of the liver: radiologic findings. Abdom Imaging 18:32–38

Sidhu PS, Dawson P, Ansell G (1997) The urogenital system. In: Ansell G (ed). Imaging drug reactions and toxic hazards, 3rd edn. Chapman and Hall Medical, London, pp 187–229

Silva EG, Tornos CS, Follen-Mitchell M (1994) Malignant neoplasms of uterine corpus in patients treated for breast carcinoma: the effects of tamoxifen. Int J Gynecol Pathol 13:248–258

Spicer DV, Ursin G, Parisky YR, Pearce JG, Shoupe D, Pike A et al (1994) Changes in mammographic densities induced by a hormonal contraceptive designed to reduce breast cancer risk. J Natl Cancer Inst 86:431–435

Spritzer CE, Norconk JJ, Sostman HD et al (1993) Detection of deep venous thrombosis by MRI. Chest 104:54–60

Steinberg KK, Thacker SB, Smith SJ et al (1991) A meta-analysis of the estrogen replacement therapy on the risk of breast cancer. JAMA 265:1985

Stomper PC, Van Voorhis BJ, Ravnikar VA, Meyer JE (1990) Mammographic changes associated with postmenopausal hormone replacement therapy: a longitudinal study. Radiology 174:487–490

Taourel PG, Deneuville M, Pradel JA, Regent D, Bruel JM (1996) Acute mesenteric ischemia: diagnosis with contrast-enhanced CT. Radiology 199:632–636

Tepper R, Cohen I, Altaras M et al (1994) Doppler flow evaluation of pathological endometrial conditions in post-menopausal breast cancer patients treated with tamoxifen. J Ultrasound Med 13:635–640

Terada T, Kitani S, Ueda K, Nakanuma Y, Kitagawa K, Masuda S (1993) Adenomatous hyperplasia of the liver resembling focal nodular hyperplasia in patients with chronic liver disease. Virchows Arch A Pathol Anat Histopathol 422:247–252

Thomas DB, Persing JP, Hutchinson WB (1982) Exogenous estrogens and other risk factors for breast cancer in women with benign breast diseases. J Natl Cancer Inst 69:1017–1025

Trotman-Dickenson B, Hansell DM, Ansell G (1997) The chest. In: Ansell G (ed) Imaging drug reactions and toxic hazards, 3rd edn. Chapman and Hall Medical, London, pp 1–86

Uggowitzer MM, Kugler C, Machan L, Groell R, Spork E, Pilhatsch A (1997) New sonographical approaches in the evaluation of the vascular architecture and resistive index (RI) in focal nodular hyperplasia of the liver. Radiology 205(P):198

Ugwumadu AH, Harding K (1994) Uterine leiomyomata and endometrial proliferation in postmenopausal women treated with the anti-estrogen tamoxifen. Eur J Obstet Gynecol Reprod Biol 54:153–156

Van Erpecum KJ, Janssens AP, Kreuning J et al (1988) Generalized peliosis hepatis and cirrhosis after long-term use of oral contraceptives. Am J Gastroenterol 83:572–575

Van Hoe L, Baert AL, Gryspeerdt S et al (1997) Dual-phase helical CT of the liver: value of an early-phase acquisition in the differential diagnosis of non-cystic focal lesions. AJR 168:1185–1192

Vandenbroucke JP, Van der Meer FJ, Helmerhorst FM, Rosendaal FR (1996). Factor V Leiden: should we screen oral contraceptive users and pregnant women? BMJ 313:1127–1130

Vogl TJ, Bergman C, Villringer A, Einhaupl K, Lissner J, Felix R (1994) Dural sinus thrombosis: value of venous MR angiography for diagnosis and follow-up. AJR 162:1191–1198

Vogl TJ, Hammerstingl R, Schwarz W et al (1996) Superparamagnetic iron-oxide versus gadolinium-enhanced MR imaging for differential diagnosis of focal liver tumors. Radiology 198:881–887

Wasenko JJ, Holsapple JW, Winfield JA (1995) Cerebral venous thrombosis. Demonstration with magnetic resonance angiography. Clin Imaging 19:153–161

Wehrli FW, Ford JC, Haddad JG (1995) Osteoporosis: clinical assessment with quantitative MR imaging in diagnosis. Radiology 196:631–641

Welch TJ, Sheedy PF II, Johnson CM et al (1985) Focal nodular hyperplasia and hepatic adenoma: comparison of angiography, CT, US and scintigraphy. Radiology 156:593–595

Wikland M, Granberg S, Karlsson B (1993) Replacing diagnostic curettage by vaginal ultrasound. Eur J Obstet Gynecol Reprod Biol 49:35–38

Wile AG, DiSaia PJ (1989) Hormones and breast cancer. Am J Surg 157:438–442

Wolman I, Jaffa AJ, Hartoov J, Bar-AM A, David MP (1996a) Sensitivity and specificity of sonohysterography for the evaluation of the uterine cavity in peri-menopausal patients. J Ultrasound Med 154:285–188

Wolman I, Jaffa AJ, Sagi J, Hartoov J, Amster R, David MP (1996b) Transvaginal ultrasonographic measurements of endometrial thickness: a reproducibility study. J Clin Ultrasound 24:351–345

Wolman I, Sagi J, Ginat S, Jaffa AJ, Hartoov J, Jedwab G (1996c) The sensitivity and specificity of vaginal sonography in detecting endometrial abnormalities in women with postmenopausal bleeding. J Clin Ultrasound 24:79–82

Zalel Y, Tepper R, Cohen I, Goldberger S, Beyth Y (1996) Clinical significance of endometrial fluid collections in asymptomatic postmenopausal women. J Ultrasound Med 15:513–515

Zimmerman HJ, Ishak KG (1987) Do estrogens cause venocclusive disease of the liver? Gastroenterology 93:384–391

Subject Index

List of Contributors

SERGE AGOSTINI, MD
Professor of Radiology
Service de Radiologie
Hôpital Sainte Marguerite
270 Boulevard Ste Marguerite
F-13009 Marseille
France

MARC ANDRÉ, MD
Service de Radiologie-Adultes
Hôpital de la Timone
264 rue Saint-Pierre
F-13385 Marseille
France

ELIZABETH BAECHLER SADOUL, MD
Service de Pédiatrie
Fondation Lenval
57 avenue de la Californie
F-06200 Nice
France

JEAN-MICHEL BARTOLI, MD
Professor of Radiology
Service de Radiologie-Adultes
Hôpital de la Timone
264 rue Saint-Pierre
F-13385 Marseille Cedex 5
France

MOURAD BELAIDI, MD
Service de Radiodiagnostic
Hôpital Pasteur
30, avenue de la Voie Romaine, BP 69
F-06002 Nice Cedex 1
France

BERNARD BENOIT, MD
Service de Gynécologie et d'Obstétrique
Hôpital de l'Archet
151 chemin de Saint-Antoine Ginestière
F-06200 Nice
France

OLIVIER BERNARD, MD
Service de Radiologie
HIA Percy
101 avenue Henri Barbusse, BP 406
F-92141 Clamart Cedex
France

ANTOINE BLEUSE, MD
Service de Radiologie
Centre Antoine-Lacassagne
33 avenue de Valombrose
F-06189 Nice Cedex 2
France

LOUIS BOYER, MD
Professor of Radiology
Service de Radiology et d'Imagerie Médicale
Hôpital G. Montpied
30 Place Henri Dunand, BP 69
F-63003 Clermont-Ferrand
France

PATRICE BRET, MD
Professor of Radiology
Service de Radiologie
Hôpital Général de Montréal
1650, avenue Cédar
H3G - 1A4 Montreal (PQ)
Canada

JEAN-MICHEL BRUEL, MD
Professor of Radiology
Service d'Imagerie Médicale
Hôpital Saint-Eloi - CHU de Montpellier
F-34295 Montpellier Cedex 5
France

JEAN NOEL BRUNETON, MD
Professor of Radiology
Centre Antoine-Lacassagne
33 avenue de Valombrose
F-06189 Nice Cedex 2
France

Philippe Brunner, MD
Service de Radiologie
Centre Hospitalier Princess Grace
Avenue Pasteur
MC-98000 Monaco

Françoise Bussière, MD
Professor of Nuclear Medicine
Service de Médecine Nucléaire
Centre Antoine-Lacassagne
33 avenue de Valombrose
F-06189 Nice Cedex 2
France

Jean Noel Buy, MD
Professor of Radiology
Service de Radiologie
Hôtel Dieu
Place du Parvis Notre Dame
F-75004 Paris
France

Francesco Calabro, MD
Radiologia
Ospedale S. Corona
I-Pietra Ligure (S.V.)
Italy

Christophe Calvet, MD
Service d'Imagerie Médicale
Hôpital Saint-Eloi - CHU de Montpellier
F-34295 Montpellier Cedex 5
France

Stéphane Chanalet, MD
Service de Radiodiagnostic
Hôpital Pasteur
30, avenue de la Voie Romaine, BP 69
F-06002 Nice Cedex 1
France

Patrick Chevallier, MD
Service de Radiodiagnostic
Hôpital de l'Archet
151 chemin de St. Antoine de Ginestière
F-06200 Nice Cedex
France

Jean Michel Cucchi, MD
Centre d'Imagerie Médicale
Rue du Gabian
MC-98000 Monaco

Isabelle Damarey, MD
Service de Radiologie et d'Imagerie Médicale
Hôpital Jeanne de Flandre
2, avenue Oscar Lambert
F-59037 Lille Cedex
France

Alan Daneman, MD
Department of Radiology
Hospital for Sick Children
555 University Avenue
Toronto, Ontario M5G1X8
Canada

Jacques Darcourt, MD
Professor of Nuclear Medicine
Service de Médecine Nucléaire
Centre Antoine-Lacassagne
33 avenue de Valombrose
F-06189 Nice Cedex 2
France

Thierry de Baere, MD
Service de Radiologie Interventionnelle
Institut Gustave-Roussy
39–53 avenue Camille Desmoulins
F-94805 Villejuif Cedex
France

Jacques Drouillard, MD
Professor of Radiology
Service de Radiodiagnostic
Hôpital du Haut Lévèque
Avenue de Magellan
F-33604 Pessac
France

François Durand, MD
Service de Radiologie et d'Imagerie Midicale
Hôpital Jeanne de Flandre
2, avenue Oscar Lambert
F-59037 Lille Cedex
France

Olivier Durieux, MD
Service de Radiologie
Hôpital de Sainte Marguerite
270 Boulevard Ste Marguerite
F-13009 Marseille
France

Afshin Gangi, MD
Service de Radiologie
Hôpital de Hautepierre
Avenue Molière
F-67098 Strasbourg Cedex
France

Véronique Gense, MD
Service de Radiodiagnostic
Hôpital du Haut Lévèque
Avenue de Magellan
F-33604 Pessac
France

Anne Geoffray, MD
Service de Radiologie
Fondation Lenval
57, avenue de la Californie
F-06200 Nice
France

Michel Ghossain, MD
Service de Radiologie
Hôtel Dieu
Place du Parvis Notre Dame
F-75004 Paris
France

Myriam Gray, MD
Institut Arnault Tzanck
Avenue du Docteur Monot
F-06700 Saint Laurent du Var
France

Anne Grimaud, MD
Service de Radiologie
Hôpital de l'Archet
151 chemin de St. Antoine Ginestière
F-06200 Nice Cedex
France

Daniel Jeanbourquin, MD
Professor of Radiology
Service de Radiologie
HIA Percy
101, avenue Henri Barbusse, BP 406
F-92141 Clamart Cedex
France

Valérie Juhan, MD
Service de Radiologie
Hôpital de la Timone
264 rue Saint Pierre
F-13385 Marseille Cedex 5
France

Robin Lecesne, MD
Service de Radiodiagnostic
Hôpital du Haut Lévèque
Avenue de Magellan
F-33604 Pessac
France

Tito Livraghi, MD
Unita Radiologia
Ospedale Civile
Via C. Battisti, 23
I-20059 Vimercate (MI)
Italy

Olivia Louis, MD
Radiologie en Medische Beeldvorming
Academisch Ziekenhuis
Vrije Universiteit Brussels
Laarbeeklaan 101
B-1090 Brussels
Belgium

Catherine Maestro, MD
Service de Radiologie
Centre Antoine-Lacassagne
33 avenue de Valombrose
F-06189 Nice Cedex 2
France

Antoine Maubon, MD, PhD
Imagerie Médicale
CMC Beau Soleil
119, avenue de Lodève
F-34000 Montpellier
France

Pierre Yves Marcy, MD
Service de Radiologie
Centre Antoine-Lacassagne
33 avenue de Valombrose
F-06189 Nice Cedex 2
France

Jean-François Merrer, MD
Service de Radiologie
HIA Percy
101, avenue Henri Barbusse, BP 406
F-92141 Clamart Cedex
France

Giulano Michelozzi, MD
Radiologia
Ospedale S. Corona
I-Pietra Ligure (S.V.)
Italy

Michel-Yves Mourou, MD
Service de Radiologie
Centre Hospitalier Princesse Grace
Avenue Pasteur
MC-98000 Monaco

Michel Osteaux, MD, PhD
Professor of Radiology
Radiologie en Medische Beeldvorming
Academisch Ziekenhuis
Vrije Universiteit Brussels
Laarbeeklaan Brussels
B-1090 Brussels
Belgium

Bernard Padovani, MD
Professor of Radiology
Service de Radiodiagnostic
Hôpital Pasteur
30, avenue de la Voie Romaine, BP 69
F-06002 Nice Cedex 1
France

Jean G. Pradel, MD
Service de Radiologie
Centre Hospitalier
F-10000 Troyes
France

Charles Raffaelli, MD
Service de Radiodiagnostic
Hôpital Pasteur
30, avenue de la Voie Romaine, BP 69
F-06002 Nice Cedex 1
France

Anne Ravel, MD
Service de Radiologie et d'Imagerie Médicale
Hôpital G. Montpied
30 Place Henri Dunand, BP 69
F-63003 Clermont-Ferrand
France

Yann Robert, MD
Professor of Radiology
Service de Radiologie et d'Imagerie Médicale
Hôpital Jeanne de Flandre
2, avenue Oscar Lambert
F-59037 Lille Cedex
France

Alain Roche, MD
Professor of Radiology
Service de Radiologie Interventionnelle
Institut Gustave-Roussy
39–59 avenue Camille Desmoulins
F-94805 Villejuif Cedex
France

Nathalie Rocourt, MD
Service de Radiologie et d'Imagerie Médicale
Hôpital Jeanne de Flandre
2, avenue Oscar Lambert
F-59037 Lille Cedex
France

Jean Pierre Rouanet, MD
Professor of Radiology
Imagerie Médicale
CMC Beau Soleil
119, avenue de Lodève
F-34000 Montpellier
France

Catherine Roy, PhD
Professor of Radiology
Service de Radiologie B
Hôpital Civil
1 Place de l'Hôpital
F-67091 Strasbourg Cedex
France

Jean Louis Sadoul, MD
Service de Diabétologie et d'Ondocrinologie
Hôpital Pasteur
30 avenue de la Voie Romaine, BP 69
F-06002 Nice Cedex 1
France

DENIS SAMANA, MD
Service de Radiologie
Hôpital de la Timone
264 rue Saint Pierre
F-13385 Marseille Cedex 5
France

SILVANO SCHIAVONI, MD
Radiologia
Ospedale S. Corona
I-Pietra Ligure (S.V.)
Italy

JEAN TRAMALLONI, MD
Cabinet de Radiologie
25 rue de Docteur Paul Bruel
F-95380 Louvres
France

FRANÇOIS TRANQUART, MD
Médecine Nucléaire et Ultrasons
INSERM U 316
CHU Bretonneau
F-37044 Tours Cedex
France

DOMINIQUE VADROT, MD
Professor of Radiology
Service de Radiologie
Hôtel Dieu
Place du Parvis Notre Dame
F-75004 Paris
France

JEAN FRANÇOIS VIALLET, MD
Professor of Radiology
Service de Radiologie et d'Imagerie Médicale
Hôpital G. Montpied
30 place Henri Dunand, BP 69
F-63003 Clermont-Ferrand
France

Medical Radiology
Diagnostic Imaging and Radiation Oncology

Titles in the series already published

Diagnostic Imaging

Innovations in Diagnostic Imaging
Edited by J.H. Anderson

Radiology of the Upper Urinary Tract
Edited by E.K. Lang

The Thymus - Diagnostic Imaging, Functions, and Pathologic Anatomy
Edited by E. Walter, E. Willich, and W.R. Webb

Interventional Neuroradiology
Edited by A. Valavanis

Radiology of the Pancreas
Edited by A.L. Baert, co-edited by G. Delorme

Radiology of the Lower Urinary Tract
Edited by E.K. Lang

Magnetic Resonance Angiography
Edited by I.P. Arlart, G.M. Bongartz, and G. Marchal

Contrast-Enhanced MRI of the Breast
S. Heywang-Köbrunner and R. Beck

Spiral CT of the Chest
Edited by M. Rémy-Jardin and J. Rémy

Radiological Diagnosis of Breast Diseases
Edited by M. Friedrich and E.A. Sickles

Radiology of the Trauma
Edited by M. Heller and A. Fink

Biliary Tract Radiology
Edited by P. Rossi

Radiological Imaging of Sports Injuries
Edited by C. Masciocchi

Modern Imaging of the Alimentary Tube
Edited by A. R. Margulis

Diagnosis and Therapy of Spinal Tumors
Edited by P. R. Algra, J. Valk, and J. J. Heimans

Interventional Magnetic Resonance Imaging
Edited by J. F. Debatin and G. Adam

Abdominal and Pelvic MRI
Edited by A. Heuck and M. Reiser

Orthopedic Imaging
Edited by A.M. Davies and H. Pettersson

Radiology of the Female Pelvic Organs
Edited by E.K.Lang

Magnetic Resonance of the Heart and Great Vessels
Clinical Applications
Edited by J. Bogaert, A. J. Duerinckx, and F. E. Rademakers

Modern Head and Neck Imaging
Edited by S. K. Mukherji and J. A. Castelijns

Radiology Imaging of Endocrine Diseases
Edited by J. N. Bruneton in collaboration with B. Padovani and M. Y. Mourou

Radiation Oncology

Lung Cancer
Edited by C.W. Scarantino

Innovations in Radiation Oncology
Edited by H.R. Withers and L.J. Peters

Radiation Therapy of Head and Neck Cancer
Edited by G.E. Laramore

Gastrointestinal Cancer – Radiation Therapy
Edited by R.R. Dobelbower, Jr.

Radiation Exposure and Occupational Risks
Edited by E. Scherer, C. Streffer, and K.-R. Trott

Radiation Therapy of Benign Diseases - A Clinical Guide
S.E. Order and S.S. Donaldson

Medical Radiology
Diagnostic Imaging and Radiation Oncology

Titles in the series already published

Radiation Oncology

Interventional Radiation Therapy Techniques - Brachytherapy
Edited by R. Sauer

Radiopathology of Organs and Tissues
Edited by E. Scherer, C. Streffer, and K.-R. Trott

Concomitant Continuous Infusion Chemotherapy and Radiation
Edited by M. Rotman and C.J. Rosenthal

Intraoperative Radiotherapy – Clinical Experiences and Results
Edited by F.A. Calvo, M. Santos, and L.W. Brady

Radiotherapy of Intraocular and Orbital Tumors
Edited by W.E. Alberti and R.H. Sagerman

Interstitial and Intracavitary Thermoradiotherapy
Edited by M.H. Seegenschmiedt and R. Sauer

Non-Disseminated Breast Cancer
Controversial Issues in Management
Edited by G.H. Fletcher and S.H. Levitt

Current Topics in Clinical Radiobiology of Tumors
Edited by H.-P. Beck-Bornholdt

Practical Approaches to Cancer Invasion and Metastases
A Compendium of Radiation Oncologists' Responses to 40 Histories
Edited by A.R. Kagan with the Assistance of R.J. Steckel

Radiation Therapy in Pediatric Oncology
Edited by J.R. Cassady

Radiation Therapy Physics
Edited by A.R. Smith

Late Sequelae in Oncology
Edited by J. Dunst and R. Sauer

Mediastinal Tumors. Update 1995
Edited by D.E. Wood and C.R. Thomas, Jr.

Thermoradiotherapy and Thermochemotherapy
Volume 1:
Biology, Physiology, and Physics
Volume 2:
Clinical Applications
Edited by M.H. Seegenschmiedt, P. Fessenden, and C.C. Vernon

Carcinoma of the Prostate
Innovations in Management
Edited by Z. Petrovich, L. Baert, and L.W. Brady

Radiation Oncology of Gynecological Cancers
Edited by H.W. Vahrson

Carcinoma of the Bladder
Innovations in Management
Edited by Z. Petrovich, L. Baert, and L.W. Brady

Blood Perfusion and Microenvironment of Human Tumors
Implications for Clinical Radiooncology
Edited by M. Molls and P. Vaupel

Radiation Therapy of Benign Diseases. A Clinical Guide
2nd revised edition
S.E. Order and S.S. Donaldson

Carcinoma of the Kidney and Testis, and Rare Urologic Malignancies
Innovations in Management
Edited by Z. Petrovich, L. Baert, and L.W. Brady

MIX
Papier aus verantwortungsvollen Quellen
Paper from responsible sources
FSC® C105338

If you have any concerns about our products,
you can contact us on
ProductSafety@springernature.com

In case Publisher is established outside the EU,
the EU authorized representative is:
Springer Nature Customer Service Center GmbH
Europaplatz 3, 69115 Heidelberg, Germany

Printed by Libri Plureos GmbH
in Hamburg, Germany